THE

MEDICAL PROFESSION

IN

UPPER CANADA

1783-1850

Reprint Edition

The Medical Profession in Upper Canada 1783-1850

Reprint Edition

WILLIAM CANNIFF, M.D., M.R.C.S. ENG.

WITH A NEW INTRODUCTION BY CHARLES G. ROLAND, M.D.

The Hannah Institute for the History of Medicine

First published by William Briggs, Toronto, 1894.
Reprint Edition published 1980 for The Hannah Institute for the History of Medicine by Clarke, Irwin & Company Limited.

CANADIAN CATALOGUING IN PUBLICATION DATA

Canniff, William, 1830-1910.
The medical profession in Upper Canada 1783-1850

Reprint of: Toronto: W. Briggs, 1894.
ISBN 0-7720-1295-4

1. Medicine—Ontario—History. 2. Medical societies—Ontario—History. I. Title.

R463.06C36 1981 610.9713 C81-094081-7

Printed in Canada

Preface to the Reprint Edition

Associated Medical Services, Inc. and the Hannah Institute for the History of Medicine are pleased to present this reprint edition of a Canadian classic in the history of medicine. It may be said confidently that such a reissue is long overdue.

The initiative for this venture has come largely from Charlotte Erichsen-Brown, to whom sincere thanks are extended. Charles G. Roland has undertaken the writing of an introduction, the purpose of which is to put the work of Canniff in the perspective of the 1980s. Heather MacDougall and S. E. D. Shortt provided helpful comments on this introductory material, though they bear no responsibility for factual error or faulty interpretation. Gratitude is expressed to all four.

Here then is Canniff once more, almost a century after the book's first appearance, still most relevant in the history of Canadian medicine.

G. R. Paterson, Ph.D.
Executive Director,
The Hannah Institute for the History of Medicine

Introduction to the Reprint Edition, 1980

Born on June 20, 1830, William Canniff came of Loyalist stock, though he was not technically a United Empire Loyalist, his father, James, having moved to Canada from the United States in the 1790s. The family settled near Belleville, where James engaged in farming and milling. Although medicine was not a traditional family profession, Canniff began studying at the Toronto School of Medicine under John Rolph and completed his studies in New York, graduating in 1854. He travelled to Europe, became a member of the Royal College of Surgeons (London), and was appointed to the medical staff of the British Army in 1856. When the Crimean War ended, Canniff resigned his commission and continued his studies in several hospitals in England and on the continent.

This education abroad made him unusually well-trained for the time, and perhaps over-trained for life as a general practitioner in Belleville. The big city beckoned. He joined the faculty of the medical school of Victoria College, to become a colleague of his old teacher, Rolph. At Victoria he taught surgery and pathology, and from this time on until his death on October 18, 1910, most of his career was fixed in Toronto. He continued to teach, and to practise, and in 1866 his first book was published, *A Manual of the Practice of Surgery*, probably the first surgical textbook published by a Canadian.

Canniff's interest in military surgery continued. He served briefly with the Army of the Potomac during the American Civil War, and he went to Ridgeway as a militia medical officer when the Fenians invaded Canada.

In 1867, the year of Confederation, the Canadian Medical Association was founded. Canniff's election as secretary for Ontario, and his appointment to four of the Association's eight standing committees, acknowledged his reputation in the profession. At about this same time he also became politically active, chiefly through the Canada First movement. He eventually became president of an offshoot of this organization, the North-West Emigration Aid Society, which aimed to promote white, anglophone, protestant, Canadian emigration to the prairies.

In a sense, Canniff's second book can be seen as one manifestation of his outspoken Canadianism. *History of the Settlement of Upper Canada, (Ontario,) with Special Reference to the Bay Quinte* was published in Toronto in 1869. Although intended as a general history of the province, an unmistakable emphasis on Loyalist settlement reflects his continuing interest in this topic. The book is a valuable collection of material based heavily on interviews with early settlers in Ontario and their descendants.

Canniff's medical career continued during all these activities. In 1883 he became the first full-time medical officer of health for Toronto. And in 1894 he published *The Medical Profession in Upper Canada*, the book that is reprinted here.

Canniff was not always in the front rank. He pooh-poohed the idea of antisepsis in surgery, and does not seem to have ever used carbolic acid in practice, but this did not prevent him from writing scathing and sarcastic denunciations of Lister's theories. Meanwhile, other surgeons, particularly Archibald Malloch of Hamilton, quietly continued to spread the gospel that would, along with anesthesia, make modern surgery possible. Canniff remained unrepentant on this subject even when the rest of the profession had accepted its importance.[1]

William Canniff's loyalism, his strong sense of Canadian identity, his respect for successful struggles by the pioneers, his interest in military medicine, his admiration for things British and his corresponding disdain of things American, are all reflected throughout his writings. Nevertheless, *The Medical Profession in Upper Canada* is much more than a vehicle to permit the author to display his interests and beliefs.

II

When the United Empire Loyalists came to what is now Ontario in 1784, they faced a difficult and heartbreaking task. In support of their king, they had abandoned or had been forced to leave established homes and farms in settled communities in the thirteen colonies. Now they had to begin again. Before their arrival, white settlement in Upper Canada[2] had consisted only of very small settlements at Niagara and along the Detroit River—a few dozen families plus the garrisons.

Homes and farms had to be claimed from the forest. Most families had left essentially everything behind. The government supplied basic necessities such as axes, hoes and kettles, plus some rough clothing, and it promised food for one or two years until the primitive farms began to be fruitful. Except for their own small group of settlers, these pioneers were far from family and friends. They worried about finding good land, and clearing it, and erecting shelter; and inevitably they worried about their health.

The effect of illness or injury, particularly to either of the parents of a young family, could be catastrophic. Only unremitting toil could wrest a homestead from the ubiquitous forest, and unremitting toil was impossible if one had to lie abed with a continued fever or a fractured thigh. Britain supplied tools and food, but provided little in the way of medical care.

Although a surgeon to the loyalists was appointed at Cataraqui, most care came incidentally (though not unimportantly) through the services of regimental surgeons in the environs of their posts. As loyalists began to come into the country by thousands, and were followed by even more thousands of Americans, English, Scots, Irish, and Germans, the number of settlements increased and the tiny centres grew into villages and towns.

In the first section of his book Canniff has described briefly, though unfortunately somewhat superficially, how the medical needs of these new Canadians were met. He reproduces portions of the early medical licensing legislation, quotes anecdotes about quackery, its evils, and its ubiquity, and lists some of the earliest practitioners.

As population grew, the appurtenances of society also came into being. Dances and fetes were held, town meetings called, clubs and societies created, masonic lodges came into being, and various trade and professional groups made tentative efforts to organize. After the War of 1812, many doctors came to Upper Canada both as immigrants and as half-pay surgeons who remained behind when their regiments were withdrawn or disbanded. The first Canadian-born physicians began their professional careers during this period, too, although they all had to be educated elsewhere because there was no true medical school in the province until 1843.

As the number of physicians rose, civil hospitals were founded in the two largest towns, Kingston and York (Toronto), boards of health were created during epidemics, and the first attempts at formal organization were made. Medical licensing legislation had existed intermittently and ineffectually until 1818, when a law was passed that was designed to combat the large numbers of ill-trained practitioners who operated in the province. Part Two of *The Medical Profession in Upper Canada* provides a description of the licensing process, the laws behind it, and early efforts to secure a medical school.

The real importance of Canniff's history, however, lies in the final section, the biographies. In the first two parts there is little that is original and a large proportion, especially in the long description devoted to the Upper Canada Medical Board, consists entirely of lengthy direct quotations from sources that are available to the historian in their primary form (though perhaps, not so easily accessible). But in Part Three, Canniff has gathered whatever information he could locate, in some instances only tantalizing shreds, about nearly 300 practitioners active in Upper Canada at some time in the years between 1783 and 1850. In many instances Canniff had interviewed or corresponded with these physicians to gather data for his biographical essays.

The biographical essays contain much material that is now lost or is difficult to obtain. In this, as in *History of the Settlement of Upper Canada*, he has performed a great service; we would know far less about the lives of these early pioneers—in some cases we would not know of their existence—without Canniff's history.

III

In *The Medical Profession in Upper Canada*, Canniff has written a limited type of narrative history, not interpretive history. And it is Whig history (how he would have bridled at the designation!), secure in its belief in steady progress to a better, wiser state. But the most obvious deficit in Canniff's book is the lack of any attempt to provide an account of medical *practice*, of the medical conditions that existed and the way they were treated. Canniff claimed only to write a history of the medical *profession* in Upper Canada; and his narrative sections do attend largely to matters that we would consider part of the story of medical professionalization—particularly the laws governing practice and the activities of the Medical Board created to examine candidates for the license. But he does fail to place his account of these affairs within a broader context.

The Medical Board of Upper Canada, for example, was not hailed by everyone in the province as a progressive innovation. Within the profession, jealousies arose with regard to membership and to the enormous power wielded by the Board. While Canniff does mention (p. 86) a protest meeting held by practitioners at Toronto in 1836, he does not attempt to provide reasons for this dissatisfaction. Nor does he point out that John Rolph, Charles Duncombe, and T. D. Morrison were serving on the Board, less than two years before the 1837 rebellion, in which Rolph, Duncombe, and Morrison figured so largely. Was the protest meeting a manifestation of reform politics impinging on the medical profession? The question remains unanswered.

Other serious issues are not considered by Canniff, including the contentious business whereby the graduates of British universities received their licenses without examination, whereas graduates of American and other foreign schools had to pass a substantial oral examination (portions of which, at least, were conducted in Latin). A second subject that merits attention is the fact that a surprising number of prominent and powerful members of the Medical Board, such as R. C. Horne, Grant Powell, and W. W. Baldwin, were not active practitioners when they served the Board. Although these are a few examples of questions we might have hoped that Canniff would discuss, we must also consider that medical history was being written in a different fashion a century ago.

IV

If we cannot expect Canniff to write history with a "modern" approach, we can expect him to be factual and accurate, and on that score I believe he ranks high. I have made detailed studies of several physicians who are "in Canniff," such as William Case, Robert Douglas Hamilton, Robert Charles Horne, Robert Kerr, Gerald O'Reilly, and Alexander Thom. On the basis of my examination of the existing primary and secondary sources, I can testify that Canniff's accounts have been substantially accurate in every instance. They are not complete (no biographical account is), but they are reliable.

Given some confidence in these data, the large number of individuals included suggests the possibility of demographic studies. There are 271 primary entries. It is not difficult to discover, for example, that 22% are English-born, 15% Scots, 17% Irish, 22% Canadian, and 20% American. Of Canniff's physicians 84% are university-trained and 16% seem to have had only apprenticeships. The possibilities of such manipulations are numerous, and represent another useful dimension for the book.

While the biographical portion of the book is its strongest feature, inevitably, several names are missing from the sketches. Although Canniff only claims to present "some brief biographies," a few of the omissions are surprising. William Lyons and John Shortt, for example, are recognized as having served on the Medical Board, yet their biographies are not included. Other omissions include E. Aspinwall and Amasa Stebbins who practised in York until about 1814, and R. Q. Short, who practised in Kingston in the 1790s. And perhaps the most prominent omission is Robert Richardson, a busy magistrate who also practised medicine along the Detroit River for several decades and was active in the War of 1812. Richardson married the daughter of the prominent trader John Askin, and was the father of John Richardson, the author of *Wacousta.* Such omissions do not diminish the value of the work in general, but it may be beneficial to remind the reader that there were medical practitioners active in Upper Canada between 1783 and 1850 in addition to those mentioned by Canniff.

The Medical Profession in Upper Canada remains a valuable document in Canadian medical history, particularly in its mass of biographical data on pioneer practitioners. It is, in fact, the only substantial work on the subject, and many later efforts are largely derivative. Its reprinting makes it generally available at a time when interest in Canadian medical history is expanding rapidly.

Charles G. Roland, M.D.
Jason A. Hannah Professor of the History of Medicine,
McMaster University, Hamilton, Ontario

References

1. See "The Early Years of Antiseptic Surgery in Canada," *Journal of the History of Medicine and Allied Sciences* 22 (1967), pp. 380-391.

2. The term "Upper Canada" refers to the geographical area of what is now Ontario falling within the southern boundaries of Lakes Ontario and Erie, the eastern boundary of Lake Huron, and bounded on the north by the Ottawa River. Before 1791 this area was part of the Province of Quebec, from 1791 till 1841 it was called Upper Canada, from 1841 till 1866, Canada West, and from 1867, Ontario.

THE

MEDICAL PROFESSION

IN

UPPER CANADA

1783-1850

Reprint Edition

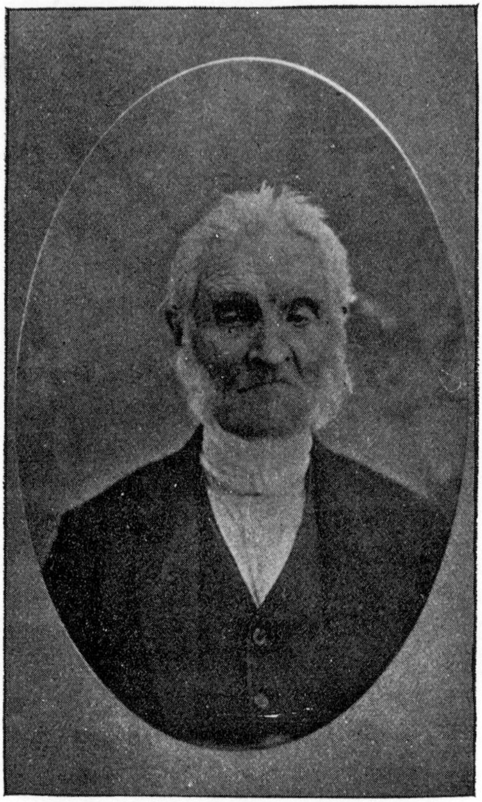

DR. HENRY TAYLOR.

In practice when one hundred years old.

THE

MEDICAL PROFESSION

IN

UPPER CANADA

1783-1850.

AN HISTORICAL NARRATIVE, WITH ORIGINAL DOCUMENTS RELATING TO THE PROFESSION,

INCLUDING

SOME BRIEF BIOGRAPHIES.

BY

WM. CANNIFF, M.D., M.R.C.S. ENG.,

AUTHOR OF "THE PRINCIPLES OF SURGERY," "SETTLEMENT OF UPPER CANADA," ETC., ETC.

ILLUSTRATED.

TORONTO:

WILLIAM BRIGGS.

1894.

The Medical Profession in Upper Canada,

1783-1850.

This Volume is Dedicated to the Descendants of the Pioneer Medical Men.

FOR CONVENIENCE OF REFERENCE, THIS WORK IS DIVIDED INTO THREE PARTS :

First Part.

THE PIONEER MEDICAL MEN, AND THE SEVERAL STEPS TAKEN TO ESTABLISH THE PROFESSION ON A LEGAL BASIS.

Second Part.

THE PROCEEDINGS OF THE UPPER CANADA MEDICAL BOARD FROM ITS ORGANIZATION, IN 1819, TO 1850; AND OF THE COLLEGE OF PHYSICIANS AND SURGEONS OF UPPER CANADA, 1839-41, WITH REFERENCES TO HISTORICAL EVENTS SHOWING THE GROWTH AND DEVELOPMENT OF THE PROFESSION.

Third Part.

BIOGRAPHICAL SKETCHES OF EARLY PHYSICIANS OF THE PROVINCE, WITH MANY REFERENCES TO EARLY EVENTS IN THE HISTORY OF UPPER CANADA.

PREFACE.

THE following pages contain the result of long-continued effort by the writer, to collect and arrange everything available relating to the early history of the Medical Profession of the Province of Ontario. Books, documents, newspapers, and letters, public and private, have been consulted, and facts appropriate to the work put to use. It may be stated that not a few historical matters recorded would have been lost, had not the writer gathered them up and embodied them in this work. It is believed that this volume supplies a valuable contribution to Canadian history. Although the number of pages is greater than intended and was promised in the prospectus, it has been found impossible to include all the material collected. This, however, shall be preserved for future use.

It will be seen by the observant reader, that the Medical Profession of Upper Canada has contributed a fair quota to the distinguished men who have taken an active part in the government of the country, and in laying the foundation of the Dominion of Canada that they were men of high education, and possessed of noble qualities which fitted them to fill various positions of public trust.

The writer must acknowledge his indebtedness to very many, not only for information, but as well for encouraging words, while he was devoting much time and labour to this work. He especially thanks the several hundred subscribers, distinguished representatives of various classes of society, who so cordially gave their names in advance.

To the publisher, the writer is under more than ordinary obligation for his considerate kindness and assistance.

W. C.

May, 1894.

CONTENTS.

PART I.

CHAPTER I.

CHAPTER II.

CHAPTER III.

CHAPTER IV.

PART II.

CHAPTER V.

CHAPTER VI.

CHAPTER VII.

CHAPTER VIII.

CHAPTER IX.

CHAPTER X.

CHAPTER XI.

CHAPTER XII.

CHAPTER XIII.

CHAPTER XIV.

CHAPTER XV.

CHAPTER XVI.

CHAPTER XVII.

CHAPTER XVIII.

CHAPTER XIX.

CHAPTER XX.

CHAPTER XXI.

CHAPTER XXII.

CHAPTER XXIII.

CHAPTER XXIV.

CHAPTER XXV.

CHAPTER XXVI.

PART III.

CHAPTER XXVII.

THE MEDICAL PROFESSION

IN

UPPER CANADA.

1783–1850.

FIRST PART.

THE PIONEER MEDICAL MEN, AND THE SEVERAL STEPS TAKEN TO ESTABLISH THE PROFESSION ON A LEGAL BASIS.

CHAPTER I.

PHYSICIANS AMONG THE U. E. LOYALISTS.

CANADA had become a British possession by the conquest of General Wolfe in 1759. In 1763, a royal proclamation was issued declaring the limits of the Province to include a portion of territory westward, which now forms part of Ontario. In 1774, the British Parliament passed an Act by which the limits were still further extended, including all of the territory now forming the Province, as well as certain parts now forming part of the United States.

In 1776, the thirteen British colonies in America raised the standard of revolt, and in 1783, after a bloody struggle, their independence was acknowledged by the British Government. The American rebellion had become a revolution. At the same time a very large number of British-Americans who would not join the rebels had become destitute wanderers and outcasts from their homes, while their property was confiscated. Ten thousand of these found an asylum in Canada. During the war some refugees had escaped to the Niagara frontier, and clustered around Fort Niagara. Likewise a few were refugees at Detroit and at Carlton Island, near Fort Frontenac, now Kingston. But the majority at first entered Lower Canada, and awaited the allotment of land in Upper Canada after the survey had been made. Up to this time the territory which now forms the Province of Ontario was a dense wilderness. The survey began in 1783, and the settlement by the Loyalists in the following year.

The medical men who gave professional attendance to the English-speaking people living in Canada after the conquest, were at first mostly, if not altogether, British surgeons attached to the army or navy. As the number of English in the Province increased, the doctors connected with the service could not give the medical attention required. Some surgeons retired from the service and engaged in civil practice; and a few came from the Old Country to settle as private practitioners. The stamp of Englishmen who thus first practised medicine in Canada was as good as British medical education could at that time produce. That they were not wanting in knowledge, and a desire to introduce the latest discoveries in medicine, is sufficiently attested. One instance of this may be given. The Quebec *Gazette*, Sept., 1768, contains the following reference to the inoculation of small-pox, which was then receiving in England a good deal of attention:

"*To the Inhabitants of Quebec.*

"Mr. Latham, surgeon to the King's (or Eighth) Regiment of Foot, acquaints the inhabitants of Quebec that before he left England he entered into partnership with Mr. Sutton for inoculation. The great success, and the many thousands Mr. Sutton has inoculated by his invention and new method, induced Mr. Latham to become his partner, in order that he may be of some use to mankind in this part of the world. Mr. Latham, some days ago, inoculated some soldiers belonging to the regiment to which he has the honour to be surgeon, by which means he has procured sufficient infection for those who *chuse* to be inoculated. All poor persons, who are not able to pay, and who are desirous of being inoculated, may apply to Mr. Latham, who will inoculate, attend, and give them medicine gratis. Mr. Latham practises midwifery. He is to be spoken to at his house, upon the Battery, Upper Town." On the 3rd of November following, Dr. Latham announced "that as there may be some individuals willing to be inoculated and who are cautious concerning the quality of infection, that he designs to inoculate in a few days one of his daughters, a child between two and three years old."

Strangely enough, nearly thirty years later the following reference to the practice of inoculation appeared in a paper published at Newark, Upper Canada:

" As the inoculation for the *small-pox* is this day commenced at Queenston, and the season of the year very favourable, the subscribers propose inoculating *immediately* in the town of Newark, and throughout the county of Lincoln, on the most reasonable terms. The poor inoculated gratis.

" ROBERT KERR,
" JAMES MUIRHEAD.

" Newark, Jan. 25th, 1797."

The *Journal* of Feb. 1st, 1797, editorially says:

" We learn from every settlement the determination of a general inoculation for the small-pox. This resolution is highly commended by persons of prudence. This country being young, and growing more exposed to that disorder, a general inoculation every one or two years will forever render its prevalence in any way of very little concern, there being then none, or but few, excepting young children, to be affected by it. This season of the year is highly favourable to it; to defer it until warm weather, or summer, is highly dangerous. The blood is in a state then easily to become putrid, fever may set in with it, and beside these, . . . to place it in the most favourable situation, . . . must sustain infinite injury. To enact a law to enforce a general inoculation looks arbitrary; but the writer of this, who can in no wise be interested by himself nor friends, is of opinion that such a law in any country, more particularly in a new one, would operate to the greatest possible benefit of the country, and justifiable on the principles of public and private good. But a so beneficial law he expects never to see so long as there remains a blindness in so many to their own safety and welfare, and a delicacy in our rulers to compel a man to throw off old prejudices and to do those things that are taught by the simple and natural laws of self-defence."

While disbanded soldiers formed a portion of the first settlers of Upper Canada, there was a larger portion of non-combatant United Empire Loyalists who entered the wilds of Upper Canada. But among them was found no qualified medical man. Not that there were no physicians among those who adhered to the Crown in the rebellious States. On the contrary, as with the other learned professions, the cream of the medical men in the several revolting colonies remained loyal to the British flag. Sabine, a writer of the United States, in his work on the "Loyalists of the American Revolution," says:

"The physicians who adhered to the Crown were numerous, and the proportion of Whigs (rebels) in the profession of medicine was less, probably, than in either that of law or theology. But unlike persons of the latter callings, most of the physicians remained in the country and quietly pursued their business. There seems to have been an understanding that though pulpits should be closed and litigation be suspended, the sick should not be deprived of their regular and freely chosen medical attendants. I have been surprised to find, from verbal communication and various other sources, that while the 'Tory doctors' were as zealous and as fearless in the expression of their sentiments as the 'Tory ministers' and 'Tory barristers,' their persons and property were generally respected in the towns and villages, where little or no regard was paid to the bodies and estates of gentlemen of the robe and the surplice." This may have been due to "the exigencies of the ladies."

"A few of the Loyalist physicians were banished; others, and those chiefly who became surgeons in the army or provincial corps, settled in New Brunswick or Nova Scotia, where they resumed practice."

From this it may be understood that the advent of the U. E. Loyalist settlers to Upper Canada in 1784, and for many years after, was attended with a want of medical aid. The number of settlers on the Niagara is uncertain; but being in close proximity to the garrison they could more readily obtain the services of the surgeon stationed there. At the eastern part of Upper Canada, we learn from the Haldimand Collection at Ottawa, the exact number of settlers. In a return signed by

Sir John Johnson, "of men, women and children settled on the new townships, St. Lawrence River and Cataraqui and Bay of Quinte," it is stated there were "1,568 men, 626 women, 1,492 children, and 90 servants," the total being 3,776.

The first settlements in Upper Canada were made under military order. There was no civil law until 1788, when Western Canada was divided into four districts, namely, Lunenburg, Mecklenburg, Nassau and Hesse, and to each district was appointed a judge, sheriff, and other necessary officers for civil government.

As we have seen, the provision for medical and surgical relief of these exiles was of the most scanty kind. At Kingston, Niagara and Detroit were garrisons with a limited number of soldiers and one or two surgeons. For many years, the pioneers were dependent upon these army surgeons, who were rarely willing to go any distance from the garrison. Some of the settlements were made by disbanded soldiers, and those who settled along the St. Lawrence had as fellow-pioneers a few surgeons who had been attached to their respective corps, and continued to enjoy their medical services. These surgeons were numbered among the U. E. Loyalists, and were on what is called the "U. E. List." As the meaning of this term is not generally understood, the following is inserted :

AT THE COUNCIL CHAMBER AT QUEBEC,

MONDAY, 9th *November*, 1789.

PRESENT :

His Excellency the Right Honourable Lord Dorchester,
The Honourable William Smith, Esquire, Chief Justice,

Hugh Finlay, Esquire,	George Powell, Esquire,
Thos. Dunn, Esquire,	Henry Caldwell, Esquire,
Edw'd Harrison, Esquire,	William Grant, Esquire,
John Collins, Esquire,	François Baby, Esquire,
Adam Mabane, Esquire,	Chas. DeLanaudiere, Esquire,
J. G. C. Delery, Esquire,	Le Cte. Dupré, Esquire.

"His Lordship intimated to the Council that it remained a question, upon the late regulation for the disposition of the waste lands of the Crown, whether the Boards constituted for that purpose were authorized to make locations to the sons of Loyalists on their coming to full age, and that it was his wish to put a marke of honour upon the families who had adhered to the unity of the empire and joined the royal standard in America before the Treaty of Separation in the year 1783.

"The Council concurring with His Lordship, it is accordingly ordered:

"That the several Land Boards take course for preserving a registry of the names of all persons falling under the description afore-mentioned, to the end that their posterity may be discriminated from future settlers, in the parish registers and rolls of the militia of their respective districts, and other public remembrancers of the Province, as proper objects, by their persevering in the fidelity and conduct so honourable to their ancestors, for distinguished benefits and privileges.

"And it is also ordered, that the said Land Boards may, in every such case, provide not only for the *sons* of those Loyalists, as they arrive to full age, but for their *daughters* also of that age, or on their marriage, assigning to each a lot of two hundred acres, more or less; provided, nevertheless, that they respectively comply with the general regulations, and that it shall satisfactorily appear that there has been no default in the due cultivation and improvement of the lands already assigned to the head of the family of which they are members.

"(Signed), J. WILLIAMS, C. C."

It may be mentioned that Adam Mabane was a surgeon, and had been in charge of the Quebec Garrison Hospital. In the Haldimand Collection is found ample evidence that he occupied a conspicuous place in the government of the country at that period.

Those whose names are found in the "U. E. List" are properly regarded as the fathers of Upper Canada. Among them the following were evidently medical men; but as surgeons at that time were rarely designated as doctor, not unlikely there were others who were not recognized as doctors or surgeons:

Solomon Jones, Eastern District, Surgeon's Mate, Loyal Rangers.

Dr. Sparham, Eastern District, Hospital Mate reduced, had served in war of 1763. Provision List, 1786.

James Stuart, Eastern District, S. G. Surgeon's Mate, Royal Rangers, New York. Provision List 2nd, 1786.

James Walker, Eastern District, Augusta, Surgeon Jessup's S. G.

Subsequently, after Upper Canada had been erected into a province, the Executive Council added from time to time other names to the "U. E. List." Among them were the following medical men:

Dr. Charles Austin, Surgeon, R. R. N. Y.
Patrick Burk, Surgeon's Mate, Butler's Rangers.
Dr. Charles Blake, Surgeon, 34th Regiment.
David Burns, Surgeon, 71st Regiment.
James Connor, Surgeon, Hospital Mate.
Robert Guthrie, Surgeon, Butler's Rangers.
John De Courcy, Hospital Mate, Canada.
John Gamble, Hospital Mate, last war.
Williams, Surgeon.
James Muirhead, Surgeon's Mate, 60th Regiment.
James Muirhead, Surgeon, 60th Regiment.
James McAulay (Macaulay), Surgeon's Mate, Queen's Rangers
George Smythe, Surgeon, Loyal Rangers.
Thomas Wright, Surgeon, 1st Battalion, 60th Regiment Hospital Mate during the war.

Among the non-combatant refugees there were few, if any, possessing skill in the practice of medicine, and the further the settlements extended from the garrisons, the greater was the want of a physician. At first anyone offering his services as a doctor among the English-speaking people of Canada was able to show some evidence of qualification from the parent country. But after a time, in Upper Canada, there came, now and then, persons from the United States professing to possess medical skill They came generally, not for attachment to the British flag, but to turn a penny. Sometimes they had a degree of medical education which had been acquired in the United States medical schools; sometimes they knew a little about the use of drugs; but too frequently they only knew how to deceive the people by arrant quackery. This class of doctors, being natives of the United States, managed to make themselves agreeable to the U. E. Loyalist settler, who was also generally a native of America. For many years only a few with qualifications from British colleges settled in Upper Canada, and only in places where there was an aggregation of settlers. As villages were formed and grew into towns, the number of doubtful practitioners increased, and as a natural result of this state of affairs, it became necessary to protect the settlers from impostors.

As we have seen, until 1788, the Loyalists who had settled in Upper Canada lived under martial law. English laws were in force, and executed by the officers of regiments stationed in the new settlements. These officers had a general oversight of the settlers, superintended the granting of lands, and bestowed such assistance as was practicable, by supplying them with food and implements for their pioneer life. But in the year mentioned, when Canada was divided into four districts, competent courts of justice were created for each district, and a judge, sheriff, and other necessary civil officers appointed.

CHAPTER II.

FIRST ACTS RELATING TO PRACTICE OF MEDICINE.

THE first step toward regulating the practice of medicine in Canada after the conquest was taken in 1788. The following is taken from a copy of old statutes in the Toronto Public Library, "A collection of the Acts passed in the parliament of Great Britain and of other public Acts relative to Canada." Printed at Quebec, 1800 (Robert Armour, jun., was the former owner of this volume. It is now owned by the Public Library):

"An Act or ordinance to prevent persons pråctising physic and surgery within the Province of Quebec, or midwifery in the towns of Quebec and Montreal, without license." (It will be remembered that Upper Canada was yet a portion of the Province of Quebec.)

"Whereas many inconveniences have arisen to His Majesty's

subjects in this province from unskilful persons practising physics and surgery; be it enacted by His Excellency the Governor and the Legislative Council, that after the first day of November next, no person whatsoever shall on any pretence sell, vend, or distribute medicines by retail, or prescribe for sick persons for gain, or practise physic or surgery within the Province, or practise midwifery in the towns of Quebec and Montreal, or the suburbs thereof, without license first had and obtained from His Excellency the Governor, or the Commander-in-chief of the Province, for the time being, which license shall not be granted but upon certificate of the person applying for the same, having been examined and approved by such persons as the Governor or Commander-in-chief, for the time being, may have appointed for the purpose of examining and inquiring into the knowledge of such persons in physic, or skill in surgery, or pharmacy, or midwifery, a copy of which certificate is to be annexed to the license, which is to be enregistered in the office of the Clerk of the Peace of the district where the practitioner resides.

"And every person acting in any of the professions aforesaid without such license, shall forfeit the sum of twenty pounds for the first offence, fifty pounds for the second, and one hundred pounds and three months' imprisonment for every subsequent offence committed against the true intent and meaning of this ordinance, to be recorded in the Court of Common Pleas of the district where the offence shall have been committed; a moiety of such forfeitures to be paid to the Receiver-General of the Province, and applied to the use of His Majesty's Government here, to be accounted for by him to His Majesty, his heirs and successors, or to the commissioners of His Majesty's treasury, for the time being, and audited by His Majesty's Auditor-General for the plantations, or his deputy, and the other moiety to be paid to the person or persons who shall sue for the same.

"Provided always, and it is hereby enacted, that nothing in this ordinance shall extend or be construed to extend to the subjecting such persons as shall have taken a degree in any university, or who have been commissioned or warranted as surgeons in His Majesty's army or navy to any examination previous to obtaining a license: but to which license, to be enregistered as above, a copy of the degree or certificate of the commission or warrant shall be annexed; and that no physician or surgeon doing duty in the army or navy within the Province be obliged to have a license; provided also, that nothing in this ordinance shall be construed to prevent retailers or others from selling such drugs for which a royal patent has been obtained.

"DORCHESTER."

"Be it therefore Enacted and Ordained by the authority aforesaid, and passed in Council under the Great Seal of the Province, at the Council Chamber in the Castle of St. Louis, in the city of Quebec, in the thirtieth day of April, in the twenty-eighth year of the reign of our Sovereign Lord George the Third, by the grace of God, of Great Britain, France, and Ireland, King, Defender of the Faith, and so forth, and in the year of our Lord one thousand seven hundred and eighty-eight.

"April 30, 1788."

Wishing to record every step or movement to secure medical relief for the pioneer, the following is inserted, as doubtless civilians as well as soldiers had the benefit of hospital treatment:

On Sept. 4, 1790, application was made by Capt. Park Porter for a hospital at Kingston. "He reminds Capt. Le Maitre that during his former command there, he was directed to give up the hospital as a place for Indian presents, which at that time could be very well spared as all the navy and greater part of the garrison were resident at Carlton Island; but at present the exigency seems to point out the necessity of having that place again as an hospital. I mentioned to Sir John Johnson my intended application and he made answer, he understood he was to give it up when required for the purpose it was originally built."

In the early part of 1791, in compliance with the request of the U. E. Loyalist settlers, the Imperial Parliament granted a distinct autonomy to Upper Canada with British laws and customs, the Province of Quebec being divided into Upper and Lower Canada. On July 8th, 1792, the first Lieutenant-Governor of Upper Canada, Col. John Graves Simcoe, assumed office, and on the 16th of the same month he issued his first proclamation. The population of Upper Canada at this time was about 20,000. The first session of the First Parliament of Upper Canada met in a house on the west bank of the Niagara River, on the 17th September, the same year. It was three years later before any legislation took place with respect to the Medical Profession.

The Duke de la Rochefoucault, who was a guest of Governor Simcoe, 1795, at Newark (Niagara), in speaking of his visit and the Indians, says: "Intermittent fevers are very frequent in this village. The Indians frequently take the advice of the physician whom the English Government appoints and pays on their account, but they far more frequently take draughts which they prepare themselves."

That surgeons of regiments quartered in the Province discharged the function of uniting parties in marriage, in the first days of Upper Canada, seems clear, from the following extract from an Act passed at the second session of the First Parliament in 1793. The Act declares "that the marriages of all persons, not being under any canonical disqualification to contract matrimony, that have been publicly contracted before any magistrate or commanding officer of a post, adjutant or surgeon of a regiment, acting as chaplain, or any other person in any public office or employment, before the passing of this Act, shall be confirmed and considered, to all intents and purposes, as good and valid in law."

On July 6, 1795, the Parliament met at Navy Hall, Newark, now Niagara-on-the-Lake. The first Act passed at this session was one to regulate the practice of physic and surgery.

The following is taken from a volume in the library of Osgoode Hall, entitled

"THE STATUTES OF HIS MAJESTY, PROVINCE OF UPPER CANADA.

"CHAP. I.—An Act to regulate the practice of physic and surgery.

"Whereas many inconveniences have arisen to His Majesty's subjects in this province from unskilful persons practising physic and surgery therein,

"Therefore be it enacted by the King's Most Excellent Majesty, by and with the advice and consent of the Legislative

Council and Assembly of the Province of Upper Canada, constituted and assembled by virtue of and under the authority of an Act passed in the Parliament of Great Britain, entitled 'An Act to repeal certain parts of an Act passed in the fourteenth year of His Majesty's reign, entitled "An Act for making more effectual provision for the government of the Province of Quebec in North America, and to make further provision for the government of the said province, and by the authority of the same."'

"That no person who shall or may have come into this Province since the passing of the above-mentioned Act, and before the passing of this Act, nor any person who shall or may hereafter come into this province, shall be permitted to vend, sell, or distribute medicines by retail, or prescribe for sick persons, or practise physic, surgery or midwifery within the Province, for profit, until such person or persons shall be duly examined and approved of by a board of surgeons, who shall be constituted and appointed (as hereinafter mentioned) with full powers to grant licenses for the practice of physic, surgery and midwifery within the Province, and has received a license under the hands of and seal of the President of the said Board and such members thereof as may be present at his or their examination.

"II.—And be it further enacted by the authority aforesaid, That it shall and may be lawful to and for the Governor, Lieutenant-Governor, or person, etc., etc., by license under his hand and seal, to order and appoint the surgeon of His Majesty's hospital for the time being, together with the surgeons of His Majesty's regiment doing duty within the Province, and all other surgeons and practitioners resident within the same, authorized to practise physic and surgery by some lawfully constituted power or board in His Majesty's dominions, or any two of them (of which the surgeon of His Majesty's hospital shall be one), from time to time, and as often as occasion may require, to hear and examine all persons that may apply for a license to practise physic, surgery and midwifery, or either, within the said province; who shall, when they have examined and approved of any person so applying as aforesaid, grant him such license under their hands and seals, for which license he shall pay the sum of two pounds lawful money and no more.

"III.—And be it further enacted by the authority aforesaid: That if any person having come into this province since the passing of the said Act in the thirty-first year of His Majesty's reign, and before the passing of this Act; or shall come into it after the passing of the same, and shall vend, sell or distribute medicines by retail, or prescribe for sick persons, or practise physic or surgery as aforesaid, until such person shall have been duly examined and licensed by two or more members of the Board, constituted and appointed as aforesaid; such persons shall for every offence forfeit and pay the sum of ten pounds, to be recovered in any of His Majesty's courts of this province by action of debt, till, plaint or information, wherein no essoin, privilege, protection, or wager of law shall be allowed, and only one . . . ; and a moiety whereof shall be given to the informer, and the other moiety paid into the hands of the Receiver-General of this province, to and for the use of His Majesty, his heirs and successors, and to and for the use of this Province and the support of the civil government thereof, to be accounted for to His Majesty through the commissioners of his treasury, for the time being, in such manner and form as it shall please His Majesty to direct.

"IV.—Provided always that nothing in this Act shall extend or be construed to extend, to any person who shall have taken a degree in any university in His Majesty's dominions, or to any person who shall have been or may hereafter be commissioned or warranted as a surgeon or surgeon's mate in His Majesty's army or navy, or to any person vending, selling or distributing drugs or compounded medicines for which a patent hath been obtained, or to any other who shall, or may have settled, and shall or may have practised physic, surgery or midwifery within this province before the passing of the said Act, in the thirty-first year of His Majesty's reign as aforesaid; provided that such person last above-mentioned do not take an apprentice or person under pretence of tuition in any branch of physic or surgery, with an intent that such person shall present himself for examination and approval as aforesaid; hereby repealing all former Acts or ordinances made for the regulation of the practice of physic or surgery within this province."

It must be admitted that this was a very comprehensive Act; and it would be interesting to know who the originator and framer was. Not unlikely, however, the author was Attorney-General John White, who came to Canada in 1792 to fill that position. The Quebec Ordinance of 1788, no doubt, formed the ground-work of this Act. "The surgeon of His Majesty's hospital for the time being" has reference most probably to the principal medical officer of the military hospital at Kingston, who was, doubtless, Dr. Jas. Macaulay. Although this Act might seem to be well adapted to the infant province, it was found to be impracticable. There is no record as to whether an Examining Board was organized under the Act, but there is reason to believe that one was convened when necessary. There is some light thrown upon the matter by Robert Gourlay in his Sketch Book. Referring to the law which required an examination before "certain regular-bred surgeons appointed by the Governor," and to the penalty of £10 for each offence against the law, he says: "Now the fact is that few men who could stand the examination of such as were regular-bred and well educated, and fewer still had received a degree at a university, *would* practise. Nobody above the rank of a common cowherd would travel round a circle of forty or fifty miles in the wilderness for the pittance which could be collected long after this law was made; and save in the larger villages—Kingston, Niagara and York—nothing like a genteel subsistence could be obtained. How absurd, then, to think of preventing the remotely scattered people from choosing whom they liked to draw their teeth, bleed, and blister them! How absurd, how cruel, how meddling that a poor woman in labour could not have assistance from a handy, sagacious neighbour, without this neighbour being liable to be informed upon and fined! This absurdity was not sufficiently perceived for ten years, and then the Act was repealed in 1806."

Rochefoucault, in his narrative, 1795, in speaking of Kingston, says: "There are but very few surgeons in this district; they who assume this appellation contrive to get well paid for their trouble." From this it might be inferred that anyone might, whether qualified or not, assume the title; it might almost be inferred that all the doctors were such, merely by assumption.

In Gourlay's translation of Rochefoucault, we find the following: "But few surgeons reside in the country; they are not suffered to practise till after having undergone an examination by a physician appointed by Government. This prevention, which may prove very beneficial in future times, is at present of avoid. For, as very few apply for leave to practise, the most ignorant are admitted without difficulty, if they will only present themselves for admission. By one of them I was informed that the inferior classes of the inhabitants dread their advice in intermittent fevers, because they always prescribe bark, and that poor people, instead of following their advice, have recourse to a sort of magic charm, in which universal confidence is placed in this country. If seized with the ague, they go into the forest, search out a branch of an elm or sassafras, of the last year's growth, fasten to this branch, without breaking it off the tree, a thread, which must be quite new, tie as many knots as they think they shall have 'spells' of the fever, and then return home perfectly convinced that they shall not experience more fits than they have bound themselves to sustain by the number of knots they have tied. The first discoverers of this arcanum used to make so few knots that the ague would frequently disappoint their hopes; but they who at present practise this superstition tie so many that the febrile matter is generally carried off before the number of fits come up to that of the knots."

CHAPTER III.

QUESTIONABLE STANDING OF MEDICAL MEN.

THE second Governor of Upper Canada was Peter Hunter, who came to Canada in 1799. He was a brother of the great Dr. Hunter. He died at Quebec, August 25, 1805, aged 59 years. His ashes lie in the English cathedral there. Over them is a marble tablet, erected by his distinguished brother. It was in the year following Governor Hunter's death that the second Act relating to medicine was passed, which repealed the former Act, as follows:

"Whereas the provisions of an Act in thirty-fifth year of His Majesty's reign, etc., etc., are inexpedient in the present state of the Province: For remedy whereof, Be it enacted by the King's Most Excellent Majesty, by and with the advice and consent of the Legislative Council and Assembly of the Province of Upper Canada, constituted and assembled by virtue of and under the authority of an Act passed in the Parliament of Great Britain, entitled 'An Act to repeal certain parts of an Act passed in the fourteenth year of His Majesty's reign, entitled 'An Act for making more effectual provisions for the government of the Province of Quebec in North America, and to make further provision for the government of the said province, and by the authority of the same,' that the said Act, entitled 'An Act to regulate the practice of physic and surgery,' be and the same is hereby repealed."

(The foregoing is taken from a volume in Osgoode Hall library, in which is the signature of W. W. Baldwin, himself a doctor, by whom it was presented to the library. "One of the Benchers of this Society, and several times Treasurer thereof." Dated 1832.)

As stated, no records have been found of any Medical Board existing prior to the repeal of this Act. But the writer has been informed by an old physician, Dr. Smith, practising in Belleville, that he was examined by a Board in 1805, and procured a license under the Quebec Ordinance. The names of his examiners, he said, were "Drs. James Macaulay, Surgeon-General Rush (?), and Baldwin." His belief was that the Act of 1806 made the practice of medicine free in the Province. That a Medical Board did meet from time to time seems likely. (See Biographical Sketch of Dr. Sumner.) Unskilful persons continued to come into the country and to engage in the practice of medicine in all its branches. But, from an editorial article which appeared in the York *Gazette* October 8, 1808, it is learned that an effort was made in the House of Parliament to procure legislation to protect the public from incompetent practitioners. The article is as follows, and gives an excellent sample of the style of writing in those days:

"It is fresh in our recollection, that a Bill to regulate the admission of individuals as physicians and surgeons in this province, was last winter brought into the House of Assembly by a distinguished member of the honourable body. We also remember that the merits of the Bill were suggested, and that they underwent discussion and investigation, and experienced several necessary amendments. We are not insensible to the mover's honourable motives in bringing so laudable a measure forward at this juncture, as the necessity of something to improve the irregular systems on which physic and surgery are now conducted, is fully obvious. By this sense of the subject the gentleman was impelled to a warm and active support of its spirit and a laudable wish for its speedy promotion.

"We cannot, however, but regret that it was dropped in the House, whilst the opinions of several gentlemen in the House were so specifically different from any we can entertain. How far we, as incompetent judges, are warranted in this different view of a common subject, remains not for us to determine, but our general impression of its necessary utility is not lessened or defeated. The principal reason, we venture to assign, for its suspension or its failure, rises from the variety of business to which the attention of the members was devoted, or that unweighed as the matter in question might be, or not familiarized to superior judgments. The opinion we maintain of such a public want arises from the conviction we feel and the knowledge we possess, that the health, nay, frequently the existence of a fellow-creature, is lost, being too often sacrificed to the pretensions or cannibal ignorance of empirics, quacks and impostors. It is an incontestible fact that we are all created patients, but few of us are born physicians, and that education and studious practice, as well as a just judgment of diagnostics and the efficient operative qualities of prescriptions, form the necessary parts of fortunate and conspicuous practitioners.

"To qualify the ordinary professors of medicine by the attainment of this necessary and ornamental part of human knowledge, and to bar the avenues to gross public impositions were the leading principles in this laudable Bill; at least, it thus forcibly impressed us, when we heard it repeatedly read.

As medicines frequently possess the properties of extending and curtailing the duration of existence, they require to be prescribed and administered with much judgment and caution, and not as in many cases by ignorant and unsparing hands. In indulging no unreasonable, no blamable, hope we really wish and anticipate the introduction of this encircling distended measure, and benevolently passed on the very spirit of promoting the safety of health and public good."

It was thought that by the repeal of this Act of Upper Canada, there existed no restrictions, and that anyone might engage in the practice of medicine, but it was found that such was not the case. Robert Gourlay, writing in 1818, respecting Upper Canada, says: "Many physicians and surgeons have gone into practice without any provincial license, supposing there was no prohibition and not suspecting that an old ordinance of the former Province of Quebec, which was not executed and had not been published among the laws of this province, was revived by a repeal of the Provincial Act, so as to be in force here."

The state of the medical profession at this period may be understood from newspaper articles which appeared from time to time. On March 3, 1812, a letter appears in the Kingston *Gazette*, from Jeremiah Freedling, complaining of a doctor who, having no one to practise upon, induced one of his daughters to be inoculated for small-pox, by which the disease devastated the neighbourhood.

At this period, the Rev., afterwards Bishop, Strachan, contributed from time to time articles on various subjects which have been compared to Addison's in the *Spectator*, under the pseudonyme, *Reckoner*. Referring to the letter of Mr. Freedling, he makes the following remarks: "I participate most sincerely in the distress of Mr. Freedling and his amiable daughter; the Province is overrun with self-made physicians who have no pretensions to knowledge of any kind, and yet there is no profession that requires more extensive information.

"They comprehend not the causes or nature of diseases, are totally ignorant of anatomy, chemistry and botany; many know nothing of classical learning or general science. Where shall you find one among them attending particularly to the age, constitution and circumstances of the patient, and varying his prescriptions accordingly. It is, indeed, preposterous to expect judgment and skill, a nice discrimination of diseases or a proper method of cure from men who have never been regularly taught, who cannot pronounce, much less explain, the terms of the art they profess, and who are unable to read the books written upon the subject. The welfare of the people calls aloud for some legislative provision that shall remedy this increasing evil; any examination, however slight, would terrify nine-tenths of the present race. Were it only enacted that no other trial than that of reading two pages of Blackstone's Commentaries or Burns' Justice, without missing lines, spelling long words, or forgetting the stops in the presence of the justices of the Quarter Sessions (after showing their credentials that they had served a regular apprenticeship). It would be of singular benefit and stop the greater number. Their gross ignorance appears in the medicines they use, which are much less innocent than Dr. Sangrados' hot water. They cure all diseases with two specifics, opium and mercury. Is a patient in great pain, he must swallow a large pill of opium. Is a practitioner in doubt about his disease, a dose of calomel is the remedy. I was lately visiting a young woman ill of a fever. The Doctor came in, felt her pulse with much gravity, pronounced her near a *crisis.* 'She must take this dose,' said the gentleman, pouring out as much calomel on a piece of paper as would have killed two ploughmen. 'Pray, what is this?' said I. Doctor: '*A febrifuger!*' 'Is it not calomel?' 'Yes.' 'You mean to divide this into several doses?' 'Not at all.' 'But the patient is weak.' 'No matter, I likes to scour well.' 'Do you not weigh carefully so powerful a medicine before you give it?' 'No, sir, I knows exactly.' As the woman was evidently getting better, I threw the calomel out of the window after his departure and sent her some bark and wine. On another occasion I found, on going to see a man ill of a bilious complaint, that the doctor (not the same practitioner) had left a large dose of calomel, and ordered three large blocks of wood heated in boiling water, one for his feet and one for each of his sides. The poor man was sweating himself to death. I commanded the blocks to be removed, ventilated the room, sprinkled the room with vinegar, washed his head and hands with it, and he began to breathe—another hour would have killed him, for you could hardly discern life in him when I entered. I mixed a little of the calomel with some toasted rhubarb to be given him when he got cool, and he recovered. I was called to a young man whose disease, a dysentery, had been much aggravated by the gross ignorance of his physician. This profound doctor had the audacity to say, after my arrival, that the youth was getting better when he was in the very agony of death, and actually expired in a few minutes. Many more cases might be stated, but every reader's memory will furnish him with plenty. Let the law check this growing evil and do justice to regular practitioners who have gone through a course of studies in order to qualify themselves for this arduous profession. At present they are elbowed out of their practice by men who can neither read nor write so as to be understood."

That illiterate and incompetent persons found their way into Upper Canada during the first fifteen years of this century may be gathered from letters which appeared in the Kingston *Gazette*.

In the *Gazette* of June 2nd, 1812, is a letter from Gananoque, signed "Candidus," giving a copy of an account sent to Mrs. John Gould by a "self-taught physician of this province."

"The estate of Mrs. John Gould, Dr.

"To Dr., For medsin and attendants whene he was chokd with a large peas of Butter no of meat, £3."

A second letter, signed "Credulus," refers to "certain medical gentlemen who have, out of pure charity, come into this country from the neighbouring States to cure us of all our maladies." They do not use opium, or calomel, but charms. He gives an account of the treatment of a tumour by stroking and using certain words to drive away "the devil's swelling."

A third letter is about a shoemaker who went where unknown, to practise, and who being called to see a case of dropsy pronounced it pleurisy, and declared that "fleglottomy" was demanded to reduce the body to natural size; but on being exposed took a hasty departure.

A fourth letter refers to a bill sent in by a doctor, with a deduction of £6, for "killing your son." This was because the doctor had carried the small-pox to the son, who died of it.

The following is an indication that at Kingston, in 1815, the more intelligent public saw the necessity of protection against incompetent men. Kingston *Gazette* contains the following:

"To the public. *Facilis descensus Averni.*

"The Parliament of this province, during the last session, provided, in part, against the imposition of empirics in medicine. This was not more necessary for the safety of the diseased than the reputation of the faculty." Then follows an earnest appeal to the public and Parliament against quacks, their danger, "without one ray of science," who "presume to thrust the created into the presence of the Creator." Signed "W." ("Not of the profession," he says.)

At the capital, York, at this period strenuous and persistent efforts were put forth, not only to place and retain the profession in a state consistent with its noble attribute, but to afford proper medical skill and care to all classes in need of hospital relief. This extract, from a current journal, gives some interesting information in connection with this and other matters:

"YORK GENERAL HOSPITAL.

"The Loyal and Patriotic Society of Upper Canada was organized at York, 1812. The object was 'to afford relief and aid to disabled militia men and their families, to reward merit, excite emulation, and commemorate glorious exploits by bestowing medals and other honourary marks of public approbation and distinction for extraordinary instances of personal courage and fidelity in defence of the Province.' The Society had only been formed a few days before the subscription of York to the fund had amounted to the respectable sum of eight hundred and seventy-five pounds (three thousand five hundred dollars), to be paid annually during the war with the United States. Medals were also struck in London, by order of the Loyal and Patriotic Society. These medals, however, never reached the intended recipients, from the fact that there were so many candidates for the coveted honour that the difficulty of deciding who was to receive them was found to be too great. The medals were finally broken up and the bullion, augumented with what remained of the funds of the Society, devoted to benevolent objects. A considerable donation from the funds was made to the York General Hospital, an institution well deserving of the favour shown to it, and the foundation of the present Toronto Hospital, which enjoys more than a provincial reputation. As a reminder of the time of the war, and the loyalty which inspired the old Canadians of that day, it will not be out of place to give a short description of this medal. It was two and one-half inches in diameter. On the obverse, within a wreath of laurel, were the words, 'For Merit;' on this side was also the legend, 'Presented by a grateful country.' On the reverse, was the following device: A strait between two lakes; on the north side, a beaver (emblem of peaceful industry), the ancient cognizance of Canada; in the background, the British lion slumbering; on the south side of the strait, the American eagle poising in the air, as if checked from seizing the beaver by the presence of the lion; legend on this side, 'Upper Canada preserved.'"

CHAPTER IV.

QUALIFIED AND UNQUALIFIED PHYSICIANS.

AFTER the repeal of the Act, nothing was done in the way of legislation until the year 1815, after the close of the war. The Act then passed, although somewhat lengthy, possesses sufficient interest, it is thought, to give it here *in extenso*:

"An Act to License Practitioners in Physic and Surgery, passed 14th March, 1815.

"Whereas, many inconveniences have arisen to His Majesty's subjects in this province from unskilful persons practising physic and surgery therein,

"Therefore, be it enacted by the King's Most Excellent Majesty, by and with the advice and consent of the Legislative Council and Assembly of the Province of Upper Canada, constituted and assembled by virtue of and under the authority of an Act passed in the Parliament of Great Britain, entitled 'An Act to repeal an Act passed in the fourteenth year of His Majesty's reign, entitled "An Act for making more effectual provision for the government of the Province of Quebec, in North America, and to make further provision for the government of the said Province,"' and by the authority of the same, that no person who shall or may have come into this province since the passing of the above-mentioned Act, and before the passing of this Act, nor any person who shall or may hereafter come into this province, shall be permitted to prescribe for sick persons, or practise physic, surgery or midwifery within the Province, for profit, until such person or persons shall be duly examined and approved of by a Board of Surgeons, who shall be constituted and appointed (as hereinafter mentioned) with full powers to grant licenses for the practice of physic, surgery and midwifery within the Province, and has received a license under the hand and seal of the President of the said Board, and countersigned by the Clerk of the said Board, which clerk the President of said Board shall and may nominate and appoint.

"2. And be it further enacted by the authority aforesaid, that it shall and may be lawful for the Governor, Lieutenant-Governor, or person administering the government of this province, by license under his hand and seal to order and appoint the senior military medical officer for the time being, together with the surgeons of His Majesty's regiment, and all staff-surgeons doing duty within the Province, and the surgeons of His Majesty's navy and all other surgeons and practitioners resident within the same, authorized to practise physic, surgery and midwifery by some lawfully constituted power or Board in His Majesty's dominion or any two of them, of which the senior medical officer from time to time, and as often as time requires to hear and examine all persons that may apply for a license to practise physic and surgery, or either, within the said province, who shall, when they have examined and approved of any person so applying as aforesaid, grant him a license under the hand and seal of the President and countersigned by the Clerk of the Board aforesaid, for which license he shall pay the sum of two pounds lawful money, and no more; provided always, that nothing in this Act contained shall extend or be construed to extend to prevent any female from practising midwifery in any part of this province, or to require such female to take out such license as aforesaid.

"3. And be it further enacted by the authority aforesaid, that if any person having come into this province since the passing of the said Act of the thirty-first year of His Majesty's reign, and before the passing of this Act, or shall come into this province after the passing of the same, shall prescribe for sick persons or practise physic, surgery or midwifery as aforesaid, until such person shall be duly examined and licensed by two or more members of the Board constituted and appointed as aforesaid, such person shall for every such offence forfeit and pay the sum of one hundred pounds, to be recovered in any of His Majesty's courts in this province, by action or debt, plaint or information, wherein no ensurer privilege, protection or wager of law shall be allowed, and only on imparfance, a moiety whereof shall be given to the informer, and the other moiety paid into the hands of the Receiver-General of this province, to and for the use of His Majesty, his heirs and successors, and to and for the use of this province and the support of the civil government thereof, to be accounted for to His Majesty through the Lords Commissioners of his treasury for the time being, in such manner and form as it shall please His Majesty to direct.

"Provided always, that nothing in this Act shall extend or be construed to extend to any person who shall have taken a degree in any university in His Majesty's dominions, or to any person who shall have been or may hereafter be commissioned or warranted as a surgeon or surgeon's mate in His Majesty's army or navy, or to any other who shall or may have practised physic, surgery or midwifery within the Province before the passing of the said Act of the thirty-first year of His Majesty's reign as aforesaid, hereby repealing all former Acts or ordinances made for the regulation of the practice of physic or surgery within this province."

The number of medical men in Upper Canada (1815) possessing some qualification, was in the neighbourhood of thirty-six or forty; but doubtless there were many others, with little or no qualification, who professed to possess medical skill.

In 1817, Robert Gourlay addressed the resident landowners of the several townships, submitting a number of questions relating to the township to be answered by them. The fourth question on the list was: "How many medical practitioners in the township?" Although a large proportion of the townships replied to the other questions, comparatively few answered this one. The following are those from which answers were supplied: Sandwich, 2; Malden, 2; Raleigh, none; Dover, East and West Chatham, Camden, Oxford, Howard and Harwich, on the River Thames (one each), summary, 5; Windham, "No medical practitioner in the township, but can generally get one within eight or ten miles"; Norwich, "One regular-bred practitioner of physic and surgery"; Blenheim, 1; Burford and its Gore, 1; Woodhouse, 1; Yarmouth, 2.

The townships of the London District, with a population of about 8,907, had six medical practitioners.

District of Gore (population, 8,543), Nelson, 1; Wellington Square, part of Nelson, 1; Ancaster, 1; total, 3.

Niagara District, with a population of about 12,548, had six medical practitioners. Of these Berlin had 1; Stamford, 2; Grantham, 2.

Midland District is stated as having ten practitioners—Thurlow, 2; Sophiasburg, 1; Hallowell, 2; Belleville (?) 3; Kingston, 4. (Not unlikely the ten given to the district does not include the town of Kingston.)

Johnston District—Walford, 1; Lansdowne, none.

Eastern District—Charlotteburgh, 2.

A table showing township reports of the Newcastle, Midland, Johnston, and Eastern districts, gives a total of fifteen practitioners.

"For the reported population of 26,977 in the Western, London, Gore and Niagara districts," there are given twenty medical practitioners.

"While I was in Canada," Gourlay writes, "men of education, talent, and experience, came from home to settle there, but it would not do, and many of them have left the Province. A country surgeon at home has hard work of it. What may he be supposed to have where the population does not amount to seven *bodies* to the square mile (?) and where fees must be received per the barrel, or the bushel; perhaps in lumber. For my part, I see no occasion to have any restraining law as to the practice of physic or surgery in any country." He then advocates free trade in medical practice. The state of the

Province with respect to medical matters, and the character of those administering to the public in the healing art—at least in Midland District—are well set forth by a writer in the Kingston *Gazette*, of May 25, 1816, who was evidently well qualified to form and express an opinion on the matter:

"MR. MILES.

"SIR,—It is a subject of deep regret to many that the executive or magistracy should show such a sluggishness in enforcing the laws of the Province. It is particularly to be deplored so far as those laws relate to persons calling themselves doctors; not only our fortunes, but also our lives are in the hands of those despicable quacks. How does it happen that an Act of the session of 1815 is not acted upon? Is it because that Act is unwise, or is it because the executive does not think it of sufficient importance to put it in opperation? If the first, why not expunge it from the laws of the Province? If the latter, what is the use of a house of assembly at all?

"Perhaps, Mr. Editor, you and other respectible gentlemen living in town, who have access to, and knowledge to value the merits of those practising medicine, may not feel so much as I do the miserable situation of the country; but, Sir, if the health of the subject is not a matter of sufficient importance to rouse the morbid sensibility of those whose duty it is to administer the laws, I should imagine that in a political point of view it would be a matter of great importance to look after those quack spies who are daily inundating the Province. Those men (most brutal, generally speaking, in their manners, and in their conduct immoral in the highest degree) go from house to house like peddlars, dealing out their poisonous pills and herbs, and holding out to the gaping ignorant the advantages of a republican government.

"But to give you an instance of the contemptible conduct of one of those animals nearer yourself. During the last session of the peace I had occasion to be in Kingston, and, although I lodged in a private house, I had occasion to call one morning at a tavern. While speaking to the landlady in the bar, in comes a doctor and called for a gill of brandy. He drank it, in the course of which he put a great many questions to her about the health of her customers, and finally said he would leave some fever powders, as it was likely the country people would be getting drunk (as he termed it) and would require medicine. The lady thanked him, and said if she wanted any medical aid she knew where to send for it.

"To conclude, Mr. Editor, the consequences of the present system will be, in the first place, to prevent native merit entering into the profession; secondly, those few respectable and regularly educated men whom we have amongst us will either leave the Province or get a miserable subsistance if they remain; and, lastly, though not the least, the Province will be in some degree revolutionized by those emissaries of a licentious republic.

"VERITAS.

"Adolphustown, May 14, 1816."

We give another phase of the matter, concerning which the reader will be able to form his own opinion:

"Notice to all unlicensed Practitioners of Medicine and Quacks in and about Kingston:

"Doctor Scott will indiscriminately and impartially make known to the Attorney-General's Office, in this province, and prosecute with the utmost rigour of the law, all and every person whom he may hereafter discern practising any branch of the medical profession under the above denomination.

"JAS. SCOTT, M.C.S., etc., etc., etc.

"Kingston, July 10th, 1817."

This card informs us who Doctor Scott was:

"Mr. Scott, late Surgeon of His Majesty's Ship 'Montreal,' on Lake Ontario, M.R.C.S., Dublin, formerly one of the Attendants at the Dublin Lying-in Hospital," . . . "long attention will be paid to patients on the reasonable terms."

Dr. Scott has in the *Gazette* an article about a child that was brought him, and to which he gave medicine, etc., "when a coil of worms passed. These may be seen at Dr. Scott's office," etc. This same Scott was prosecuting Quacks.

The following advertisement is copied *verbatim* from a manuscript bill, posted up at a public place. It was probably more taking than Dr. Scott's card:

"RICHMOND, *Oct.* 17th, 1817.

"ADVERTISEMENT.—This is to Certify that I, Solomon Albert, is Good to cure any sore in word Complaint or any Pains, Rheumaticks Pains, or any Complaint what so ever the Subscriber doctors with yerbs or Roots. Any Person wishing to employ him will find him at Dick Bells.

"SOLOMON ALBERT."

From the foregoing it is quite evident that some action by the Government was necessary to protect the public, and the necessity was duly recognized.

The Act passed in 1815 was repealed in 1818. "The provisions . . . have been found to be impracticable," it is stated in the preamble of the new Act. And further provisions for licensing practitioners in medicine were made. It reads: "That it shall and may be lawful for the Governor, Lieutenant-Governor, or person administering the government, to constitute and appoint, under his hand and seal at arms, five or more persons legally authorized to practise physic, surgery or midwifery in this province, to be a board, whereof any three to be a quorum, to hear and examine all persons desirous to apply for a license, to practise physic, surgery and midwifery, or either of them, within this province, and being satisfied by such examination that any person is duly qualified to practise physic, surgery and midwifery, or either, to certify the same under the hands and seals of two or more of such board, whereupon the Governor, Lieutenant-Governor, or person administering the government, being satisfied of the loyalty, integrity and good morals of such applicant may, under his hand and seal at arms, grant to him a license to practise physic, surgery and midwifery, or either, conformable to such certificate; provided always, that nothing in this Act shall extend to prevent any female from practising midwifery in this province, or to require such female to take out a license as aforesaid."

"And be it further enacted by the authority aforesaid,—That if any person, not excepted as aforesaid, shall practise physic, surgery, or midwifery within this province, without such license, he shall for every such offence forfeit and pay the sum of one hundred pounds; to be recovered in any of His Majesty's Courts of King's Bench, by action of debt, bill, plaint or information, one moiety whereof shall be given to the informer, and the other moiety paid into the hands of the Receiver-General of this province, to and for the use of His Majesty, his heirs and successors, and to and for the use of this province and the support of the civil government thereof, to be accounted for to His Majesty through the Lords, Commoners of His Majesty's treasury, for the time being, in such manner and form as it shall please His Majesty to direct. Provided always,—That nothing in this Act shall extend to any person who has been resident, practising physic, surgery and midwifery before the first of January, one thousand eight hundred and twelve, until twelve months after the constitution of such Board as aforesaid, and notice thereof, and of the time and place of its assembling, be given in Upper Canada *Gazette.*

"Sec. V.—And be it further enacted by the authority aforesaid,—That the said Board shall be held and kept in the town of York, in the Home District, twice in each and every year—the first Monday in January and the first Monday in July."

This Act of 1818 was the first effectual step to open a proper portal to the ranks of the medical profession·

Although the Act specifies that the Board shall meet twice a year, it will be seen that the Board met every three months.

SECOND PART.

THE PROCEEDINGS OF THE UPPER CANADA MEDICAL BOARD FROM ITS ORGANIZATION, 1819 TO 1850; AND OF THE COLLEGE OF PHYSICIANS AND SURGEONS OF UPPER CANADA, 1839-41, WITH REFERENCES TO HISTORICAL EVENTS SHOWING THE GROWTH AND DEVELOPMENT OF THE PROFESSION.

CHAPTER V.

PROCEEDINGS OF THE MEDICAL BOARD.

NO time was lost in creating a Medical Board in accordance with the Act. It came into force on November 27, 1818, and on January 4, 1819, the Board was convened at York—now Toronto.

The records of the Medical Board are contained in two volumes now in the custody of the Registrar of the College of Physicians and Surgeons of Ontario, through whose kindness these minute books have been at the writer's service. The contents of the first pages are given in full, subsequently the record is condensed so far as could be done without impairing the account of the proceedings of the Board. On the first page of the first volume are given two forms, no doubt prepared for supplying the successful candidates with the necessary certificate.

"We certify that , of , in the District of , Gentleman, hath appeared before the Medical Board, and being examined touching his qualifications to practise Physic, Surgery and Midwifery, the Board is perfectly satisfied by his Examination, and find him duly and fully qualified to practise in the above branches.

"Given under our Hands and Seals this day of"

A COPY.

"At a meeting of the Medical Board, held this day, Mr. , of , in the District of , appeared, and having been examined touching his qualifications to practise Physic, Surgery and Midwifery, the Board find him fully qualified to practise these several branches, and grant him this their certificate accordingly.

"Signed."

"PROCEEDINGS OF THE MEDICAL BOARD APPOINTED UNDER THE AUTHORITY OF AN ACT OF THE PARLIAMENT OF UPPER CANADA, PASSED IN THE FIFTY-NINTH YEAR OF THE REIGN OF OUR SOVEREIGN LORD KING GEORGE THE THIRD, ENTITULED, 'AN ACT,' ETC., ETC., ETC.

"YORK, 4th *January*, 1819.—The Board met. Present: James Macaulay, Christopher Widmer, William Lyons and Grant Powell, Surgeons. The Board adjourned till 12 o'clock to-morrow.

"YORK, 5th *January*, 1819.—The Board met pursuant to adjournment. Present as above. The Commission was read.

"Mr. John Gilchrist, of the township of Hamilton, in the district of New Castle, appeared, and being examined and found duly qualified to practise Physic, Midwifery and Surgery, he received a certificate to that effect accordingly.

"Mr. John S. Thomas, of Markham, in the Home District, likewise appeared, and on examination was found totally unqualified to practise in either branch. The Board adjourned to the first Monday in April next.

"YORK, 5th *April*, 1819.—The Board met. Present: James Macaulay, Christopher Widmer and Grant Powell, Surgeons.

"Mr. Nathaniel Bell, of the township of Nelson, district of Gore, appeared, and being examined was found fit to practise Physic, Surgery and Midwifery, and received a certificate to that effect.

"Mr. Daniel Brenaird appeared, and being examined was found unfit to practise, and was rejected. The Board adjourned to the first Monday in July next.

"YORK, 5th *July*, 1819.—The Board met. Present: James Macaulay, Christopher Widmer and William Lyons, Surgeons.

"Mr. Edward W. Armstrong, of Hallowell, appeared, and being examined was found fit to practise Physic, Surgery and Midwifery, and received a certificate to that effect.

"Mr. Anson Ladd, of Sydney, appeared, and being examined was found unfit to practise, and was rejected.

"Mr. Pitkin Gross, of Murray, appeared, and being examined was found fit to practise Physic, Surgery and Midwifery, and received a certificate to that effect.

"Mr. Horace Yeomans, of Waterloo, Kingston, appeared, and being examined was found unfit to practise, and was rejected. The Board adjourned to 12 o'clock to-morrow.

"YORK, 6th *July*, 1819.—The Board met pursuant to adjournment. Present, as above.

"Mr. Anson Heyden, of the Midland District, appeared, and being examined was found unfit to practise, and was rejected.

"Mr. Ansalon Gutherie, of Dover, Western District, appeared, and being examined was found unfit to practise, and was rejected.

"Mr. Augustus Miller, of Gainsborough, Niagara District, appeared, and being examined was found fit to practise Physic, Surgery and Midwifery, and received a certificate to that effect. The Board adjourned to the first Monday in October next.

"YORK, 4th *October*, 1819.—The Board met pursuant to adjournment. Present: James Macaulay, Christopher Widmer and Grant Powell, Surgeons. The Board adjourned to 12 o'clock to-morrow.

"YORK, 5th *October*, 1819.—Mr. Salmon King, of Oxford, London District, appeared, and being examined was found unfit for practice, and was rejected.

"Mr. Charles Dunscombe, of Delaware Town, London District, appeared, and being examined was found fit to practise Physic, Surgery and Midwifery, and received a certificate to that effect.

"Mr. H*a*rma*n*nus Smith, of Barton, district of Gore, appeared, and being duly examined was found fit to practise Physic and

Midwifery only, and received a certificate to that effect. The Board adjourned to Thursday, the 7th October.

"YORK, 7th *October*, 1819.—Mr. Anthony Morton, of Prescott, district of Johnstown, appeared, and being examined was found fit to practise Physic, Surgery and Midwifery, and received a certificate to that effect. The Board adjourned to 1 o'clock to-morrow.

"YORK, 8th *October*, 1819.—The Board met pursuant to adjournment.

"Mr. Charles Martin, of Niagara, appeared, and being examined was found unfit to practise, and was rejected. The Board adjourned to the first Monday in January, 1820."

This was the work done by the Board during the first year of its existence. Altogether eight gentlemen were admitted into the ranks of the profession.

Of these pioneer members of our profession in Upper Canada, all have passed away. Dr. Gilchrist, the first to pass the Board, died only a few years ago.

That the profession led by the Medical Board was alive to the interest of the public, as well as to their own, is shown by the following announcement:

"Proposals for building by contract, a Brick Hospital in the Town of York, will be received at the Post Office, by William Allan, Esq., where a Plan, Elevation, and particular description of the intended Building, may be seen, and any information respecting it obtained.

"Proposals to be given in within one month from this date.

"York, 24th November, 1819."

—*Upper Canada Gazette,* Nov. 25th, 1819.

How soon thereafter the hospital was erected is uncertain; but reference is made to the hospital in the weekly register for 1822. With regard to this building, Dr. Scadding records that "the old hospital was a spacious, unadorned, matter-of-fact, two-story structure, of red brick, one hundred and seven feet long, and sixty-six feet wide. It had, by the direction of Dr. Grant Powell, as we have heard, the peculiarity of standing with its sides precisely east and west, north and south. At a subsequent period it consequently had the appearance of having been jerked round bodily, the streets in the neighbourhood not being laid out with the same precise regard to the cardinal points. The building exhibited recessed galleries on the north and south sides, and a flattish hipped roof. The interior was conveniently designed.

"When the Houses of Parliament at the east end of the town were destroyed by fire in 1824, the Legislature assembled for several Sessions in the General Hospital."

Talbot, writing in 1824, says: "The York Hospital is the most extensive building in the Province, and its external appearance is very respectable."

The writer walked the wards of the old hospital in the beginning of the fifties. Its quaint appearance, as described by Dr. Scadding, is readily recalled.

At the meeting of the Board, January, 1820, Drs. Macaulay, Widmer, Lyons and Powell, being present, Mr. Geo. Baker, of Bath, "received a certificate to practise Physic and Midwifery, and the lesser operations in Surgery." Six others were examined, but rejected with a recommendation to "further study and attendance on a course of lectures at New York."

By this it may be inferred that the Board considered the medical instructions given at New York were of a satisfactory nature. That the Board was careful in their duties is shown by the limitation in the certificate granted to practise.

The Board met daily from Monday to Saturday inclusive.

At the meeting in April, 1820, the same members were present. There was only one candidate examined, Mr. R. L. Cockcroft, who received a certificate of qualification to practise.

It would seem that the rejection of six candidates at the previous meeting had a deterring effect upon aspirants for a place in the profession.

At the July (1820) meeting, the same members were present. Mr. Hiram Weeks, of Fredericksburg, Midland District, passed his examination, also Mr. Samuel Throckmortin, of Norwich, London District. One was rejected and "recommended to attend to the same line of study as pointed out on the 4th of January, 1820." More candidates were evidently expected, as the Board adjourned from day to day until Saturday.

The same members were present at the October meeting. "No candidates for examination appearing, the Board adjourned" on Monday, and on each day for the same reason, until Thursday, when one candidate was rejected, but "recommended to further study." Adjourned until Saturday, but no more candidates appeared.

Altogether, during the second year of the Board's existence, four persons were admitted to practise. Eight were rejected, four for the second time. The Board, no doubt, discharged its duty conscientiously; but it was, we can understand, with some of the rejected candidates, a very serious matter. Travelling, at that period, was exceedingly laborious and expensive, and took much time; and we find that some of the applicants came from the borders of Lower Canada and from the extreme west of the Province.

In January, 1821, the Board, consisting of the same members, met, and Mr. John Vanderpoel, of Fredericksburg, Midland District, passed his examination. It met finally on the Saturday but "no medical character appearing for examination, the Board adjourned."

At the April meeting, the Board examined one candidate who failed to pass.

At a special meeting of the Board in July we find it assuming other duties.

"YORK, 4th *July*, 1821.—The Board met. Present: Christopher Widmer, William Lyons and Grant Powell, Esq., Surgeons. The following letter was received from His Excellency the Lieutenant-Governor's Secretary:

"GOVERNMENT HOUSE,
"2nd *July*, 1821.

"SIR,—By command of His Excellency the Lieut.-Governor I have the honour to transmit to you the copy of a Circular Letter addressed by me to certain officers of the Militia drawing Pentions on account of wounds, for the information and guidance of the Medical Board, which is requested to act herein as required.

"I have the honour to be, Sir,

"Your most obedient humble servant,

"(Signed) GEORGE HILLIER,

"James Macaulay, Esq., "*Secretary.*

"Etc., Etc., Etc."

"[Circular Copy.]

"GOVERNMENT HOUSE,

"YORK, *June* 5th, 1821.

"SIR,—I have received the commands of the Lieut.-Governor to inform you that no provision has been made by the Provincial Legislature for the payment of the Pention granted to you on account of the wound you received during the late War for the current year, but as His Majesty has been pleased to sanction this allowance to you, His Excellency will not hesitate to direct a Warrant to issue for it on the funds of the Crown.

"In order, however, to do this it will be necessary that you should undergo inspection by the Medical Board, which holds its quarterly meeting at York, in the first weeks of January, April, July and October, and present a certificate at this office that the disability on account of which your Pention was granted still continues. This being the rule of His Majesty's Service and having been conformed to in the Provincial Statute lately passed with regard to the Militia Pentions.

"Without such certificate payment cannot be made.

"I have the honour to be, etc.,

"(Signed) GEORGE HILLIER."

Although the details of the examination of those asking a pension may not be considered as a part of the history of the medical profession, yet they constitute a fragment of the unwritten history of the veterans of 1812, which it is believed will be acceptable to the medical and general public. Consequently the account regarding them will be given as found in the record. It will be observed that the Board met between the periods of the regular quarterly meetings to suit the wishes of certain veterans.

"Major T. G. Simons having appeared before the Board, and being duly examined, received the following certificate:

"We certify that we have personally examined Major T. G. Simons, and are of opinion that no material alteration has taken place in the disability described in the proceedings of the Medical Board held upon his case, July 31st, 1815.

"Given under our Hands at York, this 4th day of July, 1821.

"(Signed) CHRISTOPHER WIDMER.
WILLIAM LYONS.
GRANT POWELL.

"Entered: W. Lee, *Secretary.*"

No candidates were examined at this quarterly meeting.

The name of Mr. Lee appears for the first time as secretary of the Board. (See biog. Dr. Wm. Lee.)

At the meeting of the Board on July 2, 1821, we find the name of James Macaulay, the senior member of the Board, mentioned for the last time. Christopher Widmer's name stands next, and after this, for many a year, and, invariably present, we find his name appearing as the senior member.

The next record is as follows:—

"YORK, 10th *September*, 1821.—The Board met in consequence of the following communication:

"OFFICE OF GOVERNMENT,
"YORK, 8th *September*, 1821.

"SIR,—I am directed in the absence of Mr. Secretary Hillier to signify to you that, under the circumstances stated by you, His Excellency has no objection to such meeting of the Board, providing you can prevail on the Gentlemen composing it to assemble.

"I am, Sir, your most obedient, humble servant,

"(Signed) EDWD. MCMAHON.

"To LIEUT. DANIEL MCDOUGAL,
"Late Incorporated Militia."

"Present: Christopher Widmer, William Lyons and William W. Baldwin, Esq. Lieut. Daniel McDougal appeared before the Board, and, being duly examined, received the following certificate:

"We certify that we have personally examined Lieutenant Daniel McDougal, of the Late Incorporated Regiment of Militia, and are of opinion that the disability on account of the wounds for which his pension was granted still continues.

"Given under our Hands at York this 10th day of September, 1821.

"(Signed) CHRISTOPHER WIDMER.
WILLIAM LYONS.
WILLIAM W. BALDWIN.

"Entered: WM. LEE, *Secretary*."

It will be noticed that the name of Wm. W. Baldwin, Esq., appears for the first time as a member of the Board. The members of this meeting are designated in the minutes as "Esquires," whereas previously they were called "Surgeons."

"The under-mentioned Pensioners, having appeared and being duly examined as to their labouring under the Disability of wounds, received the following certificate:

"This is to certify that the Medical Board hath personally examined   , late in the   , and that from being wounded they are of opinion the said   is incapable of earning his livelihood by hard labour.

"By order of the Board,

"(Signed) WM. LEE, *Secretary*."

"George Hutchinson, Provincial Marine; Jacob Snider, Incorporated Militia; Andrew Borland, Flank Company; William Laughton, 2nd Essex Regt.; John Bathron, Incorporated Militia; Richard Hull, Incorporated Militia. The above-mentioned received a certificate of Disability."

"YORK, 4th *October*, 1821.—Joseph Shephard, of the 3rd York Militia, received a certificate of Disability.

"YORK, 5th *October*, 1821.—The following Pensioners appeared, and being duly examined, Isaac Ball, Artillery, approved. A person by the name of Lee was rejected. Nath. Bell, 4th

Lincoln Regt., rejected; Elijah Mudge, 1st Oxford Regt., approved; John Ryan, Artillery, approved.

"YORK, 6th *October*, 1821.—Mr. Peter McDougal, late of the Indian Department (a pensioner), appeared, but was rejected." There was no examination of candidates for license to practise at this session.

"YORK, 7th *January*, 1822.—The Board met. Present: Christopher Widmer, Wm. Lyons, Grant Powell. The following certificate was granted:

"We certify that having examined Peter Miller, late private in the 3rd Regiment of York Militia, we find him incapable of earning his living in consequence of disease contracted in service in June, 1813.

"(Signed) C. WIDMER.
WILLIAM LYONS.
GRANT POWELL.

"Entered: A. L. LEE, *Secretary*."

"YORK, 8th *January*, 1822.—Joseph Boot, Aran Lester and Nathan Coho, of the 4th Lincoln Militia; John Coat, Artillery Provincials, not on the pension list.

"Lieut. Henry Ruttan, Incorporated Militia; Lieut. George Ryerson, 1st Norfolk Militia; Capt. James Gordon, 1st Essex Regt. Militia; Jacob Smith, 3rd York Militia. The above-named, having presented themselves for examination before the Board, they were rejected, as not labouring under any Disability. Andrew Kenady, 3rd York Militia; Thomas Major, 3rd York Militia; Charles McKenan, 2nd Glengarry Militia, having presented themselves, received a certificate of Disability, from wounds received in action with the enemy. Ebenezar Every, of 2nd Leeds Militia, having presented himself for examination, received a certificate of Disability, from wounds received in action with the enemy."

At this meeting Chancy Beedle, of York, and Olivor G. Tiffany, of Gore District, Gentlemen, passed Medical examination. One "was found disqualified and recommended for further study."

"1st *April*, 1822.—Drs. Widmer, Lyons and Powell present. The Commission was read appointing James Sampson, Esq., late Assistant-Surgeon in His Majesty's Service, to be a member of the Medical Board, in the room of James Macaulay, Esq., deceased.

"Lewis Clement, 2nd Regiment Lincoln Militia, and Daniel Stewart, 1st Regiment Lincoln Militia, having been examined, were rejected and discontinued from the Pension list, as labouring under no Disability from wounds."

"John Ryan, Artillery . . . appeared. The Board revise their opinion of the 5th October, 1821. Reject him as labouring under no disability from wounds, and recommend his being struck off the Pension list."

"The Board proceeded to the examination of John Bertrand, Incorporated Regiment of Militia, and are of opinion that he is incapable of earning his living by hard labour, in consequence of wounds received in action with the enemy."

The only medical candidate at this session was Alex. Burnside, who received his certificate to practise.

July 1, 1822.—Christopher Widmer, Wm. W. Baldwin, Grant Powell, Esquires, present. (Appeal.) The Board proceeded in the Examination of Farquhar McBian, late private in the 1st Glengarry Regiment of Militia, and are of opinion that he is incapable of earning his living by hard labour, in consequence of wounds received in action with the enemy.

The Board also proceeded in the examination of Samuel Randolph, 2nd Grenville (Appeal); Angus McDougall, Incorporated Regiment; John Cornell, 1st Lennox Regiment Militia; William T. Stotes, not on the list; John Mitchel, Kent Volunteers, not a militia man, but teamster, when wounded; Robert McNaughton, 1st Glengarry, not a militia man, but teamster, when wounded. "The Board reject the above from the Pension list. The Board also examined Zacharias Warner, private in the 2nd York Regiment of Militia, but suspend their opinion until he produces the necessary certificate, as being the person and where wounded. The certificate being produced, the Board are of opinion that he is incapable of hard labour."

The Board then proceeded in the examination of J. Adamson, of Toronto (township), in the Home District, Gentleman, in the practice of Physic, Surgery and Midwifery, who was found qualified to practise in the above branches, and received a certificate to that effect.

October, 1822.—Present: Drs. Widmer, Baldwin and Powell. There was no business at this quarterly meeting.

The composition of the Medical Board is thus given in Charles Fothergill's almanac for 1822:

MEDICAL BOARD, 1822.

Under 58th and 59th George III.

Christopher Widmer,	Wm. Warren Baldwin,
William Lyons,	Grant Powell,
Robert Kerr,	James Sampson, Esquires.

Secretary—Wm. Lee, Esquire.

CHAPTER VI.

PENSIONERS, CANDIDATES, MEDICAL EDUCATION.

YORK, *January* 7, 1823.—Present: Christopher Widmer, William W. Baldwin, and Grant Powell. The Board proceeded in the examination of Anthony Salls, late private in the 1st Oxford Militia; Reject him from the Pension list; Stephen Barber, late private in the 2nd Lincoln Militia; Reject him from the Pension list. John Mitchel, late private in the Kent Volunteers, who was rejected last July for want of a necessary certificate to prove him a militia man, and not a teamster, when wounded, was again rejected, the certificate produced having been found insufficient.

January 11, 1823.—Present as before. "John Mitchel, private in the late Kent Volunteers, appeared and having produced the necessary certificate as to his being a militia man when wounded, the Board recommended him to be continued on the Pension list, as he labours under the disability of earning his livelihood in consequence of wounds."

Horace Yeomans and Andrew Austin, both of Midland District, received certificates of qualification to practise.

April 7, 1823.—Christopher Widmer, Robert Kerr, Grant Powell, Robert Charles Horne, present. A commission was read appointing Robert Charles Horne, Esq., Member of the Royal College of Surgeons, London, and Assistant-Surgeon of the late Glengarry Light Infantry, as member of the Board. It is then recorded that Captain James Seacord, 1st Regiment Lincoln Militia, and Ensign Kirkpatrick, 2nd Regiment Lincoln Militia, appeared, and being duly examined, received the following certificate each:

"This is to certify that Captain James Seacord, 1st Lincoln Regiment of Militia, and Ensign Robert Kirkpatrick, 2nd Lincoln Regiment of Militia, both presented themselves before the Medical Board, at their sitting in April, 1823, and upon personal examination they are of opinion that the said Captain James Seacord and Ensign Kirkpatrick are incapable of earning their livelihood in consequence of wounds received in action with the enemy. By order of the Board.

"(Signed) A. L. Lee, *Secretary*."

[Doubtless the Seacord here mentioned refers to James Secord, the husband of the historic Laura Secord, who made the famous night journey to warn Lieut. Fitzgibbon.]

"The Board proceeded in the examination of Captain James Kerby (now Lieut.-Colonel), and upon personal examination Reject him from the Pension list."

On the same day seven medical candidates were examined; only one, Freeman Riddle, of Hallowell, Midland District, succeeded. The others were "rejected by the Board as being incompetent to practise"; but were "admonished" and "recommended further study." The Board adjourned until Saturday, when Widmer, Baldwin and Powell were present. Probably the other two gentlemen could not remain away so long from their practice. Nothing was done at this meeting.

July 7, 1823.—Present: Christopher Widmer, Grant Powell and Robert C. Horne. The Board proceeded in the examination of Joseph Long, late private Incorporated Regiment of Militia, and Reject him from the Pension list as not labouring under any disability. They also proceeded in the examination of

Adam Stull, 1st Lincoln Regiment of Militia. The Board recommend the extraction of a musket-ball from the outside of his right leg, which they are of opinion would remove the Disability complained of, and Reject him.

Elam Stimson, of Saint Catharines, Niagara District, received a certificate to practise, the Board being "perfectly satisfied."

July 11, 1823.—Present: Robert Kerr, Grant Powell and Robert C. Horne. "George Adams, Lieut. 1st Regiment Lincoln Militia, appeared for Examination as a Pensioner, and after due examination the Board are of opinion that he labours under no Disability to earn his livelihood and Reject him from the Pension list."

October 6, 1823.—Present: Widmer, Powell and Horne. One candidate examined, who was found "totally ignorant of Pharmaceutical knowledge and rejected as unqualified to practise." Met again on Saturday; same present; nothing done.

January, 1824.—Present: Widmer, Powell and Horne. The first candidate was found "deficient in Anatomy and Pharmaceutical Chymistry," and rejected with recommendation to "further study and a course of lectures."

Samuel Gilchrist and Matthew Gilchrist, of New Castle District, were examined. "The Board is perfectly satisfied by their examination and grants each of them a certificate."

Samuel Woodruff, of Saint David's District, was not quite so fortunate. He was "found deficient in Anatomy, but granted a certificate to practise Physic and Midwifery only."

At the April meeting, Widmer, Powell and Horne were present. "John Ryan, late Artillery Service, having appeared, and being duly examined, the Board are of the same opinion as 2nd April, 1822, that he labours under no disability from wounds to earn his livelihood."

At the July meeting the same members were present. The Board was "perfectly satisfied by the examination" of Stephen W. Avery and Thomas David Morrison, both of York, and gave each a certificate. One candidate was rejected.

The Board seems to have adopted the rule of adjourning

until Saturday, to allow candidates time to reach the capital. Travelling then was uncertain.

Drs. Widmer, Powell and Horne were present at the October meeting. There were no medical candidates; but "Lieut. J. McGregor, late Kent Volunteers, appeared, and being duly examined the Board does not find him so disabled by his wounds as to render him incapable of earning his livelihood."

The meeting in January, 1825, was attended by Widmer, Powell and Horne. There was no business of any kind.

The same members at the April meeting examined one candidate, Jabez Kellogg, of Mid. District, and were "perfectly satisfied."

In July, the same members examined a candidate "in the practice of surgery only," but "find him unqualified to practise, admonished him, and recommended further study and a course of lectures." Frederick L. Converse received a certificate; another candidate failed.

The same members met in October. James McAuley, of Cornwall, received a certificate of qualification. The next two candidates were found "deficient in Pharmaceutical Chymistry and classical education." Another candidate, who had been rejected the previous quarter, was found "totally unqualified to practise." The next two candidates were "deficient in Pharmaceutical Chymistry and classical education, and recommended a course of lectures." The next was found "totally unqualified to practise."

January, 1826. — Members present: Drs. Widmer, Powell and Horne. One candidate was examined and rejected.

April, 1826.—Present: Widmer, Baldwin and Horne. James Hunter and David I. Bowman, of Niagara District, received their certificates to practise. One rejected.

July 5, 1826. — Present as above. "Reuben Alward, 2nd Norfolk Militia, having presented himself for examination in consequence of wounds received in action with the enemy, the Board are of opinion that the said Reuben Alward is incapable of earning his livelihood in consequence of said wounds and have granted him a certificate to that effect."

October, 1826.—Present: Widmer, Powell and Horne. Wm. Bruce, of Cornwall District, was examined and gave "perfect satisfaction."

In concluding the record of the year 1826, it is to be stated that the matter of education in the Province of Upper Canada was receiving considerable attention, with regard to the medical profession. Dr. Strachan, writing to Sir Peregrine Maitland on the subject of education in Upper Canada, March, 1826, says: "In regard to the profession of Medicine, now becoming of great "importance in the Province, it is melancholy to think that "more than three-fourths of the present practitioners have been "educated or attended lectures in the United States; and it is "to be presumed that many of them are inclined towards that "country. But in this colony there is no provision whatever "for attaining medical knowledge, and those who make choice "of that profession must go to a foreign country to acquire it."

At this time steps were being taken to build up an efficient medical school in Lower Canada at Montreal. This important action was fraught with interest, not only to the profession of that Province, but of Upper Canada as well. Because the evil and danger of the young men of Upper Canada going to the United States for a medical education, pointed out by Dr. Strachan, would be obviated by the existence of a properly equipped medical school in the Sister Province; and as a matter of fact in the course of years, medical students from Upper Canada did go to Montreal instead of to the United States. Not a few of the medical men of Upper Canada received their medical education at McGill College. It is therefore desirable to relate the manner in which that medical school originated. This can best be done by producing a memorial article of the founder, Dr. Holmes:

"Died, 9th October, 1860, Andrew Fernando Holmes, M.D., LL.D., Professor of Medicine and Anatomy. Born in Cadiz, his parents being prisoners of war captured by a French frigate. Reached Canada in 1801, became a pupil of Dr. Arnoldi, 1811. Completed studies at Edinburgh and Paris. In August, 1819, graduated, having previously, in March, 1818, obtained M.R.C.S. Ed. Returning to Canada in 1819, he entered into partnership with Dr. Arnoldi for a time.

"About the year 1823 or 1824, conscious of the want experienced in this Province (Quebec) by medical students, of lectures on the different branches of medical study, Dr. Holmes, together with Drs. Robertson, Stephenson and Caldwell, organized themselves into a body, and under the name of the 'Medical Institute of Montreal,' they delivered lectures for the first time in 1824, forming the session of 1824-25 a course of lectures which were recognized by the University of Edinburgh afterwards, on the principle of two courses for one of that University. These early courses of an Institute which became in 1828 merged into the University of McGill College, and was the means of retaining to the Institution the benevolent bequest of its founder, were delivered as follows:

"Dr. Holmes on Chemistry and Materia Medica; Dr. Stephenson on Anatomy, Physiology and Surgery; Dr. Robertson on Midwifery and the Diseases of Women and Children; and Dr. Caldwell on the Principles and Practice of Medicine. The death of Dr. Caldwell in 1832 necessitated a change, and Dr. Robertson was appointed Professor of Medicine, the late Dr. Racey, of Quebec, was annexed as Professor of Surgery and Midwifery. In 1835 Drs. Campbell and Hall were associated. In 1844 we find the additional names of Drs. Charles Sewell, Bruneau, Hall, Crawford, McCullough and Fraser.

"In every sense of the word Dr. Holmes was a Christian gentleman. High as was the position he attained in his profession, he was not less distinguished as the Christian gentleman, ever actively employed in the service of his Divine Master."

The following extract from Morgan's "Celebrated Canadians" will be acceptable, we doubt not, to many of the older doctors in Upper Canada, many of whom were his pupils:

"At the reorganization of the Faculty (of McGill College) in 1854, Dr. Holmes became and continued to his death Dean of the Faculty, discharging the duties of his office with a zeal, diligence and alacrity beyond praise, also holding the chair of the Theory and Practice of Medicine. He was, we believe, the oldest professor in Canada. Dr. Holmes was also the founder, with a few others, of the Natural History Society, and pursued for many years the study of the natural sciences with great zeal and success, winning for himself reputation as a naturalist.

His herbarium, consisting of a very complete collection of the plants of Canada, he presented a few years ago to the museum of the University. . . . Dr. Holmes was one of the most talented *savants*, as well as one of the most estimable gentlemen in this country."

January, 1827.—Present at the Board meeting, Drs. Widmer, Powell and Horne. Andrew Van Dyck and Thomas Moore, of the Midland District, received certificates to practise medicine.

"Pursuant to an order from His Excellency the Lieut.-Governor, dated 26th inst., the Medical Board having carefully examined Charles Spinard, late an Interpreter of the Indian Department, find that he is not disabled from earning his livelihood in consequence of wounds received during the late War."

Before the quarterly meeting of the Board in April, further legislation had taken place.

April, 1827.—Present, the same as at last meeting. James Fairfield, Midland District, was examined. The Board was "perfectly satisfied by his examination, find him duly qualified."

July, 1827. — Present: Widmer, Powell and Horne. One candidate presented himself for examination. Advised "to pursue further study and a course of lectures."

October, 1827. — Same members present. Robert Ironside presented himself. "The Board is satisfied by his examination" and grant certificate to practise Physic and Surgery. Thomas Fraser MacQueen, of Edwardsburg, also obtained a certificate.

January, 1828.—Drs. Widmer, Powell and Horne present. James McCague, of York; John E. Tims, of York; David Duncombe, of London, and Alexander Wylie, of Matilda, passed their examination satisfactorily. Two candidates were found to be "incompetent to practise."

April, 1828.—Present: Widmer, Powell and Horne. Francis Ellis, of Niagara; John Porter Daily, of York, and Thomas Black, of Midland District, passed their examination. Two candidates were found "totally deficient."

July, 1828.—Present: Widmer, Baldwin, Powell and Horne. John B. Crouse, of London; Basil R. Church, of Johnston District, and Stephen H. Van Dyck, received certificates for license. One candidate was found "deficient in Chemistry, Anatomy, etc.," another the same, but "recommended further study and a course of lectures." The next was "totally unqualified to practise, as he never attended a medical school or had any advantages of acquiring his profession but from reading books."

October 28, 1828.—Present: Widmer, Powell and Horne. No business.

January 5, 1829.—Present: Chris. Widmer, Grant Powell and Robert C. Horne. A commission was read appointing Peter Deihl, Esq., member of the Royal College of Surgeons of London, to be a member of the Medical Board, at York, U.C.

At this meeting the Board granted certificates to John Thomson, of New Market, and George C. Rankin, of the Rideau Canal.

April, 1829.—Present: Widmer, Powell, Horne and Deihl. John Crumbie, of Niagara, passed his examination. With regard to another candidate: "The Board taking his serious Disability into consideration cannot proceed in his examination, he being so deaf as not to comprehend such questions as was proposed. The Board was, therefore, unanimously of opinion that they could not in justice to the Public proceed in his examination."

July, 1829.—Present: Widmer, Powell and Deihl. Peter Schofield, of Johnston District; J. E. Rankin, of Ottawa District; Wm. McMahon, of Hallowell; Marcus Whitman, Niagara District, and John Hutchison, of Port Hope, received certificates. One candidate was rejected.

October, 1829.—Present: Widmer, Powell and Deihl. Hamilton D. Jessup, of Johnston District, and Josiah C. Goodhue, of York, received certificates. Another candidate was rejected for the second time. He "having no satisfactory proof to offer to the Board that he has engaged further opportunities of qualifying himself, they decline to proceed in his examination."

January, 1830.—Present: Widmer, Powell and Deihl. William Beamish, of Cobourg; Marcus Merrick, of York; William Rees, of York; John Warner Leonard, of Sidney, Midland District, and Benjamin Walton, of Belleville, passed their examination with "perfect satisfaction." Two were rejected; of one of them, it is recorded that "the Board was surprised to find that he had no document to produce of his ever acquiring a Medical Education, that he was totally deficient in his answers to such questions as was proposed to him, and was, therefore, obliged to reject him as unqualified to practise, but recommended study at some medical university and a course of lectures to enable him to appear before the Board at some future time."

April, 1830.—Present: Widmer, Powell and Deihl. Wm. W. Howard, of Johnston District, Jiva Skinner, of the same District, passed. Two candidates were rejected; one because he was "deficient in Anatomy," and was "recommended to attend a course of lectures at some medical university"; another because he was "totally deficient in Medical Science."

Although the Medical Board was established in 1819, no official recognition by the Governor is observable in the official *Gazette* for some years. The following, however, appears in the Upper Canada *Gazette*:

"GOVERNMENT HOUSE,
"YORK, 5th *May*, 1830.

"The undersigned gentlemen having received certificates from the Medical Board of this Province of their qualifications to practise Physic, etc., His Excellency has been pleased to grant a License.

"Marcus Merrick, of York.
"Wm. Beamish, junior, of Cobourg."

These gentlemen had passed the Board at the January meeting.

July, 1830.—Present: Widmer, Powell and Deihl. Benjamin S. Cory, of Hillier, and Robert Gilmour, of Brockville, who had a diploma from Glasgow, passed. One was rejected, as "totally ignorant as a classical scholar, as well as being entirely deficient in Pharmacy and Pharmaceutical Chymistry, etc., and reject him as unfit to practise; he never attended any Medical School."

October, 1830.—The same members present. Jonathan Foot, of Whitby, passed a "perfectly satisfactory examination." Three were rejected. One of these had a diploma from the Faculty of Physicians and Surgeons of Glasgow, but was "quite ignorant of Chymistry and Pharmacy." The next "had no knowledge of the same subjects." The next, "in consequence of an attack of fever and very delicate health, was recommended to postpone his examination until next session." The next "had no testimonials to produce of his having attended Lectures, and does not remember the names of the lectures or college." He was, therefore, rejected.

In 1830 an Act was passed "to grant a sum of money to His Majesty, in aid of the York Hospital." The preamble says: "Whereas, the Lieut.-Governor has been pleased to put the building lately occupied by the Provincial Legislature into useful and beneficial operation as a public hospital, wherein members of your Majesty's sick, destitute and unfortunate subjects and emigrants have received medical and surgical assistance." The sum granted was £100, and the same amount in 1831.

A public meeting was held at Kingston, 16th September, 1830, to take steps to build a public hospital.

CHAPTER VII.

AN APPEAL TO PARENTS AND THE PUBLIC.

YORK, *January*, 1831.—Present: Widmer, Powell, Horne and Deihl. No examination.

"GOVERNMENT HOUSE, 14th *February*, 1831.

"SIR,—I am directed by the Lieut.-Governor to request that you will assemble the Medical Board at 12 o'clock, 19th February, for the purpose of examining the wounds of Mr. Nathaniel Bell, late a Militia Pensioner of this Province.

"I have the honour to be, Sir,

"Your most obedient, humble servant,

"(Signed), Z. MUDGE.

"Dr. LEE, Secretary to the Medical Board."

For report of the Board, see Biography of Dr. Nathaniel Bell.

April, 1831.—Present: Widmer, Powell and Deihl. Donald McGittis, of Williams Town; Elijah E. Duncombe, of Saint Thomas; Elias Banthan Smith, of Burford, London District; Abraham V. V. Pruyn, of Bath; Ephraim Cook, of Saint Thomas, and Japez P. Powers, of Haldimand District, received certificates. Five were rejected.

July, 1831.—Present: Widmer, Baldwin and Powell. James Cairns, of York, "produced a diploma from the University of Paris and a License from the Lower Province of Canada," and succeeded in getting his certificate. John Grant, of Williamsburg, who had a diploma from Glasgow, also passed. Likewise David Scanlan, of Brockville, and Joseph Lister, of York, who produced a certificate from the Apothecaries' Co., London, and had "most ample testimonials of his Professional Education" Henry Meade, of Prince Edward Co., "passed a good Examination and produced testimonials of having studied one course of Lectures at Fairfield." One candidate was rejected.

October, 1831.—Present: Widmer, Powell, Deihl and Baldwin. Luther Cross, of York, "produced testimonials of having attended two courses of lectures at Baudoin and Berkshire," also a diploma from Baudoin College; the Board was perfectly satisfied by his examination. A candidate produced tickets of attendance for "two courses of medical lectures at Dartmouth, also a diploma from the Medical Society, Jefferson County," but "was found deficient, so much so as not to be competent to translate a sentence from the London Pharmacopœia," and was rejected. The next had tickets of attendance at two courses of Medical Lectures "as well as a diploma from Fairfield," but he was likewise found wanting. Of the next, "the Board are of opinion that he is totally unfit to practise, he never having attended a Medical School as well as no Document to produce of his Medical knowledge."

January, 1832.—Present: Widmer, Deihl, John King and Charles Duncombe, when "Commissions from the Lieut.-Governor appointing additional members were read." James Eikin Gilchrist, of New Castle, passed; and Isaac Stephenson, of York, passed a "perfectly satisfactory examination." Two candidates were found "totally incompetent and rejected." Murray Nesbitt appeared for examination in Midwifery only and received a certificate of qualification.

April, 1832.—Present: Widmer, Baldwin, Deihl, King and John Rolph. David M. Black, of Gore District, and Hiram Uriah Gilbert, of Long Point, with testimonials from Fairfield College, received their certificates. A candidate appeared "but from his total ignorance of the Latin language, so highly necessary in the profession, could not proceed in his examination. The Board admonished him and recommended further study preparatory to his coming before them at any subsequent sitting." Another candidate was found "inadequate to answer the questions put to him in his Profession, as also being deficient of the Latin language." Another was rejected who produced a "diploma from the Apothecaries" Hall, but lost all other documents of his acquiring a Medical Education on his passage to America." He was "deficient in classical knowledge and ignorant of Chymistry and Pharmacy."

"His Excellency the Lieutenant-Governor having authorized the examination of Silas V. York, a Discharged Soldier, and to Report thereon for his information, he received the following certificate by Order of the Board: 'This is to certify that Silas V. York, a corporal in the late Incorporated Regiment of Militia of Upper Canada, appeared before the Medical Board at their sitting in April, 1832, and being duly examined touching the nature and extent of wounds received in action with the enemy, last American War, are of opinion that the above-named Silas V. York, labours under no Incapacity from earning his livelihood.'"

At the meeting of the Board on April 4, the Board unanimously elected Christopher Widmer, Esq., President, and William Warren Baldwin, Esq., Vice-President, for Life.

July, 1832.—Present: Christopher Widmer, Esq., President; Wm. W. Baldwin, Esq., Vice-President; Peter Deihl and John King, Esquires, members. James Cattermole, of York, passed his examination. Three candidates failed to pass at the outset for want of "classical attainments."

The following appears next in the minutes:

"MEDICAL BOARD,

"YORK, 6th *April*, 1832.

"The Medical Board are deeply impressed with the conviction that the success of the medical candidate must especially depend upon the proper direction of his early studies, and the systematic pursuit of the various branches of science belonging to his profession.

"Under this conviction, they wish earnestly to impress on the minds of parents and others, how very important it is to the interest of the public, and to the future credit and respectability of the practitioner, that all who desire to become candidates for the profession should avail themselves of the increasing advantages afforded by the Province for a liberal education.

"The public, it is hoped, will fairly appreciate their anxiety to improve the education and qualifications of those who are hereafter to have the care of the health of the community committed into their hands, while the student who is actuated by honourable and conscientious motives must feel that the due observance of the regulations and advice urged upon him is necessary to enable him to enter upon the duties of his profession with credit to himself and justice to the public.

"They are inclined to hope that medical practitioners in every part of the Province will be disposed to second their endeavours by encouraging the young men who are placed under their care, or who may apply to them for advice in the study of the languages and of general science, the high character which the profession has acquired in the world, and the arduous duties imposed upon its members, justify the expectation of the Board and of the public, that the future qualifications of candidates will be commensurate to the means of education within their reach.

"The Board, therefore, must hereafter require that each candidate at the commencement of his examination shall translate into English some portion of a Latin author, that they may be satisfied he has acquired a competent knowledge of a language in which the formula of medical authors and extemporaneous prescriptions of practitioners are written and from which are derived so many terms used in all the sciences with which he must be conversant.

"That for the attainment of a Science to Practise Medicine, the candidate will be required to understand Anatomy, Physiology, the practice of Physic, Chymistry, Materia Medica and Pharmacy, Medical Botany and Medical Jurisprudence.

"The candidate for Surgery will be required to understand Relative and Surgical Anatomy, Physiology, the principles and practice of Surgery, Materia Medica and Pharmacy, and Medical Jurisprudence.

"The candidate for Midwifery will be required to understand the Anatomy of the Pelvis, its contents and their appendages, and Physiology, as far as it is connected with the same, a knowledge of the nature and treatment of diseases of parturient women, and of children, and the necessary acquaintance with Materia Medica and Pharmacy.

"The York Hospital is now in successful operation, and affords to students daily opportunities of observing diseases and their treatment, and they feel it a duty to point out to students that it is at such institutions they can best acquire, at the bedside of the patient, under experienced practitioners, the practical information most essentially befitting them to render professional services to their fellow-creatures.

"(Signed) C. WIDMER, *President.*

"By order of the Board.

"A. L. LEE, *Secretary.*"

This was sent out in the form of a circular.

CHAPTER VIII.

STATE OF THE MEDICAL PROFESSION.

YORK, *October*, 1832.—Present: Widmer, Baldwin, Powell, Deihl, King and Rolph. "John Keogh, of York, a Licentiate of the Royal College of Surgeons, Ireland, as well as having other vouchers as to his medical education highly creditable," was found "duly and fully qualified." John Anderson, of York, a Licentiate of the Royal College of Surgeons, Edinburgh, "being examined, was admonished by our President, but received his certificate." Robert Stewart, of York, received his certificate. John Stoddart, of Toronto (township), applied for examination in midwifery only, and received a certificate. James Coleman, of Toronto (township), with license from the Apothecaries' Co., succeeded in passing. Three were rejected for want of classical knowledge, and two for being "very deficient in all the branches of the profession."

"A letter to Doctor Widmer from Doctors Muirhead, Telfer and Porter, of Niagara, with a copy of communication from them to the Attorney-General, and his answer":

[Copy No. 1.]

"NIAGARA, 22nd *October*, 1832.

"SIR,—From the intercourse you have doubtless had with members of the Medical Profession in various parts of the Province, you must have been struck with the want of that liberal information and of those respectable attainments that should characterize members of a learned body, and which are absolutely necessary to inspire the people with confidence in the healing art; and, moreover, the information coming to you as Attorney-General of the Province, and your own observation, must show you that everywhere there are ignorant pretenders to science, who, besides practising Physic in open defiance of the law, bring an obloquy on the profession.

"Upon first coming to this Province we certainly felt these things. Very powerfully the fact was forced upon us that the profession of Physic here was degraded from the position it should occupy.

"Physicians of proper attainments were seldom to be met, being thinly scattered about the country surrounded by empirics (licensed or not) who generally succeeded better than the former in obtaining practice, because they would adopt habit and cunning that respectable men could not think of; that these were, and continue to be facts, we at present barely assert, but if proof be required we are ready to furnish it abundantly.

"We could not any otherwise account for this state of the profession than by attributing it to a defect in the Laws, and much reflection since has confirmed us in the opinion.

"We know of no man more alive to the public welfare than yourself, nor of any more capable of furthering it; we are consequently induced to address you in order if possible to engage your services in the attempt, during the ensuing Session of Parliament, to obtain some amendment in the enactments that at present regulate the practice of Physic, Surgery and Midwifery in this Province; and we doubt not that where so much good may be done, you will spare no effort to place the medical profession in this Province on the respectable rank that it should occupy. We would take leave to suggest to you, that if medical men were organized into a society resembling your Law Society, with power to regulate their own affairs, it would be the best arrangement, and particularly as it would still keep the Licentiate of our own art under a jurisdiction that could remove or suspend him from practice, if he should be guilty of acts which he may now commit with impunity, and which are derogatory to the profession; acts which though they cannot be foreseen by a written law, may be properly appreciated and judged of by a Corporate Body, and this is particularly necessary here, because the greater number of Licentiates are strangers (many of them aliens) who do not bring a character with them to support, and who too frequently follow a course of life degrading to any situation.

"We have now said enough perhaps to attract your attention to the subject of this letter, and if you think it worthy of consideration, and are willing to take the matter in hand, we shall be happy, if you wish it, to communicate further with you, and put you more fully in possession of our opinions, and of what we can adduce to support them.

"We have the honour to be, Sir,

"Your most obedient, humble servants,

"(Signed) JAMES MUIRHEAD, *Surgeon.*
WALTER TELFER, *Surgeon.*
F. W. PORTER, M.D.

"HENRY T. BOULTON,
"Attorney-General, York."

[Copy No. 2.]

"YORK, 28th *October*, 1832.

"MY DEAR SIR,—I received your letter of the 22nd October inst., in which Drs. Telfer and Porter joined, and fully participate with you in the sentiments expressed, and shall be very happy to aid the medical profession in any way they may point out as likely to be most advantageous to them.

"Before anything, however, should be brought before the Legislation, I think the opinion of the principal medical men in the different parts of the Province should be taken, and that the application to meet any probable success should be from the general body; a petition should be presented to Parliament setting forth the intended alterations, and it should be signed by as many medical gentlemen as possible. A Bill should likewise be proposed for carrying those objects into effect.

"I am, my dear Sir, yours very faithfully,

"(Signed) H. T. BOULTON.

"DR. MUIRHEAD, Niagara."

"NIAGARA, 2nd *November*, 1832.

"SIR,—We beg leave to transmit to you a copy of a letter addressed by us to the Attorney-General and his answer thereto. You in particular must be acquainted with the state of the profession in this Province, and we think you must with us mainly attribute its degradation to the causes pointed out in our letter to the Attorney-General, who in reply coincides with us, and indicates the course most proper to pursue in order to accomplish the object before us, and if that should meet with your concurrence, we know that your influence and assistance would be valuable. We would be glad if you would communicate this matter to the profession in York, and afterwards that a meeting of the medical men in the Province (in order to draft the petition recommended) should be called at York by immediate public advertisement, to take place as soon as possible, and perhaps a great many could be collected eight or ten days after the advertisement.

"You are aware that if the Bill is to be brought into the House this session, this petition must be got with the least possible delay.

"We have the honour to be, Sir,
"Your obedient and humble servants,

"(Signed) J. MUIRHEAD, *Surgeon.*
WALTER TELFER, *Surgeon.*
F. W. PORTER, M.D.

"DR. WIDMER, York."

"Reply of the Medical Board to Drs. Muirhead, Telfer and Porter's communication to the Attorney-General through Dr. Widmer":

"SIR,—I took an early opportunity of submitting the subject of your letter of the 3rd inst. to the Medical Board, and I am requested by them as their President to communicate to you the result of their consideration.

"It may be equally true of this as of all other countries, that a few exceptionable characters clothed with all the necessary legal qualifications will descend to empiricism, but the Medical Board in the discharge of an important and often anxious duty, have at all times endeavoured to protect the interests of the public amid the just expectations of candidates, as far as was compatible with the peculiar condition of the country and the means of professional education afforded by it.

"Two points are mentioned in your letter to the Attorney-General: first, that ignorant pretenders to science practise physic in open defiance of the law; and secondly, that they bring an obloquy upon the profession. As a remedy, you propose a corporation.

"Your own statement of the evil discloses a sufficient remedy if such persons practise against the law. The law which is violated affords redress; it is not defective because it is not enforced in behalf of the community for whose welfare it was enacted; it is enough that such impostors upon the public are denounced by the law and made obnoxious to its punishment.

"Other laws, however framed in wisdom or multiplied in number, would prove equally unavailing if unenforced; it appears, therefore, to the Board, that the existing law provides a sufficient remedy for the matter for which you complain—the obloquy which in the second place you allege is brought upon the profession will be effectually prevented by the impartial prosecutions of those who impose upon the public; the profession could not in that case desire to stand upon a better foundation than its known general character for devotion to science and humanity.

"A corporation invested with the powers you propose appears to be of doubtful propriety, if not of dangerous tendency. In the first place it cannot be assumed that the due operation of laws which have been provided, not for the protection of those private rights, the illegal invasion of which often gives rise to a prosecutor, but for the protection of the health of the general community, would be more faithfully insured by a corporation than by the executive authority whose peculiar care it is to carry into beneficial operation the laws enacted by the Legislature.

"If it be true in the second place, that any regular licentiate descend to unworthy professional practices not within the redress of the laws of the land, the evil must be left, as in other countries, to the corrective influence of public opinion.

"It must be admitted that the public suffer much from the want of suitable opportunities of medical education, but it is hoped that the ample endowments long since provided by the British Government for such essential purposes will not allow this want to be much longer a matter of reproach.

"(Signed) C. WIDMER, *President.*

"York, November 10th, 1832.

In connection with the preceding correspondence the following will be appropriate:

"(*For the Western Mercury.*)

"QUACKERY.

"No greater imposition exists in Upper Canada then Quackery—its every-day use makes it appear tolerated by the laws of the land; it is an existing evil under which this Province has long groaned, but to which public attention should be directed. The regular practitioner meets it in every day's travel, is perplexed with its impudence, and with horror views its ravages and its influence.

"The character of the real Quack is the same in all countries. These persons have generally been so degraded by their vices as to render themselves odious to society, or too ignorant and indolent to gain a living by any honest means. Aware of the credulity of the people upon this subject, they suddenly and without any study, pretend to supernatural powers conferred upon them by God himself. They profess to cure diseases which the experience of two thousand years has proved to be irremediable. Their drugs are of the most active kind, it excites horror when we contemplate the freedom of their use. They cure all by one remedy! Their course of crime is supported by many minor vices, deception, effrontery, and the robbery of their victims, who, fascinated by the relation of pretended cures, often borrow money to buy their remedies and are finally left in extreme want and misery and a prey to confirmed maladies, which by proper means might have been relieved. From the attack of the robber, defence, release or escape is possible: from the Quack who gains the confidence of the people, death is too frequently the consequence.

"Another sort of practitioners are what may be denominated Licensed Quacks; these are men who have studied but one part of the profession and have obtained license to practise that part only. These men are generally the most impudent, and set up for the great doctor! They practise all parts of the profession without distinction, and thus the Licensed Quack grows rich by imposition and a knowledge of a small part of his profession. He will gravely tell you that 'he has his license,' and people not acquainted with the deception will take it for granted he is regularly authorized to practise physic, surgery and midwifery, when he has been licensed to practise one of these branches only.

"If these things are known and not remedied, we shall, ere long, be overrun by such men. The student may study a favourite branch, and in one or two years may become the *great doctor!* whilst the honest man who has devoted all his time and most of his money to obtain the necessary information, is doomed to endless defamation, indigence, and an humble walk in life. Thus impudence and ignorance triumphs over humility and education, whilst vice and roguery tramples under feet virtue and honesty.

"Will the public any longer allow such gross impositions? Or, will honest men suffer their rights to be thus invaded? I trust not. Would some gentleman of the law confer a favour by making known to the public by what means and with what expense we can detect these impostors and bring them to justice. For one, I am not content to acknowledge a Quack my superior or contend with him for my bread, but will, if possible, make an example of the nearest when the necessary information is obtained to accomplish it.

"A PHYSICIAN.

"Gore District, 31st May, 1832."

The Rev. Isaac Fidler, in his "Observations" on Canadian matters, published in 1832 (he lived at Thornhill three years), draws a comparison between the medical profession of the United States and Canada. He says:

"Some medical gentlemen emigrate from the States into Canada; but I believe they are never employed where one from Great Britain or Ireland can be procured. American physicians do not commonly place themselves in any situation in which competition with Europeans is hazarded. If any professional gentleman from the States be found in such neighbourhood, he forms an exception from the general rule. There was one such at Thornhill, but his skill was not considered as entitling him to much patronage. His practice was very limited, and chiefly to the lower orders.

"A medical man who cannot ride much on horseback ought not to go into that country. So highly are doctors paid in some places densely populated that towns and villages are generally well supplied. Medical men from the States are often found wandering up and down; and, where European physicians are not found, take possession of the practice. In some remote places a doctor has frequently to ride fifteen or twenty miles to many of his patients. The English medical gentleman near us was often sent for to the above distance. His charge for an ordinary journey was a dollar a mile. He was making a rapid fortune. There are many places upon Yonge Street and in the district around, and, I believe, in every district in the country, which are very populous, and where any respectable practitioner might settle his family in certain affluence."

He tells of a physician, who had emigrated to Canada a short time before and had purchased a farm near Niagara Falls. He had been following his profession, however, and told Mr. Fidler he had fallen into a practice which would realize him £1,100 a year (?). "This is almost as large an income as any medical man, except one or two of the most eminent in New York." He did not expect, however, to be paid altogether in money.

We find that the York General Hospital had at this time become an institution of importance and value, as will be seen by the following:

The Medical Board, at its meeting in April, 1832, in addressing the public, spoke of the Hospital as follows:

"The York Hospital is now in successful operation, and affords to students daily opportunities of observing diseases and their treatment, and they feel it a duty to point out to students that it is at such institutions they can best acquire, at the bedside of the patient, under experienced practitioners, the practical information most especially befitting them to render professional services to their fellow-creatures."

Mrs. Jameson says at this time of the Hospital: "It is a large brick building, yet too small for the increasing city."

"YORK STUDENTS' MEDICAL SOCIETY.

"At a meeting of the medical students of this town, held on Saturday, December 7, at the York General Hospital, the following resolution was unanimously adopted:

"'That the present meeting of medical students do hereby constitute themselves into a permanent society, to be hereafter designated The York Students' Medical Society, whose sole object shall be to impart reciprocally, for the purpose of general improvement, the knowledge of the various branches of the medical science.'

"The following officers were then appointed: Mr. Park, Mr. Orr, *Presidents;* Mr. Steers, *Secretary;* Mr. O'Hare, *Treasurer;* Mr. Mitchell, *Librarian.*

"Any medical gentleman wishing to become a member of the above society, is requested to send his name and place of residence, in writing, to the Secretary, who shall propose him at the next meeting of the Committee, when, if admitted as such, he will be required to pay the sum of four dollars, as an entrance fee, to defray the expenses contingent to the Society, and assist in procuring books for the Society's library, etc.; he will also be presented by the Secretary with a copy of the laws, and informed of all further particulars.

"D. STEERS, *Secretary.*

"York, December 24, 1832."

The "York Dispensary" was established August 30, 1832, Drs. W. W. Baldwin, Morrison, and Tims were the physicians. It lasted only one year, on account of the want of necessary funds.

As a matter of history, it may be well to give a brief account of a medical sect which sprang into existence about this time. In 1832 there was published at Hamilton, by Samuel Thompson, a book entitled "New Guide to Health; or, Botanic Family Physician, containing a complete system of practice upon a plan entirely new, with a description of the vegetables made use of, and directions for preparing and administering them to cure disease." The quotations given are *verbatim et literatim.* In the preface, "written by a friend," it is stated that "Dr. Thompson began his practice, as it were, by accident, with no other view than an honest endeavour to be useful to his fellow-creatures, and had nothing to guide him but his own experience. He not having had an education has received no advantage from reading books, which left his mind unshackled by the visionary theories and opinions of others. His whole studies have been in the great book of nature, and his conclusions have all been drawn from that unerring guide; by this he was enabled to form correct opinions of the fitness of things. . . . His apothecary shop was the woods and the fields."

Dr. Thompson says of himself, that "after thirty years' study and repeated successful trials of the medicinal vegetables of our country in all the diseases incident to our climate, I can, with well-grounded assurance, recommend my system of practice and medicines to the public, as salutary and efficacious. . . . Being born in a new country, at the time almost an howling wilderness, my advantages for education were very small; but possessing a natural gift for examining the things of Nature, my mind was left entirely free to follow that inclination by inquiring into the meaning of the great variety of objects around me.

"Possessing a body like other men, I was led to enquire into the nature of the component parts of what man is made. I found him composed of the four elements—Earth, Water, Air and Fire. The earth and water I found were the solids, the air and the fire the fluids. The first two I found to be the component parts, the last two kept him in motion. Heat I found was life; and Cold, death. . . . I shall now describe the fuel which continues the fire, or life of man. This is contained in two things—food and medicines, which are in harmony with each other, often grow in the same field to be used by the same people. . . . Our life depends on heat; food is the fuel that kindles and continues that heat. The digestive power being correct, causes the food to consume; this continues the warmth of the body by continually supporting the fire. The stomach is the deposit from which the whole body is supported. The heat is maintained in the stomach by consuming the food; and all the body and limbs receive their proportion of nourishment and heat from that source, as the whole room is warmed by the fire which is consumed in the fireplace. The greater the quantity of wood consumed in the fireplace, the greater the heat in the room." After speaking of the stomach as sometimes failing to digest, he declares that "all disease is caused by clogging the system, and all disease is removed by restoring the digestive powers so that food may keep up that heat on which life depends. I have found by experience that the learned doctors are wrong in considering fever a disease or enemy; the fever is a friend, and cold the enemy. . . . It is true that the study of anatomy or structure of the human body and of the whole animal economy is pleasing and useful, nor is there any objection to this however minute and critical, if it is not to the neglect of first great principles and the weightier matters of knowledge. But it is no more necessary to mankind at large to qualify them to administer relief from pain and sickness, than to a cook in preparing food to satisfy hunger and nourishing the body. There is one general cause of hunger and one general supply of food; one general cause of disease and one general remedy. . . . No person ever yet died of fever, for as death approaches the patient grows cold, until death, the last spark of heat is extinguished." Again, he says: "In all cases called fever, the cause is the same in a greater or less degree, and may be relieved by one general remedy. The cold causes canker, and before the canker is seated the strife will take place between cold and heat. . . . The truth is the canker is fixed on the inside, and will ripen and come off in a short time, if the fever is kept up so as to overpower the cold. This idea is new; never was known till my discovery. . . . The higher the fever runs the sooner the cold will be subdued, and if you contend against the heat, the longer will be the run of the fever, and when killed, death follows." One more statement is that "there is a power to produce death, which are of course directly opposed to each other; and whatever tends to promote life cannot cause death, let its power be ever so great. In this consists all the difference between my system of practice and that of the learned doctors."

Dr. Thompson was very fond of steaming his patients, the water being heated by putting into it red-hot stones. The medicines employed by him were classed under numbers, there being six in all. Thus there were No. 1, No. 2, No. 3, No. 4, No. 5, No. 6. These, he says, "form my system of practice. The first three are used to remove disease and the others are restoratives." We cannot make room to give the several constituents of these six preparations; but No. 1 was "to cleanse the stomach"; No. 2, "to retain the internal vital heat of the system, and cause a free perspiration"; No. 3, "to scour the stomach and bowels, and remove the canker"; No. 4 consisted of "bitters to correct the bile and restore digestion"; No. 5, was "syrup for the dysentery, to strengthen the stomach and bowels"; No. 6, "Rheumatic drops, to remove pain, prevent mortification and promote a natural heat."

Dr. Thompson's assortment consisted of some thirty vegetable productions. The following are "directions for preparing and using vegetable medicines."

STOCK OF MEDICINES FOR A FAMILY.

1 oz. of the Emetic Herb (Lobelia).
2 oz. of Cayenne.
½ lb. of Bayberry root bark in powder.
1 lb. of Poplar bark.
1 lb. of Ginger.
1 pt. of the Rheumatic Drops.

These rheumatic drops consisted principally of high wines or "fourth proof brandy," gum myrrh and cayenne. He says: "This stock will be sufficient for a family one year, and with such articles as they can easily procure themselves when wanted, will enable them to cure any disease, which a family of common size may be afflicted with during that time."

Thompson was, we believe, a subject of the United States; but he found in Canada a somewhat fruitful field for the practice of his peculiar views of medical science, and in time, had a considerable number of followers. They were known as "Thompsonians." Not a few young Canadians, disinclined to do manual work, as their fathers had done, cast aside their home-spun clothes, donned a broadcloth suit and kid gloves, hung up a shingle and announced themselves to be "Doctors," according to the doctrine by Thompson. Little or no preparation was required for this change of occupation, and money was generally made by the change. For many years the Thompsonians practised without a license and in defiance of law. But later on they assumed the name of "Eclectics," and commanded sufficient influence to secure from Parliament the right to grant licenses to practise medicine. They ultimately became absorbed in the general profession after the incorporation of the Ontario Medical Council.

CHAPTER IX.

PROGRESS IN THE MEDICAL PROFESSION.

YORK, *January*, 1833.—Present: Widmer, Deihl and King. Paul Darling, of Newmarket, Licentiate Royal College of Surgeons, Edinburgh, passed.

April, 1833.—Present: Widmer, Deihl, King and Rolph. John Flynn, of York, passed. A candidate failed in classical knowledge.

"The Board in pursuance of His Excellency's order, have examined Mr. James Fortier, and find that the wound he received in action with the enemy on the 10th September, 1813, does not incapacitate him from earning his livelihood by labour.

"(Signed) C. WIDMER, *President.*"

July, 1833.—Present: Widmer, Powell, Deihl, King and Rolph. Robert Aberdeen produced his diploma of the Royal College of Surgeons, Edinburgh, and various satisfactory documents of his professional education. In granting his certificate he was recommended to improve his professional knowledge, by the president. Robert Murphy produced a license from the State Medical Society, of New York, and received certificate. George Dunham, Brockville, also passed. The next candidate was found "very defective, indeed, in his anatomical requirements, but give him credit for his chemical knowledge, and recommend him to pursue his studies a few months longer." The following then appears:

"Mr. Stephenson, House Surgeon of the York Hospital, is appointed by the Medical Board, the Secretary of that Body, *vice* Dr. Lee, deceased.

"(Signed) C. WIDMER, *President.*

"Dated from the 1st July, 1833."

David Cory, Midland District; "Walter Telfer, of Niagara, member of College of Surgeons, Edinboro'," John Beatty who had attended two courses of lectures and had matriculation ticket from University of New York; John Stratford, of Bathurst, member of College of Surgeons; Thomas W. Robinson, of Kingston, a graduate of New York College, and Thomas Duggan, of York, received certificates to practise.

A candidate "acknowledged himself entirely ignorant of the Latin language," and "the Board declined going on with his examination." Two other candidates were equally deficient in Latin, and two others failed in anatomy.

August 2, 1833.—By command of His Excellency the Lieut.-Governor, the Board met to examine the wounds of John Ryan, received in the late war. Present: C. Widmer, President, John King, M.D., Peter Deihl, and John Rolph, Esqs. The Medical Board assembled this day to examine and report upon the case of John Ryan, late of the Provincial Artillery, Driver, in pursuance of an order from His Excellency the Lieut.-Governor, dated yesterday.

"The Board reports that the petitioner, John Ryan, was examined before the Medical Board in April, 1822, and in April, 1824, at both of which periods the Board reported that he laboured under no disability from wounds. The Board now confirms the previous reports.

"(Signed) C. WIDMER, *President,*
J. STEPHENSON, *Secretary.*"

October, 1833.—Present: Widmer, Deihl, King and Rolph. Two candidates failed, one of them, "after a patient and tedious examination (by the President)," although he "had served five years' apprenticeship to the Army Surgeon, at Kingston." No further business at this session.

Dr. W. Henry, in "Trifles from my Port Folio," speaking of

York, where he was stationed in 1833, remarks: "One thing is much needed here, a Chartered Medical Institution, and as there are several able men, and good clinical facilities at the hospital, it is to be hoped that those parents who wish to train their children in the healing art, may not be much longer obliged to send them to the States for this purpose." He has a foot-note that "Faculties of Physic, Surgery," etc., have been organized by Statute at Toronto lately, 1839.

The following published notice indicates the healthy spirit of progress prevailing in the profession at this period:

"At a meeting of the members of the medical profession in York, held on the 18th day of May, 1833, a society was formed under the title of the 'Medico-Chirurgical Society of Upper Canada,' the primary object of which will be the interchange and advancement of professional knowledge among the members of the profession. All regular licentiates of the Province who transmit their name to Dr. Widmer, who is President, or Dr. Stephenson, who is Secretary, on or before the first day of October next, for enrolment, will be considered as original members of the institution. The enrolment of any member must be accompanied with his annual subscription of £1 5 0."

January, 1834.—Present: Widmer, Deihl, King, Duncombe and Rolph. James Miller received certificate to practise. Two were rejected. One of these was "so deficient in his general acquirements in the different branches of the profession, that they were obliged to reject him, with strong admonition to renew his studies and in a few months he might present himself with more advantage."

April, 1834.—Present: Widmer, Deihl, King and Rolph. Adolphus Williams of Gore District, G. H. Park, Charles Rolls, John Harrison Blackwell, and Jonathan Wolverton received certificates to practise. Five candidates were rejected. One "had tickets from Fairfield of two courses of lectures and a doctor's degree in medicine after four years' study, and without any knowledge of the classicks, presented himself. Being asked the meaning of the term physiology, and also the word pathology, could not define either; he was not examined further." Another "presented certificate of attending a course of lectures at Dartmouth, in New Hampshire, and of his proficiency in the Latin language. He was, however, found to be quite ignorant of Latin grammar and was therefore advised to pursue his studies."

July, 1834.—Present: Widmer, Rolph, King and Deihl. "Mr. Francis Cameron, of the *city of Toronto*," received a certificate, also John Barnhart, of Streetsville; James W. Powell, of Bathurst District, Royal College of Surgeons, Dublin; Wm. L. Badger, who had "excellent qualifications to practise"; Wm. J. Scott, of Brockville; Patrick McGarry, of Dublin R.C.S.D., likewise passed.

Seven candidates were rejected. One of them from the University of Leyden, was "exceedingly ignorant of anatomy." Another from Royal College Surgeons, Edinburgh, "could not construe a prescription written by Dr. King and declined to be further examined." The Board "resolved that in every case the examination of a candidate shall be rigidly entered upon and pursued, let his testimonials be of whatever nature they may."

"TORONTO, *September* 2nd, 1834.—The Medical Board in compliance with the order of His Excellency the Lieut.-Governor, dated 28th August, 1834, have carefully examined Mr. James George. They find the marks of a gunshot wound on his left leg, the ball appears to have passed through the muscles at the upper part of the limb producing such an effect on the motion of the leg as to render him incapable of earning his livelihood by labour. Signed, S. Widmer, President. Members present: C. Widmer, P. Deihl, J. Rolph.

"(Signed) ISAAC STEPHENSON, *Secretary*."

October, 1834.—Present: Widmer, Deihl, King and Rolph. F. S. Primrose and Wm. Ferris, members of College of Edinburgh, and Samuel S. Knight, of Kingston, received certificates. Five were rejected. Two of them had diplomas from the College of Physicians and Surgeons, Glasgow. One claimed to be a Medical College Surgeon, of Edinburgh, but was "found to be an exceedingly ignorant man."

August, 1834.—It was publicly announced that "His Excellency, the Governor, has been pleased to appoint a Board of Health for St. Thomas and its vicinity, composed of the following gentlemen: John Bostwick, Jas. C. Crysler, Dr. C. Duncombe, Bela Shaw, Dr. McKenzie, E. Ermatinger, Dr. James A. Rolls, Dr. D. Bowman, J. K. Woodward, James Givins, Esqs."

January, 1835.—Present: Widmer, King, Rolph and Deihl. The Board sat only one day. "Mr. Gerald O'Reilly, M. Coll. Surg., Ireland, Licentiate in Midwifery, Dublin Lying-in Hospital, Licentiate of the Apothecaries' Comp., London; Edward Klinckhardt, from Leipsic and Jena; John Jarron, of Dunnville, late Assistant Surgeon Hon. East India Co.; Robert McCash, received certificates."

The Board appointed Mr. F. St. George Wilkinson, resident apothecary to the hospital, to be their Secretary.

April, 1835.—Present: Widmer, King, Deihl, Rolph and Baldwin. Wm. Craigie, M.C.S. Ed., of Ancaster; David Galbraith, M.C.R. Ed., of Darlington, passed their examination, and Samuel Richardson in surgery only. "The Board took into consideration a letter from the mayor of the city, regarding the public health of the city, and the best means of preserving it from disease."

July, 1835.—Present: Widmer, Rolph and King. Walter H. Burritt, of Marlborough; John Finlayson, "Doctor in Medicine and Surgery," of McGill College, Montreal; Isaac B. Aylsworth, of Bath; Alfred Dewson, M.D., of New York; and Flint L. Keyes, of Grand River, passed. One candidate was rejected, although a member of London College of Medicine, and "a member of the London Vaccine Institution of the Royal Jennerian Society of London."

October, 1835.—Present: Widmer, Deihl, King and Rolph. Roderick McDonald, of Cornwall, M.D. McGill College; George Southwick, St. Thomas; Joseph Clark, Toronto; John K. Fairfield, of Kingston; Wm. Taylor, of Perth; Wm. Allison, Coll. Physicians and Surgeons, Glasgow; all the candidates who appeared received certificates.

During the summer of 1834, the cholera had for the second

time been epidemic in Toronto and other places in Upper Canada. The following editorial from the *Courier* and correspondence explains that the Medical Board was looked upon by the community as a body fully qualified to guard the welfare of the public in relation to the matter of public health. In April of 1835, the *Courier* says:

"The following is the report of the Board of Health of this city, accompanied by a communication from the Medical Board of Upper Canada, addressed to the President of the Board of Health, pointing out the necessity for the preservation of the health of the city during the approaching season, which, coming from an authority so competent to judge of the matter upon which it treats, is deserving of the most serious consideration of the inhabitants of the city as well as of the corporation:

"*To the Mayor, Aldermen and Commonality of the City of Toronto, in Common Council assembled:*

"The Board of Health feel it necessary at this season to communicate to the Worshipful Council the proceeding of the Board on the information obtained by them as to the present state of the health of the city, and the necessary precaution to be observed preparatory to the approaching season when the city will be more liable to suffer from contagious diseases. The Board of Health has great satisfaction in laying before the Council the accompanying communication from the Medical Board of the Province, who have, with the utmost promptitude, at the request of the Board of Health of this city, given the accompanying document, which, coming from a body possessing the science and character of the Medical Board, must be looked upon as possessing no little authority. The Board of Health, from the individual observation of its members, since the reception of the above-mentioned communication of the Medical Board, are compelled to state for the information of the Council, that the city is at present in a most deplorable state of filth and uncleanness—so much so that the Board of Health cannot dwell upon the prospect of the ensuing summer without the most serious apprehensions for the lives and health of their fellow-citizens. The Board of Health feel that they would not perform the duties reposed in them if they did not, in the strongest terms, recommend to the Council the adoption of every means within the power of the corporation which may have a tendency to cause the proper draining of the city, and the removal of the accumulating filth and nuisances which form so pregnant a source of disease.

"T. B. SULLIVAN, *Mayor*.
(Dr.) J. D. MORRISON.
GEO. GURNETT.
THOMAS CARFRAE.

"Toronto, April 7th, 1835."

"*To His Worship the Mayor:*

"SIR,—I have laid before the Medical Board your letter of the 2nd inst., and am requested by them to communicate with you on the subject of it.

"The state of the health of the city is favourable, the season not having arrived during which any diseases usually prevail to render it otherwise.

"For the preservation of the health of the city, the Board can only suggest the obvious means of cleanliness by draining, paving and removal of offal from the different dwellings.

"The population of the city is greatly increased, and is become more dense and compact. Under these circumstances the regulations which have formerly proved sufficient to preserve the public health, will now be altogether inadequate; and unless some efficient precautions are taken, the prevalence of any epidemic must be expected to be marked with particular severity.

"The Board recommend the construction, as soon as possible, of public sewers, by which all cellars may be drained. Superficial gutters, so constructed as readily to carry off the water from the surface, may be more immediately within the resources of the city, and would be conducive to the health and comfort of the inhabitants. But the Board despair of any means proving effectual till draining shall be carried to its full extent. For the removal of offal and all accumulations of animal and vegetable matter, which, on exposure to the sun, become fertile sources of disease, the Board recommend the daily employment of scavengers. For this purpose every family should be obliged to collect the kitchen offal ready for the scavengers every morning.

"Should it be apprehended that cholera will again become epidemic, it will be desirable to have in readiness such accommodations as will, under satisfactory regulations, enable the sick to be separated from those in health.

"I have the honour to be, Sir,
"Your obedient servant,

"C. WIDMER, *President.*"

By the foregoing statements it will be seen that the views of the Medical Board as expressed fifty-eight years ago, are almost what might be expressed by a sanitarian of to-day. And it is also learned that the fathers of the medical profession who constituted the Board were eminently qualified to fill the position of health officer as well as to watch the door of entrance to the profession.

For Public Health Act and appointment of Board of Health with remarks, see Appendix.

The spirit which animated the profession at this time is indicated by this notice:

"A meeting of the members of the medical profession, residing in this city (Toronto) and vicinity, will be held at the Grand Jury's room, 15th July, 1835, to consider the expediency of forming a Medical Reading Room and Library, also matters connected with the advancement of Medical Science."

CHAPTER X.

DISSATISFACTION WITH THE MEDICAL BOARD.

TORONTO, *January*, 1836.—Present: Widmer, Rolph and King. Arthur Paterson, formerly Hospital Sergeant in the 72nd Regiment, who had an "Excellent certificate from the Surgeon," and of "Attendance on Lectures in Marischal Coll., Aberdeen, and the Royal Infirmary of that city," passed his examination. Three were rejected: one, a Member of the

Apothecaries' Co., and "with ample testimonials from Grainger's School"; another had a "diploma from College of Physicians and Surgeons, Glasgow, and an abundant supply of Tickets"; the other had certificates from Glasgow and Edinburgh.

The following letter then appears in the minutes:

"GOVERNMENT HOUSE,
"30th *January*, 1836.

"SIR,—I am directed by the Lieutenant-Governor to inform you, for the information of the Members of the Medical Board, that His Excellency will receive those gentlemen for the purpose of presenting an Address on Monday next, 12 o'clock.

"I have the honour to be, Sir,
"Your most obedient, humble servant,
"(Signed) J. LOVELL.

"To the Secretary of the Medical Board."

"*February* 1st, 1836.—The Board met for the purpose of waiting on His Excellency and presenting a congratulatory Address:

"*May it please Your Excellency:*

"The Medical Board of Upper Canada congratulate Your Excellency on your safe arrival in this Province, and beg leave to commend to Your Excellency's favourable consideration the interests of the profession."

"*Gentlemen:*

"I thank you for your obliging congratulations upon my arrival in this Province.

"I consider that your character and the interests of the inhabitants of this Province are so far identical that for the welfare of both I shall always be desirous to afford you every proper encouragement."

The Lieutenant-Governor was Sir F. B. Head.

"*February* 15th, 1836.—The Board met pursuant to an order from His Excellency the Lieutenant-Governor to examine and report upon the case of Private David Van Volkenbergh, late of the Glengarry Light Infantry. Present: C. Widmer, President;

Dr. King, John Rolph. The Board report that he is incapable of earning his livelihood by labour in consequence of a gunshot wound of the right foot."

April 4, 1836.—The Board met. Members present: C. Widmer, Esq., P. Deihl, Esq., John Rolph, Esq., Dr. Latham, Dr. Baldwin, Dr. King, Dr. Hornby, T. D. Morrison, Esq., and Dr. Chas. Duncombe.

"It was moved by Dr. King, and seconded by Dr. Baldwin, that the President do take the Chair, and that the Board do proceed to business, which was carried."

Dr. Winder sent a message by the Secretary that he had communicated to His Excellency the Lieutenant-Governor his resignation as a member of the Medical Board, and that His Excellency had accepted of the same.

"The commission was then read—as also the letter accompanying it from Mr. Secretary Joseph, addressed to C. Widmer, Esq., senior member of the Medical Board, which was as follows:

"'SIR,—By command of the Lieutenant-Governor I have the honour to transmit to you the accompanying Instrument reconstructing the Medical Board of this Province,

"'And to be, Sir,
"'Your most obedient and humble servant,

"'(Signed) J. JOSEPH.

"'To Christopher Widmer, Esq.,
"'Senior Member of the Medical Board.'

"It was then proposed by Dr. Duncombe, and seconded by Dr. Deihl, that it be *Resolved*, That Drs. Baldwin, King and Morrison be a committee to inquire into the legality of the terms of the new commission, which purports, in conjunction with Mr. Secretary Joseph's letter, to reconstruct the Medical Board, and subject its members to hold their office during pleasure, which was carried.

"The President reported to the Board that he had been informed by His Excellency the Lieutenant-Governor that the Barrister's room in the public building might be occupied by the Board for holding its sitting.

"It was then moved by Dr. Rolph, seconded by Dr. Baldwin, that the Secretary be directed to put himself in communication with Mr. Secretary Joseph to procure the necessary accommodation for the Board in the apartment appointed by His Excellency for their sitting, which was carried.

"It was then moved by Dr. King, and seconded by Dr. Morrison, that it be *Resolved*, That the examination of candidates before the Board be conducted as hitherto under the direction of the President, which was carried."

April, 1836.—Henry Rolls, of Toronto; James Edward Burton, of Paris, Canada; Cyrenus Hall, Fort Erie; William Bulmer Nicol, of Toronto, with tickets from King's College, received certificates. Two were rejected: one because his answers generally were indifferent, and "in midwifery profoundly ignorant"; the other was favoured with an examination on two days before being rejected.

July, 1836.—Present: Drs. Widmer, Deihl, King, O'Brien, Hornby and Morrison. Chas. McCosker, with a diploma from Glasgow; Daniel Macintyre, with Glasgow diploma; James Meagher, of Kingston, from McGill College, received certificates. Two were rejected; one of them was "from the United States, educated at the University of Maryland and Pennsylvania. He exhibited a total ignorance of the Latin language, and seemed to be as uninformed of English Grammar."

October, 1836.—Present: Widmer, King, Rolph, Morrison, Hornby and Deihl. James Mitchell, "a pupil of Dr. Rolph's," appeared for examination; he had been one winter at Jefferson College, Phil., and an attentive pupil of Toronto Hospital, and "underwent a severe examination with credit," and received certificate. Matthew Campbell, Member College of Surgeons, Edinburgh, and had served in East India Company's Service, also passed. Three were rejected. One "knew nothing of anatomy beyond books, never having dissected in his life."

During the year 1836, no little feeling existed on the part of a portion of the medical profession against the Medical Board and those who had the management of the General Hospital. To what extent this feeling had grounds of justification is uncertain. It culminated, however, in the calling of a public meeting of the profession. The meeting was called by this:

"NOTICE.—A meeting of the medical profession of this city (Toronto) will take place at the Court House, 4th January, 1836, to consider the propriety of petitioning the Lieutenant-Governor upon subjects connected with the Hospital and the Medical Board," which was accordingly held. An account of the proceedings were published by the *Patriot:*

"MEDICAL EDUCATION.—A meeting of the medical practitioners of the city of Toronto, pursuant to public advertisement, was held at the Court House, on the 14th inst. (January, 1836), when the following resolutions were unanimously adopted:

"I. *Resolved,*—That it is the opinion of this meeting that no institution has been devised better calculated to lighten the afflictions of the poorer portion of society labouring under disease, or suffering from accident, than an hospital constituted on wise and liberal principles and conducted by an adequate number of skilful practitioners.

"II. *Resolved,*—It being a subject of general notoriety that there exists in the minds of the poorer classes in all countries a prejudice against such institutions, that it is the opinion of this meeting that this prejudice, partly natural, arises principally from an ill-grounded apprehension that medical men requite themselves for unpaid services by the extensive field of experimental practice thus opened to them, remote from the observation of the public and of the friends and relations of the patient.

"III. *Resolved,*—That it is of the utmost importance to remove this prejudice, as far as may be, and that it appears to this meeting that nothing is better adapted to this end than the precautions of such institutions at home, viz., appointing particular days in the week for important operations that admit of delay, when medical men and their pupils, and all persons interested, are at liberty to attend—publishing periodically full statements of the number of persons admitted, their ailments, recovery or death, etc.,—and generally by affording to visitors such easy access to the wards as is consistent with the comfort and accommodation of the patients.

"IV. *Resolved*,—That it is the opinion of this meeting that over the hospital of this city a veil of obscurity impends which it is highly advantageous to have removed. No appointed days invite the attendance of medical men in connection with the institution; no published reports inform the public of the number of those who have been restored to their friends, cured of their diseases or healed of their infirmities; the passing bier alone affords a melancholy proof that the institution still exists in active operation.

"V. *Resolved*,—That a respectful application be made to the Lieutenant-Governor of this Province, requesting information upon the following points: The Original Constitution of the Hospital, the number and mode of election of the medical attendants, whether there exists a Board of Control. If so, of whom composed; whether a periodical statement of patients admitted, their ailments, treatment, recovery or death, is submitted to the Lieutenant-Governor or any board authorized to receive or demand such statement.

"VI. *Resolved*,—That it is the opinion of this meeting that the Medical Board of this city, consisting as it does, for the most part, of members who, from the remoteness of their residences and being devoted to other pursuits, cannot attend to the important duties intrusted to them,

"VII. *Resolved*,—That it is contrary to the practice in other countries and manifestly inexpedient, that *two* or *three* medical practitioners holding their inquisition in utter darkness should have from year to year the power of pronouncing *without appeal*, on the professional merit of *their own* pupils, or those of others with whom they may possibly be at variance.

"VIII. *Resolved*,—That a respectful petition be presented to the Lieutenant-Governor, praying him to introduce such changes into the constitution of the Medical Board as may seem to His Excellency best calculated to restore to it the confidence of the medical men of this country, and of those who are to submit to their decision, their future prospects in life.

"IX. *Resolved*,—That an immediate application be made to

the Provincial Legislature to extend to the Licentiates of the Colleges of Surgeons of Dublin, Edinburgh and Glasgow, those privileges which they have already conceded to that of London —making thereby an invidious distinction insulting to those colleges, and to the countries to which they belong.

"WM. C. GWYNNE, *Chairman.*
WM. REES, *Secretary.*"

Dissatisfaction with the Medical Board and the Executive authority still further manifested itself by the following editorial remarks. How far they were in accordance with facts we are not in a position to judge. Of course, jealousy and intrigue are not confined to any time or place:

"The *Courier*, March 5th, 1836: By the last official *Gazette* we observe that the Medical Board of the Province has been re-organized and enlarged, and now consists of the following gentlemen, viz., Drs. Widmer, Baldwin, Grant, Powell, Horne, Sampson, Deihl, King, Rolph, Ridley, Stratford, C. Duncombe, Harnley, Latham, Winder, O'Brien and Morrison; the first eleven gentlemen being the members of the former Board, and the latter five being new members added thereto by the present Lieutenant-Governor.

"We think that an addition to the number of members residing in the capital is a proper measure, as the duties of the Medical Board had, for some time past, devolved on three or four gentlemen only; but His Excellency, we think, has not been very happy in the selection of those additional members." The article goes on to say that Dr. Gwynne should have been the first in selection. The following tribute is paid to Dr. Gwynne: "It is commonly known in this neighbourhood that Dr. Gwynne's professional attainments, talents, practice and personal character and weight in society, are equal to those of any of the gentlemen who constitute the Medical Board; while those qualifications are greatly superior (as admitted even by themselves) to a majority of those who have just been added to the Board."

"There are other medical gentlemen in town whose claims to the appointment in question are also admitted to be very superior to those of some of the gentlemen who have now been added to the Board; we allude to Dr. Egan, Dr. Telfer and others. Who would think of comparing Dr. Winder or Dr. Latham with Dr. Gwynne, or indeed, either of those gentlemen whom we have named as being left out. The first time the existence of such a person as Dr. Winder was known to ninety-nine-hundredths of the city was the appearance of his name in the last official *Gazette*, while the other gentleman (Dr. Latham) is understood to be on the eve of emigrating to Texas, there to take up his residence, and which gentleman is himself quite astonished at his appointment to the Medical Board of Upper Canada, and is ascribed to motives which we will not just now mention.

"We have alluded to the secret springs of intrigues which have evidently been employed to effect the proscription of the gentlemen in question; particularly of Dr. Gwynne, towards whom great professional jealousy and envy are known to have been long entertained by certain medical practitioners—one of whom has very recently been elevated to the Executive Council—and it is to the influence of the secret intrigues in question that the exclusion of Drs. Gwynne, Egan, etc., and the appointment of persons of inferior professional qualifications is now universally ascribed."

CHAPTER XI.

CONCERNING KING'S COLLEGE.

TORONTO, *January*, 1837.—Present: Widmer, Deihl, O'Brien, Hornby and Rolph. James Campbell, M.D., of Kingston, from University of Burlington, Vermont, and Licentiate in Medicine and Surgery of Lower Canada, passed. One was rejected.

April, 1837.—Present: Widmer, Rolph, Deihl, King and Hornby. Thomas Chamberlain, of Bath, passed his examination in physic and surgery only. Two were rejected.

July, 1837.—Present: Widmer, King, Deihl, Rolph and Hornby. John Turquand, of Toronto; Robert McLean, of

Kingston, received certificates. Three rejected. Some of those rejected had been students at Fairfield College.

August 8, 1837.—The members of the Medical Board met this day to take into consideration the interests of the medical profession involved in the proceeding of the Council of King's College, lately made public, regarding the university.

Present: C. Widmer, President; Dr. Baldwin, Dr. Hornby, Dr. King and Dr. Rolph. "It was moved by Dr. Rolph and seconded by Dr. Hornby, that a committee consisting of Drs. King, Hornby, Baldwin and O'Brien, be appointed to draw up resolutions regarding the constitution of the Council of King's College, and other matters connected with the interests of the medical profession, and that the Committee be requested to report on Thursday next at 12 o'clock."

August 10, 1837.—The members present at this meeting were: C. Widmer, President; Drs. Baldwin, Deihl, Horne, King, Hornby, Morrison and Rolph.

"The Committee appointed to draw up resolutions reported the following:

"1st. *Resolved*,—That, by the Charter of the University of King's College it was intended to provide for 'the Education, and Instruction of Youth and Students in Arts and Faculties.' Carried. Dr. Deihl dissenting because the Charter provides accordingly.

"2nd. *Resolved*,—That the usefulness of such an institution in an eminent degree consists of preparing those youths who have already received an elementary education for the practical discharge of the duties of the learned professions. Carried.

"3rd. *Resolved*,—That of those professions, the healing art has at all times been justly ranked among the most honourable, the most learned and the most useful. Carried.

"4th. *Resolved*,—That the members of the Medical Board have noticed with surprise and regret that in the composition of the Council of the University of King's College there is not, since the necessary retirement of Messrs. Powell and Widmer, one member of the medical profession to guard and advance its interests, although it is evident that this department will furnish a large proportion of the students at the University should it be provided with teachers of acknowledged talent. Carried.

"It was ordered that the Secretary do enclose a copy of the foregoing resolutions to Mr. Secretary Joseph, for the information of His Excellency, as Chancellor of the University of Upper Canada.

"MEDICAL BOARD, U.C.,
"TORONTO, 22nd *August*, 1837.

"SIR,—I have the honour to transmit to you, for the information of His Excellency the Chancellor of the University of King's College, a resolution passed at a meeting of the members of the Medical Board, on the 10th inst.

"*Resolved*,—That the President of the Medical Board be requested to obtain from His Excellency, the Chancellor of the University of King's College, U.C., information respecting the arrangements which have been and are intended to be made for the organization of the Medical Department.

"In performing the duty assigned to me by the foregoing resolution, I am induced to represent to His Excellency the anxiety with which the members of the medical profession throughout the Province are waiting for the development of an effective plan of medical instruction for the numerous class of students within it; and here, long from causes perhaps unavoidable, the first claims of these young men to participate in the benefits of the University, have been delayed.

"The Medical Board having been in frequent correspondence with His Excellency's predecessor, Sir John Colborne, on the subject of establishing a school of medicine in anticipation of the opening of the University, I am enabled to state that Sir John was strongly impressed with the imperious necessity of preventing so many youths of the Province from resorting to a foreign country for the means of instruction, where their early political principles were exposed to an influence not likely to prove advantageous to themselves or their country.

"Now that the period is at hand when the most important and beneficient results may be derived from the operations of King's College, it becomes the duty of the Medical Board to afford all the aid which their experience may enable them to give, in furtherance of the completion of such a plan of professional education as shall ensure to the medical students of the Province all the advantages that a University can bestow; and that shall be so attractive to the public generally as to invite not only the Canadians as aspirants to professional honour, but the medical students of all the North American provinces and even of neighbouring States of the Union. These results, if an enlarged and liberal course of professional instruction be adopted, will no doubt be realized—for it is a fact that no university enjoying a desirable celebrity for medical education exists north of Philadelphia; it may therefore be reasonably expected that if the Medical Faculty of King's College is established on a footing of respectability, it will be thronged with students.

"The members of the Medical Board, I am warranted in declaring, are actuated solely in this communication to His Excellency the Chancellor, by a desire to obtain such information as may enable them to correct, if necessary, any erroneous views that may be taken by those whose official duty it is become to make the arrangement for the Medical Department of King's College.

"(Signed) C. WIDMER, *President.*"

"MEDICAL BOARD,
"*August* 28th, 1837.

"Copy of a letter in reply to the letter of the President of the Medical Board from His Excellency the Lieutenant-Governor's Civil Secretary, received this day, concerning the arrangements and appointments made and about to be made in the Council of the University of the King's College:

"GOVERNMENT HOUSE,
"*August* 26th, 1837.

"SIR,—Having laid before His Excellency the Lieutenant-Governor your letter of 22nd inst., I have the honour by His Excellency's command to inform you, that in compliance with the wish expressed by the Resolution passed at a meeting of the members of the Medical Board, His Excellency will always be happy to communicate to the President of the Medical Board, any information which the Board may desire respecting such arrangements as may have been made by the King's College Council for the organization of the Medical Department.

"I have the honour to be, etc.,

"(Signed) J. JOSEPH."

October, 1837.—Present: Widmer, King, Rolph, Morrison, Duncombe, Deihl and Hornby. One candidate was rejected. The Board passed the following:

"*Resolved*,—That the Medical Board have been anxiously expecting the information desired by their resolution of the 10th August from His Excellency the Chancellor of the University of King's College, and as the applications from the Medical Students of the Province to the Members of the Board are frequent and urgent for the establishment of a public institution for their instruction in medicine, that the Board, through their President, do again respectfully renew their application for such information.

"(Signed) C. WIDMER, *President*.

W. W. BALDWIN, M.D.	R. C. HORNE.
PETER DEIHL.	JOHN KING, M.D.
CHAS. DUNCOMBE.	ROBT. HORNBY, M.D.
D. MORRISON.	JOHN ROLPH."

"The following letter was received this day in reply to the above resolution from Mr. Secretary Joseph, addressed to the Secretary of the Medical Board, 14th October, 1837:

"GOVERNMENT HOUSE,
"*October* 13th, 1837.

"SIR,—I have the honour to acknowledge the receipt of your letter of yesterday's date, transmitting a copy of a Resolution passed at a meeting of the Medical Board on the 7th inst., and having laid the same before the Lieutenant-Governor, I am directed by His Excellency to refer you to the letter which, on the 26th August, I had the honour by His Excellency's commands to address to the President of the Medical Board, expressing His Excellency's readiness at all times to communicate to the President any information which may be desired respecting such arrangements as may have been made by the King's College Council for the organization of the Medical Department.

"His Excellency, however, is not aware that any arrangements for that object have yet been made.

"His Excellency further directs me to state that any information or suggestions which the Medical Board may deem it advisable to lay before him, he will receive with attentive consideration, and will lose no time in communicating to the College Council.

"I have the honour, etc.,

"(Signed) J. JOSEPH."

October 24, 1837.—Present: C. Widmer, President; Drs. Baldwin, Rolph and King.

Dr. King stated to the Board that he, in conjunction with the President, had been sent for by His Excellency the Chancellor, who, in conversation, stated that if a case strong enough to convince him of the necessity of establishing a course of medical instruction before the general operations of King's College were commenced, were presented to him, His Excellency would feel it to be his duty to take the same into his serious consideration.

It was then moved by Dr. Rolph, and seconded by the President, that Dr. Baldwin and Dr. King be a committee to draw up a representation on the foregoing subject and submit it to the Board on Tuesday next.

CHAPTER XII.

RECOMMENDATION TO FORM MEDICAL FACULTY.

TORONTO, *November* 2, 1837.—Present: C. Widmer, President; Drs. Baldwin, Deihl, King, Rolph and Hornby. Dr. Baldwin, of the Committee, read a report to His Excellency the Chancellor of King's College, for the consideration of the Board. The Board unanimously adopted the report and ordered it to be engrossed and transmitted to His Excellency.

"MEDICAL BOARD,
"*November* 12th, 1837.

"SIR,—At a special meeting of the members of the Medical Board, convened by the President on the 2nd inst.,—present: The President, Drs. Baldwin, Deihl, King, Rolph, Hornby and Morrison—Dr. King informed the members present 'that His Excellency the Lieutenant-Governor (through his secretary) requested the attendance of the President (Dr. Widmer) and himself at Government House; that they accordingly had the honour of waiting upon His Excellency, and during their interview His Excellency was pleased to say that "if the Medical Board could make out a case sufficiently strong to convince him of the necessity of establishing at once a medical faculty in King's College, he would take the matter into his serious consideration."'

"I have the honour, by order of the Board, to inclose you, for the information of His Excellency the Chancellor, 'a case' (representing the present state of the medical profession in this Province with their claims, etc., etc., etc.,) which was unanimously agreed upon in behalf of the Board by the members present.

"I have the honour to conclude, Sir,

"Etc., etc.,

"F. WILKINSON, *Secretary.*

"*To* JOHN JOSEPH, ESQ.,
"Etc., etc., etc."

"*May it please Your Excellency.*

"In answer to their communication of the 7th October, the Medical Board have been honoured by a reply through Your Excellency's Secretary, repeating the assurance of your willingness to receive their suggestions on the subject of a medical faculty to be formed in the new University of King's College.

"The Board will not doubt this willingness, not only in respect to Your Excellency's assurances, but also because the matter of this correspondence is of deep public interest. Under these circumstances, and as incidental to the duty of a public body invested by the law of the Province, during its infancy (as it were), with the guardianship of the medical profession and practice, the Medical Board feel themselves imperiously called on to repeat to Your Excellency, but with some amplification, their views on the subject.

"In the first place, therefore, premising, with due deference to Your Excellency, that however education and professional reputation might naturally, and without call for apology, induce the Board to hope that, in the appointment of some of its members to professorships in the Medical Department of this University, to Your Excellency as Chancellor would have been conceded the opportunity of giving some worthy testimonial of public gratitude to those gentlemen who not only discharge the duties of the Board, consisting of minute scientific and practical examination of medical candidates, and occupying a large portion of valuable time without any adequate remuneration, but who also most humanely and gratuitously attended the general hospital in this city, it may be said from its very foundation to the present moment. Yet, as no suggestion of this nature appeared in the previous communications of the Board with Your Excellency, it is with some degree of surprise that they now have occasion to observe themselves called upon 'to make out a case sufficiently strong to convince Your Excellency of the necessity of establishing at once the medical faculty in King's College,' as if private interest alone dictated their interference.

"The Board trusts this could not have been so meant, inasmuch as no case can be offered to Your Excellency, but that of the public interests of the community throughout the Province without exception of persons, place, condition of life, religion or politics. The people of the Province, like mankind generally, are subject to all the variety of disease, accident and their consequences; all in their turn receive their share of pain and anguish, to assuage or remove which is the object of the physician's and surgeon's united science and skill, and thus it is that if there be any one object of human knowledge of more importance to society than another, it is that of the healing art. The Board means not to deny the value of moral and religious instruction, nor to take from general science its just praise; but being called on 'to make out a case,' the Board are constrained to bring before Your Excellency's consideration the relative position which the wants of the public give to the respective departments of education at the promised university, the means of which at present (as it is said) are unequal to the complete organization of the whole.

"The prior claim of a medical department rests not merely in the general interests of the community, as before very briefly mentioned, but on many other circumstances, of which the following should fairly be weighed well with it:

"1st. That the moral education of youth, always in a large degree supplied by the care which parents most generally feel and take in the direction of their children's principles and conduct, is further promoted by the religious supervision and preaching of the numerous pastors chosen or appointed to the various congregations of Christians throughout the Province, to which may be added, that the prosperous progress of the Upper Canada College and (as it may be hoped) the improving course of the district and common schools, all conspire not only to enlarge the sphere of moral and religious education, but also by a very favourable foundation for literature, the profession of the law, too, is largely provided for, and thus, while morals, religion, literature and law are greatly, if not adequately provided for, medical education may be said to be totally disregarded in this Province; truly some medical gentlemen (to their honour be it mentioned) do give instruction to their own pupils, yet they feel and complain of the deficiency of adequate means, means beyond their reach, and which nothing can supply but the appropriate institution of a university.

"2nd. The rising youth whose parents are able and desirous of devoting their sons to this useful and honourable profession are debarred by the apprehension of sacrificing their time and talents to a pursuit for the honours of which they cannot be fitted within the Province. Some, therefore, have been sent to Great Britain and Lower Canada, many to Philadelphia, New York, Fairfield, and other Colleges of the neighbouring States, there to procure even partially what is denied them here altogether; and from these seminaries they often return unqualified. How grievous, then, is the injustice to them and their parents in the unavoidable rejection to which they are often exposed in their examinations before the Medical Board—rejections very seldom induced by want of talent or assiduity, but by the lamentable want of some collegiate institution suited to the great objects of medical science. Well may these candidates say of the Board, ''Tis cruel to reject us for ignorance when you supply us not with the sources of knowledge,' to which the Board can as well reply, 'The law has imposed upon us (till better establishments be formed) the duty of protecting the lives and health of the public from the desolation and plunder of empiricism'—and this can only be done by rejecting at the Board all the unqualified. So sensible of this was Your Excellency's late predecessor, Sir John Colborne, that he frequently called upon the Board to attend him in consultations on this subject, and more than once on these occasions assured the Board that he 'saw that a medical school could not be delayed without manifest injury to the Province,' and intimated frequently his readiness to appoint professors immediately, but the confirmation of the charter having been suspended for causes not here necessary to be alluded to, he was unable to carry his intentions into effect.

"3rd. With a view to the private hopes and interests of medical students, it is fair to state that the establishment of a medical faculty in a university in this Province would afford the student of physic the great advantage of allowance of time in foreign universities, not only in England, but in the continent of Europe, where very probably most of those who could afford the expense would wish to resort for one or two years though unwilling to subject their parents to the expense of an entire education abroad.

"One or two years' study in those universities where numerous hospitals attended by the most eminent men of the profession afford a source of instruction unattainable on this side of the Atlantic; this advantage the student cannot attain by attendance on mere lectures, however able to instruct.

"The Medical Board cannot think it necessary to spread before Your Excellency any further the circumstances of interest and importance that envelop the consideration of this subject; and yet after all, notwithstanding the public demand for a medical school in a provincial university; notwithstanding the lively hopes of students and parents in the public announcement of King's College Charter; notwithstanding the late Lieut.-Governor's conviction of the necessity and his approbation of a prompt establishment of an adequate medical school; this Board (forbearing to express the extent of their surprise) fear they discover an intention of postponing this necessary department of the university to objects of minor importance, or, if not of minor importance, at least of far less urgency as to priority of commencement, and as called upon 'to make out a case' the Board take the liberty for Your Excellency's information, of adverting to a printed paper which appeared about April last purporting to be a plan or arrangements of the several departments of science in King's College; shortly, however, after its appearance, it was mentioned with some sort of mysterious reserve amongst those who ventured to speak of it, that it was to undergo some new modification; the Board therefore on the occasion of requesting Your Excellency as Chancellor to inform them of the arrangements, if any had been made, forbore every allusion to that paper; as obviously just towards the college authorities, to this hour, nevertheless, the Medical Board are uninformed of any determinate plan adopted, or to be adopted by the College Council as regards a medical faculty therein; and it is therefore still left to the Board to ask Your Excellency as Chancellor if it be possible that nothing is as yet done? In the meantime, while uninformed, in order to make out the case required the Board can only revert to the printed paper before mentioned; by which it would appear to have been proposed that professorships or lectureships should be established in the following branches of science and literature, viz.:

"1st. Classical and Modern Literature—two professors.

"2nd. Medical Physics—two professors.

"3rd. Medical Mental Philosophy—one professor (the President).

"4th. Medical Theology—in abeyance.

"5th. Medical Jurisprudence—one lecturer (no professor). One Professor of Chemistry.

"6th. Medicine—(subservient to other departments as well as medicine) and three lecturers.

"Thus the medical department, last as least in the estimation of this extraordinary proposal, was to be all concentrated in one chair to be filled by a Professor of Chemistry (subservient to other objects as well as medicine), furnished, as it were, with out-door servants under the appellation of lecturers. How does it happen that thus in Upper Canada, Medical Science, of such universal interest that every individual of the community must experience its bane or blessing according to its barbarism or its culture, should be so degraded, and the tenderest sympathies of human nature so outraged; a Professor of Chemistry forsooth!!! with out-door lecturers in medicine, surgery and anatomy; Your Excellency surely knows that a Professor of Chemistry may be very little versant in the most necessary branches of medicine,—nay, if the professor be a chemist worthy of the chair, it is next to impossible that he should be capable of commencing medical instruction; this it may be answered is not intended; if so, then it remains manifest that the object of the arrangement in the printed paper was to exclude a medical professor from the College Council. (See note in the Appendix.) How then, it may be asked, can it be possible for a Council composed of men altogether ignorant of medicine and its manifold scientific sub-divisions, to make suitable arrangements for medical classes, or distribute the courses between the lecturers; moreover, first attempts will unavoidably be found more or less faulty; time only can mature a smooth working of the whole; during such time, who are to direct the out-door servants? The printed paper in effect, answers: men ignorant of the work in their servants' hands.

"What dissatisfaction may be anticipated to arise between masters and servants—the Council and their lecturers! What disgust with the pupils! What despair with parents! Finally, what degradation will await this highly necessary and honourable profession by such ill-judged measures? If there be at present in the Province any gentleman legitimately honoured with the profession and fitted for the task, willing to accept the office of an out-door lecturer, the Board can only regret it for the sake of the profession and the public at large. Very true it is, that most of the large cities having universities have also independent lecturers, highly learned and honourable men, and deriving an honourable reward from their useful labours; but these learned men, however able and worthy, cannot confer the honours nor the privileges of a faculty in a university. Finally, the Board respectfully beg leave to urge upon Your Excellency's consideration as Chancellor, the crying want of the Province, and the paramount importance of making the medical faculty a prominent feature of King's College at its very commencement. Such a faculty cannot well be imagined to exist or be formed with less than six professors. The Board suggest the following:

"I.—Anatomy.

"II.—Materia Medica and Pharmacy.

"III.—Practice of Physic and Medical Pathology.

"IV.—Chemistry.

"V.—Principles and Practice of Surgery and Surgical Pathology.

"VI.—Midwifery and Diseases of Women and Children.

"These six may be considered the most necessary to be at once established; and it will also be necessary for each of these professors to lecture on one or other of the following subjects until the university should afford the expense of separate professorships therein, that is to say, Botany, Medical Jurisprudence, Institutes of Medicine, Natural History, Clinical Medicine, Clinical Surgery.

"Of the professors forming the faculty of medicine in the university, two at least should belong to the College Council, where their presence and a knowledge of their proper duties will enable the Council safely to devise and arrange all matters connected with the interests of the Medical School. It is very far from the intention of the Medical Board to recommend to Your Excellency's consideration anything unreasonable or impracticable. If the funds at present at the disposal of the College Council require a narrower sphere in the commencement of the institution, surely the requisite construction should not be such as totally to exclude the profession most required by the community. With a view to the narrow finances of the King's College, the Board respectfully submit to Your Excellency that there can be no reasonable objection raised to the hiring of apartments in the city for the delivery of medical lectures. This course is frequently taken in the universities of Europe, as Your Excellency without doubt well knows, and even in Dublin at this day the university affords accommodation only to three of the medical professors, the others lecture in Sir Patrick Dunn's Hospital.

"Before closing the case to Your Excellency, the Board have directed an examination of their records to be made as to the number of medical candidates presenting themselves for admissions, and the proportion rejected for the causes above explained; and by this it appears that since the year 1830, down to the last term inclusive of both, the number presenting themselves were one hundred and sixty-four, of whom sixty-four were rejected; for a detail of which they respectfully refer Your Excellency to the statement in the appendix annexed. Thus Your Excellency will be enabled in some degree to measure the magnitude of the evil inflicted on the students, and the still more painful evil on the community at large by admission of candidates but partially educated.

"Trusting that they have sufficiently, if not as amply as the subject admits, made out the case required, the Medical Board have the honour to submit this their view of it to Your Excellency's consideration; and the members present in behalf of the Board beg leave to subscribe themselves,

"Your Excellency's Most Obedient Servants,

"C. WIDMER, *President*.

W. W. BALDWIN, M.D.	JOHN ROLPH.
PETER DEIHL.	ROBERT HORNBY, M.D.
JOHN KING, M.D.	T. D. MORRISON."

"APPENDIX.

"NOTE 1.—And that the members of the College Council, including the Chancellor and President, shall be twelve in number, of whom the speakers of the two Houses of the Legislature of the Province, and His Majesty's Attorney and Solicitor-General for the time being shall be four, and the remainder shall consist *of the five senior professors of Arts and Faculties* of said College, and the Principal of minor or Upper Canada College (see an Act to amend the Charter of the University of King's College).

"Total number of candidates who presented themselves for examination since 1830 to the last term inclusive, 164; of whom finally passed, 100; rejected, 64.

"Of the 64 rejected, 7 were rejected twice; 1 rejected three times.

"Of the number passed at first examination, 83; second examination, 15; third examination, 2; total, 100.

"Of the 100 finally passed, there were members of Colleges of Surgeons of Dublin, Edinburgh, Glasgow and foreign universities, 64; Canadians, 36; total, 100.

"Of the above number, 2 passed for midwifery only; 2 for surgery, and 1 for physics and surgery.

"Of the 36 Canadians, not one was educated in the Province without resort to foreign institutions; of the 64 rejected, 47 have not returned for examination, and consequently remain unqualified, by reason of the deficient means of instruction in the Province."

"GOVERNMENT HOUSE,
"*November* 17th, 1837.

"Sir,—I am commanded by the Lieut.-Governor to inform you that he has read with attention the report dated the 10th inst., which has been addressed to him by the Medical Board, in which it is stated 'that it is with some degree of surprize that they now have occasion to observe themselves called upon "to make out a case sufficiently strong to convince Your Excellency of the necessity of establishing at once the Medical Faculty in King's College" as if private interest alone dictated their interference.' As the assertion by the Medical Board of its having been by the Lieut.-Governor 'called upon to make out a case' is several times repeated throughout the report, His Excellency feels it necessary to inform the Board that in a conversation which he had the pleasure to hold with Dr. Widmer and Dr. King, he assured those gentlemen how completely he concurred with them in the propriety of giving every proper encouragement to medical science in this Province—that he was desirous to do so with as little delay as possible—at the same time His Excellency observed that it might be questionable whether it would not be for the interest of the Medical Faculty that it should delay commencing its operation until the other branches of the University were prepared to support it.

" His Excellency, however, observed to Dr. Widmer and Dr. King that he was quite disposed to bring before the College Council any arrangements in favour of their object which the Medical Board might deem it advisable in writing to submit to him. And His Excellency added that if the Medical Board should succeed in making out their case, he could assure them it would be taken into serious consideration. The Lieut.-Governor has now received the report of the Board, coupled, His Excellency regrets to observe, with animadversions on His Excellency's intentions, which His Excellency desires me to inform you he cannot in justice to himself think of submitting for the consideration of the College Council.

" His Excellency, however, desires me to inform you that, should the scientific matter of the report be divested of the uncalled-for observations to which I have alluded, His Excellency will be happy to bring the suggestions of the Medical Board under the immediate consideration of the College Council.

" I have the honour to remain, Sir,

" Etc., etc., etc.,

" (Signed) J. JOSEPH.

" F. WILKINSON, Esq.,

" *Secretary, Medical Board.*"

At a meeting of the Medical Board held on the 24th day of November, 1837 (present: C. Widmer, President; W. W. Baldwin, M.D.; John King, M.D.; Peter Deihl, John Rolph), the following resolution was adopted:

Resolved,—That after His Excellency the Chancellor of King's College had been pleased to intimate to Dr. Widmer and Dr. King, that if the Medical Board should succeed in making out their case, he could assure them it should be taken into serious consideration; the Medical Board proceeded to the execution of that duty by their communication of the 12th November, and should they in doing so have used any expressions which, most contrary to their intentions, may admit of a construction they cannot themselves discover, implying animadversions on His Excellency's intentions, they trust the public interests will not be allowed to suffer from such inadvertency.

This year an Act was passed granting £750 in aid of the Toronto Hospital. From Kingston a petition by the clergy was received, and other inhabitants, in which it was stated that the "bedding, furniture, and store belonging to the hospital had been destroyed by fire, and stating the necessity for immediate furnishing and fitting up the new hospital, and praying for a grant of £500, which petition was granted by Act of Parliament.

January, 1838.—Present: Widmer, King and Deihl. No business.

April, 1838.—Present: Widmer, Deihl, King and Hornby. Harvey Ross passed, "also Wm. Hope, from Kingston, appeared with tickets of attendance on two courses of lectures at Fairfield. He has been a pupil of Dr. Wm. Adamson, of Kingston, and Dr. Samson, of the same place, for upwards of four years. He passed a very good examination"; also, George Burnham, of Port Hope, who had attended two courses at University of New York. "George Gwynne Bird, a practitioner from England of upwards of forty years, without tickets of any kind, gave satisfaction," and received certificate. Two were rejected; one had two courses, tickets from Fairfield and the Berkshire Medical Institution, Massachusetts.

"*April* 11th, 1838.—By command of His Excellency the Lieut.-Governor, the undermentioned members of the Medical Board of this Province proceeded to the examination of John Ryan, late of the Provincial Artillery Drivers, and make the following report, viz.:

"That the said John Ryan was examined before the Medical Board in April, 1822, in April, 1824, and in August, 1833, and reported by the Board not to be disabled. That he has this day been carefully examined by them, and they are of opinion that he is not incapable from earning his livelihood by labour in consequence of the wound in his foot.

"(Signed) C. WIDMER.
JOHN KING, M.D.
ROBERT HORNBY, M.D."

July, 1838.—Present: Widmer, Deihl, Hornby and King. George R. Grassett, of Amherstburg, "Licentiate of Lower Province, ample certificates and testimonials of a regular course of education," passed. Wm. M. Smith, Port Hope, pupil of Dr. G. N. Ridley, of Belleville, and M.D. of New York, also passed.

October 1, 1838.—The following members of the Board met this day, viz.: C. Widmer, Dr. Deihl, Dr. Gwynne, Walter Telfer, Esq.

"A new commission dated 25th ultimo having been received by Dr. Widmer, and now produced, it is ordered to be read, and the following is a copy thereof:

"UPPER CANADA.

"By His Excellency Sir George Arthur, Knight Commander of the Royal Hanoverian Guelph Order, Lieut.-Governor of the Province of Upper Canada, Major-General Commanding Her Majesty's Forces, etc., etc., etc.

"To Christopher Widmer, Member of the Royal College of Surgeons of London, and Staff-Surgeon on half pay of His Majesty's forces; William Warren Baldwin, Doctor of Medicine, of the University of Edinburgh; Robert C. Horne, Member of the Royal College of Surgeons, London, and late Assist.-Surgeon of the Glengarry Regiment of Fencible Light Infantry; James Sampson, late Assist.-Surgeon on half pay of Her Majesty's forces; Peter Deihl, member of the Royal College of Surgeons in London; John King, Doctor of Medicine, of the University of Edinburgh; George Neville Ridley, Member of the Royal College of Surgeons in London; Samuel John Stratford, member of the Royal College of Surgeons in London; Robert Hornby, Doctor of Medicine, of the University of Edinburgh; Lucius O'Brien, Doctor of Medicine, of the University of Edinburgh, and Member of the Royal College of

Surgeons in London; William Durie, Assist.-Inspector of the Ordnance Medical Department, on half pay; Joseph Hamilton, Doctor of Medicine, of the University of Edinburgh; Walter Telfer, Surgeon of the Royal College of Surgeons of Edinburgh; James Hamilton, Doctor of Medicine, of the University of Edinburgh; William C. Gywnne, Bachelor of Medicine, of the University of Dublin, and Robert Douglas Hamilton, late Surgeon Royal Navy.

"Whereas in and by an Act of the Parliament of this Province, passed in the fifty-ninth year of the reign of His Majesty George III., entitled 'An Act to repeal an Act passed in the fifty-fifth year of His Majesty's reign, entitled "An Act to license practitioners in physic and surgery throughout this Province, and to make further provision for licensing such practitioners,"' it is among other things enacted that it shall and may be lawful for the Governor, Lieut.-Governor, or person administering the government for the time being, to constitute and appoint under his hand and seal five or more persons legally authorized to practise physic, surgery and midwifery in this Province, to be a Board, whereof any three to be a quorum, to hear and examine all persons desirous to apply for a license to practise physic, surgery and midwifery or any of them within this Province; and being satisfied by such examination that any person is duly qualified to practise physic, surgery or midwifery, or any of them, to certify, as the case may be, the same, under the hands and seals of three or more of such Board, in order that the person so applying may obtain a license to practise as in the said Act is provided.

"Now know ye, that being well assured of your integrity and ability, I do hereby, under and by virtue of the abovementioned Act, nominate, constitute and appoint you, the said Christopher Widmer, William Warren Baldwin, Robert C. Horne, James Sampson, Peter Deihl, John King, George Neville Ridley, Samuel John Stratford, Robert Hornby, Lucius O'Brien William Durie, Joseph Hamilton, Walter Telfer, James Hamilton, William C. Gwynne, and Robert Douglas Hamilton, to be a Board, whereof any three of you are to form a quorum, to hear and examine all persons desirous to apply for license to practise physic, surgery and midwifery, or any of them, within this Province, and being satisfied by such examination that any person is duly qualified to practise physic, surgery and midwifery, or any of them, to certify the same under the hands and seals of any three or more of you; and, moreover, to do all such acts and things as by virtue of the said Act shall be by you to be done; to have, to hold and enjoy the said office or commission unto you as aforesaid during pleasure and your residence within this Province, together with all and every the fees, profits and advantages thereunto belonging and appertaining. Thereby enjoining you that you do make at the several days and at the place in the said Act provided there and then, to do whatsoever by this commission and the said Act shall be to be done.

"Given under my hand and official seal at Toronto this 25th day of September, 1838, and in the second year of Her Majesty's reign.

"(Signed) GEO. ARTHUR,
"*Lieut.-Governor.*

"By command of His Excellency.

"(Signed) JNO. MACAULAY."

"No candidate appearing, the Board then adjourned until to-morrow at the usual hour."

October 2.—Present: Dr. King, Dr. Gwynne, Peter Deihl Esq., C. Widmer, Esq.

"Dr. King proposed, seconded by Dr. Deihl, that Dr. Widmer be re-elected President of the Board. It was then resolved *nem. con.* that he be the President accordingly.

"Dr. Deihl then proposed, seconded by Dr. Gwynne, that Mr. Wilkinson be re-elected the Secretary of the Board. Carried."

1st. *Resolved,*—Proposed by Dr. King and seconded by Dr. Hornby:

"That in the opinion of this Board the law at present in force regulating the practice of the medical profession in this Province, is very inadequate for the purpose for which it was enacted; particularly for the suppression of empiricism, so baneful to the health and morals of the community and injurious to the medical profession."

2nd. *Resolved*,—Proposed by Dr. King and seconded by Dr. Deihl:

"That a petition be presented to the Honourable, the Common's House of Assembly, setting forth the above facts and other circumstances affecting the interests of the profession; humbly praying that Honourable House to appoint a committee to take those matters into their consideration, and report upon them, with a view to their remedying the defects in the law, and adopting such measures as in their wisdom may seem most likely to place the profession of medicine, so long neglected in this Province, on a more honourable footing than it has hitherto stood."

3rd. *Resolved*,—Proposed by Dr. King and seconded by Dr. Hornby:

"That the licentiates in medicine within this Province be allowed to subscribe such petition as may be adopted by the Board upon those resolutions."

4th. *Resolved*,—Proposed by Dr. King and seconded by Dr. Gwynne:

"That the President, Dr. King and Dr. Deihl and Dr. Gwynne, be a committee to draft a petition founded on the above resolutions, and that said committee be requested to report the same to this Board on the last day of this session.

The following petition was reported by the Committee:

"To the Honourable the Common's House of Assembly of Upper Canada in Provincial Parliament assembled. The petition of the members of the Medical Board, and of certain other licensed practitioners of medicine, humbly sheweth:

"That the law now in force in this Province, regulating the practice of the medical profession, and for the prevention of persons practising without license, has been found very inadequate. That of late years the number of persons practising without license or qualification has much increased, chiefly by the influx of empirics from the neighbouring States, causing great danger to the health of the community, and in some instances the loss of valuable lives; being alike detrimental to the peace and tranquility of the country, and degrading and humiliating to the honourable and useful profession of medicine.

"That the profession of medicine, ranking, as it does, amongst the first for science and literature in every part of the world, has been overlooked and neglected in this Province. That the youth intended for the profession have great reason to complain of the lamentable deficiency of the means of instruction within the Province, thereby imposing upon them at much inconvenience and expense, the necessity of having recourse to foreign countries for their education. That by the law amending the Charter of the University of King's College, lately passed by your Honourable House, the appointment of a Council is provided for without at the same time making it imperative that such Council should be so constituted as that certain members thereof (appointed for that purpose) should be capable of fairly and fully representing the interests of certain faculties therein, in consequence of such inadvertency and deficiency in the law. That in the Council of King's College, as at present constituted, whilst the interests of the other departments in the University are more than efficiently guarded, the Medical Faculty alone stands unrepresented. We therefore pray your Honourable House may appoint a committee to inquire into the present state of the medical profession, that they may report thereon to your Honourable House, with a view to such alterations and amendments being made in the existing laws as may be most conducive to the interests of the medical profession and the public at large; and also to cause such enactments to be made as in your wisdom may seem best fitted for placing the profession upon a more honourable and favourable footing than it has hitherto stood in this Province. And your petitioners, as in duty bound, will ever pray, etc.

"Medical gentlemen wishing to sign the above petition will please to call at the office of the Secretary of the Medical Board, at the General Hospital, where the petition now lies for signature, and those living at a distance may have their names attached by sending authority to the Secretary, or any of the members of the Medical Board residing at Toronto (if by letter post-paid).

"(Signed) C. WIDMER, *President.*
F. T. WILKINSON."

The Toronto *Patriot*, after giving the resolutions and petition, says editorially:

"*October* 12th, 1838. Quacks are an intolerable nuisance in any and every country, but especially in this, where empiricism and radicalism go hand in hand. It is a monstrous grievance that our Government should allow the Province to swarm, as it does, with these pestilent vagabonds, every one of whom is a Yankee loafer, and makes his occupation a cloak for inculcating Jacobinical principles. All know how numerous have been the self-styled 'doctors' implicated in the rebellion, but perhaps all may not know that they were almost one and all Yankee Quacks. We are truly glad to see that the Medical Board are active in setting about means to annihilate the dirty birds, nest and all; we trust the Legislature will second their efforts."

At the October session, Francis Clarke Mewburn, after an apprenticeship with his father of five years, and a full course of lectures at Philadelphia, received certificate. Two were rejected —"one of whom was from the Belfast Institution and the other from the Andersonian University of Glasgow."

January, 1839,—Present: The President, Drs. Gwynne, King, Hornby and O'Brien. William Clark, M.R.C.S.I., received certificate. One rejected.

February 11.—At a special meeting of the Medical Board, held this day (present: The President, Drs. Hornby, Gwynne, O'Brien, King and Baldwin), the subject of adopting a tariff of fees being offered to the consideration of the Board by Dr. Gwynne, after discussion, the following was the tariff approved of, viz.:

"TARIFF:

"Medical opinion,
"Visit within the city in the day, } To be determined.
"Night visit,

"Visit in the country, 5s. per mile from market house, in addition to fee for opinion.

"Consultation fee, single opinion,
"Consultation for a continuance, per visit, } To be determined.
"Midwifery, attendance in town,

"Midwifery, attendance in country, 5s. per mile, for nine days in addition.

"Vaccination, 5s., in addition to regular fee.

"Introduction of catheter, 2s. 6d., in addition to regular fee.

"Venesection, 2s. 6d., in addition to regular fee.

"Cupping, 5d., in addition to regular fee.

"Letter of advice,
"Reducing a fracture of the extremities, including fractures of the clavicle,
"Capital operations, } To be determined.
"Regular fee for after-attendance,
"Attendance for one hour and for any period over that time in ordinary cases, per hour,

"Professional debts are expected to be paid quarterly."

April, 1839.—Present: The President, Drs. King, Hornby, Gwynne and O'Brien. John W. Hunter, of Grimsby, passed his examination. Two failed. One stated that "his trunk having been stolen, his testimonials of education are lost, but that he has been ten years in the study of his profession." He underwent a protracted examination, which was so unsatisfactory that the Board could not grant him a certificate.

The Medical Board of Upper Canada did not meet again until May, 1841. This hiatus was the result of a Provincial Act of Incorporation of the College of Physicians and Surgeons of Upper Canada, a body clothed with authority to examine candidates for a provincial license to practise medicine in the Province, and to confer a diploma which entitled the holder to practise Physic, Surgery and Midwifery. The Act was passed May 11th, 1839. Its scope and the ambition of its promoters can only be fully estimated by perusing the somewhat lengthy Act of forty-four sections, which is given in the Appendix. The proceedings of the College of Physicians and Surgeons of Upper Canada are recorded in a volume now in the custody of the

Registrar of the Ontario College of Physicians and Surgeons. It forms a connecting link, and affords an interesting chapter in the history of the medical profession of the Province.

CHAPTER XIII.

COLLEGE OF PHYSICIANS AND SURGEONS OF UPPER CANADA.*

TORONTO, *May* 13th, 1839.—At the first meeting of the Fellows of the College of Physicians and Surgeons held this second Monday in May, pursuant to the 7th clause of the Act incorporating the said College, there were present: Dr. Widmer, Dr. Stratford by proxy, Dr. Baldwin, Dr. O'Brien, Mr. Horne, Mr. Durie, Mr. Deihl, Mr. Telfer, Dr. King, Dr. Hamilton, of Flamboro', by proxy, Dr. Ridley by proxy, Drs. Gwynne and Hamilton, of Scarboro', by proxy. Dr. Baldwin was called to the chair.

Resolved unanimously,—That Dr. Widmer be President for the remainder of the current year; that Dr. King be Vice-President for the remainder of the current year.

Dr. Widmer having taken the chair,

Resolved unanimously,—That the thanks of the meeting be given to Dr. Baldwin for his conduct in the chair.

Resolved unanimously,—That Dr. O'Brien be appointed Secretary and Registrar; that Mr. Horne be elected Treasurer. (Dr. Hornby enters.)

Resolved unanimously,—That the Fellows of the College of Physicians and Surgeons avail themselves of the earliest opportunity of tendering to Henry Sherwood, Esq., Q.C., and M.P.P., their unanimous thanks for the presevering efforts he has made in procuring the passage through the Legislature of the Act of Incorporation, a measure so well calculated to raise the character of the profession and benefit the public at large.

Resolved unanimously,—That Dr. Baldwin and Dr. Gwynne be a committee to adopt a design for the common seal of the College.

---

* In this and the chapters immediately following are given *verbatim ct literatim* the Minutes of the meetings of the College of Physicians and Surgeons of Upper Canada.

That the Secretary be authorized to provide forthwith, such books and stationery as may be necessary for registering the proceedings of the College.

That a committee consisting of the President, Dr. Hornby, the Secretary and Dr. Gwynne, be appointed to draw up a code of by-laws for the government of the College, which rules shall be submitted at the earliest convenience of the committee.

That the Secretary be authorized to provide for the use of the Fellows of the College 200 copies of the Act of Incorporation with marginal notes.

Resolved,—That whereas one of the prominent reasons for the establishment of the College of Physicians and Surgeons in Upper Canada is the promoting the respectability and usefulness of the profession therein; and whereas it is evident such object cannot be better forwarded than by affording the youth of the Province adequate means of instruction in the various branches of the profession, the establishment of a school of medicine within the Province as soon as possible, be considered a paramount duty of this College.

Therefore,—That an humble address be presented by this College to His Excellency the Lieut.-Governor, laying before him the degraded state in which the practice of the profession of medicine existed in this Province hitherto, and the various causes producing such a state; praying His Excellency's favour and protection, and that he will be graciously pleased to assist this College in their endeavours to form, as soon as possible, an efficient school of medicine, the want of which has been so long felt in this Province.

Resolved,—That Drs. King, Durie, Telfer, Gwynne and O'Brien be a committee to draft an address founded on the above resolutions, and that the committee be requested to report the same at the next meeting of the College.

Resolved,—That this meeting do now adjourn until the call of the Committee on By-laws. Adjourned accordingly.

May 21st, 1839.—Present: Dr. King, Vice-President, Mr. Horne, Mr. Telfer, Dr. Hornby, Dr. Gwynne, Dr. O'Brien. The minutes were read. The President entered and took the chair.

An application was read from John Shortt, M.D., and Member of the Royal College of Surgeons in London, Assistant-Inspector of Hospitals in Upper Canada, to be admitted a member of the College, and enclosed the fee of £5. Admitted.

Resolved,—That the Secretary and Treasurer be authorized, until the by-laws of the College shall be in force, to receive such moneys as may be paid into the College by applicants for licenses, membership or Fellowship.

Resolved unanimously,—That John Shortt, M.D., be admitted to Fellowship in this College, upon his complying with the provisions of the Act incorporating the College.

The Committee for preparing an address to His Excellency the Lieut.-Governor, reported one accordingly, which being taken into consideration,

Resolved,—That the following address to His Excellency be adopted :

"To His Excellency Sir George Arthur, K.C., Lieut.-Governor of the Province of Upper Canada, and Major-General Commanding Her Majesty's Forces therein.

"*May it please Your Excellency.*

"We, the President, Vice-President and Fellows of the College of Physicians and Surgeons of Upper Canada, take this early opportunity of approaching Your Excellency, to tender our grateful acknowledgments that under Your Excellency's favourable auspices the Act incorporating the College has become the law of the land, a measure we confidently anticipate will confer incalculable benefits upon the profession of medicine and the public generally in this Province.

"Being well aware that without Your Excellency's favour and patronage the sphere of our usefulness must necessarily, for the present, be very limited, we, therefore, humbly commend to Your Excellency's protection, our infant institution, hoping that you will be pleased to allow us easy access to Your Excellency at any time that the interests and welfare of our College may require that its affairs should be brought before your notice.

"Among the many objects the College must ever have in view, it will be our first and paramount duty to cherish and cultivate loyalty and devotion to the person and Crown of our beloved Monarch, which we will always endeavour to render characteristic of our institution.

"It will be our next duty (and certainly second only in importance to that which we owe our Gracious Sovereign) to promote the respectability, learning and usefulness of the medical profession, and to raise it to that dignified position which it holds in other countries.

"The establishment at once of an efficient school of medicine with an ample library and museum is intended by us, as the first step towards the accomplishment of this desirable object; this will, by affording within the Province the means of instruction in medical science, prevent hundreds of our youths resorting to the neighbouring States for their education, from whence they too often return with little addition to their information, and most commonly with principles at variance with the allegiance due to their Sovereign.

"His Excellency Sir John Colborne was so deeply impressed with the baneful effects of an education acquired in the United States upon the morals of our youths intended for the profession of medicine, that he upon many occasions stated that he saw that 'a medical school could no longer be delayed without manifest injury to the best interests of the Province.'

"As it is not in our power, without assistance, to carry our intentions into effect at as early a period as might be desirable, and as we have no representatives in the Council of King's College, who could bring so important a matter before that body, we therefore humbly and most earnestly pray Your Excellency's attention to the subject, as Chancellor of the University, with the view to Your Excellency's recommending the Council to make such arrangements as may be best calculated to second our endeavours in bringing into full operation by the ensuing winter an efficient school of medicine.

"Wishing Your Excellency a continuance of good health and a prosperous administration of the affairs of this Province, we beg leave, on the part of the College of Physicians and

Surgeons of Upper Canada, to subscribe ourselves Your Excellency's devoted servants.

"(Signed) C. WIDMER, *President.*
JNO. KING, M.D., *Vice-President.*
W. W. BALDWIN, M.D.
ROBERT HORNE.
ROBERT HORNBY, M.D.
LUCIUS O'BRIEN, M.D.
WALTER TELFER.
WM. CHAS. GWYNNE, M.B.
JOHN SHORTT, M.D."

Resolved,—That the Secretary be requested to transmit a copy of the foregoing address to the Secretary of His Excellency with a request to know at what time it may be convenient to His Excellency to receive the College with such address.

Application was made by Mr. Henry Sullivan, M.R.C.S.L., Licentiate Accoucher of the Dublin Lying-in Hospital, and Licentiate in Physic, Surgery and Midwifery of the Province of Upper Canada, to become a member. £5 paid into the hands of the Treasurer. Admitted.

Application from Mr. John Turquand, of Woodstock, Licentiate in Physic, Surgery and Midwifery of the Province of Upper Canada. £5 paid to the Treasurer. Admitted.

Resolved,—That the Secretary procure from the Government Office a certified list of all the licensed practitioners up to the close of the late session of the Provincial Parliament.

Dr. Gwynne reported that the Committee upon By-laws had drawn up a code which they submitted for the consideration of the College.

Resolved,—That the College do meet to take into consideration the above-mentioned report at the house of the President, on the 23rd instant, at 6 p.m.

Resolved,—That the President be empowered to call special meetings of the College to examine into diplomas or other qualifications of individuals applying for license under the 12th clause of the Act of Incorporation, at any time, until the by-laws shall come into force.

The President read a letter from Doctor Rees, offering a box of books for sale to the College.

Resolved,—That the College declines Dr. Rees' offer, having, as yet, no available funds. The College adjourned.

May 23, 1839.—Present: C. Widmer, President; Mr. Horne, Dr. King, Vice-Presidents; Dr. Hornby, Mr. Telfer, Dr. O'Brien, Dr. Gwynne. The Secretary reported an application from Mr. Henry Rolls, Licentiate in Physic, Surgery and Midwifery, to become a member of the College, and that £5 had been paid into the hands of the Treasurer. Admitted. Also a letter from the Honourable J. Macauley, stating that His Excellency the Lieut.-Governor would be pleased to receive the College with their address at 11 o'clock a.m., on Friday, 24th inst. (to-morrow). Also a letter from the Honourable J. Macauley stating that he had directed a certified list of all licensed practitioners to be prepared for the use of the College. Doctor Shortt was introduced and took his place as a Fellow of the College. The report of the Committee on the By-laws was taken up.

Resolved,—That the College do adjourn till Saturday next, 25th inst., at the house of the Vice-President. Adjourned.

May 24, 11 a.m.—Present: C. Widmer, Esq., President; Mr. Horne, Dr. King, Vice-Presidents; Dr. Hornby, Dr. O'Brien, Mr. Telfer, Dr. Gwynne, Dr. Shortt. The College proceeded to present their address to His Excellency the Lieut.-Governor, who was graciously pleased to return the following answer:

"GENTLEMEN,—In thanking you, as I most cordially do, for this address, I take the opportunity of congratulating you upon the formation of your College, under the Act of Incorporation recently passed, which, I am confident, will be found equally as useful in elevating the general character of the medical profession, as in conferring upon the people of the Province many important benefits.

"The care with which you propose to blend the cultivation of a loyal spirit with the extension of a sound system of medical instruction, commands unqualified commendation; and I assure you that I shall always find it most gratifying to afford you any reasonable aid within the means of the executive authority for the advancement of your institution and the promotion of its welfare.

"The Council of King's College, in which I discover that your profession is not at present represented, are engaged in a close inquiry into the state of its endowment, and they will soon be required to carry into effect the Act which has lately received the royal assent for the advancement of education in the Province.

"I shall request the immediate attention of the Council to the desire which you express for their co-operation with your College in the speedy establishment of an efficient school of medicine, and shall, with much pleasure, concur in any measure which the Council may feel safe in recommending for the attainment of that object without prejudice to other interests.

"(Signed) GEORGE ARTHUR, L.-G."

May 25, 1839.—Present: Doctor King, Vice-President; Mr. Horne, Dr. O'Brien, Mr. Telfer, Doctor Gwynne, Dr. Shortt.

The report of the Committee on the By-laws was taken up. (C. Widmer, Esq., President, enters, takes the chair.)

Resolved,—That the College do adjourn to Monday, 27th inst., at 6 p.m., at Mr. Horne's house. Adjourned.

May 27, 1839.—Present: C. Widmer, Esq., President; Mr. Horne, Dr. King, Vice-Presidents; Mr. Telfer, Dr. Shortt. A letter to the President from Mr. J. Wilson, of Perth, enclosing £5, and requesting to be admitted a member of the College. As his name does not appear in the published lists, the Secretary is directed to inquire at the Government Office, or to wait for the certified list, before answering the letter.

The President made the following communication, viz.: The President of King's College having waited on him this day, stated that His Excellency the Lieutenant-Governor having referred the address of the College of Physicians and Surgeons of Upper Canada to him, he is desirous that the College should transmit to the Council of King's College, a plan in detail of the objects of the College alluded to in the said address; and that it be furnished before Saturday next.

Resolved,—That a committee consisting of the Vice-President, Dr. Shortt, and Mr. Telfer, draft a plan to be laid before the College on Wednesday evening next. (Doctors Hornby and O'Brien enter.) The Report of the Committee on By-laws was taken up. (Dr. Gwynne enters.)

Resolved,—That C. Widmer, R. C. Horne, Esq., Drs. Hornby and Shortt be a committee to revise our by-laws, embody them and submit them to a meeting of the College as soon as convenient. Adjourned.

May 29, 1839.—Present: C. Widmer, Esq., President; Mr. Horne, Dr. King, Vice-Presidents; Dr. O'Brien, Mr. Telfer, and Dr. Shortt. Dr. King presented a report from the committee to whom the communication from the President of King's College was referred. Mr. Telfer, therefrom, presented another report on the same subject. (Drs. Gwynne and Baldwin enter.)

The Secretary presented an application from Dr. Geo. Herrick, M.D., T.C.D., M.R.C.S.L.'s, to become a member of the College. Fee £5, paid. Admitted. (Dr. Hornby enters.)

An amended report on the communication from King's College was received, but ordered to be taken into consideration to-morrow. Adjourned.

May 30, 1839.—Present: C. Widmer, Esq., President; Drs. Hornby, O'Brien, Gwynne, Shortt.

The amended report relative to the communication from the President of King's College was taken up. (Mr. Telfer enters.)

The following report was adopted:

"*Report upon a communication from the President of King's College, to the President of the College of Physicians and Surgeons of Upper Canada:*

"The College of Physicians and Surgeons, desirous of removing as soon as possible, the great evil of obliging medical students to resort to the neighbouring States for their education, and desirous to afford them, within this Province, the means of instruction in medical science, respectfully invite the co-operation of the Council of King's College in the accomplishment of so desirable an object.

"It being obvious that the College of Physicians and Surgeons have not at their disposal means to defray the expenses of an efficient school of medicine, and it being evident that the Council of King's College are not prepared to set on foot an establishment equal to the wishes or wants of the medical community, this College therefore propose to the Council the propriety of meeting the wants of the medical youth of the Province, by conjointly establishing a school of medicine.

"Such a course was adopted with success, when the School of Physics in Ireland was perfected conjointly by the University of Dublin and the King and Queen's College of Physicians in Ireland; the former providing for four Professors and one Lecturer, and the latter, three Professors and one Lecturer, as follows: By the University of Dublin,—Regius Professor of Physics, Professor of Anatomy and Surgery, Professor of Chemistry, Professor of Botany; Lecturer on Natural History; By King and Queen's College,—Professor of Materia Medica, Professor of Institutes of Medicine, Professor of Practice of Medicine, Lecturer on Midwifery.

"The medical profession of both Institutions form conjointly the faculty of medicine of the University; and the examinations of all matters connected with the medical department, as well as that of candidates for degrees in medicine, are conducted by them.

"The College of Physicians and Surgeons, aware of the great advantages that would accrue to the public and the medical profession from a similar establishment, respectfully submit the following outline for the formation of a medical school:

"For the formation of an efficient school of medicine adapted to the necessities of this Province, it is necessary that professors shall be appointed to teach the following branches of medical science: 1. Anatomy and Surgery. 2. Chemistry and Pharmacy. 3. Materia Medica and Botany. 4. Practice of Physic and Medical Pathology. 5. Surgery and Surgical Pathology. 6. Midwifery and diseases of Women and Children. 7. Medical Jurisprudence.

"Together with the above it will be necessary that the professors shall lecture upon the following subjects, Clinical Medicine, Clinical Surgery. It is therefore proposed that three

9

professors shall be appointed by the Chancellor of the University, and shall enjoy all the privileges of other professors of King's College; that three other professors be appointed by the College of Physicians and Surgeons of Upper Canada; that the several professors shall receive not less than the following salaries to be paid by the University, exclusive of all fees accruing from their respective classes:

"The Professor of Anatomy and Physiology	£200	per annum
"Theory and Practice of Physic -	200	"
"Theory and Practice of Surgery, etc.	200	"
"Theory and Practice of Midwifery, diseases of Women and Children -	200	"
"Theory and Practice of Materia Medica and Pharmacy - - - -	200	"
"Medical Jurisprudence - - -	200	"
"And a Demonstrator of Anatomy, who shall be appointed by the College of Physicians and Surgeons - -	150	"

"A sum will be required for the hire of the necessary accommodation for lecture rooms, etc., until convenient buildings be erected by the University. This sum may be estimated at £100 per annum.

"It is further necessary to state, that as a library and museum will be absolutely necessary to the successful operations of the proposed institution, the sum of one thousand pounds be appropriated by the University to the College for the purchase thereof.

"The conjoint medical professors of both institutions, with the President of the College of Physicians and Surgeons, for the time being, shall be the faculty of medicine of the University.

"The College of Physicians and Surgeons would urge on the College Council that though they have not placed a professor of chemistry on the list of medical professors, they consider that it ought to be a University chair immediately established, because the knowledge of chemistry is essential to medical science, because it is one of the studies most essential to the promotion of useful arts as well as to medical science, and because the students of chemistry will probably include a very large number independent of the medical students."

Resolved,—That the Secretary forward the above report (being first signed by the President) to the President of King's Council.

The Committee to revise the by-laws submitted the code to the meeting which being read,

Resolved unanimously,—That the report be received, and that the code now presented be adopted as the by-laws of the College.

Resolved,—That the code of by-laws be signed by the President and countersigned by the Secretary, on behalf of the College, and that the seal of the College be affixed thereto as soon as it shall be procured. Adjourned.

CHAPTER XIV.

COLLEGE OF PHYSICIANS AND SURGEONS OF UPPER CANADA—(*Continued*).

TORONTO, *June* 8, 1839.—(Special.) Present: C. Widmer, Esq., President; Dr. King, Vice-President; Dr. Gwynne, Dr. Baldwin, Dr. Shortt, Dr. Hornby, Dr. O'Brien, Mr. Telfer. A letter was read from Mr. Telfer to the President, containing charges against Dr. Hornby of an unprofessional character. Dr. Hornby having heard the letter read, declined the interference of the College on the ground that the operation of the by-laws had not commenced. The College concurred in the objection of Dr. Hornby to its interference. Adjourned.

June 10, 1839.—Present: C. Widmer, Esq., President; Dr. King, Vice-President; Dr. Gwynne, Dr. O'Brien, Dr. Shortt, Mr. Telfer, Dr. Hornby.

The by-laws as now revised, were directed to be published in the Upper Canada *Gazette.*

Resolved unanimously,—That James Wilson, Esq., Surgeon of Perth, Member of the College, be elected a Fellow thereof, on his complying with the provisions of the Act.

The Secretary laid Dr. Herrick's license before the College in consequence of his name not appearing in the certified list of licentiates. Adjourned.

June 11, 1839.—Present: C. Widmer, Esq., President; Dr. Jno. King, Vice-President; Dr. O'Brien, Dr. Hornby, Mr. Telfer. Proceeded to examine James Orland De la Hooke, a member of the Royal College of Surgeons of London, who being found duly qualified to practise Physic, Surgery and Midwifery, was granted a license to practise accordingly.

June 14, 1839.—At Dr. Baldwin's house. Present: C. Widmer, Esq., President; Dr. King, Vice-President; Dr. O'Brien, Dr. Baldwin, Mr. Telfer, Mr. Horne, Dr. Shortt, Dr. Hornby.

A set of regulations in regard to apothecaries and druggists was proposed and referred to Dr. Shortt and the Secretary to revise.

Resolved,—That Dr. King, Vice-President, be appointed Inspector of Apothecaries and Vendors of Drugs in the Province, and that he have the power to nominate a Deputy to act in each of the corporate towns within the jurisdiction of the College.

June 28, 1839.—Present: C. Widmer, Esq., President; Dr. King, Vice-President; Mr. Telfer, Dr. O'Brien, Dr. Shortt, Dr. Hornby.

Mr. Henry Hover Wright was called up for examination for license, he having complied with the requisite preliminaries. He passed a very satisfactory examination in all of his profession, and a license to practise Physic, Surgery and Midwifery was granted accordingly.

July 5, 1839.—Present: C. Widmer, Esq., President; Dr. King, Vice-President; Mr. Horne, Dr. O'Brien, Dr. Baldwin, Dr. Shortt.

Resolved,—That the Secretary do inquire of the Secretary of King's College, whether the communication from the College of Physicians and Surgeons of Upper Canada has been taken into consideration by the College Council, and if any steps have been taken thereon.

Resolved,—That as several instances of the appointment of persons not qualified by law to practise the profession of medicine, to be Surgeons and Assistant-Surgeons of Militia, has come to the knowledge of the College of Physicians and Surgeons, the Secretary be therefore requested to inform His Excellency the Lieutenant-Governor through his Civil Secretary, of the fact, that such steps may be taken by His Excellency as may be necessary to prevent the continuance of a practice alike derogatory to the profession and injurious to the public service.

Resolved,—That the Secretary do address the Mayor of this City, pointing out the fact of unlicensed persons within its bounds, performing the practice of the Profession of Medicine and Surgery, and requesting that proper steps may be taken to suppress the same.

Resolved,—That the following books be procured by the earliest opportunity: Edinburgh Medical and Surgical Journal, Johnson's Medico-Chirurgical Journal, Dublin Medical Journal, British and Foreign Medical Journal, Medico-Chirurgical Transactions, London Pharmacopœia, last editions.

Resolved,—That the two following committees be appointed to examine candidates for licenses:

No. 1.—The President, Drs. Baldwin, Gwynne, Hornby, and Shortt.

No. 2.—The Vice-President, Dr. O'Brien, Messrs. Horne and Telfer and Dr. Durie.

Resolved,—That in case either of said committees shall on examination of a candidate, report him to be deserving of a license, the Secretary shall provide him with such license properly signed and sealed, according to the by-laws on that subject. Adjourned.

July 16, 1839.—Present: C. Widmer, Esq., President; Dr. King, Vice-President; Dr. O'Brien, Dr. Baldwin, Mr. Telfer, Dr. Hornby, Dr. Gwynne, Dr. Shortt.

Mr. William Nicholson Ross having applied for license to practise Surgery and Midwifery, his documents were laid before the College, viz.: A Diploma from the College of Surgeons of Edinburgh, and a Certificate from Drs. McIntosh and

Russell, of Edinburgh, of his fitness to practise Midwifery. But not appearing in person, it was

Resolved,—That he do not obtain a license without a personal attendance. (Mr. Telfer withdraws.)

The Secretary was directed to furnish the Mayor with a list of the licensed practitioners in Toronto.

Resolved,—That the fees paid for inspection and registration of the documents of candidates for the license of the College be allowed to the Secretary, Dr. O'Brien, for the present, as a small consideration for his services.

Mr. Russell's account for Books (viz.: Minute, Register, Letter, and Account Books) presented, and being audited for £5 13 3 was signed by the President and directed to be paid. Adjourned.

QUARTERLY MEETING, *Monday, August* 5, 1839.—Present: C. Widmer, Esq., President; Dr. King, Vice-President; Dr. O'Brien, Dr. Baldwin, Mr. Telfer, R. D. Hamilton, Esq., Dr. Shortt.

The Committee of Examination, No. 1, reported that Mr. George Graham Upton, from Brockville, had presented himself for examination, but from his ignorance in Materia Medica and Pharmacy, they had not proceeded in his examination. The Treasurer's books examined. Balance available £55, and deposit £10.

Mr. Robert Winchester Clarke, of Whitby, applied for a license. He exhibited a Diploma from the Faculty of Physicians and Surgeons of Glasgow, to practise Surgery and Pharmacy. The proper affidavit of identity being produced, the Secretary was directed to issue a license on the payment of the fees.

Resolved, unanimously,—That Sir James McGrigor, Bart., M.D., be elected an Honorary Fellow of this College.

Resolved, unanimously,—That Joseph Skey, M.D., etc., Inspector-General of Hospitals, be elected an Honorary Fellow of this College. Moved and seconded,—That Geo. Herrick, M.D., etc., a Member of the College, be elected a Fellow thereof. To be balloted for at the Quarterly Meeting in October. (Dr. Hornby enters.) A letter from Alexander Smith, M.D., Assistant-Surgeon of 1st Dragoon Guards, Member Royal Asiatic Society, M.R.C.S. London, and Licentiate R.C.S. Edinburgh, to Dr. Shortt, requesting to be enrolled as a Member of this College, was read. The fee, £5, being paid, he was admitted accordingly. A letter from James Wilson, Esq., Perth, dated July 5, 1839, was read. A letter from the Hon. Wm. Morris to James Wilson, Esq., dated July 3, was also read. The Secretary was directed to write to Mr. Wilson to say that the College is obliged to follow the obvious meaning and plain construction of the Act in regard to the fees as well as in other matters.

A letter from the Hon. John Macauley, "for the Bursar" of King's College, dated July 28, 1839, stating "that the application of this College has been referred to a committee to report thereon," was read.

Resolved,—That the President, Vice-President, and Dr. Hornby be a committee to inspect certain premises proposed as a hall for meeting, and a library. And that they be authorized to take the same for one year, if deemed eligible, not exceeding the annual rent of £25, and to procure certain furniture for the same. Adjourned.

August 6, 1839.—Present: C. Widmer, Esq., President; Dr. King, Vice-President; Dr. O'Brien, Robt. D. Hamilton, Esq., Mr. Telfer.

The Secretary laid before the College a letter from Mr. Boys, the Bursar of King's College, enclosing the following report from a committee of the King's College Council as a reply to the communication made to the King's College Council by this College on the establishment of a joint School of Medicine:

"The committee appointed to report on the application of the College of Physicians and Surgeons for assistance to carry into effect the design of establishing a School of Medicine, have the honour to submit the following recommendation:

"That the Registrar be instructed to communicate to the President of the College of Physicians and Surgeons, that the Council of King's College, although fully impressed with the importance of the object which the College of Physicians and

Surgeons propose, yet feel that they would not be justified in extending assistance to any other corporation until they shall have first endeavoured to attain the objects for which they have themselves been incorporated, and on which they are at present engaged in maturing plans which they trust will be the means of ultimately affording efficient instruction in all the branches of an University Education.

"(Signed) JOHN McCAUL, *Chairman.*

"King's College Council Office,
" *July* 31st, 1839."

(Dr. Gwynne and Dr. Hornby enter.)

Resolved,—That Drs. King and O'Brien, and R. B. Hamilton, Esq., be a committee to take into consideration the above "recommendation" and communication from the King's College Council, and to draw up a rejoinder thereto.

Resolved,—That the medical journal edited by Dr. Dunglison, of Philadelphia, be ordered from the commencement and continued henceforward. Adjourned.

August 29, 1839.—Present: C. Widmer, Esq., President; Dr. King, Vice-President; Dr. Baldwin, Dr. O'Brien, R. B. Hamilton, Esq., Mr. Telfer, Dr. Hornby.

The report of the committee to whom the communication from the King's College Council was referred, was taken up. It was referred back to the committee to be presented again on Saturday next, the 31st.

Resolved,—That a solicitor be appointed to the College forthwith, and that Henry Sherwood, Esq., Q.C., be the solicitor.

The Committee of Examination, No. 1, reported that Mr. Wm. Nicholson Rose applied for a license to practise. He produced a diploma for Surgery and Pharmacy from the Faculty of Physicians and Surgeons in Glasgow, and being examined, was recommended to obtain a license to practise Surgery and Midwifery. License granted accordingly, dated August 14.

The Committee of Examination, No. 2, reported that Mr. Wm. McPherson had applied for a license to practise. He produced a diploma from the Faculty of Physicians and Surgeons of Glasgow, and, declining an examination, was recommended to obtain a license to practise *Surgery* only. License granted accordingly, dated August 14.

The Secretary laid before the College a letter from Mr. Ewing, of Hawkesbury, applying to be admitted a member of the College. Refused, not being a licentiate, and to be informed that application for license cannot be entertained unless on personal appearance and production of original documents. Adjourned.

SATURDAY, *August* 31, 1839.—Present: C. Widmer, Esq., President; Dr. Baldwin, Dr. O'Brien, Mr. Telfer. There not being a quorum, adjourned.

TUESDAY, *September* 3, 1839.—Present: C. Widmer, Esq., President; Dr. King, Vice-President; Dr. Baldwin, Dr. Horne, Dr. O'Brien.

The Secretary informed the College that he had received a letter from S. B. Harrison, Esq., Secretary to His Excellency the Lieut.-Governor, enclosing a copy of the communication from the Council of King's College, which had been already sent by the Bursar to this College.

The committee to whom the communication from King's College was referred, report they recommend the following letter to be sent by the Secretary to the Council of King's College:

"Your Committee, after a deep consideration of the subject, feel that they cannot with any propriety recommend any answer that does not enter fairly into the matter in question for the purpose of avoiding all misapprehension:

"SIR,—I have the honour to acknowledge the receipt of your letter of August 3rd, enclosing the report from a committee of the Council of King's College upon a communication from the College of Physicians and Surgeons, recommending the formation of the Faculty of Medicine of the University, and the immediate establishment of a School of Medicine. I am directed by the College to forward to you the following to be laid before the Council of King's College:

"The College of Physicians and Surgeons regret much that the Council of King's College has misunderstood them in supposing that they require assistance from the King's College for their corporation or for carrying any of the exclusive objects of the College into operation.

"It being more than twelve years since a charter was granted to the University of King's College, an institution so munificently endowed, the College of Physicians and Surgeons (as the guardians of the medical profession in Upper Canada) considered it their duty to invite the attention of the University of King's College to the baneful effects of a further delay on their part of the performance of a paramount duty, and to the expectations of the medical public that the long promised opportunity of acquiring medical science should be afforded to the youth of the Province by the University.

"In establishing that faculty and an efficient School of Medicine which (if the University go into operation at all) must be the most prominent department of it, the College of Physicians and Surgeons tendered their co-operation and advice, and lest at any future period both parties should form rival establishments which might interfere with the harmony and good feeling that ought to subsist between them, the College of Physicians and Surgeons proposed that a School of Medicine should be formed conjointly.

"The College of Physicians and Surgeons submitted as a precedent, the School of Medicine in Ireland, established conjointly by the University of Dublin and the King's and Queen's College of Physicians in Ireland, and following that precedent, proposed the following bases for the formation of a joint School of Medicine:

"That this School shall consist of six Professors, or seven if the Professor of Chemistry be included;

"That three Professors, besides the Professor of Chemistry, shall be appointed by the University, with rights and privileges the same as the other Professors of the University;

"That three Professors shall be appointed by the College of Physicians and Surgeons;

"That these six Professors (with the Professor of Chemistry if considered advisable), together with the President of the College of Physicians and Surgeons, for the time being, shall form the Faculty of Medicine of the University, and as such, shall have the management of all matters belonging to that department, and hold the examinations of all candidates for degrees in medicine.

"As the College of Physicians and Surgeons are as yet without funds, it was proposed that the King's College should pay certain salaries to the several Professors, as also to a Demonstrator of Anatomy, to be appointed by the College of Physicians and Surgeons. Also, that the sum of one thousand pounds should be appropriated by King's College, to the foundation of a library and museum devoted to medical and surgical science, which library and museum shall remain the property of King's College, but be under the control and superintendence of the faculty of medicine as above proposed to be constituted, and be available for the use and instruction of the students of the profession.

"The College of Physicians and Surgeons conceive that the granting assistance to another corporation has been the only grounds upon which the University might decline to join the College of Physicians and Surgeons in the matter proposed, and that the Council of King's College misunderstood the College of Physicians and Surgeons on that ground, and they confidently anticipate that the Council of King's College will see the advantages of coalescing with the College of Physicians and Surgeons, so as to attain their common objects.

"Should the proposition of the College of Physicians (which they hope will now be better understood) not meet with the approbation of the Council of King's College, they respectfully request that the Council will intimate to them any other plan they may deem advisable, so as to establish a School of Medicine in this city without further delay.

"But if no such plan is in contemplation by the Council, in order to obviate further difficulties as far as possible, the College of Physicians and Surgeons respectfully invite the Council of King's College to appoint a committee of three of their body to confer with an equal committee of this College, which joint committee might be authorized to propose some plan by which the common object of both Colleges might be speedily and successfully attained.

"I have the honour to be,

"Etc., etc., etc."

(To be signed by the Secretary.)

Resolved,—That the report now read be adopted.

Resolved,—That the President, Vice-President and R. C. Horne, Esq., be a committee to provide proper accommodation for the meetings of the College, which may be suitable for a library and museum.

Resolved,—That Mr. Mulock's letter dated Lloydtown, be laid before Mr. Sherwood, and his opinion requested thereon, and on the following questions:

1. Can the College of Physicians and Surgeons legally take upon themselves the prosecution of those who, offending against the law by practising medicine, surgery or midwifery without lawful authority, are subjected by the law to certain fines?

2. Can the College of Physicians and Surgeons lawfully appropriate any portion of those fines, or of their other funds to the purposes of such prosecutions?

Adjourned.

CHAPTER XV.

COLLEGE OF PHYSICIANS AND SURGEONS OF UPPER CANADA—(*Continued*).

TORONTO, MONDAY, *September* 30.—Present: C. Widmer, Esq., President; Dr. King, Vice-President; Dr. Hornby, R. C. Horne, Esq., Dr. Baldwin, Dr. O'Brien, Dr. Shortt. The Secretary laid before the College a letter from Henry Sherwood, Esq., Q.C., Solicitor for the College, which was directed to be entered on the minutes as follows:

"TORONTO, *September* 20th, 1839.

"SIR,—In answer to your letter of the 11th inst., I beg to state that I cannot discover any ground upon which it can be urged that the College of Physicians and Surgeons cannot legally take upon themselves the prevention of those who, offending against the law by practising physic, surgery and midwifery without lawful authority, are subjected by the law to certain fines. Nor can I see upon what principle it can be contended, that they cannot lawfully appropriate any portion of those fines, as of their other funds, to bring such offenders to justice. I consider the College as a body incorporated for the purpose of placing the medical profession upon a more respectable and efficient footing. It is the only body which now legally has any control over the members of the profession. From the College the right to practise the various branches of the profession can now only be obtained, and it does appear to me there would be great reason for complaint against the Fellows of the College, not only by its members but by the community generally, if knowingly they suffered unauthorized persons openly to practise the various branches of the profession, without any exertion on their part to stop the evil of barretry. What is termed a common barretor is a common quarreler, a common exciter or maintainer of quarrels and suits in courts—a person who invents or disperses false rumours whereby discord arises—but to insist that an incorporated body established by law to regulate and control one of the learned professions, would be guilty of barretry by appointing a person to prosecute before a proper tribunal persons who are practising contrary to law, who are, in fact, guilty of misdemeanours, would, in my humble judgment, be extending the meaning of the term beyond any reasonable limit.

"The matter contained in Mr. Mulock's letter is peculiarly for the consideration of the College, and it is for the Fellows to determine what means shall be adopted to prevent the great and increasing evil of which Mr. Mulock complains.

"I am, Sir, your Obedient Servant,

"(Signed) HENRY SHERWOOD.

"LUCIUS O'BRIEN, ESQ., M.D.,
"*Secretary, College Physicians and Surgeons, Toronto.*"

Mr. Mulock's letter was again taken up by the College, and the Secretary's answer (see letter book) having been read, no further proceedings were directed to be taken thereon.

The Secretary laid before the College a letter from Joseph Skey, M.D., Inspector-General of Hospitals, dated Montreal, September 2, 1839, acknowledging the receipt of the communication of his being elected an Honorary Fellow of the College, and returning thanks for the same.

An application for membership was made by Alexander Burnside, Esq., Licentiate, Upper Canada, and the fee having been paid he was admitted accordingly. A similar application was made from James Campbell, M.D., Licentiate, Upper Canada, Brockville, and the fee being paid he was admitted accordingly.

The Committee of Examination, No. 1, reported that Mr. William Adams having exhibited a License in Surgery from the Faculty of Physicians and Surgeons of Glasgow, and having undergone an examination in Physic and Midwifery, was recommended to obtain a license to practise Physic, Surgery and Midwifery. The license was granted accordingly.

WEDNESDAY, *October* 2, 1839.—Present: C. Widmer, Esq., President; Dr. King, Vice-President; Dr. O'Brien, R. C. Horne, Esq., Dr. Hornby, Dr. Shortt.

Mr. D. R. Bradley appeared for examination for a license to practise Physic, Surgery and Midwifery, and after a patient examination on Pharmacy, Anatomy, Surgery and Practice of Physic, was found so deficient that he was rejected.

Resolved unanimously,—That no application for examination for license to practise from D. R. Bradley be received in less than twelve months from this date.

The Secretary presented a diploma as Master in Surgery, and other documents, from Mr. Archibald Pass, at Barrie, with an application for license. Refused till Mr. Pass appears personally. (The President goes out, Dr. King takes the chair.)

Resolved,—That Messrs. Black & Armstrong be authorized in the event of a favourable opportunity occurring to purchase the earlier numbers of the Dublin *Medical Journal*, and that they forward a catalogue of French medical books.

Resolved,—That the Treasurer be authorized to purchase a Bill of Exchange for £36 13 0 sterling, to be remitted to Mr. Wenham in payment of Black & Armstrong's (booksellers) account, dated August 24, 1839, and that he be authorized to pay charges for the inlaid expenses upon the same.

Resolved,—That the College recommend sending for the following works at the earliest opportunity: Dr. Bright's Medical Works, Paris & Foublangue's Medical Jurisprudence, Gordon's Medical Evidences, Medical Jurisprudence, etc., Guy's and St. Thomas' Hospital Reports. Adjourned.

QUARTERLY MEETING, *November* 4, 1839.—Present: C. Widmer, Esq., President; R. C. Horne, Esq., Dr. Gwynne, Dr. O'Brien, Dr. Shortt, Dr. Hornby.

The Treasurer's accounts were laid before the College, found correct and audited, presenting a balance of £40 0 6, subject to a repayment to Mr. Rolph, of Ancaster, of £5, leaving a real balance of £35 0 6.

The motion made on the 5th day of August last, that Dr. Herrick be admitted to Fellowship, was taken up, when it was

Resolved,—That George Herrick, M.D., be admitted to Fellowship in this College on his complying with the provisions of the Act of Incorporation.

A letter from Mr. Thos. H. Mulock, dated October 13, was read.

Resolved,—That the meetings for the examination of candidates for license shall be held in future on the first Thursday of every month, at 6 p.m.

The Committee of Examination, No. 2, reported that Mr. Wm. Thistle had produced a diploma from the Faculty of Physicians and Surgeons of Glasgow, and had been examined in Midwifery. They recommended that he be granted a diploma in *Surgery* only. They report also that Mr. Wm. Henry Dalton had been examined in Physic, Surgery and Midwifery, and having acquitted himself to their satisfaction, they recommend that he be granted a license to practise all *three* branches.

The two licenses granted accordingly to be dated November 1, 1839.

Moved by Dr. Gwynne, seconded by Dr. Hornby, that whenever an extraordinary meeting be called, the subjects to be discussed be stated. *Lost.*

Moved by Dr. O'Brien, seconded by Dr. Shortt, that John Turquand, Henry Sullivan, Alex. Smith, M.D., and James Campbell, M.D., being Members of the College, be elected to Fellowship therein to be balloted for at the January meeting, which motion being put to the vote was *Lost*.

SPECIAL MEETING, *November* 28, 1839.—Present: C. Widmer, Esq., President; Dr. King, Vice-President; Dr. O'Brien, R. C. Horne, Esq., and Dr. Shortt.

The Secretary laid before the College a letter from Mr. John Allanby with his answer thereto. Nothing ordered until the documents alluded to be produced.

Resolved,—That the officer alluded to in the nineteenth clause of the Act of Incorporation shall be designated the collector of the College, and that it shall be his duty to collect evidence and lay information before the proper authorities against all persons practising any branch of the profession who have not been legally licensed. That the said officer shall receive the sum of £2 10 as a remuneration for his trouble, on all convictions arising from his information, and that he shall receive the sum of one and a half per cent. on all other fines collected.

Resolved,—That Mr. William Higgins, High Constable of the Home District, be appointed collector.

Resolved,—That a notice be inserted in the Toronto *Patriot*, *Commercial Herald*, Kingston *Chronicle*, Hamilton *Gazette*, Cobourg *Star* and Niagara *Chronicle* newspapers, requesting all magistrates convicting any offenders against the Act incorporating the College of Physicians and Surgeons of Upper Canada, to remit the amount of all fines to the collector of the College appointed under the nineteenth clause of the Act of Incorporation.

Resolved,—That a committee be appointed to prepare an address to His Excellency the Governor-General, relative to the deficient means of medical education in the Province, and to pray that His Excellency may be pleased to assist us in providing a remedy for so great an evil.

Resolved,—That a committee be appointed to prepare a petition from the College to each branch of the Legislature, to request that steps be taken to form at once an efficient medical school in this city.

ADJOURNED MEETING, *December* 4, 1839.—Present: C. Widmer, Esq., President; Dr. King, Vice-President; Dr. O'Brien, Dr. Baldwin, W. Telfer, Esq., R. C. Horne, Esq., Dr. Shortt, Dr. Gwynne.

Resolved,—That the College having reconsidered the propriety of addressing the Governor-General in compliance with the resolution of last meeting, do not now deem it expedient to do so.

The committee appointed to draw up a petition to the different branches of the Legislature presented a draft of one accordingly. After discussion it was

Resolved,—That the following petition be presented to each branch of the Legislature:

" *To the Honourable the Legislative Assembly, Commons House of Assembly, in Provincial Parliament assembled:*

"The Petition of the President and Fellows of the College of Physicians and Surgeons of Upper Canada humbly sheweth:

"That one essential and prominent point set forth in a petition presented to your Honourable House during last Session from the Medical Practitioners of this Province, was the deficiency of Medical Education therein.

"That your Petitioners, since the Incorporation of the College, have assiduously applied themselves to remedy this evil, more especially by representation to the Council of King's College, therein pointing out a code of establishing a Faculty of Medicine in the said College, which your Petitioners have no doubt, if carried into effect, would have proved successful in its results; but it is with deep regret they are compelled to acknowledge that their efforts hitherto have proved wholly unsuccessful, and they have no prospect, for a long period, of any beneficial change by any means within their own power.

"The fact that large sums have been from time to time appropriated for the support of general education, induces your Petitioners to hope that your Honourable House will devise some measures whereby the students of a branch of education of such importance as that of medicine may be reduced from the degrading necessity of resorting to a foreign country for that knowledge which ought to provided within the Province.

"Your Petitioners earnestly represent to your Honourable House, that in consequence of having no representative in the Council of King's College, they have no means of bringing fairly before that body the just and urgent claims of the Medical Profession, whilst other Faculties are amply represented in that Council.

"Your Petitioners therefore humbly pray that your Honourable House will take the premises into your favourable consideration and so alter and amend the late Act, amending the Charter of King's College, as to provide that certain members of that College Council shall be appointed to represent the Medical Faculty therein, and that your Honourable House will afford such other relief in the premises as may be deemed advisable."

Resolved,—That Henry Sherwood, Esq., Q.C., be requested to present the above petition to the Commons House of Assembly; and the Hon. William Morris to the Legislative Council.

Resolved,—That the Secretary be directed to write to the Clerk of the Peace, H.D., informing him that a fine of two pounds had been imposed by — Snook, Esq., and requesting him to direct that this fine may be remitted to the Treasurer.

In 1839 an Act was passed, granting £500 for the maintenance of the Toronto General Hospital.

ANNUAL MEETING, *January* 6, 1840.—Present: C. Widmer, Esq., President; Dr. King, Vice-President; Walter Telfer, Esq., Dr. O'Brien, R. D. Hamilton, Esq., R. C. Horne, Esq., Dr. Shortt, Wm. Durie, Esq., Dr. Herrick.

The Secretary laid before the College a communication from T. W. C. Murdock, Esq., Secretary to His Excellency the Governor-General, acknowledging the receipt of the petition of the College to His Excellency, and that it will receive His Excellency's consideration.

Resolved unanimously,—That Christopher Widmer, Esq., be elected President for the ensuing year.

Resolved unanimously,—That John King, M.D., be elected Vice-President for the ensuing year.

Resolved unanimously,—That Lucius O'Brien, M.D., be elected Secretary and Registrar for the ensuing year.

Resolved unanimously,—That Robt. C. Horne, Esq., be elected Treasurer for the ensuing year.

Resolved,—That the following Fellows be elected as Censors for the ensuing year: John King, M.D., Vice-President; Lucius O'Brien, M.D., Walter Telfer, Surgeon; W. C. Gwynne, M.B., George Herrick, M.D.

Resolved,—That the Committee of Finance do consist of W. W. Baldwin, M.D., Robert Hornby, M.D., and George Herrick, M.D.

Resolved,—That John King, M.D., Vice-President, be appointed Inspector of Apothecaries' Shops, etc.

The names of Apothecaries and Vendors of Drugs who have registered their names, was then read, viz.: C. H. Peck, Prescott; Rufus Holden, Belleville; J. W. Brent, Toronto; Joseph Beckett & Co., Toronto; Richard Tuton, Toronto; Leslie Bros., Toronto; Gravely & Jackson, Cobourg.

The Secretary laid before the College a letter from Sir James McGrigor, Director-General of the Army Medical Department, dated London, Oct. 9, 1839, acknowledging the receipt of the Secretary's letter of August 5, 1839, and returning thanks for the high honour conferred upon him, etc.

Ordered, that the Secretary do direct the back numbers of the "American Medical Library and Intelligencer" to be forwarded forthwith in reply to a letter from A. Waldie, Philadelphia.

The Treasurer's books were examined, showing a balance of £14 4 9 due to the College to Dec. 31, 1839, were audited and approved.

Moved by Wm. Durie, Esq., seconded by the Vice-President, that Sir John Webb, K.C.B., Director-General of the Ordnance Medical Department, be elected an Honorary Fellow of this College, to be taken into consideration at the next regular meeting. (Dr. Hornby enters.)

The Committee of Examination reported that Mr. John Stewart, of Tecumseth, had produced a diploma from the

Edinburgh College of Surgeons and been examined in Physic and Midwifery, and they recommended a license be granted to him to practise all three branches. License ordered to be dated December 26, 1839.

Moved and seconded, that Dr. Herrick having presented a diploma from Alex. Robinson from the College of Surgeons of Edinburgh, accompanied by an affidavit, that said Alex. Robinson is the person therein mentioned. It be

Resolved,—That the same be deemed satisfactory by the College, and that he receive his license accordingly, which, being put to a vote, was *Lost.*

Moved and seconded, that no application for license be entertained unless on the personal appearance of the applicant, and that a "statute" to that effect be adopted; to be taken into consideration at the next regular meeting.

Moved and seconded, "That the opinion of the Solicitor of the College be obtained on the construction of the 12th clause of the Act of Incorporation," which, on being put to the vote was *Lost.*

Moved and seconded, that James Campbell, M.D., of the University of Edinburgh, of Brockville, being a member of the College, "be admitted to Fellowship therein;" to be taken into consideration at the next regular meeting.

Moved and seconded, that Mr. Henry Sullivan, Mr. John Turquand and Alexander Smith, M.D., etc., etc., being members of this College, be elected to Fellowship therein; to be considered at the next regular meeting.

Resolved,—That a committee be appointed to frame "rules" for the library. Adjourned *sine die.*

CHAPTER XVI.

SUGGESTIONS TO THE LIEUT.-GOVERNOR BY THE COLLEGE.

TORONTO, *February* 3, 1840—First Monday in February (Quarterly Meeting).—Present: C. Widmer, Esq., President; Doctor King, Vice-President; Doctors Hornby, O'Brien, Shortt, Herrick, Gwynne and W. Telfer, Esq.

The motion, "That Sir John Webb, etc., etc., be elected an Honorary Fellow of this College," was adopted unanimously.

Dr. James Campbell, Brockville, Mr. Henry Sullivan, Mr. John Turquand, Alexander Smith, M.D., were elected to Fellowship.

Resolved,—That the opinion of H. Sherwood, Esq., be taken upon the question—"Whether, under the clause of the Act of Incorporation, it be lawful to enact a Statute or By-law requiring the personal appearance of applicants for license before such license shall be granted."

Resolved,—That the motion, "That no application for license be entertained unless on the personal appearance of the applicant," be postponed until the regular meeting in May.

Moved and seconded, that Henry Boys, M.D., be elected to Fellowship on his complying with the terms of the Act of Incorporation. Ordered to be taken into consideration at the next regular meeting. Adjourned.

February 4, 1840.—Present: C. Widmer, Esq., President; Dr. King, Vice-President; Dr. O'Brien, Dr. Baldwin, Dr. Gwynne, Dr. Hornby, Dr. Shortt and Dr. Herrick.

Mr. R. Coucher presented an application for license; referred to the censors. (N.B.—Mr. Coucher presented a diploma from the London College of Surgeons only, and was informed that to obtain a license to practise Physic, Surgery and Midwifery, he must undergo an examination in Physic and Midwifery —on which he withdrew, saying he would not trouble the College any further.)

Dr. Hornby presented from the Library Committee a report and code of regulations.

Moved and seconded, that the examination of candidates for license be open to any person introduced by a Fellow, which motion being put to the vote was *Lost.*

Resolved,—That Thomas Rolph, Esq., of Ancaster, be requested to act as agent of this College while he is in Great Britain, in the transaction of such matters as the College may deem expedient. Adjourned.

February 5, 1840.—Present: C. Widmer, Esq., President; Dr. O'Brien, and Dr. Herrick. No quorum. Adjourned *sine die.*

SPECIAL MEETING, *March* 3, 1840.—Present: C. Widmer, Esq., President; Dr. Hornby, Dr. O'Brien, Dr. Herrick, Mr. Sullivan, and Mr. Telfer.

The Secretary reported to the College that the case of books from Black & Armstrong, London, had arrived, and that the contents were much damaged by water; that Mr. Rowsell had surveyed them and estimated the damage as follows: "15 volumes of the bound volumes will require to be taken to pieces and cleaned and entirely new bound at 4s. 3d. per volume. 9 volumes cleaned and repaired at 1s. 10½d. per volume. 24 numbers in paper covers repaired at 6d. each. N.B.—If the loose numbers are half bound calf same as the others, the price per volume will be 3s. 9d."

Resolved,—That the Secretary be authorized to employ Mr. Rowsell to repair the 15 volumes of bound books at 4s. 3d. per volume; the 9 volumes at 1s. 10½d. per volume, and to procure the loose numbers to be bound at 3s. 9d. per volume.

SPECIAL MEETING, *April* 18, 1840.—Present: John King, M.D., Vice-President; Dr. Hornby, Dr. O'Brien, Dr. Gwynne, Dr. Herrick, Walter Telfer, Esq., and Henry Sullivan, Esq.

The Secretary laid before the meeting the following letter from the commissioners for erecting a lunatic asylum:

"TORONTO, *April* 16, 1840.

"SIR,—The commissioners for erecting a lunatic asylum in this Province, have resolved to ask the opinion of the College of Physicians and Surgeons regarding the eligibility of a certain site north of the city, whereon to erect the building, as to salubrity.

"The commissioners respectfully request the attention of the College to this matter at its earliest convenience, and will point out the spot alluded to whenever the College shall be pleased to give them notice of its intention to view it.

"We have the honour to be, Sir,

"Your Obedient Servants,

"(Signed) C. WIDMER, ALEXANDER WOOD, } *Commissioners.*

"*To* LUCIUS O'BRIEN, M.D.

"*Secretary, College of Physicians and Surgeons of Upper Canada.*"

The above letter being taken into consideration, a committee was appointed to enquire into the subject of it.

ADJOURNED SPECIAL MEETING, *April* 25, 1840.—Present: John King, M.D., Vice-President; Dr. O'Brien, Dr. Herrick, W. Telfer, Esq., and Dr. Shortt.

The committee to whom the subject of the salubrity of certain sites for a lunatic asylum was referred, presented their report:

"The committee to whom was entrusted the investigating the subject of the eligibility of certain sites as to salubrity, etc., upon which to erect a lunatic asylum, respectfully beg leave to report as follows:

"Your committee have visited the different situations pointed out to them by the Commissioners, Messrs. Widmer and Wood, viz., three lots north of the city and lying contiguous to each other, the most easterly of which is the property of John Scadding, Esq.; the middle, of James Small, Esq., and that most towards the west, of the Hon. Wm. Allen.

"The elevation of the land generally, the expanded and varied view of the country and the lake in front; the distance (about a mile and a half) from the marsh being far beyond the limit within which marsh miasmata are known usually to have a noxious influence, incline your committee to the opinion that any one of those situations would be in point of salubrity and scenery, an eligible site for the intended asylum. But your committee at the same time beg leave to add that they decided to prefer the site, the property of James Small, Esq., as possessing from its superior elevation, all the above advantages in an eminent degree.

"All of which is most respectfully submitted.

"(Signed) JOHN KING, M.D., *Chairman.*
WM. C. GWYNNE.
GEO. HERRICK, M.D.

"College of Physicians and Surgeons, April 25, 1840."

Resolved,—That a copy of the report be transmitted to the said commissioners. Adjourned.

QUARTERLY MEETING, *May* 4, 1840.—Present: C. Widmer, Esq., President; Dr. King, Vice-President; Dr. Baldwin, Dr. O'Brien and Mr. Sullivan.

Resolved,—That the sum of five pounds deposited by Thos. Rolph in the hands of the Treasurer, be refunded, he having exhibited no qualification for being elected a member.

Resolved,—That Mr. Wm. Clarke, of Guelph, having laid before the College a certificate of examination in Physic, Surgery and Midwifery before the late Medical Board of this Province, dated January 11, 1839, and praying for the license of the College thereon, the College consider that this testimonial is sufficient to justify the College in granting him its license.

Resolved,—That the license recommended by the College to be granted to Mr. Wm. Clarke, shall issue upon the payment of the further sum of one pound ten shillings, and upon his conforming with the regulations of the College.

Resolved,—That the Treasurer do remit the sum of two pounds ten shillings to Adam Waldie, Philadelphia, in payment of subscription for the fourth year of the "American Library and Intelligencer," commencing April 1, 1840.

The following gentlemen have appeared before the censors for license since February 3:

February 6.—Archibald Pass, M. C. Glasguens, Barrie, license for Physic, Surgery and Midwifery.

March 5.—James McCarthy, Toronto, license for Physic and Surgery.

March 24.—William Burgess, Licentiate of the Royal College of Surgeons of Edinburgh, Port Talbot, license for Physic, Surgery and Midwifery. Adjourned.

ADJOURNED MEETING, *May* 5, 1840.—Present: Christopher Widmer, Esq., President; Dr. Hornby, Dr. Gwynne, Dr. O'Brien, Dr. Shortt, Dr. Herrick and Mr. Telfer.

The following communication was laid before the College:

"SIR,—We have the honour to request you to lay the enclosed communication before the College at its meeting this day.

"(Signed) JOHN KING, *Vice-President.*
LUCIUS O'BRIEN.

"C. WIDMER, ESQ.,
"*President*, etc., etc."

"The undersigned consider it their duty to lay before the College of Physicians and Surgeons the following report of circumstances connected with the disallowance of the Act of Incorporation of the College, and beg leave to observe that the present is the first opportunity which they have had of making the communication.

"On the Wednesday immediately preceding the departure of the Governor-General from Toronto, we heard that a despatch had been received disallowing the Act of Incorporation of the College, and considered that some steps ought to be taken immediately to obviate it if possible. Accordingly, Dr. O'Brien called on the President, but not finding him at home, sent him a message, and was favoured with a call from him next morning (viz.), Thursday, when Dr. O'Brien proposed that we should wait on His Excellency to ascertain the facts and request a postponement of the promulgation of the disallowance. This the President declined.

"Having consulted with Mr. Sherwood, and conceiving that

no time was to be lost in a matter of such moment, he, Mr. Sherwood, very readily agreed to accompany us to His Excellency, and we three accordingly waited on him that afternoon, not as a deputation from the College, but as individuals feeling deeply interested in its welfare. His Excellency informed us that such a despatch had been received, entered courteously and attentively into the subject, gave us an order to see the despatch, said he would be glad to see us again either next day or on Saturday, and receive any arguments we might have to bring forward against the disallowance, and that in the meantime he would postpone its publication.

"It being then too late to call at the office of the Secretary, Mr. Murdock, we called next day, Friday, accompanied by Dr. Widmer, and read over the despatch.

"Saturday afternoon, Dr. Widmer, Dr. King, Dr. O'Brien and Dr. Gwynne, accompanied by Mr. Sherwood, waited according to appointment on the Governor-General, with whom Mr. Sherwood entered very fully into the subject, and the interview resulted in His Excellency expressing himself strongly in our favour, and requesting that Mr. Sherwood would embody our arguments in a memorial to him, which he would make the foundation of a despatch to the Imperial Government and support by his favourable recommendation.

"Early on Monday morning His Excellency left Toronto for Montreal.

"N.B.—His Excellency informed us that the disallowance was to have been published in the *Gazette* the following Thursday.

"We cannot in justice close this report without bringing under the notice of the College the very handsome and prompt manner in which Mr. Sherwood afforded us his advice and assistance in this very urgent and critical conjuncture.

"(Signed) LUCIUS O'BRIEN.
JOHN KING, *Vice-President.*"

Thereon it was

Resolved,—That the Secretary be requested to write to Mr. Secretary Murdock, requesting that the College may be furnished with a copy of the despatch containing the objection to the Bill incorporating the College of Physicians and Surgeons.

The regulations for the library were then taken into consideration, when it was

Resolved,—That until a suitable room for the library can be obtained, the books of the College now in possession of the Secretary shall be allowed to circulate among the Fellows of the College under certain restrictions :

RESTRICTION No. 1.—Every Fellow receiving a book from the Steward of the Hospital shall deposit with him as a pledge for its safety and return within fourteen days, the sum of "two dollars." No. 2.—Every book shall be returned when done with, to the Steward, and not transferred from Fellow to Fellow.

Resolved,—That at every quarterly meeting a committee of three be appointed to examine and report upon the state of the books.

Resolved, — That the President, Vice-President and Dr. Gwynne be the Committee for the present quarter.

Resolved,—That the books of the College be for the present deposited in the Hospital, and that the key of the case be left in charge of the Steward, who shall give the books to the Fellows, receive the deposit, and enter the name of the Fellows, between the hours of 12 and 1 o'clock, daily.

Resolved,—That the Secretary be authorized to procure a case with shelves, lock and key, capable of containing all the books of the College.

Resolved,—That the Secretary be authorized to procure Stencil Plates with the words "Coll. Phys. and Surg. U.C." for the purpose of marking the books and plates.

Resolved,—That a suitable book be procured for the library in which shall be entered the name of the person taking out any book, the title of the book and number of volume, with the dates of issuing and returning it, with any remarks which may be required as to the state it may be in when issued or returned. Adjourned.

SPECIAL MEETING, *June* 9, 1840.—Present: C. Widmer, Esq., President; Dr. King, Vice-President; R. C. Horne, Esq., W. Telfer, Esq., Dr. Herrick.

A communication from Mr. Hopkirk, Acting-Secretary to His Excellency the Lieut.-Governor, to the President, announcing his determination to fix the site of the intended Lunatic Asylum at Kingston, having been read, it was

Resolved,—That a memorial to His Excellency the Lieutenant-Governor, be forthwith prepared and forwarded without delay, stating the injurious effects of such a measure upon the best interests of the profession, as well as the rising members thereof, and praying that His Excellency will be pleased to locate the asylum in the immediate neighbourhood of this city. And that the President, Vice-President, the Secretary and Dr. Herrick be a committee to draw up the same memorial. Adjourned.

ADJOURNED SPECIAL MEETING, *June* 10, 1840.—Present: C. Widmer, Esq., President; Dr. King, Vice-President; Dr. Herrick, Dr. O'Brien, W. Telfer, Esq., H. Sullivan, Esq.

The President presented a draft of a memorial to His Excellency the Lieutenant-Governor, which being taken into consideration, was adopted as follows:

"*To His Excellency Major-General Sir George Arthur, K.C.H., Lieutenant-Governor, etc.*

"We, the President, Vice-President and Fellows of the College of Physicians and Surgeons of Upper Canada, respectfully beg leave to address Your Excellency on a subject of vital importance to the College and the Profession generally throughout the Province.

"Having understood that Your Excellency has recently come to the determination that the asylum to be erected in this Province for the receptacle of insane and lunatic persons, in pursuance of the provisions of the Statute of the 2nd Victoria, chap. xi., shall be located at Kingston, we would earnestly but most respectfully offer to Your Excellency, many cogent reasons upon which we hope Your Excellency may be rendered to alter your determination thereon.

"It certainly could not have escaped Your Excellency's penetration, that such an establishment as a lunatic asylum should be so situated that it would afford to the friends of the pitiable objects, for whose accommodation, protection and cure it is founded, the assurance of their receiving the most efficient and popular professional aid that could be obtained in the Province; and without detracting at all from the merits of the respectable practitioners of our art in Kingston, we would humbly submit that, as is the case in other countries, the description of talent most likely to be highly estimated by the public, is generally to be found in the dense and wealthy population of a metropolitan city. In looking forward to the future, the period we hope is not far distant, when the beneficial operations of the ample endowment of an University in this city, will be available for the instruction of medicine.

"The pressure of an institution for the cure of mental diseases as an adjunct to the present practical benefits offered by the General Hospital, will present to the student of medicine, advantages of an importance that he should not, for trifling considerations, be deprived of. The rapid strides with which the science of mental pathology has of late years advanced, would lead to the hope that the opportunities for observation in so large a field as this asylum would present, will not be lost to the medical student of our future University, through an error which, when once consummated, cannot be remedied.

"We shall not be deemed visionary when we declare to Your Excellency that the first fruits of an effective organization of a school for medical instruction of which the projected lunatic asylum should form a part, will afford results of an immensely valuable nature, both politically and morally, to the inhabitants of this favoured Province.

"If we are deprived of the important addition which we pray for, and the asylum is removed without the pale of the University, we consider that it will be shorn of a most valuable and important feature in its usefulness.

"Having pointed out the reasons which more immediately concern us as a professional body, we would suggest to Your Excellency, one of a character which, as citizens, we cannot allow ourselves to pass over unnoticed. The House of Assembly in its last session was moved to address His Excellency the Governor-General for reasons then brought forward, praying that His Excellency would cause the asylum to be located in Kingston.

"This motion being negatived by a large majority of the House is a proof that the feelings of the representatives of the people were opposed to the measure now about to be adopted by Your Excellency, and cannot fail to strike us as a proof that it would be highly unpopular generally in the Province.

"In the hope that Your Excellency will consider the importance of the subject submitted to Your Excellency in this address as a sufficient excuse for trespassing upon Your Excellency's valuable time, we conclude by earnestly entreating Your Excellency to reconsider the determination which Your Excellency has arrived at."

Resolved,—That a copy of the said memorial be transmitted to His Excellency the Governor-General. Adjourned.

CHAPTER XVII.

THE LEGALITY OF THE COLLEGE CALLED IN QUESTION.

TORONTO, *August* 3, 1840 (Quarterly Meeting).—Present: C. Widmer, Esq., President; Dr. King, Vice-President; W. Telfer, Esq., Dr. O'Brien, Dr. Shortt, and Henry Sullivan.

The Secretary stated that no answer had been received from Mr. Murdock relative to the application made for copy of the despatch containing the disallowance of the Act of Incorporation of the College.

The Secretary laid before the College, Mr. Secretary Harrison's reply to the address of the College, relative to the location of the lunatic asylum.

"THE CENSORS' REPORT.—Since last quarterly meeting the following gentlemen have applied for license:

"Mr. John Robinson Dickson, from Peterborough, not having certificate of hospital attendance, his examination was not proceeded in.

"Mr. Wm. Clarke, of Guelph, having the certificate from the late Medical Board, dated January 11, 1839, a license was issued accordingly.

"Mr. Wm. Henry Cuddy produced a diploma from the London Royal College of Surgeons. In consequence of his extremely defective answering in the practice of Physic, a license in Surgery and Midwifery was directed to be granted, which, however, Mr. Cuddy refused to receive."

Resolved,—That with reference to the communication made to the College by Drs. King and O'Brien, entered on minutes of May 5, a committee be appointed to take into consideration the disallowance of the Act of Incorporation of the College and report thereon to the College.

Resolved,—That the foregoing committee do consist of the Vice-President, Secretary and Dr. Telfer.

Resolved,—That a committee be appointed to prepare an address to His Excellency the Governor-General, relative to the delay in establishing a Medical School in King's College; such address to be submitted to the College when prepared.

Resolved,—That the foregoing committee do consist of Dr. King, Vice-President, and Dr. Sullivan.

The Secretary laid before the College a letter from Sir John Webb, Director-General of the Ordnance Medical Department, dated Woodstock, May 17, 1840, acknowledging the receipt of the Secretary's letter enclosing the Resolution electing him an Honorary Fellow of the College, and returning thanks for the honour done him. Adjourned.

SPECIAL MEETING, *August* 24, 1840.—Present: C. Widmer, Esq., President; R. C. Horne, Esq., W. Telfer, Esq., Henry Sullivan, Esq., Dr. O'Brien.

The committee to whom the subject of the disallowance of the Act of Incorporation of the College was referred, submitted a report which was adopted as follows:

"Your Committee find that the proposed disallowance of the Act of Incorporation of this College has been founded on the following grounds:

"1st. A petition from the Royal College of Surgeons of London, which recites that part of the 18th of George II., cap. 15, which confers on the members of that body the right to practise freely and without restraint the act and science of surgery throughout all and every part of His Majesty's dominions.

"2nd. This petition represents that this Act (of Incorporation) confers on the College powers greater than any ever granted to any existing body or college, that such powers are not clear and defined, and that several clauses of the Act infringe the rights and privileges conferred by the Charter of the London College of Surgeons.

"3rd. The opinion of the Attorney and Solicitor-General, viz., that several provisions of the Act encroach on the privileges of the College and of several other bodies in this country, and have a tendency to establish a monopoly which might be found highly inconvenient to the inhabitants of that Province.

"On these several sections your Committee would remark *seriatim:*

"Section 1. Our Act of Incorporation acknowledges in the fullest degree the right of the members of the Royal College of Surgeons of London to practise the art and science of surgery throughout this Province as part of Her Majesty's dominions, as the Act makes it imperative on the College to issue its license on the production and verification of a diploma from that College.

"But the College also feels that it is imperative on them not to grant its license to practise other branches of the medical profession except on proof of further qualification, especially as the examinations on which the diplomas of the London College of Surgeons are granted, do not embrace an inquiry into a knowledge of the practice of medicine or midwifery. And your Committee regret to say that the records of the College and of the Medical Board afford instances of the ignorance of some of the members of the various colleges of surgeons in the theory and practice of physic and midwifery. Your Committee does not bring this forward as applying to British surgeons generally, but simply to show that however well informed they commonly are, the few exceptions that occur render it imperative on the College, to whom this important duty is assigned, to take care that ignorant individuals shall not receive the same license as those who are fully competent.

"Your Committee are also prepared to show that the London College of Surgeons can claim no legal right to practise any branch of the profession but the art and science of surgery in any part of Great Britain or Ireland.

"By the charter of the London College of Physicians, no person is allowed to practise physic in London, or within seven miles of it without their license, and they can fine and imprison offenders.

"The Censors have the power to survey, govern, and arrest all physicians and others practising physic within their jurisdiction, and to fine, amerce, and imprison them at discretion.

"The College of Physicians of Edinburgh was 'instituted to prevent abuses . . . of foreign and illiterate quacks and impostors,' etc., and by its charter no person is allowed to practise physic, throughout their jurisdiction, without their license, under a penalty.

"The jurisdiction of the Apothecaries' Company in England is even far more extensive, embracing England and Wales, and the members of the London College of Surgeons cannot practise as Apothecaries within this jurisdiction, without being subjected to heavy penalties, unless they have a license from the Apothecaries' Company.

"These instances, which might be extended, will show that the members of the London College of Surgeons can claim a right under colour of their diplomas to practise only the art and science of surgery in any place where there is any other jurisdiction by law established.

"Section 2. The petition before alluded to represents that this Act confers on the College powers greater than any ever granted to any existing body or College, that such powers are not clear and defined, and that several clauses of the Act infringe the rights and privileges conferred by the Charter of the London College of Surgeons.

"1st. The College being in fact and truth a College of Physicians and Surgeons, has been entrusted by law with the supervision of the qualifications requisite to practise either or both of these departments, and in this respect only appears to profess greater privileges than other existing bodies, for there are none similarly constituted, as far as your Committee are aware, except the Faculty of Physicians and Surgeons of Glasgow.

"2nd. The College professes in regard to the Universities and other British Colleges, the privilege only of calling on their graduates, members and licentiates to produce and verify their several diplomas, being compelled on the production and verification of such diplomas to issue their license accordingly, which license is then an assurance to the public that the individual holds the qualification he professes to have, and simply stands in lieu of the license which, previous to the formation of the College, was issued by the Lieut.-Governor.

"3rd. The only other power or privilege possessed by the College is that of ascertaining, by actual *viva voce* examination, whether any individual not possessing any qualification from a British body legally entitled to grant one, be a fit person to be permitted to practise as a Physician, Surgeon or Accoucher, in the Province of Upper Canada.

"This duty or privilege was exercised formerly by the Medical Board, established by law, in this Province, and has been very much limited by the right now extended to all the members, etc., of the British Colleges.

"Your Committee conceive that this duty or privilege must be exercised by some authorized body, for the mutual advantage and security of the public, and of those individuals whose limited circumstances have not enabled them to avail themselves of the advantages of professional education in Great Britain, and they believe that it could be entrusted to more fitting hands than to this College.

"4th. Your Committee do not perceive to what particular part of the Act the next objection refers, viz., 'that such powers are not clear and defined.'

"On the contrary, your Committee are of opinion that the powers and duties of the College are stated so clearly and distinctly as to be available for most useful purposes, and to be clear and intelligible to all individuals who will take the trouble of perusing the Act with common attention.

"5th. It is stated 'that several clauses of the Act infringe the rights and privileges conferred by the Charter of the London College of Surgeons.'

"This point will come to be considered under the next general head, viz.:

"Section 3. The opinion of the Attorney and Solicitor-General, which may be divided into two parts:

"1st. That 'several provisions of the Act encroach on the privileges of the College (of Surgeons, of London) and of several other bodies in this country (England).'

"Your Committee regret that the wording of this opinion from the highest official law-officers in Great Britain, should have been so vague as to make it almost impossible to understand and therefore to answer it.

"Your Committee have already shown that the Members of the London College of Surgeons possess only the legal right to practise the art and science of surgery in those places where there is any local professional jurisdiction, without license or permission of the authority exercising such jurisdiction. They have also shown that this College possesses no right over these individuals, except calling on them to produce and verify their diplomas; and that obviously for the purpose of guarding against the numerous evils arising from persons pretending to possess professional qualifications, but who, in fact, are totally destitute of all such, either legally or by education.

"By the 'several other bodies' must be meant the British Universities, and the various other bodies authorized to grant diplomas or licenses in Great Britain. The arguments above adduced in respect to the London College of Surgeons will apply, *mutatis mutandis*, to the British Universities. And reference to this Act, compared to prior Acts, will show that the only effect of it in regard to the other bodies above alluded to, is to place their diplomas on a footing similar to those of the London College of Surgeons.

"Your Committee is, therefore, totally unable to understand that giving these 'several other bodies' the same rank and footing as the London College, is encroaching on their rights or privileges in any way whatever.

"2nd. That they 'have a tendency to establish a monopoly in Upper Canada, which might be found highly inconvenient to the inhabitants of that Province.'

"Your Committee can hardly imagine that this idea could

have entered into the mind of any person who had looked into the provisions of the Act.

"If this College had a discretionary power of withholding or granting licenses in every case, such a possibility might occur. But as it is absolutely imperative that a license shall be granted to any or everyone exhibiting a diploma, license, commission or warrant, as described in the Act, and as every licentiate has it in his power to become a member at any time he may choose without the College having the discretionary power to refuse him, it is an absolute impossibility that any professional monopoly can arise out of this Act.

"But if by the word 'monopoly,' allusion is made to the power granted to the Fellows to augment their number by election from among their members, it remains to be shown how, by any clause, this can produce the least 'inconvenience to the inhabitants of this Province.'

"Your Committee would ask, suppose that the Fellows be disposed to follow the example of the Council of the London College of Surgeons and make the College a close corporation, could that, under the existing Act, confine to their body the exercise of professional talent and information, so as to prejudice the health or interests of the community at large?

"The warm support which this Act received from the most respectable and influential portion of both branches of the Legislature, shows that they did not apprehend that the community at large could suffer any serious inconvenience under it.

"Your Committee would now draw the attention of the College to the following summary of the Colonial Acts, by which it will appear that the effect of disallowing this Act would be, not to place the London College of Surgeons on a more favourable footing, but to exclude the Colleges of Surgeons of Dublin and of Edinburgh, the Faculty of Physicians and Surgeons of Glasgow, and the Members of King's and Queen's College of Physicians in Ireland, and of the College of Physicians of Edinburgh, who may be graduates of British Universities from a privilege equal to them, and to subject their licentiates to examinations from which those holding London diplomas are exempt:

"SUMMARY OF COLONIAL ACTS.

"In 1818, the Legislature of Upper Canada passed a law by which all persons were restrained from practising Physic, Surgery or Midwifery within the Province under certain penalties, except persons authorized by any university in His Majesty's dominions, or by commissions, or warrant in His Majesty's Naval or Military Services.

"By this Act, the Members of the London College of Surgeons (among others) were expressly prohibited from practising in this Province (though not by name), unless they submitted to an examination before the Medical Board established by this Act, and obtained a license.

"In 1819, another Act was passed repealing part of and amending the Act of the previous year, but it extended no privilege to the Members of the College of Surgeons of London.

"In 1827, another Act passed on the subject, by which the Members of the London College of Surgeons (as also the London College of Physicians) were first named and classed with the graduates of the universities, and with them permitted to receive licenses from the Lieut.-Governor, on producing and verifying their diplomas on oath and paying certain fees. Thus from 1818 to 1827, a period of nine years, by the laws of Upper Canada, members of the Colleges of Physicians and of Surgeons of London were debarred from the privilege of practising their respective professions within this Province without a license, and, in fact, during that time they stood upon the same footing as ordinary applicants for licenses.

"When a greater privilege was extended to them in 1827, by the last named Act, the members of other colleges in Great Britain, such as the Colleges of Surgeons of Dublin and Edinburgh, and the Faculty of Physicians and Surgeons of Glasgow, expressed great dissatisfaction that they should not have equal privileges, and from that time till 1838 continual applications were made to the Legislature and elsewhere by the latter class, to have extended to them the same privileges as the Statute of 1827 extended to members of the College of Surgeons of London.

"The Act incorporating the College of Physicians and Surgeons of Upper Canada, which passed in 1839, extended the privilege which the London College enjoined, to the Members and Licentiates of every College and Faculty of Physicians and Surgeons in the United Kingdom.

"This liberal provision was well received, and was one which the ordinary rules of equal justice required.

"Until the last-mentioned Act was passed, all licenses were issued by the Lieut.-Governor, and the fees paid were given as a perquisite to his Secretary; now they are paid to the College for the general benefit and advantage of the profession.

"A member of the London College of Surgeons has now to satisfy the College of Physicians and Surgeons of Upper Canada that he is the person named in the diploma produced, instead of the Lieut.-Governor as formerly—no privilege heretofore possessed by him is abridged or interfered with in the least.

"Your Committee cannot dismiss the subject without indicating two points which have presented themselves very forcibly to the minds of all those who have been made aware of the interference of the London College of Surgeons, and of the opinion of the law-officers of the Crown, relative to this Act.

"1st. That the College has been led to interfere in consequence of misrepresentation from individuals in this Province, who either did not understand the Act, or wilfully misrepresented it.

"2nd. That the opinion referred to above, as quoted in the despatch, was given in ultra-ignorance of the Colonial Acts on the subject, and without considering what are the real and undoubted rights of the London College of Surgeons as distinguished from those it may pretend to, not distinguishing the right to practise with a certain diploma from the right of the Colonial Legislature to call for the production and verification of such diploma. And that the meaning and tendency of this Act have been taken from an *ex parte* statement of the London College, instead of the Act itself being duly considered and compared not only with the Charter of the London College but also with prior Acts of this Legislature."

Resolved,—That a copy of the foregoing report be enclosed

to the Secretary of His Excellency the Governor-General for His Excellency's information.

Resolved,—That the Secretary do apply again to the Secretary of His Excellency the Governor-General, for a copy of the despatch containing the disallowance of the Act of Incorporation.

The Committee appointed to prepare an address to His Excellency the Governor-General, relative to the delay in establishing a Medical School in King's College, reported one which was adopted as follows:

"To His Excellency the Right Hon. Charles Poulett Thompson, one of Her Majesty's Privy Council, Governor-General, etc., etc., etc.

" *May it please Your Excellency.*

"We, Her Majesty's dutiful and legal subjects, the President, Vice-President and Fellows of the College of Physicians and Surgeons of Upper Canada, most respectfully pray Your Excellency's attention to the length of time which has now elapsed since our late Munificent Sovereign endowed the University of King's College in Upper Canada, and to the fact that there is not yet a Medical School in the Province.

"It will, we are convinced, be unnecessary to urge on Your Excellency the necessity for such an institution, when Your Excellency is made aware that the medical student of Upper Canada, if he have no opportunities beyond those offered in the Province, must pursue his studies without a library, without a museum, without a botanic garden, without an hospital, without a dissecting-room, in fact without public instruction in any branch of the profession, and it must be remembered that few, indeed, have the means of seeking academical instruction in the Mother Country.

"We have waited in patient but anxious expectation, that the intentions of our Sovereign and of the Legislature of the Country, would be carried into execution by the Honourable the Council of King's College, but finding that no steps, of which we are aware, have been taken by that body (notwithstanding the full powers with which it has been invested) for the establishment of a medical school, we humbly and respectfully pray Your Excellency's interference for the promotion of this great object, and that Your Excellency will be pleased to direct such immediate consideration of the claims of the Medical Faculty as will obviate the difficulties which at present stand in the way of professional education within the Province, and the consequent necessity of students seeking the attainment essential to the knowledge of the profession by attendance on the institutions of a foreign country."

Resolved,—That the Fellows do assemble to wait on His Excellency, with the above address, whenever the Secretary shall notify His Excellency's assent.

CHAPTER XVIII.

THE ACT ESTABLISHING COLLEGE OF PHYSICIANS U. C. DISALLOWED.

TORONTO, *November* 2, 1840 (Quarterly Meeting).—Present: C. Widmer, Esq., President; Dr. King, Vice-President; Dr. Herrick, Dr. O'Brien, Dr. Gwynne, Dr. Shortt and Henry Sullivan, Esq.

Resolved,—That the Secretary do now lay before the College, a list of the persons who have come within his knowledge, as being fined for practising without license, and that he be requested to state whether the punishment inflicted has had the effect of putting a stop to the evil.

Resolved,—That a notice be inserted in the *Patriot* newspaper that an authorized list of the Fellows, Members and Licentiates of the College, together with the Registered Apothecaries and Druggists in the Province, shall be published in pamphlet form shortly after the first day of January, 1841.

Moved by Dr. King, seconded by Dr. O'Brien, that William Pulteney Alison, M.D., Professor of the Institutes of Medicine in the University of Edinburgh, be elected an Honorary Fellow of this College. To be balloted for at the next regular meeting.

Resolved,—That Henry Boys, M.D., being a member of this College, be elected to Fellowship therein.

Moved and seconded, that Robert Christison, M.D., Professor in the University of Edinburgh, be elected an Honorary Fellow of this College. To be balloted for at the next regular meeting. The Censors report that since last quarterly meeting the following gentlemen had applied for license: William H. Evatt (M.D., of Philadelphia), Toronto, license granted; H. G. Spafford, license refused.

The state of affairs at this period, with regard to the General Hospital at Kingston, is shown by an Act of Parliament:

"KINGSTON GENERAL HOSPITAL (1840).—An Act to authorize the temporary occupation of the proposed University at Kingston of the General Hospital at Kingston, upon certain terms.

"*Whereas*, a building was erected at Kingston by the voluntary contributions of certain of the inhabitants, and by a grant from the Province, for the purpose of a General Hospital which, for the want of the necessary endowment, has not been used for the object contemplated, and, in consequence thereof, the building is unoccupied and subject to damage and decay."

ANNUAL MEETING, *January* 4, 1841.—Present: John King, M.D., Vice-President; R. C. Horne, Esq., Dr. Shortt, Dr. O'Brien, Dr. Herrick, Dr. Gwynne, Dr. Boys.

The Secretary laid before the College a letter from S. B. Harrison, Esq., Private Secretary to His Excellency the Lieut.-Governor.

Resolved,—That the said letter be entered in the minutes.

"GOVERNMENT HOUSE,
"*December* 28th, 1840.

"SIR,—I have the honour, by command of the Lieut.-Governor, to acquaint you, for the information of the College of Physicians and Surgeons, that a despatch has been received from Her Majesty's Principal Secretary of State for the Colonies on the subject of the Provincial Act of 1839 incorporating that body.

"His Lordship states that the Royal Charter of the College of Surgeons in London, confirmed by the Statute 18 Geo. 2nd, C. 15, confers on the members of that body the right to practise freely and without restraint the art and science of surgery throughout all and every Her Majesty's dominions, any law or custom to the contrary notwithstanding.

"His Lordship further states that the College of Surgeons represented to him that the Provincial Act confers on the Governors of the College instituted by it, powers greater than any ever granted to any existing body or college, that such powers are not clear and defined, and that several of the clauses of the Act infringe the rights and privileges conferred by the Charter of the London College of Surgeons, and by the Statute 18 Geo. 3rd, C. 15; and that having referred this statement to Her Majesty's Attorney and Solicitor-General, they had reported to His Lordship that the objections of the College of Surgeons are well founded, and that several of the provisions of the Act encroached on the privileges of the College of Surgeons and of other bodies in Great Britain, and had a tendency to establish a monopoly, which might be found highly inconvenient to the inhabitants of the Province.

"Under these circumstances, His Lordship states that it became the inevitable, though very unwelcome, duty of Her Majesty's confidential advisers to submit to the Queen that the Act ought not to be allowed; and His Lordship encloses an order passed by Her Majesty in Council by which it is disallowed accordingly.

"In communicating this decision, His Excellency has been requested by His Lordship to say that he will endeavour to provide by an Act of Parliament, some remedy for the inconveniences which the Act was intended to meet.

"I have the honour, etc., etc., etc.,

"(Signed) S. B. HARRISON.

"LUCIUS O'BRIEN, ESQ., M.D.,
"Etc., etc., etc."

Resolved,—That, considering the present circumstances in which the College is placed, the present officers be re-elected.

An application from Mr. Thos. Shirley was read, setting forth that if he be not allowed an examination previous to next Thursday, he cannot get a license from this College, and that the Medical Board cannot meet till the first Monday in April, and he will thereby be unable to procure a license for three months to come, and thereby suffer great inconvenience.

Resolved,—That the Censors be called together this evening to proceed to the examination of Mr. Thos. Shirley. Adjourned.

ADJOURNED MEETING, *January* 5, 1841.—Present: R. C. Horne, Esq., Dr. Hornby, Dr. O'Brien, Walter Telfer, Esq. R. C. Horne, Esq. was called to the chair. There not being a quorum, the meeting was adjourned.

ADJOURNED MEETING, *January* 6, 1841.—Present: C. Widmer, Esq., President; Dr. King, Vice-President; Dr. Shortt, R. C. Horne, Esq., Dr. O'Brien, Henry Sullivan, Esq., and Dr. Boys.

The Treasurer laid an abstract of his accounts before the College, showing a balance in favour of the College of £20 18 9 in his hands.

The Censors reported that the following gentlemen had received licenses since the last quarterly meeting: Horatio Gates Spafford, Physic and Surgery; Thomas Shirley, Physic, Surgery and Midwifery.

At the request of the Treasurer, it was

Resolved,—That Dr. King, Vice-President, and Dr. Boys be requested to compare the entries in the Treasurer's books with the entries in the books of the Bank of Upper Canada, and make an entry accordingly, signed by their names, in the Treasurer's books.

Resolved,—That the various papers and other official documents belonging to the College be transferred to the Medical Board, to be received into the charge of such officer as they may appoint for that pupose.

Resolved,—That the books and furniture of the Library of the College of Physicians and Surgeons be transferred to a committee of eight, who are Fellows of the College, *in trust*, for such purposes as the Fellows generally may deem most expedient for the benefit of the profession and the continued existence of the library within this Province; and that such committee shall have power to fill up any vacancies which may occur by death or otherwise; and such committee be composed of the following persons: C. Widmer, Esq., R. C. Horne, Esq., Dr. King, Dr. O'Brien, Dr. Shortt, Dr. Herrick, Henry Sullivan, Esq., and Dr. Boys.

Resolved,—That the surplus funds remaining in the hands of the Treasurer be left in his hands, subject only to the control of the Committee appointed by the last resolution, for the uses of the Library.

LUCIUS O'BRIEN,
Secretary, College of Physicians and Surgeons.

At a meeting of the Committee appointed to take charge of the Library and other property of the late College of Physicians and Surgeons of Upper Canada, held at the Museum of King's College, a communication from the Medico-Chirurgical Society was presented, containing a request that the Committee would be pleased to permit the Library to be placed for the use of the Society, subject to such rules and regulations as the Society may deem proper to direct.

Resolved,—That a meeting of the Fellows of the late College of Physicians and Surgeons be called, to be held at the Hospital on the 15th day of October, 1844.

At a meeting of the Fellows of the late College of Physicians and Surgeons of Upper Canada, held at the Hospital, on the 15th day of October, 1844 (Present: C. Widmer, Dr. Herrick, Dr. Telfer, Dr. O'Brien and Dr. Boys),

It was moved by Dr. Boys, and seconded by Dr. Telfer, the Medico-Chirurgical Society having applied to the Fellows of the late College of Physicians and Surgeons for the use of the Medical Books in their possession, it is resolved by the Fellows now present, that it will be proper to lend the books to that Society as soon as it shall appear that the Society have provided a fit place for their reception. And that the committee named at the meeting of the 6th of January, 1841, be now empowered to carry this resolution into effect.

"ROOMS OF THE TORONTO MEDICO-CHIRURGICAL SOCIETY,
"NORTH AMERICAN HOTEL,
"TORONTO, *November* 9th, 1844.

"SIR,—I have the honour to annex an extract from the

minutes of the meeting of the Toronto Medico-Chirurgical Society, held on the sixth inst., and to request that you will be pleased to communicate the same, at your convenience, to the Trustees of the property belonging to the late College of Physicians and Surgeons of Upper Canada.

"I have the honour to be, Sir,

"Your very Obedient, Humble Servant,

"GEO. R. GRASETT,

"*Secretary, T.M.C.S.*

"DOCTOR WIDMER,

"*Senior Member of the Committee appointed by the late College of Physicians and Surgeons of Upper Canada.*"

"A report of the Committee of Management was presented by Dr. O'Brien, recommending that the Library of the late College of Physicians and Surgeons be entrusted to the Secretary, should it meet with the approval of the Trustees. The report was adopted by the meeting.

"The Secretary having signified his willingness to receive charge of the Library, and having stated that he had a proper place for its reception, it was

"*Resolved*,—That the Secretary be empowered to communicate to the Library Trustees, the Resolution of the Society relative to placing the Library under his charge, and requesting this concurrence.

"A true extract from the minutes.

"GEO. R. GRASETT,

"*Secretary, T.M.C.S.*"

At a meeting of the Trustees (members of the late College of Physicians and Surgeons) for the care of the Library of the College (Present: C. Widmer, Dr. O'Brien. Dr. Herrick, Dr. Boys),

A communication from the Secretary of the Medico-Chirurgical Society and a resolution of the said Society were read, whereupon it was

Resolved,—That the whole of the books constituting the Library of the said College, together with the book-case, shall be delivered to the custody of Dr. Grasett, the Secretary of the said Medico-Chirurgical Society, a list of them being prepared, and a receipt given by Dr. Grasett.

Resolved,—That this Committee retains the power of reclaiming the possession of the said books and book-case at any time the Committee shall see fit.

The author feels satisfied that in giving these minutes, almost unabridged to the public, he will have the approval of all lovers of Canadian history. The efforts of these comparatively early medical men to raise the character of the profession, to establish a Canadian Medical School that the young men of the Province should not be obliged to go abroad for medical instruction, are worthy of all commendation. Nor may it be supposed that their work was in vain. The seed sown by them has resulted in a rich crop, reaped by the later generations of our profession in this Province. No one can read the transactions of the College of Physicians and Surgeons of Upper Canada, without being impressed with the fact that the Governors had lofty aims and the interest of the profession fully at heart, at the same time looking to the welfare of the public; and it must not be forgotten that their work was performed more than half a century ago.

During the period of existence of the College, correspondence took place with different persons, mostly with applicants for membership. No copy exists of the letters received; but many of those written by the Secretary are of interest as containing historical reference. (See Appendix.)

CHAPTER XIX.

PROCEEDINGS OF UPPER CANADA MEDICAL BOARD.

THE last meeting of the College of Physicians and Surgeons of Upper Canada took place in January, 1841. The function of granting licenses to practise medicine in the Province was consequently suspended. The Act of Parliament, under which the former Medical Board was organized and acted, was now again in force. The revived Medical Board of Upper Canada held its first meeting, July 3, 1841. The following is the record of the proceedings found in the minutes from this date:

July 5th, 1841.—A commission from His Excellency the Governor-General, dated May 31st last, having been received by Mr. Widmer, appointing the following gentlemen members of a Medical Board for the examination of candidates, in accordance with the statute passed in the 59th year of the reign of His late Majesty George the 3rd, viz.:

Christopher Widmer, Esq., Walter Telfer, Esq., William C. Gwynne, M.B., Lucius O'Brien, M.D., Robert Hornby, M.D.

The said commission was then read as follows:

"By His Excellency the Right Honourable Charles Baron Sydenham, of Sydenham, in the County of Kent, and of Toronto in Canada, one of Her Majesty's Most Honourable Privy Council, Governor-General of British North America, etc., etc. To Christopher Widmer, member of the Royal College of Surgeons, London; William C. Gwynne, Bachelor of Medicine, of Trinity College, Dublin; Robert Hornby, Doctor of Medicine, of the University of Edinburgh; Walter Telfer, Licentiate of the Royal College of Surgeons, of Edinburgh; and Lucius O'Brien, Doctor of Medicine, of the University of Edinburgh.

"*Whereas*, in and by an Act of the Parliament of the late Province of Upper Canada, passed in the 59th year of the reign of His late Majesty George the 3rd, entitled 'An Act to repeal an Act passed in the 55th year of His Majesty's reign, entitled "An Act to license Practitioners in Physic and Surgery throughout the Province, and to make further provision for licensing such Practitioners,"' it is, among other things, enacted that it shall and may be lawful for the Governor, Lieutenant-Governor, or person administering the Government, for the time being, to constitute and appoint, under his hand and Seal-at-Arms, five or more persons legally authorized to practise Physic, Surgery, or Midwifery in this Province, to be a Board, whereof any three to be a quorum, to hear and examine all persons desirous to apply for a license to practise Physic, Surgery, and Midwifery, or either of them, within this Province, and being satisfied with such examination that any person is duly qualified to practise Physic, Surgery, and Midwifery, or either, to certify the same under the hands and seals of two or more of such Board, in order that the person so applying may obtain a license.

"*Now know ye*, that being well assured of your integrity and ability, I do hereby, under and by virtue of the abovementioned Act, nominate, constitute and appoint you, Christopher Widmer, William C. Gwynne, Robert Hornby, Walter Telfer, and Lucius O'Brien, to be a Board, whereof any three of you are to form a quorum, to hear and examine all persons desirous to apply for license to practise Physic, Surgery, and Midwifery, or either of them, within that part of the Province of Canada formerly constituting Upper Canada, and being satisfied by such examination that any person is duly qualified to practise Physic, Surgery, and Midwifery, or either of them, to certify the same under the hands and seals of any three or more of you; and moreover, to do all such acts and things by virtue of the said Act shall be by you to be done. To have, to hold and enjoy the said office or Commission unto you, the said Christopher Widmer, William C. Gwynne, Robert Hornby, Walter Telfer, and Lucius O'Brien, for and during pleasure and your residence within that part of the Province of Canada, formerly constituting Upper Canada, together with all and every fees, profits and advantages thereunto belonging, appertaining, hereby enjoining you that you do at the several days, and at the place in the said Act provided, then and there to do whatsoever by this Commission and the said Act shall be to be done.

"Given under my hand and seal at Kingston, this 31st day of May, in the year of Our Lord One Thousand Eight Hundred and Forty-One, and of Her Majesty's reign the Fourth.

"(Signed) SYDENHAM.

"By command.

"(Signed) S. B. HARRISON,

"*Secretary of the Province.*"

A letter from Dr. O'Brien was then read, of which the following is a copy:

"TORONTO, *July* 5th, 1841.

"SIR,—I beg to inform you, as senior member of the present list in the Commission of the Medical Board, for the information of the other members, that in consequence of what I deem to be an error in the position of my name in that list, I have stated to His Excellency, through the Secretary for this part of the Province, that I have declined accepting the appointment therein intended to be conferred upon me.

"I further beg leave to state that however willing I am to communicate all information in my power to gentlemen generally, I shall not feel myself justified in giving up any books papers, etc., in my charge until a person is duly appointed by a Board consisting of the number required by law.

"I have the honour to be, Sir,
"Your most Obedient Servant,

"(Signed) LUCIUS O'BRIEN.

"A true copy.
"G. E. GIVINS, *Secretary*."

Upon which it was

Resolved,—That the proceedings of this body should not be disturbed by the receipt of the above letter, and that we now proceed to the election of the officers of the Board. It was

Resolved,—That a copy of Dr. O'Brien's letter be forwarded to Mr. Harrison, Secretary of the Province.

It was then moved by Dr. Hornby, and seconded by Dr. Gwynne, that Mr. Widmer be appointed President of the Board and that the election be annual. Carried unanimously.

The Board then proceeded to elect a Secretary, when it was proposed by Dr. Gwynne, and seconded by Dr. Telfer, that Mr. George Givins be appointed the Secretary for the ensuing year. It was then

Resolved,—That the examination of candidates shall be conducted in the presence of the members only of the Board.

It was then moved by Dr. Gwynne, and seconded by Dr. Hornby, that the members of the Board be appointed, severally, to examine upon a particular subject annually. Carried *nemo con.*

It was then ordered by the Board that the Secretary do write to Dr. O'Brien, late Secretary of the College of Physicians and Surgeons, for all the records of the late Medical Board of the Province.

Copy of the letter to Dr. O'Brien :

"TORONTO, *July* 5th, 1841.

"SIR,—Having this day been appointed the Secretary of the Medical Board, I have the honour, in compliance with a resolution of the Board, to request that you will be pleased to deliver into my possession all the records of the late Medical Board of this Province, in order that the Board may be possessed of the necessary information as to the former proceedings of that body.

"I am,
"Your Obedient Servant,
"G. E. GIVINS, *Secretary.*

"LUCIUS O'BRIEN, ESQ., M.D.,
"*Late Secretary of the*
College of Physicians and Surgeons."

It was then

Resolved,—Tha tthe following subjects shall form the particular examination of each member, viz. :

Pharmaceutic Chemistry and Materia Medica, and also (for the present) the Theory and Practice of Physic—Dr. Hornby.

Anatomy—Dr. Gwynne.

Surgery—Dr. Telfer.

Midwifery—Dr. Widmer.

The following reply to the letter written by the Secretary of the Board to Dr. O'Brien, in pursuance of the resolution of yesterday, was received this morning:

"TORONTO, *July* 6th, 1841.

"SIR,—I have the honour to acknowledge your letter of yesterday purporting to be signed as Secretary to the Medical Board.

"As there are now only four members of that Board and the law requires five, I cannot acknowledge any act of theirs purporting to be acts of the Board as valid, and therefore cannot return any reply to any communication from you as their Secretary, though, individually, I shall be very happy to interchange any courtesies by letter or otherwise.

"I have the honour to be, Sir,
"Your most Obedient Servant,
"(Signed) LUCIUS O'BRIEN.

"G. E. GIVINS, ESQ."

"SECRETARY'S OFFICE,
"KINGSTON, *July* 31st, 1841.

"SIR,—I have the honour to acknowledge the receipt of your letter of the 6th instant, with its enclosures reporting the proceedings of the Medical Board, which I have laid before the Governor-General.

"In reply I am to acquaint you that on a reference to the Attorney-General, it appears that your proceedings have been legal and proper, and that His Excellency has been pleased to approve of them accordingly.

"I have the honour to be, Sir,
"Your most Obedient Servant,
"(Signed) JAMES HOPKIRK.

"C. WIDMER, ESQ.,
"*Surgeon.*"

"SECRETARY'S OFFICE,
"KINGSTON, *July* 30th, 1841.

"SIR,—I have the honour to transmit herewith a new Commission constituting yourself and others a Medical Board to examine all persons desirous of practising physic, surgery, etc., within the late Province of Upper Canada, pursuant to Provincial Act, 59 George 3rd., ch. 13.

"I have the honour to be, Sir,
"Your most Obedient, Humble Servant,
"(Signed) JAMES HOPKIRK.

"DR. WIDMER,
"Etc., etc., etc.,
"*Toronto.*"

"PROVINCE OF CANADA.

"By His Excellency the Right Honourable Charles Baron Sydenham, of Sydenham, in the County of Kent, and Toronto in Canada, one of Her Majesty's Most Honourable Privy Council, Governor-General of British North America, etc., etc., etc.

"To Christopher Widmer, Member of the Royal College of Surgeons, of London; William C. Gwynne, Bachelor of Medicine of Trinity College, Dublin; Robert Hornby, Doctor of Medicine of the University of Edinburgh; Walter Telfer, Licentiate of the Royal College of Surgeons, of Edinburgh; William Durie, late Assistant-Inspector of Ordnance Hospitals, K.H.; and Henry Sullivan, Member of the Royal College of Surgeons, of London.

"GREETING:—*Whereas*, in and by an Act of the Parliament of that part of this Province formerly known as Upper Canada, passed in the fifth-ninth year of the reign of His late Majesty King George the Third, entitled 'An Act to repeal an Act passed in the fifty-fifth year of His Majesty's reign, entitled "An Act to license Practitioners in Physic and Surgery throughout this Province, and to make further provision for licensing such Practitioners,"' it is, amongst other things, enacted that it shall and may be lawful for the Governor, Lieutenant-Governor, or Person administering the Government, for the time being, to constitute and appoint under his hand and Seal-at-Arms five or more persons legally authorized to practise Surgery or Midwifery in this Province to be a Board, whereof any three to be a quorum, to hear and examine all persons desirous to apply for a license to practise Physic, Surgery and Midwifery, or either of them, within this Province, and being satisfied by such examination that any person is duly qualified to practise Physic, Surgery and Midwifery, or either, to certify the same under the hands and seals of two or more of such Board in order that the person so applying may obtain a license.

"*Now know ye*, that being well assured of your integrity and ability, I do hereby, under and by virtue of the above-mentioned Act, nominate, constitute and appoint you, Christopher Widmer,

William C. Gwynne, Robert Hornby, Walter Telfer, William Durie and Henry Sullivan, to be a Board, whereof any three of you are to form a quorum, to hear and examine all persons desirous to apply for license to practise Physic, Surgery and Midwifery, or either of them, within that part of the Province of Canada, formerly constituting Upper Canada, and being satisfied by such examination that any person is duly qualified to practise Physic, Surgery and Midwifery, or either, to certify the same under the hands and seals of any two or more of you; and moreover, to do all such acts and things, as by virtue of the said Act, shall be by you to be done. To have, hold and enjoy the said office or Commission unto you the said Christopher Widmer, William Durie and Henry Sullivan, for and during pleasure, and your residence within that part of the Province formerly constituting Upper Canada, together with all and every the fees, profits, and advantages thereunto belonging and appertaining, hereby enjoining you that you do meet at the several days, and at the place in the said Act provided then and there to do whatsoever by this Commission and the said Act shall be to be done.

"Given under my hand and seal at Kingston, this twenty-eighth day of July, in the year of Our Lord One Thousand Eight Hundred and Forty-One, and in the Fifth year of Her Majesty's reign.

"(Signed) SYDENHAM.

"By command,

"(Signed) S. B. HARRISON,
"*Secretary.*"

July, 1841.—At this session, James Stewart, of Huntley, Bathurst District; Edward Dancey, of London District; Allen N. Wolverton, of Grimsby; Joseph Orlando Orr, of Toronto; Robert McCullough, of Gore District, who had a diploma from Geneva College, N.Y.; George Givins, of Toronto, and John Reid, R.C.S. Ed., received certificates.

October, 1841.—Present: C. Widmer, W. C. Gwynne, Walter Telfer, and Henry Sullivan.

The new commission received during the recess was ordered

to be read by the Secretary and entered on the minutes. It was then

Resolved,—That Mr. Widmer be President for the remainder of the year, and that Mr. George Givins be continued as Secretary.

In pursuance of the following resolution of the late College of Physicians and Surgeons, date January 6, 1841, viz.,—That the various papers and official documents belonging to the College be transferred to the Medical Board, to be received into the charge of such officers as they may appoint for the purpose—the Board resolved that the Secretary be empowered to receive and take charge of the said official documents and give a receipt for the same. The Board then adjourned.

One candidate was rejected at this quarterly meeting.

By an Imperial Act passed July 23, 1840, Upper and Lower Canada were united, forming the Province of Canada. At the first meeting of the Provincial Parliament, an Act was passed, September 18, 1841, authorizing qualified medical men of either Province to practise throughout the Province. (See Appendix.)

CHAPTER XX.

PROCEEDINGS OF U. C. MEDICAL BOARD—(*Continued*).

TORONTO, *January* 3, 1842.—Present: C. Widmer, Dr. Gwynne, Dr. Hornby, Dr. Telfer, Dr. H. Sullivan.

They first proceeded to elect officers for the ensuing year, when it was

Resolved,—That Dr. Widmer, be re-elected President, and Mr. George Givins be re-appointed Secretary.

It was then agreed that the subjects to be taken by each examiner for the ensuing year be as follows:

Dr. Gwynne, Anatomy; Dr. King, Pharmaceutic Chemistry and Materia Medica; Dr. Telfer, Surgery; Dr. Widmer, Theory and Practice of Physic; Dr. Sullivan, Midwifery.

January 8, 1842.—Present: C. Widmer, President; Dr. Gwynne, and Dr. Sullivan.

No candidate appearing for examination during this session, the Board terminated its sitting.

At a special meeting of the members of the Medical Board held this day, January 15 (Present: C. Widmer, President; Dr. Hornby, Dr. Gwynne, Dr. Telfer, and Dr. Sullivan), it was

Resolved,—That the following memorial to His Excellency the Governor-General as Chancellor of the University of King's College be adopted, and that it be signed by the members and forwarded to Kingston without delay:

"MEMORIAL.

"To His Excellency the Right Honourable Sir Charles Bagot, K.C.B., Governor-General of British North America, and Captain-General and Governor-in-Chief in and over the Province of Canada, Nova Scotia, New Brunswick and the Island of Prince Edward, and Vice-Admiral of the same, etc., etc., etc.

"The memorial of the members of the Medical Board in that part of the Province of Canada formerly constituting the Province of Upper Canada, respectfully sheweth that your memorialists hail with great satisfaction the arrival in the person of Your Excellency, of a statesman of superior talents and enlarged experience, whose wisdom will not fail to justly appreciate the object of your memorialists in addressing Your Excellency at this early period of Your Excellency's administration. The subject of your memorialists' present addresses had, your memorialists are well aware, excited the attention of Your Excellency's lamented predecessor, and but for the calamity which caused the death of the late Lord Sydenham, your memorialists have reason to believe, would have by this time received His Lordship's full consideration.

"Among the numerous classes of young men whose preliminary education has been completed in that excellent institution, Upper Canada College, many of course are destined for the learned professions. In those of the law and divinity no difficulty exists in following out the full completion of the necessary studies at home. But in the profession of medicine it is different; the student must resort to a foreign country to obtain his object, and unfortunately the neighbouring United States affords the only opportunity within his reach of acquiring the necessary information with economy. There, it is admitted, he may attain all the knowledge that is desired, but surely the necessity of resorting to such a source of instruction is to be deprecated, for no other result can be anticipated than the acquirement of those democratic principles which are so interwoven with the system there pursued.

"Your memorialists believe that it is unnecessary to inform Your Excellency that a munificent endowment for the education of youth has long ago been made by Royal Authority in granting the Charter of King's College in Western Canada. This endowment having lain dormant for many years, seems now to be almost forgotten.

"Your memorialists entertaining the fullest confidence in your sagacity as a statesman, approach Your Excellency now with the hope that Your Excellency will feel it necessary to take into consideration, at an early period, the useless condition into which this Royal Endowment has fallen, and make an arrangement for the commencement of a complete system of medical and surgical instruction, by establishing a Faculty of Medicine in the University of King's College.

"Deeply convinced that no greater source of satisfaction to the population of this part of the country could be effected by any measure of Your Excellency's administration, your memorialists conclude by expressing the hope that Your Excellency will discover no obstacle to the fulfilment of the prayer of this memorial.

"(Signed) · C. WIDMER, *President.*
G. E GIVINS, *Secretary.*"

"SECRETARY'S OFFICE,
"KINGSTON, *February* 11th, 1842.

"SIR,—I have the honour, by command of the Governor-General, to acknowledge the receipt of the memorial of the members of the Medical Board of that part of the Province, formerly Upper Canada, praying for the establishment of a Faculty of Medicine in the University of King's College.

"In reply, I am to acquaint you for the information of the Medical Board, that the subject will receive that early and attentive consideration from His Excellency which its importance merits.

"I have the honour to be, Sir,

"Your most Obedient, Humble Servant,

"JAMES HOPKIRK.

"G. E. GIVINS."

April, 1842.—Present : Widmer, Telfer, Gwynne and Hornby. Nathaniel E. Mainwaring, of St. George, Dumfries, a student of seven years, attended lectures at Fairfield and New York; Henry Riggs Goodman, of Grimsby; Beaumont Wilson, Bowen Dixie, of Toronto; John Robinson Dickson, of Niagara —passed. One candidate was rejected.

July, 1842.—Present: C. Widmer, President; Dr. Gwynne, Dr. Telfer and Mr. Sullivan. The Secretary, Mr. George Givins, having this day tendered his resignation of the office of Secretary, which being accepted, it was proposed by the President and seconded by Dr. Gwynne, that Mr. Edwin Henwood, the resident apothecary of the hospital, be appointed his successor, which was carried unanimously.

It was ordered, therefore, that Mr. Henwood do write to the Secretary of the Province announcing his appointment.

Horatio Yates, of Kingston (M.D., of Pennsylvania University), passed. One rejected.

October, 1842.—Present: Widmer, Hornby, Gwynne and Telfer. Patrick Trenor, R.C. Ed., and George Smith, of Flamboro', passed. One was rejected. The following letter was then read, addressed to the President:

"GODERICH, *September* 30th, 1842.

"SIR,—I have pursued the inquiry relative to the provincial license of —— ———— in the manner you suggested, and I am now able, positively, to state that he has procured it by the exhibition of a spurious diploma.

"I have communicated with Mr. Hopkirk, who says he produced a diploma from the University of Edinburgh, coupled with a strong recommendation from the Warden (Dr. Dunlop), the Sheriff, and Magistrates of this District.

"I have also received an answer from the University of Edinburgh, in which it is distinctly stated that no such person as —— ———— appears on their records as having obtained a diploma from them; a copy of these letters I will subjoin.

"As this is such a serious offence, and of so great importance to the profession generally and the community at large, it must not pass over unnoticed, and I now call upon you as the President and those who constitute the Medical Board (now you are in possession of the facts), to take such steps as will bring the matter before the proper tribunal. I am actuated by no other motive than that of maintaining the dignity and welfare of the College of which I have the honour to be a member, of protecting my professional brethren against a recurrence of a similar fraud, and of putting down these empirics.

"I beg leave to add that I have in my possession, letters from the College of Surgeons in Dublin and London, as also the Apothecaries' Hall, in which they one and all declare that this individual has never received a diploma or license from them. I have not given you a copy of these, as I do not consider it necessary; however, if requisite, I will forward one to you. I have only now to say that these letters are at any time subject to your perusal, and I will give you my personal attendance when required; from the information I have afforded you will, I am sure, see the propriety of at once proceeding against —— ————.

"Waiting your reply,

"I remain, your Obedient Servant,

"J. ACLAND DE LA HOOKE.

"*To* C. WIDMER, ESQ."

Copy of Mr. Hopkirk's letter:

"SECRETARY'S OFFICE, WEST,
"KINGSTON, *September* 24, 1842.

"SIR,—In reply to your letter of the 20th inst., I beg to inform you that a diploma was granted to —— ————, of Goderich, by authority of Provincial Statute, 8 Geo. 4, Ch. 3, he having forwarded to this office a diploma from the University of Edinburgh, dated August 1st, 1835, and made affidavit before Mr. Acland, the judge of the Huron District Court, that he was the person named therein. He also forwarded a certificate signed by the Warden, Sheriff, and several magistrates, testifying very strongly their opinion in his favour.

"I have the honour to be, Sir,
"Your most Obedient, Humble Servant,

"JAMES HOPKIRK,
"*Assistant-Secretary.*

"J. ACLAND DE LA HOOKE,
"*Goderich.*"

Copy of a letter from the University of Edinburgh:

"UNIVERSITY OF EDINBURGH, *August* 6th, 1842.

"It is hereby certified that the records of this University have been inspected, and that it does not appear that any such person as —— ———— ever received the degree of Doctor of Medicine at the University of Edinburgh.

"R. CHRISTISON, M.D., *Dean of Medical Faculty.*
"DAVID BROWN, *Sub-librarian.*"

"EDINBURGH, *August* 10th, 1842.

"It is hereby certified that, after careful inspection of the register of the Royal College of Physicians at Edinburgh, it does not appear that any diploma or license has been at any time granted to any person of the name of —— ————.

"DAVID CRAGIE, M.D.,
"*Counsellor and Secretary to the Royal College of Physicians at Edinburgh.*"

"TORONTO, *October* 4th, 1842.

"SIR,—Your letter to the President, of September 30th, has been laid before the Board, and it is a source of much regret that any individual should have adopted the course it would appear —— ———— has.

"The Board has not power, 'being only an examining body,' to pursue a prosecution, but under the flagrant circumstances of the case, feel it incumbent to address the Government on the subject.

"(Signed) E. HENWOOD,
"*Secretary.*

"*To* J. ACLAND DE LA HOOKE,
"*Surgeon, Goderich.*"

"TORONTO, *October* 4th, 1842.

"SIR,—The circumstance of a fictitious diploma having been presented to the Executive Government on a former occasion, the detection of which produced the sudden disappearance of the delinquent, combined with the fresh instance detailed in the accompanying copies of a correspondence received by the Medical Board at its present session, induces that body to press upon the attention of the Government the necessity of adopting some mode of verifying the character of all diplomas presented by candidates for a license.

"The Board suggests, as the most effectual means of accomplishing this object, that it should be incumbent on the applicant for a license to submit his diploma to the inspection of the Board, the members of which are necessarily the best judges of the true character of the signatures and seals usually appended to the various diplomas of the Universities and Chartered Bodies of Britain.

"If the power of the Government to enforce this reference is not warranted by the wording of the present statute, some further legislation on the subject becomes evidently necessary.

"In regard to the case, the particulars of which are enclosed, the Board trusts that such action will be taken by the proper authorities as will ensure the punishment of the perpetrator of so flagitious an act.

"By command of the Board,

"I have the honour to be, Sir,

"Your Obedient Servant,

"C. WIDMER, *President.*

"To the Honourable

"S. B. HARRISON,

"*Secretary*, etc., etc., etc."

George Smith, of Flamboro', passed his examination at this session. One was rejected: having presented himself at a late hour of the day, when there was not sufficient time to notify all the members of the Board to attend, it was

Resolved,—That the Secretary be instructed to notify all applicants for examination that "due notice" must be given by a registration of the applicant's name and the payment of his fees at least twenty-four hours before the day of examination.

The session then closed.

A copy of Mr. Harrison's letter to the President:

"SECRETARY'S OFFICE, WEST,

"KINGSTON, *October* 13th, 1842.

"SIR,—I have the honour to acknowledge your letter of the 4th inst., enclosing certain correspondence relating to a diploma granted to a Mr. ———, of Goderich, and in reply beg to inform you that I have called upon him, by command of the Governor-General, to transmit the original diploma by virtue of which the one for this Province was granted to him.

"I have the honour to be, Sir,

"Your most Obedient, Humble Servant,

"S. B. HARRISON.

"DR. WIDMER,

"*Toronto.*"

Strangely enough, the next letter in the minutes is on a somewhat analogous matter to the one just referred to, though the two cases have no connection the one with the other.

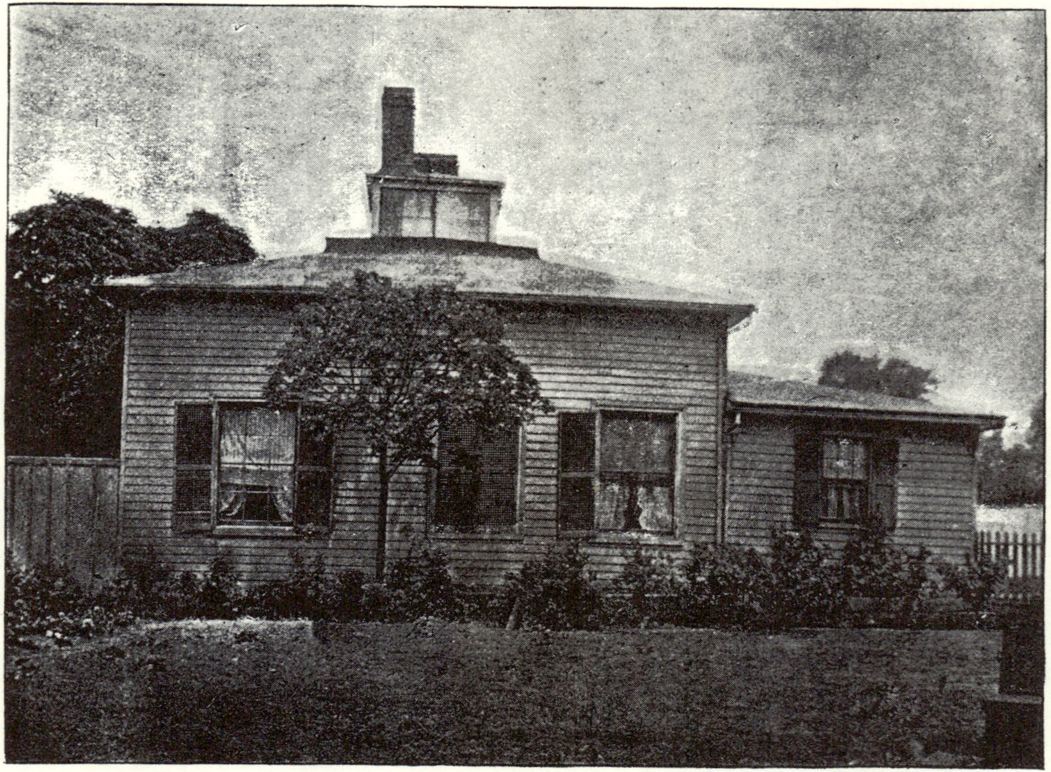

FIRST MEDICAL SCHOOL IN UPPER CANADA.

Medical Department, King's College, erected 1844.

James Hunter, jun., and John Fraser, R.C.P.S. Glas., passed. One was rejected.

The year 1843 was one of great importance to the medical profession of this Province. Repeated efforts had been fruitlessly made to establish a Medical School in Upper Canada, but now the fond hopes and aspirations of the profession to possess an establishment at home, where young men studying medicine might be fully prepared for practice without having to go elsewhere, were fully realized. An account of this important event will doubtless be acceptable to the reader.

CHAPTER XXI.

ESTABLISHMENT OF THE FIRST MEDICAL SCHOOL IN UPPER CANADA.

THE MEDICAL DEPARTMENT, KING'S COLLEGE.

THE first record we find relating to King's College is in a newspaper clipping—name of paper lost: "In 1842, the Parliament Buildings were fitted up for the use of the College, at an expense of £4,831 4 2, the larger part of this sum being expended on the College chapel, and in June, 1843, the institution was opened for education, with the following list of officers and professors: President, Bishop Strachan; Vice-President and Prof. of Rhetoric and Belles Lettres, Rev. Dr. McCaul; Theology, Rev. Dr. Beaven; Chemistry, Prof. Croft; Mathematics, Prof. Potter; Materia Medica, Prof. Nicol; Anatomy and Physiology, Prof. Gwynne; Obstetrics, Prof. Herrick; Medicine, Prof. King; Practical Anatomy, Prof. Sullivan; Surgery, Prof. Beaumont; Law, Prof. Blake."

At a meeting of the Council of King's College, September 25, 1843, a "committee for establishing the Medical School" was appointed, consisting of the Vice-President, Dr. McCaul; Profs. Potter, Croft and Gwynne. They "are requested to consult the members of the profession connected with the University, viz., Dr. King, Mr. Beaumont and Mr. Sullivan." In what way they were connected with the University does not appear. But probably it was an agreement that they should become members of the Medical Faculty. Dr. King was appointed a member of the Council, September 23, 1844, and Dr. Beaumont, September 27, 1848.

October 4, 1843.—Prof. Gwynne submitted the report of the Committee of Medical School. The report was received and discussion deferred until next meeting.

October 6.—Part of the report adopted. On the 9th the whole was adopted. The Medical Committee are of the opinion—

"1st. That in order to constitute an efficient School of Medicine in the University of King's College, it is necessary that provision should be made for adequate instruction in the following branches: Medical Science, Chemistry, Theory and Practice of Medicine, Theory and Practice of Surgery, Materia Medica and Pharmacy, Midwifery and Diseases of Women and Children.

"2nd. Also of opinion that it will conduce to the interests of the Medical School, and be more in accordance with the usages of some British universities if the designation of Demonstrator of Anatomy be altered to that of 'Professor of Practical Anatomy.'

"3rd. Lectures upon the following subjects may be instituted with advantage at some future period: Forensic Medicine and Botany.

"4th. In addition to provision for instruction in the above branches of science, a hospital capable of containing not less than eighty beds for medical and surgical cases will be required, and separate accommodation for, at least, six puerperal patients will also be necessary.

"5th. The following shall be the medical requirements for a student presenting himself at the final examination for his degree: A certificate that he has attained the age of twenty-one years; that he has passed five years in acquaintance of medical knowledge, three of which must have been occupied in attendance on medical lectures in schools recognized by the University, and one, at least, in the Medical School of this

University. That he shall produce certificates of attendance on the following lectures and hospital practice: Chemistry, one course of six months; Practical Chemistry, one course of six months; Anatomy and Physiology, two courses of six months; Medicine, two courses of six months; Surgery, two courses of six months; Materia Medica and Pharmacy, one course of six months; Midwifery and Diseases of Women and Children, one course of six months; that he has attended for, at least, eighteen months on the Medical and Surgical practice of an hospital containing not less than eighty beds, twelve months of which shall be during winter sessions, when lectures on Clinical Medicine and Surgery will be delivered.

"N.B.—Two courses of three months each will be considered equivalent to one of six months.

"6th. Having examined the scale of fees adopted in other universities, both in Europe and America, the Committee are inclined to recommend the following:

	£	s.	d.
"Chemistry - - - - - -	£4	0	0
"Practical Chemistry - - - -	2	10	0
"Anatomy and Physiology - - -	4	0	0
"Medicine - - - - - -	4	0	0
"Surgery - - - - - -	4	0	0
"Practical Anatomy - - - -	4	0	0
"Materia Medica and Pharmacy - -	2	10	0
"Midwifery and Diseases of Women and Children - - - - -	2	10	0

Hospital Attendance.

	£	s.	d.
"18 months - - - - - -	15	0	0
"12 months - - - - - -	12	10	0
" 6 months - - - - - -	7	10	0
"Or a perpetual ticket - - - -	20	00	0

(Other clauses 7th and 8th not inserted.)

"9th. The medical sessions should commence on the first Monday in November, and terminate on the last Monday in April.

"10th. It will be expedient to appropriate one of the wings

of the Parliament Buildings to the Medical Faculty, which will supply sufficient accommodation for their purposes.

"11th. It is expedient to enter into arrangement to secure the exchange of recognition of our certificates by other universities, by the Army Medical Board and the medical institutes incorporated by charter, which may be submitted by this University."

The only amendment to this report was "that it is desirable that the medical session shall commence at the same time with the Faculty of Arts."

Dr. Gwynne moved a resolution asking "His Excellency for the use of the eastern wing of Parliament Buildings, which it is understood will shortly be vacated by the Law Society and officers of the courts of law." Carried.

November 4, 1843.—The draft of the proposed salary attached to each subject, forming the committee of medical study, was submitted with the names of the professors:

Anatomy and Physiology - - - -	£200
Theory and Practice of Physic - - -	200
Theory and Practice of Surgery - - -	200
Midwifery and Diseases of Women and Children - - - - - -	200
Materia Medica and Botany - - -	200
Practical Anatomy - - - - -	250

November 29, 1843.—Wm. R. Beaumont appointed Professor of Surgery.

December 21, 1843.—Warrants of His Excellency the Chancellor, granting professorships in the University, were produced and read: Dated December 6, 1843, George Herrick, Esq., M.D., Midwifery and Diseases of Women and Children; December 7, Wm. Bulwer Nicol, Esq., Materia Medica; December 8, Henry Sullivan, Esq., Practical Anatomy and Curator of the Anatomical and Pathological Museum.

December 27, 1843.—Report of Medical Faculty said they had taken into consideration the steps necessary to be taken, in order to put the medical department into speedy and efficient operation. They recommend that the following measures should be adopted without delay:

"1st. That inaugural lectures should be delivered by each of the professors in his own department, on the first two days of term in the public hall. Regular course of lectures commencing January 15th, 1844. (It is said that Dr. Herrick found it somewhat embarrassing in delivering his introductory lecture before the ladies.) That immediate arrangements should be made with the trustees of the hospital, whereby the professors of the Medical Faculty should have either the exclusive medical superintendence thereof, or a certain number of wards reserved for their sole use.

"Arrangements should be made for procuring subjects for the use of students (students to pay for these).

"It was ordered that for the present the rooms occupied as the museum and workshop, shall be the apartment wherein the school of medicine shall be conducted, and that the business of the school shall commence there on Monday, January 15th, 1844, and that a frame building erected on the north or west side of the western wing will be sufficient for the above purposes.

"The table of lectures, plan of dissecting room and anatomical theatre were submitted. This was to be built forthwith. Tenders for dissecting room received, and work allotted to McBean & Withrow for £276, to be built within four weeks."

January 6, 1844.—A letter from Dr. Widmer, Chairman, Board of Trustees, Toronto Hospital, was read, offering to surrender the whole of the upper flat of the hospital to the Medical Faculty of the University, for their exclusive use on the following conditions:

"1st. £100 to be paid to the trustees to furnish additional equipments.

"2nd. 3s. per diem be paid monthly for each patient in the medical faculty.

"3rd. A list of medical faculty be furnished to the trustees that they may be individually appointed by them to the offices as medical attendants of the hospital.

"4th. That the members of the medical faculty be subject to the rules and regulations at present in force regarding the general economy of the hospital, etc."

"The Council after much deliberation on this matter regret they cannot accede to the proposition."

January 10, 1844.—Regulations relating to medical studies: To be two classes. 1st. Those who are candidates for degrees; 2nd. Occasional students. First class to wear academical habit.

Resolved,—That Profs. Gwynne, Beaumont and Sullivan be authorized to enter into engagement for procuring subjects; Bursar to advance requisite funds. Dr. Paget to be written to and authorized to expend the sum of money remaining in his hands, as to him may seem most advantageous for the medical department.

By this it is inferred that Dr. Paget was engaged in looking after subjects for dissection.

The Medical Faculty of King's College was composed of W. C. Gwynne, John King, W. R. Beaumont, Geo. Herrick, W. B. Nicol, Henry Sullivan.

There is no record of the number of students in attendance during this first session beginning January 15. It was only a fragment of a session and doubtless the attendance was small. It was the session of 1844-45 which marked the beginning of the regular work of a medical school. At the beginning of the lectures, 1843, there were but two matriculated students, J. H. Richardson and —. Lyons. Dr. R. was the only student in our branch, at least.

As to the equipment of the school, the records of the Council show that there had been purchased medical instruments to the value of £355 16 10, and for the medical school there had been expended £114 3 6.

The following is a list of Professors in all the departments of King's College at that time:

1843. Rev. John McCaul, LL.D., Classic Literature, Logic, Rhetoric and Belles Lettres.

1843. Rev. James Beaven, D.D., Divinity, Metaphysics and Ethics.
1843. Richard Potter, M.A., Mathematics and Natural Philosophy.
1843. H. H. Croft, Chemistry and Experimental Philosophy.
1843. W. C. Gwynne, M.B., Anatomy and Physiology.
1843. John King, M.D., Theory and Practice of Medicine.
1843. W. H. Blake, B.A., Law and Jurisprudence.
1843. W. Beaumont, F.R.C.S. England, Principles and Practice of Surgery.
1843. George Herrick, M.D., Obstetrics and Diseases of Women and Children.
1843. W. B. Nicol, Materia Medica, Pharmacy and Botany.
1843. H. Sullivan, M.R.C.S. England, Practical Anatomy and Curator of Pathological Museum.
1845. Lucius O'Brien, M.D., Medical Jurisprudence.
1839. Henry Boys, M.D., was appointed Registrar and Bursar.
1845. L. O'Brien, received M.D. (*ad eundem*).
1845. E. M. Hodder, C.M.
1849. J. H. Richardson, M.B.

The following is taken from *Fasti Academici*, from 1827 to 1850:

"King's College at York (now Toronto) was established by His late Majesty George IV., by Charter bearing date March 15th, 1827, with the style and privileges of a University. It was endowed by the same Sovereign with 225,914 acres of land, by patent bearing date January 3rd, 1828.

"In the year 1837, the two Houses of the Legislature of Upper Canada amended the Charter by a Bill to which the Lieutenant-Governor gave the royal assent, March 4th of that year.

"In the year 1842, on April 23rd, the foundation stone of the building in the University Park was laid by His Excellency the Right Hon. Sir Charles Bagot, G.C.B., M.A., Christ Church, Oxford, Governor-General of British North America, etc.

"In the year 1843, temporary accommodation having been provided in the Parliament Buildings, the first matriculation of students took place; and the inaugural addresses and lectures were delivered on June 8th and 9th.

"In the year 1849, the two Houses of the Legislature of Canada, by a Bill to which the Deputy-Governor gave the royal assent, May 30th of that year, repealed the Act of 1837, and 'so much of the said Charter so granted by His late Majesty King George IV., as aforesaid, as is contradictory with this Act or any of the provisions thereof, or as makes any provision in any matter provided for by this Act, other than such as is hereby made in such matter.'

"On October 25th, 1849, His Excellency the Right Hon. the Earl of Elgin and Kincardine, K.T., M.A., Merton College, Oxford, Governor-General of British North America, etc., presided as Chancellor at the last commencement of King's College.

"On January 1st, 1850, the new Act came into operation, and the institution is hereafter to be conducted, according to its provisions, under the designation of 'The University of Toronto.'"

In the year 1843, an important Act was passed by Parliament "to regulate and facilitate the study of Anatomy." (See Appendix.)

CHAPTER XXII.

FURTHER PROCEEDINGS OF THE MEDICAL BOARD.

TORONTO, *January*, 1844.—Returning to the proceedings of the Medical Board, the Board met. Present: Drs. Widmer, Gwynne, Telfer, Sullivan and Hornby. Dr. Widmer was re-elected President, and E. Henwood, Secretary. John Kirk, of Moulton, Niagara District, passed. One was rejected.

April, 1844.—Present: Drs. Widmer, Gwynne, Hornby, Telfer and Sullivan. Wm Tempest, Toronto, passed. Three were rejected.

July, 1844.—Present: Drs. Widmer, Telfer, Gwynne, Hornby and Sullivan. Joseph Augustus Vervay, of Amherstburg, and Thomas Moore, of Picton, passed. Two were rejected.

October, 1844.—Present: Drs. Widmer, Telfer, Hornby, Gwynne and Sullivan. Fred. Pugh, of Guelph, and Thomas Holywell received certificates.

The Board having taken into consideration the application of Dr. Crew for an opinion on certain charges made by him for attendance and medicines on the Indians of the Credit, resolve that the Statute does not empower the Board to decide on such matters.

Resolved,—That the Secretary of the Board be directed to communicate with the Civil Secretary of the Government, with a view to obtaining a correct list of the licensed medical practitioners of this Province up to the present period, in order that the Board may be in a position to give correct information upon this subject to such persons as may require it.

January, 1845.—Present: Drs. Widmer, Hornby, Telfer, Sullivan and Gwynne. The President and Secretary were re-elected. Richard Walsh Trunners and Edwin Henwood, "Resident Apothecary at the Toronto Hospital," passed. Two were rejected.

April, 1845.—Present: Drs. Widmer, Hornby, Telfer and Sullivan. Charles Jones, of Esquesing, educated "at the Borough Hospital, London," and John Moffatt, of Toronto, passed. One was rejected.

July 7, 1845.—A new Commission was read appointing Christopher Widmer, William C. Gwynne, Robert Hornby, Walter Telfer, William Durie, Henry Sullivan, John King, William Beaumont, George Herrick, William B. Nicol and Joseph Hamilton to be a Board, whereof any three are to be a quorum, to hear and examine all persons desirous to apply for a license to practise Physic, Surgery and Midwifery, or either of them, dated seventh day of May, one thousand eight hundred and forty-five.

The members present under the Commission were as follows: Drs. Hamilton, Telfer, Herrick, Nicol, Sullivan, Beaumont, Gwynne, Widmer, and King.

Resolved,—That Mr. Widmer be the President for the ensuing year; also, that Mr. Henwood be continued as Secretary.

The following resolution, proposed by Dr. Gwynne, and seconded by Dr. Beaumont, was lost, viz.:

"That not more than five members be permitted to examine any one candidate, and that the fees payable by the candidate be divided amongst the examining members."

Dr. King proposed the following resolution, seconded by Dr. Hamilton, which was carried: "That it be understood that the hour of twelve o'clock noon be the hour of the opening of the Board on all future occasions."

G. L. Beard, of Woodstock (M.D., Pennsylvania), was the only one who passed, out of six candidates. Four were rejected for ignorance of the classics. One of the rejected was an M.D. of Jefferson Medical College, and one an M.R.C.S. of Edinburgh.

October, 1845.—Present: Drs. Widmer, Hornby, Hamilton, Herrick, Nicol, King, and Beaumont.

The new broom continued to sweep clean, as all the candidates, five in number, were rejected. One was an M.D. of the Willoughby University, in the State of Ohio.

January, 1846.—Present: Drs. Widmer, Telfer, King, Beaumont, Herrick, Nicol, and Hamilton.

Moved by Dr. King, and seconded by Dr. Hamilton, that it be

Resolved,—That inasmuch as Dr. Widmer is senior in the Commission, and as such, by right, President of this Board, it is not necessary, in the opinion of the Board, that in future any election for President should take place.

Thomas C. Macklem, of Niagara, from University of Edinburgh, and McGill College, passed, and one was rejected.

April, 1846.—Present: Dr. Gwynne, President (acting) Drs. Hornby, Herrick, Beaumont, Hamilton, Nicol and King.

Reginald Henwood, of Toronto; Henry Hanson, of London; Michael George Long, of Aylmer, from Dublin and King's College, Toronto; and John Gunn, of Whitby, passed. Three candidates were rejected; one because he was "found quite ignorant of the Latin language."

The circumstance of Mr. James Atkinson having illegally

obtained a license to practise Physic, Surgery and Midwifery, from the Government, being brought under the notice of the Board by a member of that body, the Board came to the decision that the following letter upon the subject should be addressed to the Provincial Secretary:

"TORONTO, *April* 7th, 1846.

"SIR,—I have the honour, by order of the Medical Board of Canada West in quarterly session assembled, respectfully to direct the attention of His Excellency the Administrator of the Government, to the circumstance of a license to practise Physic, Surgery and Midwifery having been granted to a person of the name of James Atkinson, of Kingston, on November the 27th, 1844, upon his presenting a diploma from the Royal College of Medicine, London.

"As no such body as the Royal College of Medicine, London, is recognized by the Act of the Provincial Legislature, 8th George 4, Ch. 3, or by any Imperial Statute, the Medical Board have directed me respectfully to submit that the Government has been imposed upon, and under the influence of such imposition have, in direct violation of the law, granted a license to the said James Atkinson.

"The Medical Board are desirous also of stating that they think it a duty they owe to the public and to the profession of medicine, to make it known to His Excellency that impositions have from time to time been practised upon the Government, by which ignorant and illiterate persons have been authorized to practise, and who, as recognized medical men, are alike detrimental to the public safety, and disgraceful to an honourable and learned profession.

"I have the honour, etc.,

"E. HENWOOD,

"*Secretary*.

"*To* THE HONOURABLE D. DALY,

"*Provincial Secretary, etc., Montreal.*"

The Board adjourned with the understanding that a meeting was to be called by the Secretary for Saturday, the 11th inst., to take into consideration the propriety of addressing the Legislature in relation to a Medical Bill which is about being introduced into Parliament.

The following resolution was proposed by Dr. Herrick, and seconded by Dr. Beaumont, viz:

Resolved,—That the Medical Board having lately heard that certain Petitions have been forwarded to both Houses of Legislature, praying for the enactment of measures which if carried into effect would materially interfere with the privileges of this Board, and of the medical profession generally in Canada West. Be it resolved, that the Secretary be directed to frame a Petition addressed to each House of the Legislature praying that a copy of any Bill which may be introduced into either House having such a tendency, may be forwarded to this Board for their opinion thereon prior to any action being taken upon such Bill.

It was proposed by Dr. Beaumont, and agreed to by the Board, that a copy of the Petition alluded to in the foregoing resolution, should be forwarded by the Secretary to the Honourable John Hamilton, with a request that he should take charge of it in Legislative Council; and likewise another copy to the Honourable R. Baldwin, that he should take charge of it in the House of Assembly.

Dr. Nicol and Dr. Gwynne were deputed by the Board to superintend the carrying into effect the object of the meeting.

Copy of Petition addressed both "To the Honourable the Legislative Council and Legislative Assembly of the Province of Canada in Parliament assembled":

"PETITION.—The Petition of the Medical Board of Canada West respectfully sheweth, That the Medical Board having lately heard that Petitions have been forwarded to your Honourable House praying for some alterations in the government of the medical profession within that portion of the Province formerly constituting the Province of Upper Canada, your Petitioners therefore humbly pray that a copy of any Bill which may be introduced into your Honourable House in any manner affecting the privileges of this Board, or of the Medical Practitioners generally in that portion of the Province formerly constituting Upper Canada, may be forwarded to this Board in order to give your Petitioners an opportunity of expressing to your Honourable House their opinion upon the Provisions and subject matter of such Bill, prior to any action being taken thereon by your Honourable House, and your Petitioners as in duty bound will ever pray.

"By order of the Medical Board,

"E. HENWOOD, *Secretary.*

"Toronto, April 11th, 1846."

Copy of letter accompanying Petition addressed both to the Honourable John Hamilton and the Honourable R. Baldwin :

"TORONTO, *April* 11th, 1846.

"SIR,—At a meeting of the Medical Board, held at the City of Toronto this 11th day of April, it was resolved that a Petition should be presented to the Honourable the Legislative Council of the Province of Canada in Parliament assembled; and it was at the same meeting likewise resolved that such Petition should be forwarded to you with the request that you would be pleased to undertake the charge of presenting the same to the Honourable the Legislative Council of the Province of Canada in Parliament assembled, at an early opportunity.

"I have therefore the honour in pursuance of the order of the said Board to transmit the enclosed Petition to you, and to request upon behalf of the Board that you will be pleased to take charge of the same, and present it to the Honourable the Legislative Council of the Province of Canada in Parliament assembled, at your earliest convenience.

"I have the honour to be, Sir,

"Your most Obedient, Humble Servant,

"E. HENWOOD, *Sec. of the Med. Bd.*

"*To* THE HON. JOHN HAMILTON,

"*Legislative Councillor.*"

July, 1846.—Present: Hon. Dr. Widmer, Drs. Hamilton, Nicol, Beaumont, Herrick and Hornby. James Nichol, of Perth, R.C.S. Ed.; Gavin Russell, of Carleton; John Reid, of

Toronto; Benj. Dickey, of London, passed. One candidate rejected.

October, 1846.—Present: Drs. Widmer, Hornby, Herrick, Hamilton, Beaumont, Nicol and King. Only one candidate, who was rejected.

It was proposed by Dr. King, and seconded by Dr. Hamilton, that a committee be formed of the members present, to wait on the Hon. Mr. Draper, on the subject of the medical profession.

CHAPTER XXIII.

COMMUNICATIONS WITH THE MEDICAL BOARD OF MONTREAL.

TORONTO, *January*, 1847.—Present: Drs. Widmer, Beaumont, Nicol, Herrick and Telfer. There were no candidates.

April, 1847.—Present: Drs. Widmer, Hornby, Herrick, Nicol, Hamilton, Beaumont, Gwynne and Telfer. James Salmon, of Simcoe; "Henry Lord, of Lacolle, near Montreal, who presented a Commission as Assistant-Surgeon in the Provincial Cavalry," and John Harvey, of Kingston, received certificates. Two were rejected.

The following resolution was proposed by Dr. Gwynne and carried unanimously:

"*Resolved*,—That it has hitherto been customary with the Government to furnish this Board from time to time with a copy of the Statutes in order to facilitate their business, and that the Secretary be directed to apply to the proper authority for a copy of the Revised Statutes of the Province, recently published.

"*Resolved*,—That the Chairman be requested to correspond with the Medical Boards of Montreal and Quebec on the subject of the institution of a uniform system of examination for candidates applying for certificates of the said Boards and this Board, and of the mutual exchange of the names of rejected candidates with the reason of their rejection, and the period during which they have been recommended to continue their studies before presenting themselves for re-examination."

The following is a copy of a letter addressed to the President of the Medical Boards of Montreal and of Quebec:

"TORONTO, *April* 26, 1847.

"SIR,—The following is a copy of a resolution passed at this April session of the Medical Board of Canada West:

"The course this Board pursues in the examination of candidates is as follows:

"1st. Some acquaintance with the Latin language is required. With this view, if the candidate cannot construe some paragraphs of Gregory's Conspectus, a portion of the Pharmacopœia Londinensis or a Latin written prescription was substituted; in the event of a total failure in these, the professional examination is not proceeded in. If the Latin examination is satisfactory then follow:

"2nd. Materia Medica and Pharmaceutic Chemistry.

"3rd. Anatomy and Physiology.

"4th. The Theory and Practice of Medicine.

"5th. Practical Surgery.

"6th. Midwifery and the Diseases of Children.

"We hope for the concurrence of your Board with the spirit of the resolution transmitted: for we cannot but believe that the licensing of a candidate by a certificate from one Provincial Board after his rejection at another exhibits an anomaly productive of an unfavourable impression as regards the rules that regulate the course of the examining bodies.

"I have the honour to be, Sir,
"Your Obedient Servant,

"(Signed) C. WIDMER.

"*To the President of the Medical Board*
"*of Montreal.*"

Copy of a letter received from the Secretary of the Montreal Medical Board:

"MONTREAL, *May* 5th, 1847.

"SIR,—The President of Montreal Medical Board this day laid before the Board your favour of the 26th April, to which I have been directed to reply. The Board entirely acquiesce in the spirit of the resolution passed by the Toronto Medical Board, and have desired me to establish the communication requested, and in accordance therewith I enclose a letter to your Secretary containing our proceedings at this meeting. Our examinations are similar, with the exception of Latin, which C. R. Ogden, Esq., then Attorney-General, informed us we were not empowered to enforce an acquaintance with.

"The Quebec Board acting on the advice of Sir James Stuart, then a barrister, enforce four years' study, and a preliminary examination in Classics.

"I am, your Obedient Servant,

"S. E. SEWELL, M.D.,
"*Secretary, M.M.B.*

"C. WIDMER, ESQ.,
"*Chairman, Medical Board for Canada West.*"

"MONTREAL, *May*, 1847.

"SIR,—At the spring quarterly meeting of the Montreal Medical Board, held at the Court House, on the 4th and 5th inst., the following gentlemen were examined and were recommended for license to practise Physic, Surgery and Midwifery: Messrs. Charles Keefer, I. C. Butler, David P. Yeomans, W. C. Allen, John Clarke, J. C. Montgomery, C. H. Latour, A. Fanceuf (?) and A. B. Larocque.

"The following gentlemen were remanded to their studies for six months: Messrs. Jas. Culver, J. R. Lee, P. P. Piercy, L. E. Bardy, L. Larne, Moise Sabourise and Louis Genaud.

"I remain,
"Your Obedient Servant,

"S. C. SEWELL, M.D.,
"*Secretary, M.M.B.*

"*To the Secretary of the Medical Board*
"*for Canada West.*"

July, 1847.—Present: Drs. Widmer, Hornby, Hamilton, Herrick, King, Nicol and Beaumont.

Samuel Seager, of Walsingham; Alexander McDougall, of Niagara, Geo. Herod, of Guelph; Charles Cameron, received certificates. Two were rejected on their Latin.

October, 1847.—Present: Drs. Gwynne, Hornby, Nicol and Hamilton.

I. Duncomb, of Richmond Hill; M. Hardy, of Smithfield; Francis Armstrong, of Amherst Island, R.C.S. Dublin; James A. Whiting, of Dumfries, and John Roy Philip, of Waterloo, passed. It was then

Resolved,—That the Secretary be instructed to send to the Montreal Medical Board a list of the names of all candidates who may have presented themselves during the last and present session of this Board.

At a special meeting of members of the Medical Board, held this day (November 16), a letter published in the *Globe* newspaper of the 13th inst., was read, and the following letter written to the editor of that paper:

[No. 1.]

"SIR,—At a meeting of the members of the Medical Board held this day, a letter published in the *Globe* newspaper of the 13th inst., was read.

"As this letter contains matter of a libellous nature affecting the character and honour of the Medical Board, I am directed to call upon you, as the editor of the *Globe*, to afford me the name of the author of the said letter, to enable the Board to take such steps in the matter as it may deem necessary.

"I am, Sir,
"Your Obedient Servant,

"E. HENWOOD,
"*Secretary, T.M.B.*

"J. G. BROWN, ESQ.,
"*Editor of the 'Globe.'*"

[No. 2.]

"'GLOBE' OFFICE,
"TORONTO, *November* 17th, 1847.

"SIR,—In reply to your letter without date received this day, I have to inform you that Dr. R. Hunter, late of Markham, and now of Toronto, is the author of the communication in the *Globe* referred to.

"I am, Sir,
"Your Obedient Servant,

"GEO. BROWN.
(*Per* J. G. BROWN.)

"E. HENWOOD, ESQ.,
"*Secretary, Medical Board.*"

[No. 3.]

"TORONTO, *November* 22nd, 1847.

"SIR,—Enclosed is a copy of a letter written to the editor of the *Globe* newspaper and his reply thereto. The Medical Board of Canada West in forwarding these letters to you, request that the name of the member of the Board whom you state made you the disgraceful offer of obtaining you a license for the sum of ten pounds may be forwarded to the Board, and that if you may be in possession of any collateral evidence to substantiate your accusation, you will communicate the same for the information of the Board.

"I am, Sir,
"Your Obedient Servant,

"E. HENWOOD,
"*Secretary, T.M.B.*

"DR. R. HUNTER,
"*Church Street, Toronto.*"

November 26, 1847.—The Board met, when the following letter from Dr. Hunter was read :

[No. 4.]

"CHURCH STREET, TORONTO, *November* 24th, 1847.

"SIR,—In reply to your letter of the 22nd inst., conveying a request from the Medical Board of Canada West, to forward for the information of the Board the name of the member who offered to procure me a license for ten pounds, I have only to say that, much as I deprecate the act, I have no desire to victimize an individual. I wrote defensively, not vindictively. Indulging a hope that the learned member who proved himself so devoid of honour and so unworthy of public trust, has ere this repented his gross abuse of the confidence reposed in him, and as giving up his name can only be productive of private injury and perhaps the ruin of an individual without accomplishing any material result, the writer prefers leaving him to the renovating process of time, hoping yet to see him rise from the wreck of moral principle.

"As to the grounds of my letter in the *Globe* of the 13th inst., signed 'A Newly-Licensed Practitioner,' I am prepared to maintain all that is there put forth, though I cannot but feel that it would be more creditable to certain gentlemen to pursue the honest course of their profession than to prostitute their very high position and their superior education by uniting their energies to crush 'A Newly-Licensed Practitioner.'

"I have the honour to be, Sir,
"Etc., etc., etc.

"R. HUNTER, M.D.

"E. HENWOOD, ESQ.,
"*Secretary, T.M.B.*, etc., etc., etc."

[No. 5.]

Resolved,—That the President be authorized to forward a copy of the foregoing correspondence, together with the copy of the *Globe* of November 13, to the Secretary of the Province, with the request of the Board that he will obtain the opinion of the Law-officer of the Crown as to the steps to be pursued for obtaining a just vindication of the character and honour of this Board.

The following is a copy of the President's letter to the Provincial Secretary:

"TORONTO, *December* 1st, 1847.

"SIR,—In compliance with a resolution of the Medical Board of Canada West, passed at a meeting of the Board, held on the 26th ult, a copy of which, marked 'No. 5,' is enclosed, I have the honour to forward to you the newspaper in which the article complained of will be found (signed 'A Newly-Licensed Practitioner'), and to request that you will be pleased to lay the same, together with the accompanying correspondence, before the Attorney-General, who will, the Medical Board confidently hopes, adopt such measures either by filing an *ex-officio* information for libel against the author of this production, or such other course as in the opinion of the Attorney-General may best secure the character of the Medical Board from the effects which the publication of so malicious a libel is calculated to produce on the public mind. Moreover, the Medical Board trusts that, in the exercise of its legitimate functions for the public service, it may be considered as justly entitled to all the protection that the power of the Government is capable of affording it.

"I have the honour to be, Sir,
"Your Obedient Servant,

"C. WIDMER, M.D.,
"*President, T.M.B.*

"*To* THE HON. D. DALY,
"*Provincial Secretary*, etc., etc., etc."

"SECRETARY'S OFFICE,
"MONTREAL, *December* 11th, 1847.

"SIR,—I have the honour, by command of the Governor-General, to acknowledge the receipt of your letter of the 1st inst., as President of the Medical Board of Canada West, with its enclosures, transmitting, in compliance with a Resolution passed by that Board on the 26th ultimo, a copy of the *Globe* newspaper of the 13th ultimo, containing a certain libellous letter (signed 'A Newly-Licensed Practitioner') affecting the character of the Board, and to inform you that I have, in accordance with the request contained in your letter, submitted the same to the Honourable the Attorney-General for Canada West, with a view to his taking such steps in the premises as to him may appear advisable, in the event of the case being, in his opinion, of such a nature as to call for the interference of the Executive Government.

"I have the honour to be, Sir,
"Your most Obedient Servant,

"E. A. MEREDITH,
"*Assistant-Secretary.*

"THE HON. C. WIDMER,
"*President of the Medical Board of*
"*Canada West, Toronto.*

"A true copy.
"E. HENWOOD, *Secretary.*"

CHAPTER XXIV.

LIBELLOUS ATTACKS UPON THE BOARD.

TORONTO, *January*, 1848.—Present: Drs. Widmer, Telfer, Herrick, Beaumont and Nicol.

Doctor Godfrey H. Schmutter, of Berlin, who "exhibited a diploma of Doctor of Medicine and Surgery from Berlin, Prussia," and Joshua Fidlar, of Lindsay, passed.

Resolved,—That the Secretary be directed to communicate with the Civil Secretary of the Government, with a view of obtaining a continuation of the list of Licensed Medical Practitioners of this Province, since the last report of July 16, 1845, up to the present period.

April, 1848.—Present: Drs. Widmer, Gwynne, Hornby, Sullivan, King, Beaumont, Nicol and Herrick.

Wm. H. Wilson, of Simcoe; George Holmes, of Perth, R.C.S. Dublin, late Assistant Royal Marine Hospital, Plymouth; Wm. Scott, of Woodstock; David Farrer, of London; John Phelan, of

Toronto; and Edward Hipkins, of Richmond Hill, passed. Five candidates were rejected. It was

Resolved,—That Drs. Gwynne and Sullivan be requested to wait upon the Attorney-General, to state the correspondence that has already taken place between this Board and the Government on the subject of a libellous attack made on the Board in November last, and that Drs. Gwynne and Sullivan will be pleased to communicate to the Board before this session closes, the result of their interview with the Attorney-General. It was

Resolved,—That every member of the Board who shall be present at the time of the votes being taken as to the passing of candidates, shall sign his name to the certificate, it being understood that he signs such certificate not individually, but as the act of the majority of the Board alone; and that the names of the members voting for this resolution shall be entered on the minutes. Yeas: The President, Drs. Gwynne, King, Beaumont, Herrick, and Nicol. Nays: Dr. Hornby.

The Committee appointed on the 3rd inst. to wait on the Attorney-General reported the following letter as the result of their communication:

"FRONT STREET, *April* 7, 1848.

"MY DEAR SIR,—I have read the papers you left with me from the Medical Board, and must in the first instance ascertain from the late Attorney-General what had been done by him on the reference spoken of in the Assistant-Secretary's letter, and will take the instructions of the Government, if necessary, on the subject.

"I remain, Yours, etc.,

"ROBERT BALDWIN.

"DR. SULLIVAN.

"A true copy.

"E. HENWOOD, *Secretary.*"

July 3, 1848.—Present: Hon. Christopher Widmer, President; Drs. King, Sullivan, Nicol, Hornby, Herrick and Beaumont.

The first business was appointing a Secretary. It was

Resolved,—That whereas Mr. Henwood, late Secretary to the

Board, has changed his residence from Toronto, it is expedient that a successor be immediately appointed. It was

Resolved,—That Edward Clarke, M.R.C.S. Edinburgh, the House Surgeon to the Toronto General Hospital, be appointed Secretary.

Mr. Clarke was ordered to procure a new minute-book, and charge the members of the Board with the amount of the cost.

Dr. Sullivan produced a note from the Attorney-General, to the effect that the report of the late Attorney-General, on the subject of the papers left with him, had not been found; but, as it was understood it was not favourable to action being taken in the matter, I write you that the Board might see that the subject has not been forgotten. (Signed) R. BALDWIN.

At this session, Egerton Perry, Cobourg; Samuel Sedden Woolbank, Toronto; Horace Croft Hastings, Toronto; Wm. Case Wright, and John Clark Wasbrick received certificates for license. Two were rejected.

October, 1848.—Present: Widmer, Herrick, Hornby, Nicol, King and Gwynne.

Wm. Johnson, Sarnia, and John Nation, Toronto, passed their examination. One candidate rejected.

January, 1849.—Present: Widmer, Beaumont, Hornby, Nicol and Herrick.

George Perks, of Newboro', Johnston District, passed, the only candidate at this session.

April, 1849.—Present: Widmer, King, Gwynne, Sullivan, Nicol, Beaumont, Hornby and Herrick.

The following passed and received certificates for license to practise: Alex. Harvey, of Peterboro'; W. G. Middleton, of Guelph; W. T. Aikens, Toronto; U. Ogden, Cooksville; C. S. Askin, of London; T. McK. Ferguson, of Prescott, Johnston District; R. Mullen, of Beverley, Gore District; and J. Langstaff, Thornhill. Three were rejected.

July, 1849.—Present: Widmer, King, Gwynne, Herrick, Hornby, Telfer, Nicol and Beaumont.

These obtained certificates: A. Jackes, of Toronto; George C.

Cotter, Toronto; Wm. Markland Lyons, Niagara; James Ford Curlett, Demorestville. One rejected.

October, 1849.—Present: Widmer, Telfer, Hornby, King, Herrick, Beaumont and Nicol.

Out of four candidates, Daniel Wilson, of Norwich, was the only one who passed.

This ends the minutes of the proceedings of the Medical Board up to the beginning of the year 1850.

It continued till October 7, 1865, on which day the last meeting took place.

A Board of Health was first organized in London, June 18, 1849, the members of which were: A. Anderson, S. Morrill, L. Lawrason, J. Ashton and S. Eccles. This year Dr. Henry Going had charge of the cholera hospital at London, when a number of immigrants were patients. The Municipal Council at first refused to acknowledge Dr. Going's services, but on being referred to Drs. Phillips and McKenzie, a small remuneration was granted.

In this historical account of the profession, it was not the intention of the writer to pass beyond the year 1849; but as in the following year another Medical School was established, an account of its organization may very properly be given, and which will doubtless be acceptable to the reader, especially the large number who claim Trinity College as their *Alma Mater*.

CHAPTER XXV.

ESTABLISHMENT OF TRINITY COLLEGE MEDICAL SCHOOL.

ON the 10th April, 1850, the Bishop of Toronto, Dr. Strachan, took his departure from Toronto for Great Britain, with the object of securing a Charter for a Church of England University, to take the place of King's College, which had recently been deprived of its Charter and been superseded by the Toronto University, or as Dr. Strachan put it: "The College or University of Toronto is founded on the ruins of King's College, whose

Royal Charter it has repealed, under the pretence of amending it, and whose endowment of eleven thousand per annum, though secured by a Patent from the Crown, and guaranteed by the Pledge of three Kings, it has seized and appropriated to itself."

Dr. Melville, in his work, says: "A Provisional Council was appointed at a general meeting of the friends and supporters of the undertaking, and active measures were adopted to secure the co-operation of churchmen throughout the Province, by opening subscription lists for the collection of an endowment fund. The meetings of the Council were held at stated periods, and the progress of their exertions was duly reported to the Bishop during his stay in England.

"In the course of the summer of this year, Drs. Hodder and Bovell projected and organized a School of Medicine; the advertisement of the course of instruction to be pursued was advertised under the title of the 'Upper Canada School of Medicine.' With these were associated Drs. Badgley, Hallowell, Bethune and Melville. On His Lordship's return from his transatlantic journey a deputation from this School waited upon him and tendered their services as the Medical Faculty of the projected University, should His Lordship have contemplated extending the range of education to all the liberal arts and sciences; and viewing the difficulties necessarily attending the early progress of such an undertaking, these services were offered gratuitously until the revenues of the University should be in a condition to warrant the payment of a competent remuneration. His Lordship cheerfully and readily accepted this offer, and as the usual period for the commencement of the Winter Course of study had already arrived, he sanctioned the naming of a day on which the several teachers should begin the labours of the first session of the Faculty by delivering the customary Introductory Lectures in public, His Lordship kindly promising that he would open the proceedings in a formal manner. Accordingly, on the 7th of November, as previously announced by advertisement, the Faculty met at the hall of the Mechanics' Institute, the use of which had been very liberally granted for the occasion, and at which the public and friends of the University had been invited to attend. A most numerous and influential meeting was assembled on the occasion. At eleven o'clock, a.m., His Lordship took the chair. The Rev. H. J. Grassett, M.A., said a selection of prayers from the Morning Service, after which His Lordship thus addressed the audience:

"He experienced much gratification on his return to the Province, when a deputation called upon him to inform him that several gentlemen of the medical profession wished to establish a school of medicine, to be attached to the future church university, the principles of which, when in operation, they were disposed to adopt; the leading principle of that church university being that religion should form the basis of the whole system of education, being by far the most important part of knowledge that man could attain, and that neither the advantage of individuals nor the prosperity of the State could exist unless guided by religious principles. This being the case, and considering that an efficient school of medicine would be an advantage to the country, he felt it his duty to attend on the present occasion and to make a few observations which, however, must be few, not having had either time or opportunity to make himself acquainted with the details; but he would observe one circumstance that established a coincidence between the gentlemen now coming forward on the present occasion, and the King's College, London. He would now state to the meeting what had happened in respect of the University College of London. There had been previous complaints of the want of more moral and religious care of the medical students of that great city, that they were under no sort of discipline, exposed to all sorts of temptations and misery, and in consequence it was not to be wondered at that many went wrong. This was more conspicuous in the Medical School attached to that University, and induced great numbers, as the evil was increasing rapidly, to turn their thoughts to the remedy. With that view, they added to the course of instruction at King's College, a medical department, and the result has been that King's College is now equal, if not superior, to the University College in that branch of instruction, and this has not only produced a statutory change on the students in the School of King's College, but on the Hospital students also."

At the conclusion of His Lordship's address, Dr. Badgley

commenced his lecture on Medical Jurisprudence, and was followed by Dr. Hodder, on Obstetrics; Dr. Bethune, on Anatomy; Dr. Hallowell, on Materia Medica; Dr. Melville, on Surgery, and Dr. Bovell, on Medicine. These lectures were adapted, as much as the respective subjects would permit, to a popular assemblage, and were received with marked attention and interest. At their termination His Lordship again addressed a few remarks to his hearers, and terminated the proceedings by the benediction.

The following remarks of the church newspaper, in reporting this meeting, afford evidence of the favourable opinion entertained of this proceeding:

"On Thursday last the Lecturers of the Medical Faculty of the Church University delivered their introductory addresses in the Mechanics' Institute. Seldom have we witnessed in Toronto a more intelligent and influential assemblage than that which filled the Hall on this deeply interesting occasion.

"Seldom if ever has our Province witnessed a more interesting event than that which took place on that occasion. Generations yet unborn will keep that day in remembrance, connected as it is with the first operations of a University founded to counteract the infidel spirit of the age, and to combine the blessings of science with the far more specious blessing of Christianity.

"Regarding the ability displayed by the respective lecturers, but one opinion can be entertained. Brief and popular as the addresses necessarily were, they furnished the most solid assurance that the teachers of the newly-formed school are fully competent for the effective discharge of the duties which they have undertaken; and that, under their fostering care, the reputation of the Church University will be materially advanced by its faculty of medicine."

Thus it is seen that the Medical Faculty commenced operations in the autumn of 1850, before even the first sod was turned for the erection of the university building.

The lectures were delivered in a building on the west side of Spadina Avenue, just north of Queen Street, while the school continued to exist.

PROVISIONAL RULES TO BE OBSERVED BY STUDENTS IN MEDICINE.

1st. Students in medicine may either reside within the walls or at their respective places of abode in the city.

2nd. All students who reside in College will be amenable to the rules and regulations governing students of Arts.

3rd. Occasional students who reside without the walls will be expected to comply with the same rules when within the walls, except as regards the attendance at Chapel in the case of those who are not members of the Church of England.

4th. All students intending to graduate must either take a Degree in Arts or pass the usual examinations appointed for students at the University of Cambridge.

5th. All the students, whether matriculants or occasional, will be required to register their names with the Dean of the Faculty, at the commencement of each Michaelmas and Easter term, and to observe strictly all other rules or by-laws which may be passed by the Faculty from time to time for the regulation of their studies.

RULES TO BE OBSERVED BY CANDIDATES FOR THE DEGREE OF M.B.

1st. The ordinary period of medical study will extend over twelve terms, and the students who have kept all their terms, and acquitted themselves satisfactorily in their examinations, will then be entitled to a certificate from the College, or, in the event of the College having the power to grant degrees, to the degree of M.B. or M.D.

2nd. All candidates for the degree of M.B. must produce evidence of

(*a*) Having attained the age of twenty-two years.

(*b*) Having taken a degree in Arts in this or some other recognized College, or having passed the examination styled "The Little Go. Examination" at Cambridge.

(*c*) Having attended not less than two courses of lectures during two terms, upon each of the following branches: Anatomy and Physiology, Practical Anatomy, Institutes of Medicine, Practice of Medicine, Principles and Practice of

Surgery; and one course of two terms upon Materia Medica, Chemistry, Midwifery, Medical Jurisprudence; and a course of one term on Practical Chemistry and Botany.

(*d*) Three consecutive terms at least must be in this College; and no certificate of attendance will be recognized from any institution in which two subjects are taught by the same individual, except in the cases of Clinical Medicine and Clinical Surgery, which may be taught respectively by the teachers of the Principles and Practice of Medicine and of Surgery.

(*e*) Having attended the practice of a recognized Hospital for eighteen months, and some Obstetric Institution for six months.

(*f*) Having passed examinations in all of the above subjects.

(*g*) Having written and defended a thesis on some medical subject, chosen by the Dean of the Faculty.

N.B.—Fees for Matriculation, Attendance and Degree will be regulated by the By-laws of the Faculty.

THE DEGREE OF M.D.

This degree may be taken at the end of two years after taking the M.B. degree, on similar terms to those in force at the University of Cambridge.

OFFICERS OF THE COLLEGE.

Provost, Rev. George Whitaker, M.A., Queen's College, Cambridge; Professor of Divinity, The Rev. the Provost; Professor of Classics, Rev. Edward St. John Parry, M.A., Baliol College, Oxford; Professor of Mathematics, Rev. George Clerk Irving, B.A., St, John's College, Cambridge.

FACULTY OF MEDICINE.

Professors: Obstetrics, E. M. Hodder, Esq., M.D., M.R.C.S. Eng.; Institutes of Medicine, James Bovell, Esq., M.D., M.R. C.P. Eng.; Principles and Practice of Surgery, Henry Melville, Esq., M.D. Edin.; Anatomy and Physiology, N. Bethune, Esq., M.D., M.R.C.S. Eng.; Practice of Medicine, F. Badgley, Esq., M.D., M.R.C.S. Edin.; Materia Medica and Therapeutics, W. Hallowell, Esq., M.D., M.R.C.S. Edin.; Chemistry (subsequently), H. Y. Hind.

FACULTY OF LAW.

J. H. Hagarty, Esq., Q.C.; the Hon. J. H. Cameron, Q.C.; P. M. Vankoughnet, Esq., Q.C.

Among the benefactors to the College were the following:

	£	s.	d.
Dr. Bovell	£150	0	0
Richard C. Horne, M. D.	12	10	0
Dr. Boys	6	0	0
Dr. Hodder	50	0	0
Wm. Winchester, M.D	2	10	0
John Finlayson, M.D., Elora........	2	0	0
F. Mack, M.D., St. Catharines	5	0	0
A. Carson, M.D., St. Catharines.....	8	0	0
Morgan Hamilton, Goderich........	10	0	0
George Goldstone, Cobourg, in land..	30	0	0
G. S. Lowe, Darlington	25	0	0
Peter Deihl, Kingston, in land	100	0	0

The following is a list of the students attending the first course of lectures, who had entered to take the degree of M.B.: Everett Hastings Coleman, Arthur Henry Paget, Charles Mills, John George Gray, John Salmon, and Augustus James Thibock. But there were others in attendance who were preparing to pass the Medical Board. Of the names of these there is no record; but one at least was Covernton.

Other early students of Trinity were: Edwin Goodman, Parie Francois Corbes Desländer, Richard Paul Lewis, Isaac Ryall, David Earl Burdett, R. Leeming Ball, John Thomas Mackenzie.

CHAPTER XXVI.

STATE OF THE MEDICAL PROFESSION, 1850.

THE condition of the medical profession of Toronto, and the extent to which the public were served by its members in 1850—the period at which this historical account closes—is well set forth in the subjoined extracts from "Rowsell's Toronto and County York Directory" for 1850-51:

Provincial Lunatic Asylum.—President of Board of Directors, the Hon. C. Widmer, M.D.; John Scott, M.D., Superintendent.

Medical Board, Canada West.—President, Hon. C. Widmer, M.D., F.R.C.S. E. Members: Gwynne, Beaumont, F.R.C.S. E., Hornby, Herrick, Telfer, Nicol, Durie, King; E. Clarke, Secretary.

Medical Practitioners residing in Toronto.—Drs. Badgley, Beaumont, Bethune, Bovell, Gamble, Gwynne, Hallowell, Herrick, Hodder, Holmes, King, Macdonald, Morrison, McIllmurray, Nicol, O'Brien, Primrose, Rees, Richardson, Robinson, Rolph, Russell, Scott, Stratford, Telfer, Trainer, Widmer, and Workman.

Toronto General Hospital.—Among the Trustees, King, Widmer, O'Brien. Attending Physicans, Widmer, King, Telfer, O'Brien, Herrick, Beaumont. Resident Surgeon, E. Clarke. During winter sessions, clinical lectures twice a week, by King and Beaumont.

Toronto School of Medicine.—Opens last Monday in October. Lectures correspond to the requirements of the Medical Faculty of the University of McGill College, this school having been recognized by that Institution. Lecturers, Drs. Workman, Morrison, Langstaff, Aikens, and Rolph.

Upper Canada School of Medicine.—Lecturers, Drs. Hodder, Norman Bethune, J. Bovell, W. Hallowell, H. Melville; F. Badgley, M.D., Secretary.

Toronto Eye Infirmary. (South-east corner of Church and

King Streets.)—Hours of attendance: From 10 to 12 daily, except Sunday. Surgeon, Dr. S. J. Stratford, M.R.C.S. London.

Toronto General Dispensary and Lying-in Hospital. (Corner of Victoria and Richmond Streets.)—Established 1st June, 1848. First establishment of the kind in Toronto. Medical Officers, Hodder, O'Brien and Bovell.

Provincial Lying-in Hospital and Vaccine Institute. (30 Richmond Street West.)—Medical attendants, Hallowell, Bethune, Primrose, McIllmurray and Herrick. Open at all hours. Persons vaccinated on Mondays and Fridays, from 12 to 3; and vaccine shipped at a distance by transmitting 5s. Lectures delivered during winter months on Mondays, Wednesdays and Saturdays, on Anatomy, Physiology, etc., Natural and Unnatural Labour, and on Diseases of Women and Children, by Herrick, King, Bethune, A.B., M.D., M.R.C.S. E. Clinical instructions given daily.

Maternity Lying-in Hospital and General Dispensary. (In connection with Toronto School of Medicine. 36 Adelaide Street West.)—Medical Officers, Rolph, Morrison, Workman, Russell and Aikens.

House of Industry.—Dr. Hodder gives his medical attendance free.

The Catholic Orphan Asylum.—Daily visitor, Dr. Hayes.

Reserve Battalion, 71st Light Infantry; stationed at Old and New Barracks.—George Carr, Surgeon; U. A. Jane, Assistant-Surgeon.

University of Toronto. (Formerly King's College.) Faculty of Medicine, H. H. Croft, Esq., Chairman; Gwynne, Anatomy and Physic; King, Medicine; Beaumont, Surgery; Herrick, Midwifery and Diseases of Women and Children; Nicol, Materia Medica; O'Brien, Medical Jurisprudence; James Henry Richardson, M.B., M.R.C.S. E., Practical Anatomy.

Coroner.—Dr. James Adamson, Toronto township.

Toronto General Hospital occupies, with the ground surrounding it, nearly all the block of ground bounded by King,

Adelaide, John and Peter Streets. The site is remarkably salubrious and very pleasant, and the halls and rooms spacious and airy. The hospital itself is 107 feet long by 66 feet wide, and two stories high. There are, besides, two other buildings attached thereto, for fever patients. The number of patients in hospital may be said to generally average 100, etc., etc. This institution has acquired a deservedly high reputation, and is resorted to by invalids from all parts of Canada, and, in some instances, from the Lower Province and the United States.

Cooksville.—W. P. Crew, M.D. and J.P.

Springfield.—Dr. Beaumont, W.B. Dixie.

Streetsville.—John Barnhart, Jr., John Crombie, Surgeons.

Township of Whitby.—Dr. W. Allison, Lot 20, Con. 5.

THE MEDICAL PROFESSION IN TORONTO.

Respecting the medical men of Toronto, the statement of Mr. Clarke Gamble, so well known and respected, will be found interesting. He writes:

"My opportunities of forming a correct opinion of the medical confraternity during the period referred to are, in consequence of my position, very good, nay, excellent; and I can bear clear, unequivocal testimony to them as a class. And I assert that nowhere could be found a better educated, more skilful, kind courteous and attentive set of medical men than our community has been blessed with from 1820 to the present time."

With regard to the Toronto General Hospital, Mr. Gamble, says:

"I have lived and been brought up in a medical atmosphere, in addition to which I have been closely, very closely, connected with the Toronto General Hospital for more than fifty years. I was one of the first trustees appointed in conjunction with the late Percival Ridout and John Ewart, to carry out the necessary reforms in the management which, up to that time, had been entirely in the hands of Dr. Widmer, and had run to seed fearfully. I went through the cholera times and ship fever, and my connection with the institution has not yet ceased, as I am still Legal Adviser to the Charity."

CONCLUSION OF SECOND PART.

In taking a review of the growth and development of the medical profession during the first half of the nineteenth century, it must be admitted that the advance made, although attended with many and serious difficulties, was steady, solid and permanent. Few of the actors on the stage now remain, but they have left a record of noble work done. They planted, and subsequent generations have reaped the fruit. Pioneers in the field of medical science, they prepared the ground for their successors; and, it must be added, their successors have not been laggard in tilling the soil which the pioneers had prepared for their cultivation.

THIRD PART.

BIOGRAPHICAL SKETCHES OF EARLY PHYSICIANS OF THE PROVINCE, WITH MANY REFERENCES TO EARLY EVENTS IN THE HISTORY OF UPPER CANADA.

CHAPTER XXVII.

DR. JOSEPH ADAMSON

Was a descendant of an old Scotch family, and born in Dundee, Scotland, 1786. Was educated in Dundee and at St. Andrew's University, Edinburgh. Removed to the town of Hedron, near Hull, Yorkshire, England, in which place he practised medicine in partnership with Dr. James Campbell, father of Sir Alexander Campbell, a sketch of whom is given on another page. Dr. Adamson remained here until 1822, when he came to Canada with his wife and two sons, James and William. He passed the Upper Canada Medical Board, July, the same year, and then settled in the Township of Toronto, where he had purchased four hundred acres of land. He entered upon the practice of his profession, in which he continued up to the time of his death, 1852. A brother of Dr. Adamson had preceded him to Canada, 1821, well known in his day as the Hon. Peter Adamson, Member of the Legislative Council of Upper Canada. He had won distinction in the army. He had been Major of the 71st Highlanders and Colonel of the 6th Cavalry, also Brevet-Major-General in the Portuguese Service during the Peninsular war. He was at the capture of Ciudad Rodrigo, the storming of Jacagoy, and the battle of Salamanca. During the Mackenzie rebellion he was Colonel of the 1st Battalion Incorporated Militia, and his brother, the Doctor, was Surgeon. Dr. Adamson had previously been Surgeon to the West York Militia, 1827. His two sons, James and William, also served under their uncle during the rebellion as captain and lieutenant. Of the children of Dr. Adamson, Alfred and his sister, Mrs.

Skynner, still (1893) possess the land bought by their father. James, now dead, was well known in Toronto as a wharfinger, and William, still living, is equally well known, having been a member of the City Council for twenty-two years, and City Weigh-master for the last twenty-four years.

DR. WM. ALLISON

Appeared before the Medical Board, Upper Canada, October. 1835. He "exhibited a diploma from the Faculty of Physicians and Surgeons, Glasgow, dated March 5th, 1827," and, after examination, received a certificate to practise.

Dr. Allison was long known as a respected practitioner of Bowmanville. In 1874 he was elected a member of the Council of the College of Physicians and Surgeons, Ontario, and continued a member until 1885. He occupied the Presidential chair in 1880-81. In a letter to the writer, June, 1889, Dr. Allison modestly writes:

"There is nothing in my life worth noticing. I only tried to earn a living by my profession in the plainest manner possible. Whether I have succeeded or not, I leave my friends to judge, I have altogether retired from practice and live in obscurity; am eighty-four years of age and in rather infirm health. Thanking you for your kindness in taking notice of an old man, I hope you will succeed in your enterprise. It is rather an arduous undertaking; but there is plenty of material in the country to work upon."

The writer has a pleasant recollection of the genial old gentleman, and of his efficient assistance when performing an operation in his town, now a good many years ago. Dr. Allison died, 1890.

DR. JAMES YOUNG ALLEN

Was born, April 12, 1814, the eldest of four children of Squire Wm. Young Allen, of Cookstown, Co. Tyrone, Ireland. His mother was the daughter of Dr. James Young, Surgeon, R.N. We have before us in printed form, the document in quaint phraseology, which informs us that "This Indenture witnesseth that James Allen doth put himself apprentice to John Young, Surgeon and Apothecary, to learn his Art, and with him (after the manner of an apprentice) to dwell and serve from the first September, eighteen hundred twenty-nine, until the full end and Term of four Years from thence next following to be complete and ended," etc. (For copy of the whole of such document, see sketch of Dr. O'Reilly.)

During the winter, 1831-32, Mr. Allen was in Dublin in attendance at "Park Street School of Anatomy, Medicine and Surgery," etc. The several certificates state that he attended dissections, lectures on anatomy, physiology, surgery, etc., during the session which commenced on October 31, 1831, and terminated on April 30, 1832. "To these certificates are found the names of J. W. Cusack, Will. Hen. Porter and John Hart. He also attended lectures on Materia Medica and Pharmaceutic Chemistry, by Samuel Stratton, M.D., at his house; "Terms two Guineas." The following season Mr. Allen passed in Paris, and his certificates show that he was an "assiduous" student of the *Faculté de Médécine de Paris* for the session, 1832-33, under the instructions of Andial, Comvielier and other distinguished men. He also attended a course of clinical lectures at the Hotel Dieu.

Returning to Dublin, he studied at the "Surgical School," Royal College of Surgeons, and clinical lectures at the "City of Dublin Hospital," and "diligently attended the practice" there; also a course of lectures on diseases of the eye. To the certificates are found the names of A. Jacob, Robert Harrison, James Apjohn, Thos. Beatty, Chas. Benson, H. Marsh, A. Colles, J. Wilmot, W. H. Porter, Wm. Hargrave, Robt. William, David Hastings MacAdam, M.D., and Geo. West,—names more or less distinguished and known to the student of medicine. Mr. Allen continued his studies at the University of Glasgow, 1834-35, and attended lectures by James Wilson and Thomas Thompson, M.D., of the Faculty of Physicians, and he was granted a degree by the Senate, April, 1835. For some time after graduating, Dr. Allen held the position of Assistant-Surgeon in the Dublin Hospital. In July, 1836, he was married to Rebecca, second daughter of Capt. Wm. Cole Hamilton Walsh, of the 8th Regiment Foot, King's Regiment, which he accompanied to

Canada, 1808. It may be mentioned that Capt. Walsh served under Wellington, and was one of his aides-de-camp at Waterloo. Capt. Walsh married, 1813, Elizabeth Bissett, daughter of a wealthy merchant of Halifax, while the regiment was stationed there. In this connection we insert the following interesting statement, published 1893:

"*An Old Regiment Coming Back to Canada after an Absence of Seventy Years.*

"The King's Regiment, the 8th Regiment of Foot, is coming back to Canada after an absence of over seventy years. This regiment was formed in 1685, and in 1768 embarked for Canada. In 1775, the regiment was in Upper Canada, some companies being at Niagara, and others at Detroit. In 1776, part of the regiment was sent to Lower Canada, and in 1785 it returned to England. In 1808, the 1st Battalion landed at Halifax, and in 1810 it was quartered in Quebec. In the autumn of 1812, five companies proceeded to Fort George. Two companies (the Grenadiers) of 175 men halted east of the Don bridge, on the Kingston Road, and then marched up King Street to the Old Fort, and in April of 1813, the 8th and a few militia, and a company of the Royal Newfoundland Regiment, bravely fought the engagement that eventually ended in the capture and burning of the city. This regiment had the first Masonic Field Warrant issued by the Grand Lodge of England, granted in 1755. It was No. 156 for 1770 to 1780, and No. 124 in 1780. The Lodge held meetings in Canada and Niagara, but there is no record of the lodge after 1789. Joseph Clement, the ancester of John M. Clement, of Niagara, was made a Mason in this lodge."

Dr. Allen engaged in practice at Cookstown until 1841, when he came to Canada and commenced practice at Kingston, having obtained license from the Governor-General, Sir Charles Bagot, Jan. 21, 1842, and continued to practise at Kingston until 1852. He was commissioned Assistant-Surgeon 2nd Batt. Lennox Militia, by Earl of Elgin, July 1st, 1847. Dr. Allen was a personal friend of Sir John Macdonald, and was one of the promoters that first brought him out as a candidate for parliamentary honours, a circumstance Dr. Allen always spoke of with pride. He practised for a time at Demorestville, Prince Edward County, and then located at Bradford, County of Simcoe. In April, 1856, he was made coroner for the county, In November, 1886, he moved to Toronto, where he practised until the time of his death, Jan. 31, 1893, in the seventy-eighth year of his age. Dr. Allen was a Presbyterian, and was a regular attendant of Old St. Andrew's Church, and a personal friend of the pastor, Rev. Mr. Milligan. He left a widow, aged seventy-six, and seven children out of fourteen born to them. His son, Henry S., holds an appointment in the Post Office Department, Toronto.

DR. JOHN ARDAGH

Was born in Waterford, Ireland, 1810. He took his degree of M.D. at Edinburgh University, and his M.R.C.S. in England, 1831. Engaged in practice in his native place, and was for eight years physician to the House of Industry and the Insane Asylum. In 1842, he made a visit to Canada, where his cousin, the Rev. S. B. Ardagh (first Rector of Barrie), had come to settle. The following year Dr. Ardagh came out again and settled at Orillia, where he continued to practise till his death, August 6, 1872. Dr. Ardagh experienced all the hardships incident to the practice of medicine in the early days of this country. He was no stranger to long, lonely horseback rides through a thinly settled country, with roads at times almost impassable, and in all sorts of weather. He was highly esteemed as a skilful physician, was much beloved, especially by the poor, to whom in their sickness he never failed to pay the utmost attention, giving his professional services gratuitously, however far he might have to travel and however inclement the weather might be; insomuch that he was known in the country as the "poor man's doctor." For some years he was medical attendant to the Indians at Rama; and when the Lunatic Asylum was established at Orillia, he was appointed Medical Superintendent; and he conducted the affairs of the institution with great judgment and unremitting attention. He was a member of the Church of England; in politics, a Conservative, and was a Freemason of high standing.

Dr. Ardagh was twice married. First in 1837, to Annie, daughter of Samuel Boyce, Esq., of Waterford, by whom he had five sons and two daughters. He married his second wife, 1867, who was Virginia, daughter of W. J. Hardy, Esq., of Norfolk, Virginia, by whom he had one son.

Dr. Johnson Arthur Ardagh, son of above by his first wife, was born, 1843. He studied medicine at McGill College, Montreal, and took his M.D., C.M., 1869. Practised his profession in Orillia till his death, May 25, 1887. None of Dr. John Ardagh's sons are now living. His youngest daughter, Maude, has for some years filled the important position of Superintendent of the Hamot Hospital, at Erie, Pennsylvania.

DR. JOHN RUSSELL ARDAGH

Was born in 1808, in the city of Waterford, Ireland. His father was the Rev. Arthur Ardagh, Fellow of Trinity College, Dublin. At an early age he entered Trinity College, where he took his degrees of A.B., and M.D. Afterwards he proceeded to London, at that time quite a journey by stage-coach, where he continued his medical studies, attending the hospitals, and taking his degree of M.R.C.S. Eng. Returning to Ireland, he practised for some time near Dublin, and afterwards in the North.

In the year 1843, he decided to follow his brother, the Rev. S. B. Ardagh, A.M., who had emigrated to Canada and settled on the shores of Lake Simcoe, as Rector of Barrie and Incumbent of Shanty Bay. Shortly after Dr. Ardagh's arrival in Canada, he began practising at Holland Landing, then a thriving place, at the head of navigation on Lake Simcoe. He soon established the reputation of a skilful surgeon, and his practice became extensive, keeping three horses in constant use. He travelled over a large tract of country, at that time sparsely settled, and the roads in many places dangerous, which occasioned him frequent accidents, several of which nearly cost him his life. He used to tell many exciting stories of his long journeys and narrow escapes. Afterwards he removed to Barrie, where he practised until a few years before his death, in 1868.

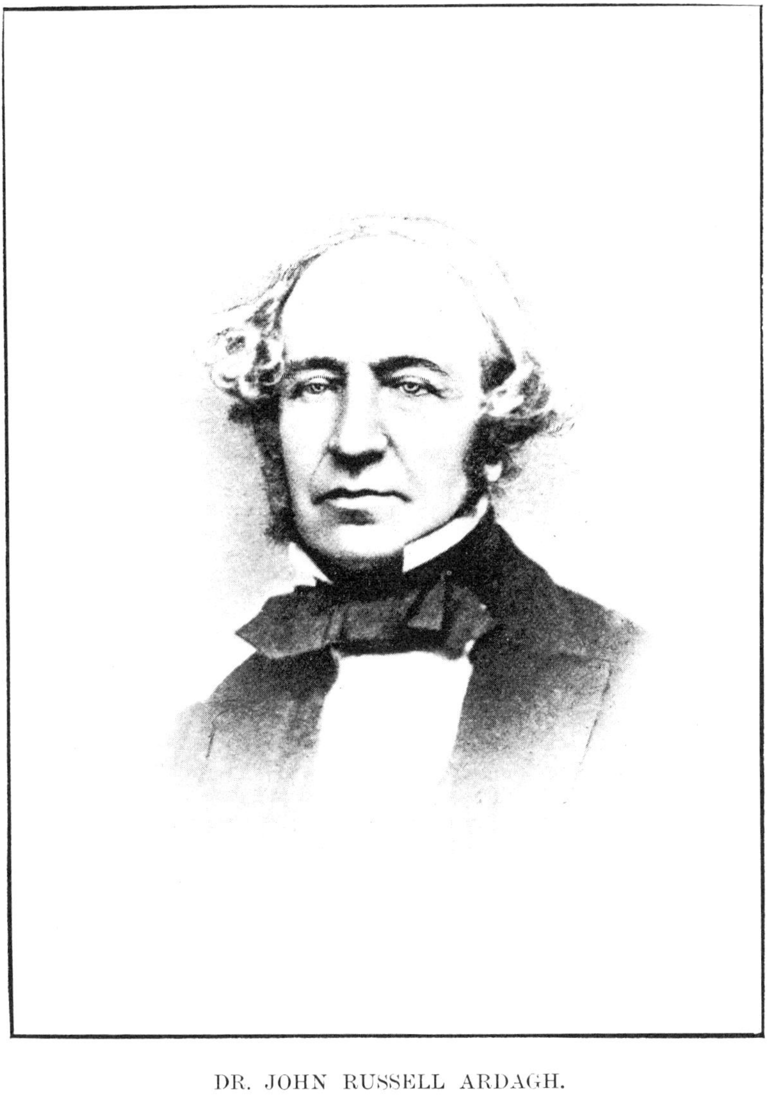

DR. JOHN RUSSELL ARDAGH.

Dr. Ardagh was a man of a very happy temperament. His genuineness and hearty manner won him many life-long friends, and the universal esteem and respect of the community in which he lived. As a practitioner he was very successful, but especially was he regarded, and deservedly so, as a very skilful surgeon. He inherited his father's talent for languages, and was looked upon by the college men of his day as a fine classical scholar. In religious matters he took an active part, especially at Holland Landing, where he did much for the Church, and acted for years as warden. In the year 1846, he married Anne, eldest daughter of Henry Hatton Gowan, Esq., and sister of the Hon. James Robert Gowan, a member of the Senate of Canada, and for many years Judge of the Judicial District of Simcoe—a talented and highly educated woman, of more than ordinary depth of character, a devoted wife and mother. She was a true helpmeet to him in times of difficulty. She survived him twenty years. He had seven children, two only of whom are at present living, Henry Hatton Ardagh, of Toronto, barrister-at-law, and Anna B. Ardagh, unmarried.

DR. EDWARD W. ARMSTRONG

Passed the Upper Canada Medical Board, July 5, 1819. His examiners were Drs. Macaulay, Widmer and Lyons. He was born in Fredricksburg, on the Bay of Quinte, August 29, 1789. His mother was the eldest daughter of the celebrated Major Rogers, whose disbanded battalion settled that township. The doctor was one of Major Rogers' legatees. He had one brother and one sister. The brother, James Rogers Armstrong, was a well-known pioneer merchant of Picton, then of Kingston. He subsequently removed to Toronto. He married a daughter of Dr. Dougal, of Picton. He at one time represented Prince Edward County in the Provincial Parliament. One of his daughters became the wife of Dr. Beatty, of Cobourg. Dr. Armstrong's parents died while the children were quite young. Edward found a home with his uncle, who removed to Little Lake in Hallowell. "Here," says Dr. Armstrong, "was the scene of my earliest recollections." In 1796, the three children were taken to Vermont to be educated, where they continued until 1806. Dr. Armstrong obtained his medical education at Dartmouth College, N.Y., and came, it is related, to Hallowell, 1817, where he continued to practise until 1820 or 1822, when he removed to Kingston and engaged in practice. In 1838 he took up his residence at Rochester, N.Y., where he remained during life.

The writer received an interesting letter from Dr. Armstrong in July, 1867, giving a great deal of information about early times, especially at Kingston. He wrote of his intimate association with the Hon. Richard Cartwright, Col. John Ferguson, Allen McLean, the first Upper Canadian lawyer, made so by Act of Parliament; also the Senior Hagerman, of Adolphustown, likewise made a lawyer by the Crown. He also mentioned Barnabus Bidwell, Archdeacon Stuart and others of note in that day, with whom he was intimate. Dr. Armstrong presided at a meeting for the suppression of intemperance at Kingston, February, 1830. He died at Rochester in 1877, aged eighty-eight.

DR. CHARLES JAMES STEWART ASKINS.

The minutes of the Upper Canada Medical Board record that Mr. Askins appeared before that body, April, 1849. He was "a matriculated student of King's College, Toronto," and his examination was "highly satisfactory." Dr. Holmes, of Chatham, has kindly supplied the following: Dr. C. J. S. Askins, son of Col. Askins, of London, Ont., graduated in Toronto and settled in Chatham about 1846. (He passed the Medical Board of Upper Canada, 1840.) He was a well-educated physician and a very popular citizen. Was a member of the Town Council many years and occupied the Mayor's chair several years. He was Surgeon to the 24th Kent Battalion, and went to the frontier at the time of the Fenian Raid, 1866. When the Medical Council came into existence, he became the first representative from the Western and St. Clair Divisions. He died in 1872.

DR. ANDREW AUSTIN

Was a native of Vermont; born, 1788. He came to Hallowell, now Picton, 1816. He had studied medicine at Middlebury

College, Vermont. January, 1820, he appeared before the Upper Canada Medical Board, but failed to pass, being "recommended further study and attendance on a course of lectures." He accordingly studied at the University of New York, and graduated, 1822. He was a pupil of the eminent surgeon and teacher, Dr. Valentine Mott. He returned to Picton, 1822, and practised for a short time before again applying for his license, January, 1823, when he was found "qualified to practise in all branches" of the profession. Dr. Austin had as a rival, Dr. E. W. Armstrong, who came to the place, it is stated, 1817. They were opponents, not only as practitioners, but in politics. Dr. Austin, although from the States, was, it is related, "a great Tory," while Dr. Armstrong was "Republican in his tendencies." In the field of practice, it is related that the "contest between them was keen, but Austin took the lead."

He was very much respected by all who knew him, and took an active part in matters affecting the public welfare. It is announced, in the Hallowell *Free Press*, of April 12, 1831, that Dr. Austin, Vice-President of the Temperance Society, would deliver a public address on Temperance. He continued to practise until his death, October, 1849, aged 61.

DR. ISAAC BROCK AYLSWORTH.

The following facts are taken from an obituary notice which appeared in the *Christian Guardian:*

"He was born near the village of Bath, in the township of Ernesttown, December 4th, 1812. His parents were of United Empire Loyalist families, and possessed in a full measure the characteristic virtues of their class—industry, frugality and steady integrity. He received a liberal education at the Bath Academy, of which Dr. Stouton was Principal, and entered upon the study of medicine in the same place. He completed his studies at New York and took the degree of M.D. Having passed the Upper Canada Medical Board, July, 1835, he commenced the practice of his profession in the vicinity of his home, achieving, for a young man, more than ordinary success. Removing to Newburgh, he continued to practise his profession until 1843. He was the leading man in the community. Possessing a large share of public confidence, popular in the positions he occupied, wealth was fast flowing in upon him, and the prospect of securing more than a competency was encouraging, but he had reached a crisis in his life—a crisis that called for a decision. There was a pressing conviction on his mind that he ought to devote himself to the work of the Christian ministry, and he entered the ranks as a minister of the Methodist Church. In 1847, he was placed on the list of supernumeraries, and returned to Newburgh, resuming the practice of medicine. In 1853, he re-entered the pastoral work. In 1874, he withdrew from connection with the Conference, but retained his ordination papers, which gave him the status of an ordained minister. For about eighteen years he resided in Collingwood, rendering efficient service to the Church as a local preacher, and sharing largely the confidence of the Methodist community of the District, and of the Annual Conference. His death was unexpected and sudden. He was proceeding with his wife to visit friends in London. At Georgetown he left the car to render assistance to a friend, and while doing so, fell on the platform. Recovering himself, he walked a few steps, then fell the second time, and before his wife could reach him life was extinct. So died Dr. Aylsworth, in the seventy-sixth year of his age.

"Dr. Aylsworth was greatly esteemed in the town of Collingwood. He was regarded by his fellow-townsmen, and that rightly so, as no ordinary man. His sterling qualities, his unceasing activities and undeniable usefulness greatly endeared him to the community. Although brusque in manner and somewhat uncourtly in address, yet he was to many a guide, counsellor and friend."

DR. GEO. BAKER,

Of Bath, before Medical Board, January, 1820, "was found fit to practise Physic and Midwifery and the lesser operations in Surgery." It is related that he had been a student of Dr. Carlile, and succeeded him in his practice at Bath. Not unlikely, before passing the Board he assisted Dr. Carlile, who

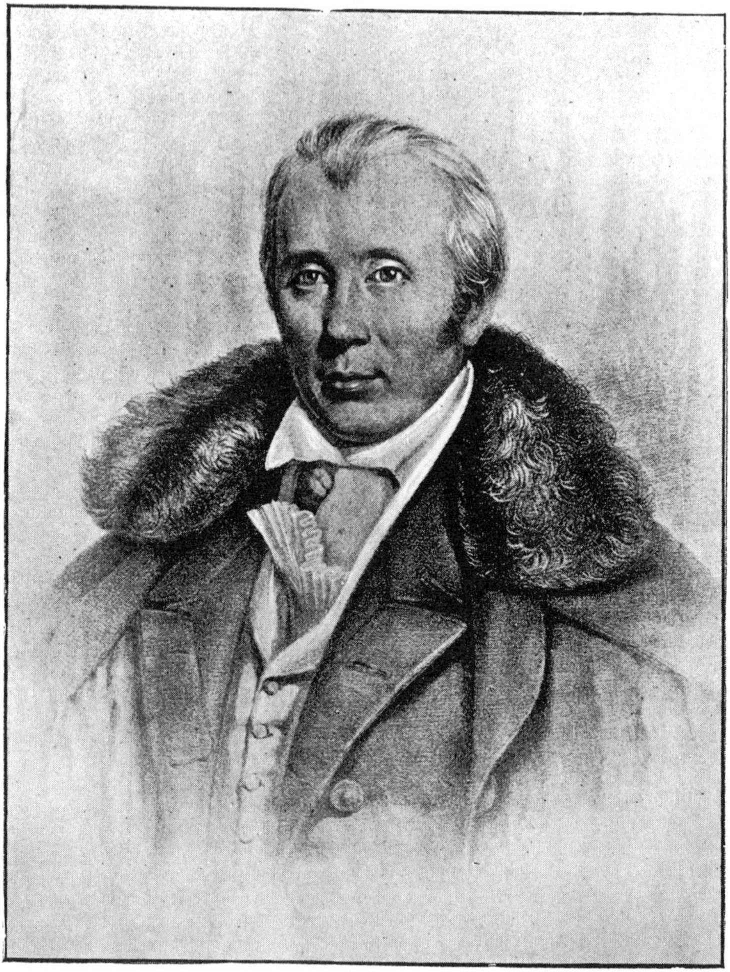

DR. WILLIAM WARREN BALDWIN.

confined himself mostly to Kingston. Dr. Baker probably came to the place near the beginning of the century. Gourlay records that at a meeting of resident land-owners at A. P. Foward's hotel, Elizabethtown, Dr. Geo. Baker was chosen clerk. He was the only practitioner at Bath for many years. The doctor is described as of medium height, a little stout, and as a very fascinating person. It will not, therefore, be a matter of surprise that he had, in the course of his life, five wives, all persons of some distinction. This notice appeared: "Married at Bath, May 10, 1830, Dr. Geo. Baker to Miss Jane Macaulay." It is stated that all of his wives were buried at Picton. Was appointed Surgeon to the 2nd Addington Regiment of Militia, November 24, 1823. We find Dr. Baker's name in the records of St. John's Church, Bath, but the time of his death is not given.

DR. WM. WARREN BALDWIN

Was the son of Robert Baldwin, who emigrated with his family from a parish near Cork, Ireland, in 1789. Besides William Warren, the eldest, there were John Spread and four daughters. After undergoing many adversities and meeting many adventures by sea and land, the family finally reached Upper Canada, and settled in the Township of Clark. Here the family remained until 1812, when they removed to York, where the father died, 1816. The pioneer life of Mr. Baldwin and his family was all the more trying from their being persons of education and refinement. The accounts we have heard of the events in connection with the several members of the family are full of interest; but only a few may be briefly referred to.

Dr. Baldwin had three brothers; John Spread, who came to Canada with him, married the daughter of Major-General Shaw, and the widow of Dr. Scott, R.N. His son Edward married Miss Grasett, by whom he had two sons, Dr. E. St. George, and Rev. Henry Grasett. Henry B. was a Captain in the Merchants' Service, from which he retired, then came to Canada and settled at Belleville, where he died, 1849. The other brother, Augustus W. Baldwin, had an eventful life. Born 1776, he entered the merchant navy as a boy. Receiving cruel treatment, he made his escape from his ship; but while doing so was seized by a press-gang. His name becoming known to the captain, he obtained a commission. In 1800, he became a lieutenant, and took part in many glorious combats and victories achieved by the British navy. For gallant conduct he received a gold medal, 1808; became a commander in 1812, and was made a post-captain in 1817. Having retired from the service as admiral, he came to Canada in 1820. He took up his abode on the Davenport Road, north of Toronto, and his place of residence was known as Russell Hill, now the home of Mr. Nordheimer. He took an active part in public affairs as a Conservative, and became a member of the Executive Council during the administration of Sir. F. Bond Head. In 1826, he married Miss Augusta Melissa, daughter of J. M. Jackson, Esq. Three children were born, who died young. Admiral Baldwin died, January 5, 1866, aged 90. "In social qualities he excelled, keeping his frank sailor bearing to the last, with a smile and pleasant word for everyone."

Dr. Wm. Warren Baldwin had been a practising practitioner for a year or two prior to his coming to America. His professional education was probably obtained mostly at Edinburgh; at least he took the degree of M.D. at the University of Edinburgh.

From what can be gleaned upon the matter, it seems that Dr. Baldwin spent but little time with his father after settling in the woods; but naturally much of his time at York, where there was, at least, a small field for the practice of his profession. But the doctor either did not find enough to do, or had resolved to enter upon the study of another profession, that of law. Says Dr. Scadding: "On his arrival at York from the first Canadian home of his father on Baldwin's Creek, Dr. Baldwin's purpose was to turn to account for a time his own educational acquirements by undertaking the office of a teacher of the youth." In the *Gazette* and *Oracle* appeared the following notice, dated December 17, 1802:

"Dr. Baldwin, understanding that some of the gentlemen of this Town have expressed some anxiety for the establishment of a Classical School, begs leave to inform them and the public generally that he intends, on Monday, the first of January next, to open a school in which to instruct twelve boys in writing, reading and classics and arithmetic. The terms are, for each boy, eight guineas per annum, to be paid quarterly or half-yearly. One guinea entrance, and one cord of wood to be supplied by each of the boys on the opening of the school.

"N.B.—Mr. Baldwin will meet his pupils at Mr. Willcocks' house on Duke Street."

About this time Dr. Baldwin was married to Margaret Phœbe, second daughter of Wm. Willcocks, a name well known in the early days of York, of which there were three persons. William Willcocks, Dr. Baldwin's father-in-law, had been Mayor of Cork, and was a cousin of the Hon. Peter Russell, who became President on the retirement of Col. Simcoe, the first Governor of the Province, in 1797. He was, in 1802, Judge of Home District Court. In 1804, Dr. Baldwin lived at the corner of Front and Frederick Streets. Here was born his son Robert, who became Attorney-General for Upper Canada in 1842, and whose name is inseparably connected with the history of the Province; who was the father of Responsible Government in Canada, and the active promoter of genuine reform.

Dr. Baldwin witnessed the exciting scenes in connection with the invasion of York, in 1813, and took some part in the capacity of Surgeon. The writer had the privilege of knowing the late Mrs. Breckenridge, a sister of Dr. Baldwin's, and mother of the late Mrs. Edmund Murney, of Belleville, and has heard from her lips a thrilling account of some of the events of the war of 1812. Mrs. Murney wrote a very interesting account, which the writer has had the privilege of seeing.

On the day of invasion, Mrs. Breckenridge's narrative says: "The ladies settled to go out to Baron de Hoen's farm. He was a good friend of the Baldwin family, whose real name was Von Horn, and he had come out about the same time as Mr. St. George, and had been in the British army. He had, at this time, a farm about four miles up Yonge Street. Miss Russell, sister of President Russell, loaded her phaeton with all sorts of necessaries, so that the whole party had to walk. My poor old grandfather, Mr. Baldwin, the father of Mrs. Breckenridge, by long persuasion at length consented to give up fighting and accompany the ladies. Aunt Baldwin, the wife of Dr. W. W. Baldwin, and her four sons, Major Fuller, who was an invalid under Dr. Baldwin's care, Miss Russell, Miss Willcocks and the whole cavalcade sallied forth; the youngest boy, St. George, a mere baby, my mother, Mrs. Breckenridge, carried on her back nearly the whole way. When they had reached about half way out they heard a most frightful concussion, and all sat down on logs and stumps frightened terribly. They learned afterwards that this terrific sound was occasioned by the blowing up of the magazine of York garrison, when five hundred Americans were killed, and at which time my uncle, Dr. Baldwin, was dressing a soldier's wounds. He was conscious of a strange sensation—it was too great to be called a sound—and he found a shower of stones falling all around him, but he was quite unhurt. The family at length reached Baron de Hoen's log house, consisting of two rooms, one above and one below. After these days, Miss Russell and my mother walked into town just in time to prevent Miss Russell's house from being ransacked by the soldiers. All now returned to their homes and occupations, except Dr. Baldwin, who continued dressing wounds and acting as surgeon until the arrival of Dr. Hackett, the Surgeon of the 8th Regiment. Dr. Baldwin said it was most touching to see the joy of the poor wounded fellows when told that their own doctor was coming back to them. My father, Mr. Breckenridge, was a student-at-law with Dr: Baldwin, who had been practising law after giving up medicine as a profession, and had been in his office about three months when he went off like all the rest to the battle of York. The Baldwin family all lived with Miss Russell after this, as she did not like being left alone. The Americans made their second attack about a month after the first. General Sheaffe had gone off some time before, taking every surgeon with him. On this account Dr. Baldwin was forced, out of humanity, to work at his old profession again, and take care of the wounded."

As has been stated, Dr. Baldwin did not find a sufficient field in the practice of medicine for his robust energies and mental strength, and consequently entered upon the study of law, in the practice of which he became an ornament to the profession; indeed, he may be called the father of the profession in Upper

Canada. He, in time, held distinguished positions in both professions; but it was in law that he could best exercise his natural endowments, where he shone, and found profitable employment. "His career is now a part of Upper Canadian history. It presents a curious instance of that versatility which we have had occasion to notice of the men who have been eminent in this country"—*Scadding.*

Besides his private means and professional income, Dr. Baldwin inherited valuable property through the Hon. Peter Russell. In his position as Administrator of the Government, Mr. Russell enjoyed the privilege of signing away grants of land to persons eligible for such favours. Among those who found favour with the Administrator, was one Peter Russell, and plenty of documentary proof is extant that Peter Russell had very valuable lands granted to him by the grace of Peter Russell, Administrator. Dr. Scadding remarks that he was designated sometimes, "the man who would do good unto himself." On his death "his property passed into the hands of his sister, who bequeathed the whole to Dr. W. W. Baldwin, into whose possession, also, came the valuable plate elaborately embossed with the armorial bearings of the Russells."

Dr. Baldwin made his home with the Russells, Russell Abbey, after the time of the war, 1813, and remained until he removed to Spadina House. The original word Spadeena is Indian, and means "*a rising ground,* or *little hill.*" Upon the summit of the hill, on a line with Spadina avenue, Dr. Baldwin built Spadina House, and subsequently laid out the magnificent way extending from Queen Street to the water's edge.

This avenue is three miles (two and three-fifths) long, and 160 feet wide. Were it not for Knox College building, interjected upon an oval widening of the avenue, it would be one of the finest avenues in the world. In speaking of this matter, Dr. Scadding remarks that "Dr. Baldwin, a Liberal in his political views, was nevertheless influenced by the feudal feeling, which was a second nature with most persons in the British Islands some years ago. His purpose was to establish a family in Canada whose head was to be maintained in opulence by the proceeds of an entailed estate. There was to be forever a Baldwin of Spadina. It is singular that the first inheritor of the newly-established patrimony should have been the statesman whose lot it was to carry through the Legislature of Canada the abolition of the rights of primogeniture. The son grasped more readily than the father what the genius of the North American continent will endure and what it will not."

As has been stated, Dr. Baldwin devoted himself to law rather than medicine, yet he did not altogether neglect his first love. He naturally took an interest in the formation of the Medical Board in 1819, and in its proceedings. In 1821 he became one of the members, and his name is rarely missing in the records of the subsequent proceedings; and in 1832 he was elected vice-president. Nor did Dr. Baldwin refuse to respond to calls for medical relief by the public. Tradition gives a number of instances of his dual professional work. The following is one: "It was no uncommon occurrence in the early days of Toronto, when surgeons were scarce in the young capital, for Dr. Baldwin to be compelled to leave court in the middle of a trial, and to hurry away to splice a broken arm or bind a fractured limb. He was once engaged in arguing a case before his father-in-law, when a messenger hurriedly arrived to summon him to attend the advent of a little stranger into the world. The circumstances were explained to the judge, and the further consideration of the argument was adjourned until the doctor's return. After the lapse of an hour, he again presented himself and prepared to resume his interrupted argument. The judge expressed the hope that all had gone well with the patient, whereupon the doctor replied, "Quite well; I have much pleasure in informing Your Lordship that a man-child has been born into the world during my absence, and that both he and his mother are doing well."

At the time Dr. Baldwin adopted the profession of law, it was passing through a stage of development. But unlike the profession of medicine, it had a sure fountain-head in officers of the Crown in the Provincial Government, the Attorney-General and the Solicitor-General.

The first session of the second Provincial Parliament met at York, June 1, 1797, and was prorogued on July 3. This was the first time for the Parliament to assemble at the new capital. Among the seventeen Acts passed was one for the better regulation of the practice of law. The Act set forth that "persons now admitted to practise in the law and practising at the bar of any of His Majesty's Courts of this Province" could form themselves into a society to be called the Law Society of Upper Canada, etc., etc. The Act provided that the six senior members of the present practitioners, including His Majesty's Attorney-General and Solicitor-General, shall be appointed as governor or bencher of said society. This Act also provided that no persons but the practitioners shall be permitted to practise at the bar unless such person shall have previously entered the said society as a student of the law, and shall have been standing in the books of the society for and during the space of five years, etc., etc., always excepting members of the bar of England, Scotland and Ireland, or of any other British Provinces in North America. The Act specified that the said practitioners, or as many as can be called together, whereof the Attorney-General and Solicitor-General shall be two, may assemble at the Town of Newark on the 17th day of July next ensuing, for the purpose of framing and adopting resolutions.

The records to be seen in the library at Osgoode Hall show under date July 17, 1797, that there met in obedience to the direction of the Act, at Wilson's Hotel, Newark, at eleven o'clock, the following gentlemen: John White, Attorney-General; Christopher Robinson, Isaac Des Gray, Solicitor-General; Allan McLean, Angus Macdonell, William Dummer Powell, James Clark, Alexander Stewart, Nicholas Hagerman and Bartholomew Crannell Beardsly. It was formally

Resolved,—That the two Crown Officers be nominated Benchers of the Law Society of Upper Canada, together with the four senior barristers, and that the benchers, according to seniority, take upon themselves the treasurership of the said society annually. Beside the gentlemen mentioned above, the following were also enrolled as members of the society at this time: Walter Roe, Timothy Thompson, Jacob Farrand, Samuel Sherwood and John McKay, sixteen in all. Thus was the Law Society of Upper Canada formed, and this was its first meeting. The next meeting took place at York, July, 1799, when Wm. Weeks was admitted. In 1801, four more were admitted, of which the third on the list was Wm. Warren Baldwin, making him the twenty-sixth on the roll of the Law Society.

It will be observed that during the six years previous, only five names had been entered on the roll, showing that the provisions of the Act of 1797 were of such a nature as to deter or prevent aspirants to the ranks of the legal profession. This led to further legislation.

On March 5, 1803, an Act was passed, the preamble of which says that "great inconvenience has arisen, etc., from want of a sufficient number of persons duly authorized to practise the profession of law, and unless the number can be speedily increased, justice will in many places be with great difficulty administered." It was therefore enacted that the Crown might grant a license to not more than six persons who, from "their probity, education, and condition in life," might be deemed "fit and proper to practise the profession of law." The only requirement was a certificate from a Judge of the King's Bench as to ability and fitness.

The first to be licensed under this Act was Dr. Baldwin.

It is recorded in the minutes of the Law Society, "that on 6th day of April, 1803, Wm. Warren Baldwin, of York, Eng., presented himself before the meeting and, produced an instrument or license under the hand and seal of His Excellency the Lieut.-Governor." This document recited the Act passed the previous month ; and stated that a certificate had been obtained from Henry Alcock, Esq., Chief Justice, that the "Court of King's Bench is satisfied of the ability and fitness of the said W. W. Baldwin to be admitted to practise as a barrister and attorney in this Province," and that Lieut.-Governor Hunter had granted the necessary license.

This account of the first days of the legal profession may seem to be a digression, but apart from giving an account of the life of Dr. Baldwin, there is supplied an interesting unpublished chapter of the early days of Upper Canada (1889).

There is yet to be added that Dr. Baldwin was made a Governor, or Bencher, of the Law Society in 1807. In 1811 he was elected the Treasurer, and continued in office during 1812, '13 and '14. Again in 1829, and in 1824, '25, '26, '27, '28, and again in 1832. As Treasurer of the Law Society he had much to do with the erection of the original Osgoode Hall which now forms the east wing.

Dr. Baldwin from time to time filled a variety of public positions of more or less importance. He was elected Member of Parliament for the Counties of York and Simcoe, and afterwards the County of Norfolk , in 1828. Was President of Mechanics' Institute, 1831. He was added to the list of magistrates for the Town of York, April 12, 1833. We find him also mentioned as Public Notary; and Gourlay, in his book, speaks of him as "Master in Chancery, attending the Legislative Council."

There is not space to speak of Dr. Baldwin as a politician; but he was unfortunate enough to incur the disfavour of the Executive. We find it recorded that official notice was issued removing Dr. Baldwin from office as Judge of the Surrogate Court of the Home District, July 16, 1836, the reason being that as an active member of the Alliance Society, "he placed himself in open hostility to the Government."

About six months before his death, he was summoned to the Legislative Council of United Canada, his son Robert being Attorney-General.

Dr. Baldwin died, January 8th, 1844, aged 69, at his residence at the east corner of Front and Bay Streets. This brick building, long known as the Baldwin Mansion, has recently (1890) been demolished, to make place for a substantial warehouse.

The following is the estimate placed upon Dr. Baldwin at the time: "Our country has lost a friend; and the country, it may be said, will follow him as mourners to the grave. By the removal of one so worthy, so disinterested, so excellent, we have sustained a loss, the magnitude of which it is difficult to appreciate, much worse in this community to repair. It is not Toronto only that will feel the privation, or drop the tears of submissive sorrow over his honoured tomb. The sad tidings, like an electric shock, the less convulsive in its effects because expected, will widely extend an awakened interest over regions sufficiently enlightened to appreciate his worth, and sufficiently grateful to deplore his loss."

Dr. Baldwin's widow died at the family residence, corner Bay and Front Streets, May 13th, 1850, aged 80.

Dr. Baldwin had five sons, three of whom died young. His eldest son, Robert, became famous as the father of Responsible Government in Canada. He was born in 1804, and died, 1858. His second son, Augustus William, died in infancy. The third son, Henry, was born in 1807, and died in 1820. The fourth son, William Augustus, was born in 1808, and died June 14th, 1883. The fifth son, Quetton St. George, was born in 1810, and died in 1839.

Dr. Baldwin's eldest son, Robert, had two sons, William Willcocks and Robert, and two daughters. One daughter remained unmarried; the other, Augusta Elizabeth, became the wife of the Hon. John Ross, of Belleville.

Wm. Willcocks, the eldest son, was well known at Osgoode Hall, having charge of the office for distributing law stamps. He was appointed to this office when first established in 1864. He died, November 19, 1893, aged sixty-four. His eldest son, Henry Yarwood, entered the medical profession, having studied in Toronto and graduated in Victoria College. He has been many years in the North-West, practising for a time at Portage la Prairie, and being some time surgeon in the Mounted Police, and for the last three years practising in Winnipeg. The second son, Robert W., is with his father in the stamp office. Stephen Y. is taking a course of military instruction. A daughter married Clarence T. Whitney, another Hamilton Cassels, and another Dr. Lesslie.

Robert, the second son of Hon. Robert B., was long known in the religious and philanthropic circles of Toronto, and died there in his fifty-first year, in 1885. He was twice married—first to Miss Jemima MacDougall, a Scotch lady, who died in 1873. Their son, W. W., bearing the honoured name of his great-grandfather, is also a member of the medical profession, and has practised in Toronto since 1890. A daughter, Katie, is married to the Rev. J. R. Shields Boyd, son of Judge Boyd, of Toronto.

In 1877 Robert married for the second time. His wife was Miss Elizabeth Walker, an Irish lady who resided in Dublin. They had four children, three of whom survive. Mrs. Baldwin takes a most active part in philanthropic work, both temporal and religious.

Referring back to the other surviving son of Dr. W. W. Baldwin, that is, Wm. Augustus, who lived at Mashquoteh (a burnt plain), he was twice married—first to Isabella Clarke, daughter of James Buchanan, for twenty-five years British consul in New York. By this union, which took place in 1834, there were seven children, five being sons—H. St. George, James B., W. Augustus, R. Russell and Æmilius. Two of these, the second and the third, joined the medical profession and now practise in Toronto (1893). The two daughters—Phœbe and Isabella—are both dead. Mrs. Baldwin died in 1850, and in 1852 her husband married Margaret, daughter of Captain McLeod, of Drinoch, York County, Ont. By this marriage there were nine children—five sons and four daughters—seven of whom survive (1893). W. Augustus died in June, 1883, aged seventy-four years.

Dr. Edmund St. George, son of Rev. Canon Baldwin, and grandson of John Spread Baldwin, is B.M., C.M. Univ. Edin., 1874, Lic. R.C.S. Edin., 1877, and practises in Toronto.

No excuse is necessary for giving so large a space to the distinguished subject of this sketch and the family. He was not only the pioneer physician of Toronto, but, as well, a pioneer in legal affairs. Moreover, he occupied a conspicuous place in the early history of the Capital of the Province; while members of the family have held and continue to hold prominent positions in the country.

DR. E. J. BARKER.

In the Kingston *Spectator* of December, 1833, this notice appeared: "PROSPECTUS.—Doctor Barker respectfully acquaints his friends and patrons that in January he will publish the first number of a new commercial and political journal (imperial size) to be called the *British Whig*, and continue to issue the same every Tuesday and Friday by eight o'clock in the morning." The following editorial appeared in the semi-centennial number of the *Whig*, January, 1884: "Mr. Barker was born in Islington,

London, England, on December 31st, 1799. In 1807, the family settled in North Carolina, where his father, an accomplished linguist, died. The subject of our sketch returned to Norfolk, England, to be educated. In 1814, he joined relatives in Smyrna, in the east, and subsequently was articled to a surgeon and apothecary in Malta for five years. In 1819, he became doctor's mate on His Majesty's sloop-of-war, 'Race Horse.' He afterwards walked the London hospitals, and for ten years practised in East Smithfield, receiving the degree of M.D. from the London College of Medicine. In December, 1832, he landed in Kingston, and engaged with Noble Palmer as editor of the *Spectator*, filling that post for a year, retiring upon its sale to John Vincent, and establishing a paper of his own. He issued it in full sympathy with its title, *British Whig*, and thus it happened that, though a Liberal organ, it became a loyal one during the Mackenzie rebellion. A breach being made in its ultra supporters in consequence, it drifted into Conservative ranks, where Dr. Barker enlisted the warm sympathies of Sir John A. Macdonald, then a young rising politician, and became his faithful follower for forty years. Though never loaded down with this world's goods, and having his full share of trials and difficulties, he managed not only to keep his journal afloat, but also to be enterprising in many ways, notably in the issue of the first daily in Upper and Lower Canada in the publication of *Barker's Canadian Magazine*, and in issuing a daily of double-royal size twenty years before any of his rivals attempted it. Though not a prolific writer, as the term goes to-day, or an industrious news-gatherer, it was through the style of his editorial work, and by the co-operation of the friends made by his social qualities, that the *Whig* outlived so many of its contemporaries. No writer upon the Canadian press has had a more characteristic pen; none have possessed his knack of compressing force and ideas into few sentences, while he always had a quick, trenchant answer for an opponent, with a ready wit to turn the effective weapon of ridicule into play. But the most robust of natures tires of work at last, and he was gradually relaxing his office cares when the exigencies of politics in Kingston in 1871 led to the enlistment of another paper as the preferred Conservative organ, and he gave up the newspaper to accept the city registrarship. He was acknowledged as the Nestor of the Canadian press."

In another column it is stated that "when the *Whig* was started, 'affairs of honour' were still in vogue. The paper exposed a military officer who had insulted a host of ladies at various times in the city, describing him as 'drumstick-legged, with red ram's-horn whiskers and goatish eyes.' The officer forthwith called with a friend and two bludgeons, which he did not dare to use. He retreated and sent a challenge. The editor of the *Whig* replied that the officer's base conduct placed him outside of the privileges of the field of honour, while his privilege remained of declining to be called out by every fool who thought himself offended. That settled the affair of honour. His first year produced two challenges and one assault, for which a late politician was convicted at the Assizes. It was a lively year."

It should be mentioned that Dr. Barker, although not in regular practice, for a few years gave attention to professional work, and was accounted an excellent physician. During the prevalence of cholera in 1834, he rendered important service.

The eldest daughter of Dr. Barker married, September 4, 1843, R. Chalmers, Esq., of Quebec. Another daughter married Mr. Pense, the son of whom, Mr. E. J. Pense, is the present proprietor of the *British Whig*. Dr. Barker died, 1885.

The following newspaper clipping may be given; at one time the inhabitants of the Bay of Quinte heard a good deal about the sea-serpent, and many believed in its appearance:

"THAT SEA-SERPENT.—Mr. Julius Baker, of Trenton, was not the discoverer of the great Bay of Quinte 'sea-serpent.' So says Dr. Barker, of the *British Whig*, and who would dare dispute such authority? The *Whig* copies the paragraph headed 'Something Like a Snake,' and says: 'Dr. Barker, not Mr. Julius Baker, was the man who discovered the great sea-serpent of the Bay of Quinte. Many years ago, full a quarter of a century, the Yankees were busy with the sea-serpent off Cohasset, and it was thought a pity that the Yankees should have a big water-snake and not the Canadians. Hence the discovery of the Bay of Quinte sea-serpent. The story was told so gravely in the *British Whig*, that Mr. Francis Hall, of the *New York*

Commercial Advertiser, then in Kingston, published the account, with additions and emendations of his own, which account went the rounds of the United States press. Somebody was wicked enough to say that Mr. Francis Hall was sold, and accused the *British Whig* of being the hoaxer; whereupon Mr. Francis Hall was very angry and stopped the exchange. That it was no sell that the big snake was discovered by Dr. Barker, is proved by what Mr. Julius Baker had seen. '*Magna est veritas et prevalebit.*' "

DR. JOHN BARNHART

Is of German extraction, and the name was formerly spelt Barnhardt. The subject of this sketch was born, we believe, in the eastern part of Upper Canada. He received his early education at the Royal Grammar School at York, while it was under the patronage of the Rev. John, afterwards Bishop, Strachan, and obtained a good ground work in classical, as well as literary education. He then became an articled student of medicine to Dr. Widmer. In consequence of there being no medical school in Upper Canada, he attended the half-yearly sessions of lectures, for three years, at the College of Physicians and Surgeons of the City of New York, during which period he was the pupil of the celebrated surgeon, Prof. Valentine Mott. In the summer of 1832, he returned to York, then known as "muddy little York," in order to render such assistance as he might be able to afford to Dr. Widmer, as his student, during the epidemic of Asiatia Cholera which had invaded the town. Notwithstanding the best forms of treatment of that dread scourge, then known to the profession, and employed by Dr. Widmer, a large number of the inhabitants perished. Having passed the Upper Canada Medical Board, July, 1834, Dr. Barnhart commenced the practice of his profession in the then rising Village of Streetsville, Peel County, where he continued to pursue it throughout the surrounding townships until 1869, when he removed to the town of Owen Sound, Grey County. In 1837, Dr. Barnhart was a Regimental Surgeon of Militia, and was present at the skirmish and rout of the rebels under Mackenzie at Gallows Hill (Dec. 7, 1837), and he claims (1894) to be the only surviving surgeon who was present on that exciting occasion. He was, as well, in the succeeding year, acting as surgeon on the Niagara frontier until the rebels vacated Navy Island. After the County of Peel had been separated from the County of York, Dr. Barnhart was honoured by being unanimously chosen by the representatives of the municipality, as first Warden of the new county. In it he also held the offices of Justice of the Peace and Coroner. "These several important and honourable positions, together with the high estimation in which he was held by the general community as an able and successful practitioner of medicine, afford adequate reasons for saying that the profession of the Province should regard him as entitled to their fraternal recognition and respect as one of their number who has upheld and maintained the honour and dignity of the profession." The foregoing has been supplied by one who designated Dr. Barnhart as an old and valued friend, and who is in turn an old friend of the doctor's.

Dr. Barnhart's family consisted of his wife (*nee* Robinson) and three daughters. The eldest is the wife of Judge Reynolds, Brockville. Another married James D. Croil, merchant, of Montreal, now dead; and the other daughter married W. E. Brown, Esq., of the Canada Life Association Company, son of Adam Brown, ex-M.P., and postmaster at Hamilton.

Dr. Barnhart, whom the writer saw but recently, continues in a large degree to enjoy vigorous health of body; while his mind is remarkably active and intellect keen (1894).

DR. JOHN BEATTY

Was born January 19th, 1810, of Protestant Irish parentage, in the City of New York. The family removed to Upper Canada, February, 1819, and settled at River Credit, on the farm where now stands the Village of Meadowvale. It was then covered with woods, and the family cleared the land for cultivation. The subject of our sketch returned to New York in the autumn of 1825, entered the Wesleyan Academy, where he remained two years, and then went to the Ohio University, Athens, pursuing his studies there for three years. He returned to New York in the autumn of 1830, and entered as medical student the office of A. T. Hunter, M.D. He attended three full courses of lectures in the College of Physicians and Surgeons, and received the M.D. degree, April, 1833. Returning at once to Upper Canada, he, with the view of obtaining the provincial license, entered the office of Dr. Rolph, and passed his examination at the July session that year—Dr. Widmer, President; Rolph, King and Deihl, principal examiners.

The same month he settled at Cobourg, and commenced practice. He left Cobourg in the spring of 1835 for Toronto, where he remained until the fall of 1844, and then returned to Cobourg and resumed practice, which he continued until 1868. Since that time he has not practised his profession.

He held the Chair of Chemistry and Natural Science in Victoria College for about eight years. It was the writer's privilege to be a student at that institution during a portion of that period, where he received his first lessons in those branches of science—lessons never forgotten.

Dr. Beatty married, October, 1833, Eleanor, second daughter of J. R. Armstrong, merchant, Toronto, a brother of Dr. Armstrong. They had ten children, six of whom survive (1889)—one son and five daughters.

The eldest daughter married John Daintry, of Cheshire, England, who is now living in Cobourg; second, Geo. K. Shoenberger, of Cincinnati; the third, the Hon. Wm. Macdougall, Ottawa; fourth, C. E. Ryerson, Barrister, Toronto, son of Rev. Dr. Ryerson; and the fifth, Desirè Girouard, Q.C., of Montreal, M.P. for Jacques Cartier.

Reference to the Medical Register will show that he is, perhaps, the only one living of the record as early as 1833.

DR. WM. RAWLINS BEAUMONT.

The greater part of the following obituary notice appeared in the medical journals:

"William Rawlins Beaumont, M.D., F.R.C.S. Eng., was born in Beaumont Street, Marylebone, London, in 1803; descended from a family established in England in the beginning of the fourteenth century, originally French. Having received a liberal education, he began at an early age and 'most assiduously prosecuted his professional studies at St. Bartholomew's Hospital for a more than ordinary length of time,' as testified by Abernethy, whose dressing pupil he was, and whose esteem he had won—as also that of Sir Astley Cooper, Lawrence, Herbert Mays, Marshall Hall, and others of renown in the medical profession. In Paris he studied anatomy during ten months under Amussat, who perceived in him '*un zele et une aptitude rare.*' He also studied in Brussels.

"He obtained the license to practise surgery and was admitted a Member of the Royal College of Surgeons, London, in December, 1826; Fellow of the Royal Med. and Chirurg. Society, London, in 1836; and was surgeon to the Islington Dispensary for some years prior to 1840.

"Before leaving England he contemplated entering the Army Medical Service, a Commission in which he expected, at the instance of Abernethy, from Sir James McGrigor, Director-General; but this being long deferred, owing to official regulations regarding appointment of army surgeons, it was abandoned. He came to Canada in 1841, accompanied by his friend Dr. Spear, and soon after obtained, by the Governor-General's Warrant, the license to practise in Canada. In 1843, he was appointed to the Professorship of Surgery in the University of King's College (now the University of Toronto), which he held for ten years, until the abolition of the Faculty of Medicine, of which he was then Dean. He was appointed Member of the Upper Canada Medical Board in May, 1845, and became a very regular attendant of its meetings.

"In 1870-71, he delivered a course of lectures on Ophthalmic Surgery to the students of the Toronto School of Medicine, besides clinical lectures at the Toronto General Hospital. In 1872, he was elected Professor of Surgery in the Medical Faculty of Trinity College, and afterwards Emeritus Professor.

"He invented and himself made several surgical instruments, some of which are of great ingenuity and utility. In 1836, he invented and described, before the Royal Medico-Chirurgical Society, an instrument for passing sutures in deep-seated parts, as in the operation for cleft palate, which was admired by

Brunel, the great engineer, and was reputed by Tiemann, the surgical instrument maker of New York, to have been the origin of the Singer sewing machine. Sir James Paget told the late Dr. Fraser, of this city, of the esteem in which Dr. Beaumont was held by all old St. Bartholomew's students; and that he believed that he was the inventor of the principle of the modern sewing machine. An account of the invention was published in the *Medical Gazette* for 1836; the original account may be found in the transactions of the Medico-Chirurgical Society for the same year; and a description of it may be found in the *Lancet*, of March 17, 1866. With it a continuous chain of stitches can be sewed—though in the operations for which it was invented but one at a time was required. He also invented instruments for tying Polypi; a Sliding Iris-forceps, a Speculum, a Probe-pointed Lithotomy Knife; and others. He was the author of Essays on the treatment of Fractures of the Leg and Forearm by Plaster of Paris, 1831; on Polypi, 1838; 'Case of Large Cartilaginous Tumour of the Lower Jaw,' 1850; and contributed 'Clinical Lectures on Traumatic Carotid Aneurism' to the *Lancet*, in 1854; 'The Several Forms of Lithotomy,' *Ibid.* 1857; 'A Deeply Penetrating Wound through the Orbit (five and a half inches deep), Recovery,' *Ibid.* 1862; papers on 'Exostosis of the Scapula'; 'Aneurism of the Femoral Artery,' etc. He made many donations of valuable preparations, casts and instruments to the Royal College of Surgeons, England, and to other collections. During the Fenian Raid of 1866, he had charge at Port Colborne of the hospital for the wounded.

"In the winter of 1865, he lost all useful sight of the left eye from acute inflammation, yet was able to perform operations requiring an unerring hand—for instance, that for artificial pupil; but at length the left eye became completely useless, and the sight of the right affected, and in 1871 greatly impaired, and by the New Year of 1873, lost entirely. Since that time he had lived in retirement with his family about him, and passed quietly away on October 12, 1875, aged 72. He was a gentleman of a quiet and retiring disposition, a sound surgeon and instructive lecturer. His memory will be held in veneration by the profession and by others who knew him well."

Dr. Beaumont was one of the distinguished teachers at Toronto, when the writer was a student and attended his clinical lectures. Several of the first operations he witnessed were performed by Dr. Beaumont at the old hospital, corner of King and John Streets.

DR. CHAUNCEY BEADLE

Was born in Connecticut, U.S., June 25, 1791. While young he removed with the family to Otsego County, New York. He received his medical education at Fairfield Medical College, and at the medical school of Dr. Joseph White, of Cherry Valley, N.Y., who enjoyed a distinguished reputation as a physician and surgeon, and whose extensive practice afforded desirable facilities to students in the days when public hospitals were few, although no formal lectures were given. He passed his examination before the Otsego Medical Society, and was licensed to practise within the State of New York, May 20, 1816. He practised in Monroe County in that State, until the summer of 1821, when he removed to Canada and passed the Upper Canada Medical Board, and January 9, 1822, received his certificate of license under the seal of the Province and bearing the signature of Sir Peregrine Maitland. He commenced practice at St. Catharines immediately thereafter, and on the fifteenth of the same month married Orinda Converse, of Randolph, Vermont, by whom he had one son and three daughters. Two of the daughters died in infancy; the second daughter married the Rev. Joshua Cooke, son of Bates Cooke, of Lewiston, N.Y., and died at Storm Lake, Iowa, December 17, 1882. The son, named after Dr. Delos White, one of the sons of his esteemed medical preceptor, did not adopt the profession of his father and his father's friend, but became widely known as a fruit-grower and horticulturist. This son is now (1893) living in Toronto, the sole survivor of the family. Doctor Beadle died at St. Catharines, March 24, 1863, and his widow, January 19, 1885.

The Doctor acquired an extensive practice, attending to calls throughout the Niagara District from the Niagara River to

Hamilton, which often necessitated his absence from home for a week or more. In those days the roads were largely of a very primitive sort, winding in and out among stumps and fallen trees, often through dense woods, where at night the darkness might be felt, and one must needs trust solely to the sagacity of his horse to find the track. Such was the incessant labour of a country practitioner at that time that it was often necessary to get someone to drive for him, especially at night, while he lay down on the bottom of the waggon and slept, a task often performed by Dr. Beadle's wife.

Notwithstanding the exacting cares and duties of his profession, he found time to take an active interest in whatever tended to improve the country and develop its resources. It is claimed that he was probably the first to suggest the building of the Welland Canal, and though unable to take any active part in its construction, was ever the staunch friend and supporter of Hamilton Merritt in carrying forward that work. He secured the passing of an Act of Parliament to form a company for the purpose of running a line of stages from Queenston to Sandwich. He was also prominently active in establishing the Grantham Academy, now the St. Catharines Collegiate Institute, where a number of the young men of that district laid the foundation of a classical education. Later in life, to save himself from loss, he acquired the nurseries, since known as the St. Catharines Nurseries, and when afterwards compelled by failing health to relinquish his medical practice, he devoted himself to the introduction and dissemination of choice varieties of fruit.

DR. NATHANIEL BELL

Was born in New Jersey, U.S., October 26, 1790. Two years later his mother, with the family, came to Canada, as graphically told in the following narrative: "In the month of September, 1792, on the banks of the Delaware River, in the State of New Jersey, near where Eastown now is, you might have seen a woman about thirty years of age preparing to leave for

Canada. She had eight children, the eldest a daughter about eighteen years of age, and the youngest also a daughter aged nine months. She had two or three horses with pack-saddles and a few articles of clothing for herself and family, together with a tent, made by sewing a few sheets together, and some provisions for the journey. The clothing, tent, provisions and smallest children were packed on the horses, and in this manner they commenced their long and tedious journey through forests and over mountains, fording rivers—for bridges were not in existence at that time in the country. There were no public houses or taverns to entertain the weary travellers. Consequently they had to erect their tent or sleep in the open air. For two or three weary weeks they pursued their way, sometimes meeting with Indians and passing their villages; but those wild savages did not molest or harm the travellers, but were kind and obliging, and would give or sell them corn or venison. In fording a stream an accident occurred; one of the horses, on putting down his head to drink, pitched one of the children, a little girl of eight years, over his head into the stream. She was nearly drowned, but was finally rescued, her shoulder being dislocated by the fall. At last they arrived at Fort Niagara, which was then occupied by British soldiers, who put them across the Niagara River on the Canadian shore, the long-expected land of promise. From Niagara they made their way along the shore of Lake Ontario to the Township of Grimsby, where this woman's husband, her two brothers and sister had settled a short time before. It was a happy meeting. The children were disposed of among their friends until a log house could be erected. It was an easy matter to obtain land in Grimsby in those days. Judge Andrew Petit was a resident of that township and an uncle to the heroine of this sketch. (He was the first magistrate in the place and often performed the marriage ceremony.) Whatever he said or did was sanctioned by the Governor of the Province at that time. This woman and her husband finally settled on the mountain near Grimsby, where the writer (their youngest son) was born. They lived to see all their children married and settled. The husband died in 1820; his wife survived him fifteen years.

She was eighty-two when she died. She could say—"Arise daughter and go to thy daughter, for thy daughter's daughter has a daughter."

Dr. Bell's general education must have been obtained under considerable difficulty, as the means of acquiring it in Upper Canada at that period were very limited.

He studied medicine at Beamsville with Dr. Sumner, and during the war of 1812, with Dr. Kerr, acting as Assistant-Surgeon. It is probable that he commenced practice by himself when the war closed, 1815. At all events, he was in practice several years before the Upper Canada Medical Board was established. He was the second person to pass the Board, April, 1819. During the war of 1812-14, Dr. Bell had a busy time. Beside acting as Assistant-Surgeon, he seems to have attended to the calls in the country. On one occasion he was taken prisoner by the U. S. soldiers, and being allowed to walk about, but not on parole, he watched for an opportunity and made for the British lines. The enemy started in pursuit, but finding they could not overtake him, sent their balls whizzing after him. One struck him in the leg, and he was recaptured and kept in prison for a long time. The wound healed but he suffered in after-life from its effects. He received a pension for a time, and when it was discontinued he made repeated applications for its renewal, which was not granted. The Doctor and his friends thought the Government treated him unjustly, but it will be seen by the following certificate of the Medical Board, which body gave him a license to practise, and by which he was examined with regard to the wound, that the Government only acted on the recommendation of the Board. This certificate said:

"*February* 19, 1831.

"SIR,—In reference to your letter of the 14th inst., desiring me to assemble the Medical Board for the examination of Mr. Nathaniel Bell, a late militia pensioner, I have the honour to acquaint you for the information of His Excellency the Lieutenant-Governor, that the Board have this day examined Mr. Bell, and have directed me to say that they do not feel themselves warranted in recommending the restoration of his name to the pension list on account of any disability from his wounds.

"I have the honour to be,

"Your most Obedient, Humble Servant,

"WM. LEE,

"*Secretary to the Medical Board.*

"Z. MUDGE, ESQ.,

"*Secretary to His Excellency*

"*The Lieutenant-Governor,*

"Etc., etc., etc."

Dr. Bell's field of practice was very extensive. He lived at St. Ann's, Halton County, where he also attended to a farm of 200 acres. He made his rounds on horse-back, often westward and northward beyond the head of the lake where now is Hamilton, and to the region where Guelph is now situated. Dr. Bell was very successful in attending to his large and extensive practice. He is described as "a bold, determined and careful operating surgeon." He many times "amputated the thigh, leg and arm, and sometimes at night by candle-light, with labourers and farm-hands only for assistants, and no chloroform. He was a good accoucher." He was appointed Surgeon of the 2nd Gore Regiment Militia, 1825, and during the Rebellion, 1837, he was Surgeon to the 8th Gore.

Dr. C. W. Flock, who married his step-daughter, Miss Nelles, describes Dr. Bell as follows:

"He was six feet high, and of large but not stout build. He had a stern, determined, commanding appearance, and was a fine-looking man in every respect. He was one of the most pleasant, agreeable, generous and jolly men I ever knew. His 'word was his bond.' He hated a lie, but pitied the liar, either by word, look or act. All who knew him placed every reliance and confidence in his statements; his word was 'yea and nay.' He was a member of the Church of England, an earnest Christian. He was one of the old-school Tories. The doctor was always proud of being called a U. E. Loyalist. He worked hard for many years, but died leaving hardly anything to his family except an honourable name, which will never be forgotten where he lived and practised. He was poor because he would not stoop low enough to secure money. He took his fees if he could get them honourably, otherwise he lost them and that was very frequently. Thousands of dollars were left unpaid which should have been paid, and would have rendered good service to him during his life, and his widow and children when he was called away from them."

He was twice married. His first wife was a Miss Cline, or Klein, of Nelson, by whom he had five sons and four daughters, four of whom survive (1890). The second wife was Mrs. W. B. Nelles, of Grimsby, a sister of Judge O'Reilly, of Hamilton. By her he had three daughters and two sons, all now living but one girl (1890). His last wife is still living in Hamilton (1890), eighty-two years old, and quite active both physically and mentally.

He died, October 26, 1859, aged sixty-nine years.

DR. WILLIAM BELL

Was born in Cumberland, Eng., 1806. His father, Abram Bell, came to Canada, 1830, and lived at Quebec until 1837, when he settled in Peterborough County. William, the youngest of the family, was a student at Guy's Hospital, and left that institution, 1836. Coming to Canada, 1837, he practised a short time at Trenton, and, 1838, settled in Otonabee, where he cultivated his farm as well as practising medicine. In 1840 he commenced the drug business in Peterborough, and carried it on for fourteen years. He then lived in the Township of Monaghan, eleven years, when he again took up his residence in Peterborough. Dr. Bell married February 7, 1844, a daughter of Capt. Spilsbury, of the Royal Navy, who took part in the war of 1812 as commander of a gun-boat.

DR. NORMAN BETHUNE

Was born at Moose Factory, Hudson Bay, 1822. His father, Angus Norman, was born at Carlton Island, 1793. His grandfather, the Rev. John Bethune, of Williamstown, Glengarry, had four sons, Angus Norman, John, who was Dean of the Cathedral, Montreal, James, resident of Cobourg, and Alexander Niel, Bishop of Toronto. Angus Norman, the eldest, the father of Dr. Bethune, was connected with the North-West and Hudson's Bay Company for fifty years. In 1840, he came to Toronto, at which time his son Norman entered Upper Canada College, where he received his general education. He began his medical studies in 1843, and was a student at Edinburgh and London, and obtained in 1848, the degree of M.R.C.S. Eng. In 1850, he received the degree of M.D. Univ. Edin., and in 1860 he became F.R.C.S. Edin. He commenced practice at Toronto in 1849. He was absent from Toronto nine years, during which time he practised at Edinburgh. Dr. Bethune was for many years professor at Trinity Medical College.

Dr. Bethune married, firstly, a Scotch lady, and secondly, the widow of Dr. Winer, of Hamilton, who was a daughter of Dr. John King, of Toronto.

Dr. Bethune continued in practice in Toronto until his death, which took place, October 12th, 1892, at the age of seventy. Among the papers left by Dr. Bethune was an account, in the form of a diary, of a voyage he made from England to Hudson Bay, shortly after he had obtained his diploma, in the summer of 1849. He probably went in the capacity of ship-surgeon. Several vessels sailed in company for the cold North. In this journal, too lengthy to find a place in these pages, Dr. Bethune exhibits fine descriptive ability and no little talent in sketching the icebergs he saw in the way, and some ship scenes. The voyage was not without danger and narrow escapes, especially in returning. After a storm the vessel had encountered, Dr. Bethune writes: "The wind began to moderate and the clouds to break, after an agreeable spell upon our backs of four days and four nights. Truly our preservation during this fearful storm among icebergs and upon a lee shore has been providential. It is wonderful how we escaped collision with the bergs during the four nights, as it was impossible to see the length of the ship from eight in the evening till four-and-a-half in the morning, eight hours and a half, as it were, blindfolded." He gives an amusing pencil sketch of an incident on board, with this account of it: "A rich scene occurred to-day (Oct. 11) at dinner. The captain was busily anatomizing a chicken, when the ship gave a heavy lurch to leeward and then another in the opposite direction. The pullet shied in the first instance into the captain's lap, and then traversing the cabin beneath the table, lodged in turn upon the mantel-top to windward. The merriment this caused, to the ladies especially, was of an extraordinary character." The time occupied in this voyage from Sheerness to Moose Fort was ten weeks and five days. The return voyage lasted six weeks and five days.

DR. CHRISTOPHER BESWICK

Was an English physician, who came first to Pennsylvania and afterward to Canada, and settled in York County, near Newmarket, 1809. He was accompanied by Gabriel Lount, father of Samuel Lount, for some time M.P. for the County of Simcoe. "For many years Dr. Beswick was the only doctor north of Oak Ridges. Dr. Reed, south of the Ridges, was his earliest compeer, followed by Dr. Birny, Dr. Primrose and Dr. Thompson, after whom came Dr. Nash and Dr. Haskett." Dr. Beswick enjoyed a high reputation as a physician and surgeon among the pioneer settlers, and shared with them the privations and hardships of pioneer life. He is described by a local writer as "a pattern of frugality, economy, industry and sobriety, yet liberal and generous." His general education was good, and he took delight in preparing the constitution and by-laws of various organizations as they were developed in the growth of the community. The preparing of annual reports in connection with different societies was a constant pleasure to him. As he never married, he was able to devote himself to these congenial and useful acts. Although not a bigot, he was a devoted member of the Church of England, which manifested itself in a practical manner. The first English church of the place was erected on Dr. Beswick's land, to a great extent through his agency and by his means; and finally the land on which St. Paul's Church stands was given to the Church.

Dr. Scadding, in "Toronto of Old," speaking of this gift, remarks that Dr. Beswick's "large white house on a knoll by the wayside was always noted by the traveller from York as he turned aside from Yonge Street for Newmarket."

For many years, up to his death, Dr. Beswick lived with George Lount, where he found a home and was cared for with tenderness and considerate kindness. He died, 1837, and it is recorded on his tombstone that he had reached the remarkable age of 118 years. A local historian affirms this was verified by records found among his papers after his death.

The above account is mainly derived from the diary of Eli Gorham, prepared by his son. This chronicler very justly remarks that, in view of the valuable gift Dr. Beswick made to the Church, it would be a fitting recognition of his munificence to place in the church a memorial window, while the town of Newmarket should recognize his liberality in providing a public cemetery, by erecting a suitable metallic railing to enclose his grave and tombstone.

DR. WM. LOCKTON BILLINGS

Was the son of a manufacturer of Nottingham, Eng., where he was born in 1805. His father had a brother, a Surgeon in the Marines at Woolwich for thirty-six years. Wm. Lockton was apprenticed in 1823 to Mr. Butlin, a Surgeon of Nottingham, with whom he remained five years. He then entered at Guy's and St. Thomas' Hospital, London. In 1827, he passed the Apothecaries' Hall. He would have taken a diploma at the Royal College of Surgeons, London, had it not been for the disparaging writings of the London *Lancet* at this period relative to the College. Among Dr. Billings' instructors were Bradley and Sir Astley Cooper. He commenced practice at once in his native place, where he continued until 1842, when he emigrated to Upper Canada and settled in Hamilton, having passed the Medical Board in January, 1843. Hamilton has been his home ever since. In later years Dr. Billings has gradually relinquished his practice, but he is an excellent specimen of a green old age (1889), with intellect unimpaired and a vivacious manner; and there is reason to believe he has many years remaining to enjoy his well-earned repose. He was at one time a member of the City Council, and for seventeen years Chairman of the Public School Board. He was the first Surgeon to the former Great Western Railroad. The writer calls to mind his first meeting with Dr. Billings at Ridgeway. He had come on to take home the body of Capt. Routh, who had been shot through and through the chest, but Capt. Routh survived, and lives to-day, 1889, in the enjoyment of fair health.

Dr. Billings married in 1842. Of four children, one remains, and is now a member of the Local Board of Health of Hamilton.

DR. GEORGE GWYNNE BIRD

Came of a family which had resided for many generations in Herefordshire, and were originally of Norman descent, bearing the name of De Bird, and collaterally connected with the Gwynnes, of Cwnhordy, an ancient Welsh family. He was born in the year 1780. After receiving the usual training of an English school, he decided upon the study of medicine, and attended lectures in London. As an evidence of his ability and attainments, he was appointed House Surgeon at St. Bartholomew's Hospital, under M.. Blick and the famous and world-renowned Dr. Abernethy, and waited upon him when he was performing some of his great operations. Here he remained one year. For many years he practised his profession in Breconshire, but owing to ill-health he resolved to leave England and try colonial climate. He selected Canada for the purpose, and made all arrangements to sail, with six of his children—four sons and two daughters—by a ship leaving Bristol. Fortunately, owing to a delay respecting the luggage, he had to postpone the date of sailing. The ship he had determined to go by sailed and was never again heard of; she was lost and all on board. His next venture was by the ship "Clio," Captain Dobson. He reached New York safely. This was in 1833. After encountering the difficulties of travelling at that time, he arrived at Little York, now Toronto, and notwithstanding the earnest entreaties of the Governor of the Province for him to remain and practise medicine in the town, he took up a grant of land near Peterboro' and tried farming. This did not prove a success, because, like too many English college-educated men, before and since his time, he discovered that trees had to be felled, fields plowed and grain reaped by tough muscle and sinew, and not by Latin, and, in his case, knowledge of the pharmacopœia.

After a trial of farming for four years, he moved into Peterboro' and opened a drug store. In April, 1838, he passed the Medical Board, and is described as "a practitioner from England, of upwards of forty years, without tickets or testimonials of any kind; gave satisfaction." He remained in Peterboro' until 1841, and then fixed upon Darlington, near Bowmanville, as a residence. In this place he practised medicine until his death, May 25, 1863; aged eighty-three years.

The Rev. Dr. Macnab, who was his Rector, gives this testimony to the worth of Dr. Bird: "He was a man of much scientific research, and was generally regarded as an authority in Botany and Geology. Complimentary of his knowledge of the latter subject, he was, late in life, honoured with a visit from the Canadian Geologist, that distinguished official, the late Sir William Logan."

Four sons of Dr. Bird were also physicians. The eldest, bearing his own name, remained in England and occupied a high position in the locality in which he lived. He was Alderman and Mayor of Swansea. Dr. Charles Bird, another son, much respected and loved, and known as a great lover of sport, died only a few weeks ago at Bowmanville (1890). A daughter married Richard Morgan, of Hamilton, and is the only survivor of the original family that came out to Canada. Of those that remained in England, only one survives (1890), Dr. Henry Bird, aged eighty-two years.

The grandson, Wm. Morgan, of Hamilton, has in his possession a stained glass window from one of the old abbeys in England, brought to Canada by his grandfather. It is said to be a thousand years old.

DR. JOHN HARRISON BLACKWELL

Was a native of New Jersey. He possessed more than the ordinary amount of education, having taken the degree of M.A. at New Jersey College, in 1829. He had the M.D. degree from the Pennsylvania University, 1829. He probably came into Canada about 1834, as he passed the Upper Canada Medical Board in April of that year. He practised for a time at Stamford, and then at Drummondville. He married the daughter of Dr. Lafferty, "a remarkably handsome person." For about forty years he practised at Drummondville, or Lundy's Lane. A contemporary says he was "a well-read and educated man; far ahead of many of his brethren; a tall, ungainly man; always rode on horseback, and made the great mistake of riding poor and badly kept horses. His way of riding was known all over; no one could mistake him on horseback for anyone else, for no living man ever rode as he did; was very arbitrary in his ways, and did not get on smoothly with others. The worst that could be said of him was, 'what he did not know was not worth knowing (in his opinion).' He was good and kind to the poor, always ready with his services." He died and was buried in Drummondville, 1867.

DR. DENIS ROBERT BRADLEY,

Of Toronto, appeared before the Upper Canada Medical Board, April, 1839. He stated that his trunk had been stolen which contained his testimonials of education, but that he had been ten years engaged in the study of his profession. He failed to satisfy the Board.

Dr. Bradley was well known as a chemist and druggist for many years in Toronto; he at the same time engaged in practice. The following obituary notice taken from *The Mirror*, shows the high estimation in which Dr. Bradley was held:

"DEATH OF DR. BRADLEY.—It is our painful duty to record the death of the above named, much esteemed gentleman, which took place on January 14th, 1850, in this city, after a lingering illness, brought on by undue exertions and fatigue during the

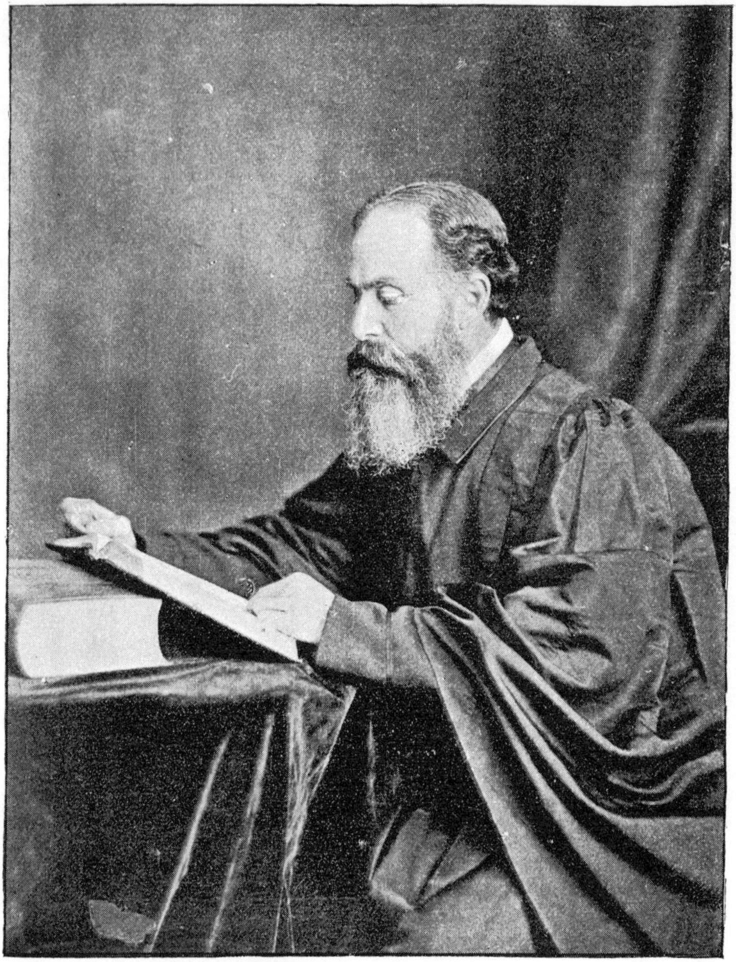

DR. JAMES BOVELL.

prevalence of cholera. In the summer of 1847, Dr. Bradley contracted typhus fever, from professional intercourse with his fellow-countrymen, to whose calls for medical aid he ever responded with promptitude, and with most self-sacrificing philanthropy. His case was one of the worst which occurred in that mournful year; and although he recovered after a very tedious convalescence, he never regained his previous bodily vigour. He suffered from a similar attack, 1849, and his case was considered hopeless. Few men have passed a more eventful life than Dr. Bradley; he has seen more of human nature in the short space of existence allotted to him than probably any other person in Canada. He had many friends; he was the poor man's friend; he knew no distinction of creed, nation or colour. The large assemblage of his fellow-citizens which followed him to his grave, attested the general respect in which he was held."

DR. JAMES BOVELL

Was son of Mr. John Bovell, banker, of Barbadoes, West Indies, and was born there in June, 1817. He died at Nevis, in the same islands, on January 16, 1880. He studied in London, Edinburgh and Dublin.

On taking his degree he returned to Barbadoes and commenced the practice of his profession. He married Julia Howard, daughter of Mr. Griffiths, of Henley, Barbadoes, when he was commencing his medical career. They had four daughters—Julia (Mrs. King), Emily (Mrs. Henderson), Alice (Mrs. F. D. Barwick), and Laura (Mrs. Connell). Of these only Mrs. Barwick survives.

Dr. Bovell came to Canada about 1848, and settled in Toronto. In 1850, he took part in establishing the Medical Faculty of Trinity College, in which he held the Professorship of the Institutes of Medicine, and was Dean of the Faculty, and after its disruption, joined the Toronto School of Medicine, where he lectured on Physiology and Pathology up to his leaving the country in 1870. In conjunction with others, in 1851, he assisted in founding the Upper Canada *Medical Journal*, the first issued in the Province. His contributions to medical scientific literature were numerous. He was also a valued member of the Canadian Institute. Of works of a theological and devotional character, he wrote: "Communion for the Sick," "Constitution and Canons of the Synod of the Diocese of Toronto," with explanatory notes and comments (1858), "Preparations for the Holy Communion" (1859), "Outlines of Natural Theology" (1859), "Outlines of the History of the British Church" (1860), "Passing Thoughts on Man's Relation to God, and God's Relation to Man" (1862). He also wrote a "Plea for Inebriate Asylums" (1862). His high attainments, not only in science but in theology, united with a character of unusual devoutness, induced the Bishop of Antiqua to urge upon him the duty of taking Holy Orders, to which, with many misgivings, he at last consented. In his character of a clergyman, as in that of a physician, he won the same deep love by the constant holiness of his life, and his absolute devotion to his work as long as life and strength were spared to him"—*Canada Lancet.*

A writer in a local Church of England magazine, in giving an account of the congregation of St. George's Church, Toronto, during its half century of existence, touchingly refers to the subject of our memoir as "the beloved and saintly James Bovell, M.D., who ended his life as a missionary in the West Indies. Speaking of him, Tennyson's lines may be aptly quoted:

" 'Sleep sweetly, tender heart, in peace:
Sleep, holy spirit, blessed soul,
While the stars burn, the moons increase,
And the great ages onward roll.

" 'Sleep till the end, true soul and sweet,
Nothing comes to thee new or strange;
Sleep full of rest from head to feet;
Lie still, dry dust, secure of change.' "

Dr. Bovell's widow, Julia Howard, died at Trinidad, West Indies, December 17th, 1891, in her eightieth year.

DR. HENRY BOYS

Was born, November 8th, 1775. His father was William Boys, M.D., the Historian and Antiquary, of Sandwich. His mother, Jane Fuller, was co-heiress of the estate of Statenborough, Kent. Henry Boys took his degree of M.D. at Aberdeen University, and M.R.C.S. London. He entered the army as surgeon, but was appointed Assistant Paymaster-General to the Duke of Wellington's forces, and served during the Peninsular War, receiving the medal and clasps. In 1833, he came to Canada and settled in Whitby, where he practised his profession. He was, also, Collector of Customs and Judge of the Court of Request, which was superseded by the Division Courts. His intention, when he left England, was to draw land, as the officers of Wellington's army had been entitled to do, but between the time of sailing and landing in Canada, the law under which he could take the land was annulled; notwithstanding, he was urged by the Governor, an old Peninsular friend, to still accept the allotment. He declined to do so, saying he could not accept what he was not legally entitled to. During the Mackenzie Rebellion, he had medical charge of two companies of the militia, viz., Capt. Macdonald's and Capt. (Dr.) Lowe's, under Col. Cox. In July, 1839, he received the appointment of Bursar of the University of King's College, and about the year 1841, he removed to Toronto, and ceased to practise his profession. But he did not lose interest in the profession, as he became a Member, and, subsequently, a Fellow of the College of Physicians and Surgeons, Upper Canada, and took an active part in its proceedings, while it continued to exist. In 1851, his increasing infirmities obliged him to accept a gratuity and resign his office as Bursar. He and his family then settled with the eldest living son in Barrie. Here he spent his remaining days in the gratuitous practice of his profession among the poor, and in the pursuit of his favorite studies in Natural History, to which he had continued to give attention. The nucleus of the collection of butterflies and insects in the museum of the University was made by him, and presented to the University when he left Toronto. He died, April 23, 1868, in his ninety-third year. A local paper, in recording the event, says: "Although physically feeble for some years past, he enjoyed good health, and retained the full possession of his faculties until his death. He was a man greatly respected for his many qualities, and was of a most kindly and gentle disposition." Dr. Boys, previous to his death, was one of the oldest, if not the oldest, living Fellow of the Linnæan Society.

Dr. Boys married Maria da Purifecacao Alves, daughter of Don Manual Alves, of Lisbon, Portugal, by whom he had a family of ten children, of whom three sons and four daughters still survive (1894). The eldest son, Henry Rammael Alves Boys, was for many years Treasurer of the County of Simcoe, but, owing to sickness in his family, had to resign his office and remove to a warmer climate. He is a resident of San Francisco, Cal. The next son, Thomas Tambs, adopted the profession of law, and is settled at Calgary, N.W.T. The youngest son, William Fuller Alves, is the Junior Judge of the County of Simcoe, and is the author of "Boys on Coroners," so well known among the members of the medical profession who are coroners. The eldest daughter married Dr. William Bulmer Nicol. The next daughter married the late Arthur Hogg, Esq., of Thornham Cottage, near Guelph. The two other daughters are unmarried.

Dr. Boys came of an ancient and distinguished Kentish family, and one which has served the State faithfully in the several departments of the Church, the Law, Medicine and the Army and Navy, receiving acknowledgments of their service from time to time by grants of knighthood and additions to their armorial bearings, and by important public appointments. It is said there are six Peninsular War medals alone held by the different members of the family.

It has been stated that Dr. Boys resigned the office of Bursar on account of increasing infirmities. But there can be little doubt these infirmities were the result of worry and continued effort to do the work laid upon him by the College Council. The writer has looked over the records of the Institution, and observed the painstaking entries of the proceedings, written with scrupulous distinctness. The present generation have little or no knowledge of the history of King's College, and into what a complicated knot its affairs were involved, which led to the appointment of a Commission to investigate the matter.

Dr. Boys did not find his duties a bed of roses. The Commissioners appointed to inquire into the affairs of King's College in 1848, made this statement with regard to Dr. Boys: "From the examination of particular cases, as well as from the general inquiry in which the Commissioners have been engaged, they have been strongly impressed with the great impolicy, if not absolute injustice, of imposing on the Bursar so heavy a weight of duty as that devolved upon Dr. Boys throughout almost the entire of his tenure of office. The Commissioners have no hesitation in attributing to this cause nearly the whole of those irregularities of official conduct in the subordinates placed under the Bursar, which appear so strikingly exemplified in one particular instance. The amount of work required of Dr. Boys was greater than could be efficiently performed by any one public officer. It is altogether impossible for those unacquainted with the general state of the University records and accounts, and the defective system of book-keeping which obtained in the University office from the commencement, to form any adequate conception of the extent of this gentleman's labours; and it should not be forgotten that, however eminently qualified he might have been as an accountant, it was impossible for him to introduce a proper system of book-keeping into the office in lieu of that which he found established. The very foundation for a set of double-entry books was wanted and could be obtained only by a reconstruction of the entire antecedent work of the accounts, on the same plan as that which the Commissioners have been obliged to pursue. Had Dr. Boys been a dishonest officer, he could have secured a very great amount of land under the confusion and obscurity of the defective system of accounts, which he found rooted in his office. That he has not only not availed himself of an opportunity so tempting to men of a different character, but, on the contrary, has preserved his important trust uninjured amidst the embarrassment and difficulties inconceivable, places his moral worth in the highest position. Unaccountable and culpable negligence has pervaded every department of the management; with the honourable exception of the case of the cash, by the late Bursar, Dr. Boys—an officer to whose industry and honesty in this part of his trust, the University is indebted to an extent which can be appreciated only by those who have thoroughly explored the defects of the system of accounts and records under which the general business was conducted."

DR. WM. HENRY BROWSE

Was born at Matilda, Dundas, June 15, 1824. His father, Col. Jacob Browse, was a U. E. Loyalist, who settled on the banks of the St. Lawrence, at the close of the Rebellion, 1776-83, when Upper Canada was a wilderness. Dr. Browse was for some time a student in Arts at Victoria College, Cobourg, and took the degree of B.A. He studied medicine with Dr. Rolph, and at McGill College, taking his degree of M.D., 1847. The same year when the ship-fever raged among the emigrants, Dr. Browse was appointed by the Government to take charge of the Fever Hospital at Port Iroquois, where there were some 300 patients.

In 1848, he commenced practice at Prescott, where he successfully laboured in his profession for about thirty years. His practice was not confined to the Canadian side of the river, as he was often called to visit patients on the opposite shore.

Dr. Browse became a prominent member of the profession He was elected a member of the Medical Council of Ontario, in 1866, '69, '72, '76, and was President of that body for 1870. Dr. Browse was not only active in relation to the profession, but as well in other departments of life. He was Reeve and Mayor of Prescott, besides holding many minor positions of trust and honour. He was a member of the Senate of the University of Victoria College. Ho was a keen politician of the Liberal type, and was elected Member of Parliament, 1872-74, and in 1878 he was made a life Senator of the Dominion. As a member of the House of Commons, and as a Senator, Dr. Browse was found actively at work in the interests of the people. He had much to do in obtaining an appropriation of $50,000 for the surviving veterans of the war of 1812. The important subject of state medicine engaged the attention of Dr. Browse, and he secured the appointment of a Parliamentary

Committee to consider the question of creating a Sanitary Bureau for the Dominion, of which he was Chairman.

It is recorded that Dr. Rolph offered him a partnership in order that he might assist as a lecturer in the Medical School, and that he was actually appointed to the Chair of Surgery; but Dr. Browse declined.

Dr. Browse removed to Ottawa, where he died.

Dr. Browse married Frances, the eldest daughter of Alpheus Jones, of Prescott, January 28, 1857, by whom he had one son and one daughter. The son, Wm. Henry, is a barrister practising in Toronto.

DR. CHARLES WILLIAM BUCHANAN.

Charles William Buchanan, M.D., was born on February 23, 1810, in Omagh, County Tyrone, Ireland. He was the son of George Buchanan, the proprietor of considerable estate near that town. He was bound as a student to Dr. Maxwell, of Omagh, for a period of five years, and many of the provisoes in his indenture would surprise and amuse the students of these days. After attending lectures in Dublin for two years, he proceeded to London, and on July 15, 1831, he passed his examination before the Royal College of Surgeons, England. His son, Dr. Charles W., of Cookstown, writes: "I have his surgical degree framed, and it is hanging in front of me as I write, and bears, in their own handwriting, the names of his examiners, who were as follows: Robert Keate, President; John P. Vincent, Geo. I. Guthrie, Vice-Presidents; Sir Wm. Blizard, Wm. Lynn, Sir Astley Cooper, Sir Anthony Carlisle, Thos. L. Thomas Anthony White, John G. Andrews. Many of these were reckoned as the most eminent surgeons of that date. This old degree I look upon as quite an interesting relic."

Dr. Buchanan then went to Glasgow, and after attending lectures there for nine months, in July, 1832, he obtained the degree of M.D. On returning home, he was appointed Assistant-Physician in the Omagh Hospital, and he, with the other medical men associated with him, had a very hard time, as in that year cholera raged with great violence in the Old Country.

In 1836, he was married to Margaret Gowan, a sister to Ogle R. Gowan: and the same year he and his wife left for Canada. Upon arriving in this country he settled in Brockville, where Mr. Gowan was then residing. The year after his arrival the Mackenzie rebellion broke out, and he was appointed Surgeon to the Leeds County Battalion, called "The Queen's Royal Borderers," of which his brother-in-law, Mr. Gowan, was Lieutenant-Colonel, and he was present with his regiment at the battle of the Windmill. After practising in Brockville for six years he came to Toronto, at which place he arrived, July 12, 1842, and resided in this city continuously until his death, October 25, 1876, a period of thirty-four years. During all that time he enjoyed a very extensive practice, and was one of the best known and most highly respected medical men in the city.

He was for many years a Coroner, and he presided at nearly all the inquests held in the city, and so thoroughly was he posted in everything relating to inquests that coroners from all over the Province were in the habit of writing to him for information in regard to such cases.

He was also Surgeon for a number of years to the Toronto Police Force. He was also Physician to the Oddfellows for many years.

Dr. Buchanan was a prominent Orangeman, and he was the first Master of, and for several years continued to fill the same office, in L.O.L. No. 501.

He was repeatedly waited on with the request to be a candidate for the position of Alderman, but he could not spare the time from his professional duties to properly fill that office.

He had a family of five children, two boys and three girls. His two sons followed in their father's footsteps and became medical men. The eldest son, Dr. Charles W. Buchanan, took the degree of M.B. at Toronto University, April, 1865, and is practising at Cookstown, County of Simcoe, where he has resided for many years. The second son, Dr. Ogle R. Buchanan, graduated at Victoria University, 1867, and practised with his father in Toronto for a number of years, and died there in June, 1871. His only surviving daughter is the wife of Mr. William Dineen, of the well-known firm of W. & D. Dineen, Toronto.

Dr. Buchanan was, all through life, a very healthy man, the only ailment from which he suffered being occasional attacks of rheumatism, but not of a severe nature. But in the fall of 1876,it developed a severe inflammatory character, and he died from the effects of it on October 25 of that year, being then nearly sixty-seven years of age. The writer has a very pleasant recollection of Dr. Buchanan, of his firm, manly form and dignified mien, and, what is more pleasant, he remembers him as a kind friend. His widow died at Toronto, January 19, 1892, aged eighty-six.

Mrs. Buchanan was a daughter of John Hunter Gowan, Esq., of Mount Nebo, in the County of Wexford, Ireland, a very wealthy and prominent man, and one who took an active part, on the Government side, in the great Irish rebellion of 1798, being present with his battalion of yeomanry at nearly all the engagements which took place between the loyalists and rebels in that part of the country.

The name of Gowan is intimately connected with the history of Upper Canada. The patriotism manifested by Mrs. Buchanan's father in Ireland was inherited in its fulness by the son Ogle R. Gowan. As a public man and member of Parliament, he was always conspicuous, diligent and useful. But it was in connection with the Orange Society that he won his greatest distinction. The following is from Morgan's "Sketches of Celebrated Canadians," published many years ago, and will doubtless be new to many of our readers, and interesting as well: "Mr. O. R. Gowan edited a political newspaper, published in the City of Dublin, styled the *Antidote*, and was the author of several pamphlets on political subjects. While in that kingdom he was a leading member of the Grand Lodge of the Orange Institution. He emigrated with his family to this country about the year 1829, and settled at Escott Park, in the County of Leeds, for which shire he has stood several severely contested elections; he was four times elected to Parliament for that county, and was subsequently elected for both the counties of Leeds and Grenville; he also contested the representation of the City of Toronto and the County of Ontario; but was defeated in both by slender majorities. For many years in succession, he was chosen Warden of the United Counties of

Leeds and Grenville, and he has also been, for many years, an alderman of the City of Toronto. He is popularly known as 'the father and founder' of Orangeism in America, and for twenty years filled the office of Grand Master of that body. Foreseeing the dawn of the rebellion in 1837, he called a meeting at Brockville, at which he made a very remarkable speech to the people, predicting the unfortunate insurrection which soon after followed. At this meeting the germ was laid of the first Volunteer Association formed in the Province; the enrolment was called the Brockville Invincibles. It gave the impetus to those noble defenders of the soil, the Canadian Volunteers. Immediately after this movement, he was appointed by His Excellency Sir F. B. Head, Bart., a captain in the 2nd Regiment of the Leeds Militia, then commanded by the Hon. Charles Jones. He was subsequently promoted by His Excellency Lieutenant-General Lord Seaton, to a company in the Queen's Own Rifles, commanded by Lieutenant-Colonel McMillan, and while serving in that capacity, was present at the capture of 'Hickory Island,' near Kingston, in 1838. While serving in the Queen's Rifles, he attracted the attention of His Excellency Major-General Sir George Arthur, then commanding the forces in Upper Canada, by whom, in the year 1838, he was appointed to the command of the Ninth Provisional Battalion of embodied militia, as Lieutenant-Colonel. At the engagement fought between the British troops and the American invaders, at the 'Windmill,' near Prescott, in November, 1838, Lieutenant-Colonel Gowan commanded the right wing, and was three times wounded: a rifle ball passed through his left leg, he was cut across the inner side of the knee by a buck-shot, and received a bayonet stab in the hip. The British loss in this engagement was eight officers and sixty-two rank and file; that of the Americans seventy-two, and 167 prisoners. For his personal conduct upon that day, Lieutenant-Colonel Gowan was publicly thanked in the military 'general orders,' dated the 19th of November, and by a 'general order,' dated the 4th of December, 1838, his regiment, the Ninth Provisional Battalion, was allowed, as a mark of special distinction and approbation, to be thereafter distinguished and known as the Queen's Royal Borderers."

With regard to his parliamentary career, this is the character of Mr. Gowan, as drawn by a pen understood not to be over friendly to that gentleman:

"This gentleman (Mr. Gowan) has for eight or nine years occupied a prominent position in the politics of the country, not only as the head of a powerful body, but in consequence of a talent he possesses of engaging the minds of popular assemblies and leading them with him. As a speaker he is fluent and energetic, very often powerful in his appeals to feeling, and evidently speaks more for the audience than the house; his sarcasm is bitter, and possessing great evenness of temper, you seldom see him ruffled at any remarks which may be made. He is an active, well-made man, rather low, with a prepossessing face and easy insinuating manners, very mild in his address, and with talents which, if rightly applied, would soon raise him to an eminent situation."

It may be well to state that Mr. Gowan did not introduce Orangeism into Canada. This distinction belongs to one Arthur Hopper, who immigrated in 1812, and had established at Montreal the first Orange Lodge soon after his arrival there. He afterwards settled in Huntly, six miles from Ottawa, and had built there an Orange Hall, the first in Upper Canada.

DR. EDWARD BULL,

Born, December, 1823, in the Township of York, near Toronto, was the son of Bartholomew Bull, Esq., who was a native of County Tipperary, Ireland, and came to York, 1819. He acquired a valuable tract of land near the town, and established his home on the Davenport Road, which is now a beautiful winding street in the outskirts of Toronto. Mr. Bull passed a long and useful life in the community, dwelling in his comfortable home with his esteemed wife, surrounded by his family of four daughters and five sons. He lived to his eighty-seventh year, and all through his life was highly respected among his wide circle of friends and acquaintances. Of his daughters, Mary died unmarried; Mrs. Shaw is also deceased; Mrs. Good, the widow of James Good, at one time well known as the proprietor of a foundry, and at which he constructed the first locomotive to run on the old Northern Railway; another daughter is the wife of Dr. Alexander Pattullo, well known as a practitioner at Brampton for many years, and latterly in Toronto. Of his sons, John P. is a Justice of the Peace; Bartholomew, jr., who was also a Justice of the Peace, and for many years Reeve of York Township, now deceased; Dr. Frank, deceased, and Thomas H., the present Clerk of the Peace for the County of York. As it is not within the scope of this work to give extended family histories apart from the subject of the sketch, it may only be added that all the sons have occupied prominent positions in their respective lines of life, and possessed the public respect.

The subject of our sketch left home at the age of seventeen to become a student at Victoria College, Cobourg, and continued there for three sessions. In 1842, he entered upon the study of medicine under Dr. John Rolph, and acquired his professional knowledge mainly from that distinguished teacher of the medical science. In 1846, he passed the Lower Canada Medical Board, and subsequently he received the degree of M.D. from Victoria University.

Dr. Bull began his career as a practitioner at the Village of Lloydtown, Township of King, County of York, 1847, where he continued in active work for eighteen years. He was appointed Coroner for the Counties of York and Simcoe, 1850, and he served two years in the Municipal Council of King, removed to the Village of Weston, 1865, where he pursued his practice for twelve years, and led a very busy life. While there he was appointed President of the High School Board of Weston. Dr. Bull took up his residence in Toronto, 1876, not so much to practise medicine as to enjoy a well-earned rest and the advantages which Toronto affords. He with his wife and daughter made a tour of two years' duration, visiting the Pacific Coast States and Canada, and Honolulu. Dr. Bull is well known in the moneyed circles of Toronto.

He married, 1852, Miss Mary Ida, daughter of Stewart Grafton, of Dundas, a granddaughter of the Rev. John Beatty. They have two children, a son, of the firm of Kerr, Bull and Rowell, barristers, and a daughter who lives at home. It may

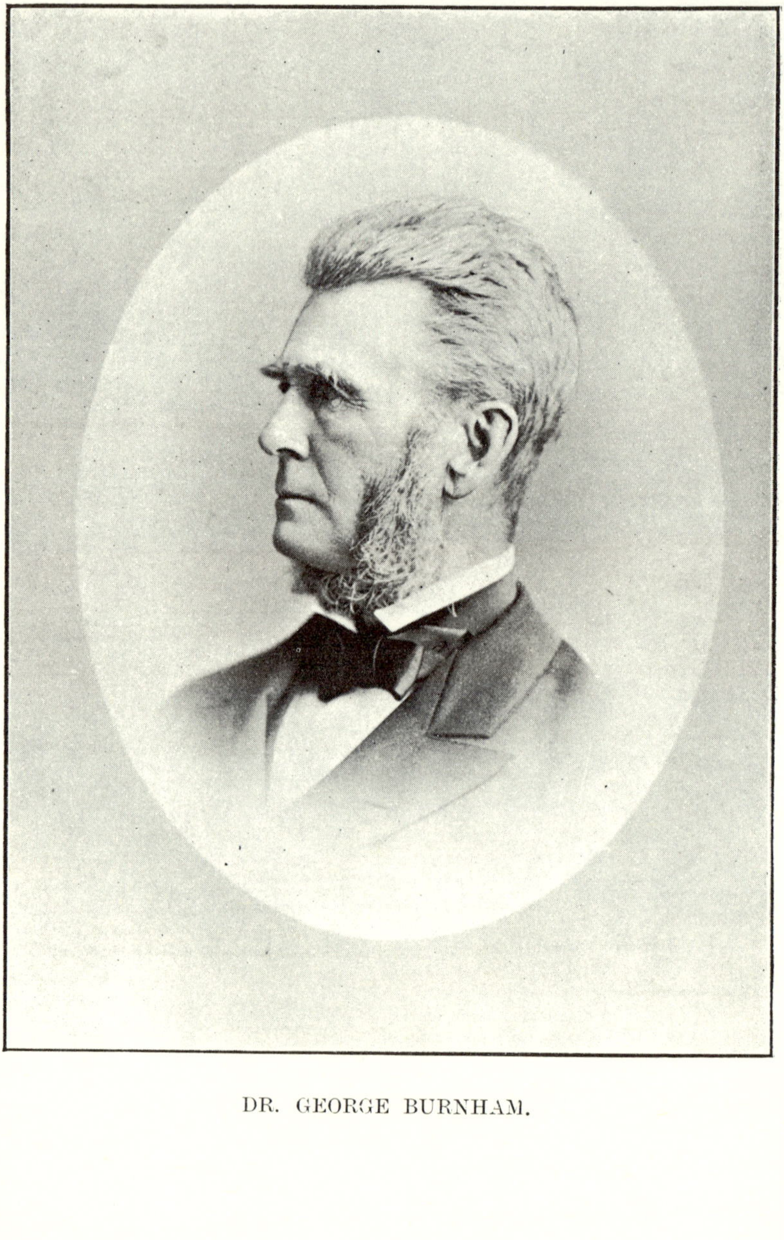

DR. GEORGE BURNHAM.

be mentioned that Dr. Bull has been a keen politician, and had he been so disposed, might have had the nomination as candidate for parliamentary honours.

Dr. Frank Bull was born at the family residence, Springmount, July 25, 1831. He received his literary training at Victoria College, Cobourg, and pursued his professional studies in the medical department of that institution in Toronto. Procured his license to practise from the Upper Canada Medical Board, October, 1854. Attended the University of New York the following winter, and received the degree of M.D., also the same degree from Victoria University, 1855.

Dr. Frank Bull engaged in practice at Brampton for some time and then removed to Toronto, where he continued to practise until his illness which resulted in death, January 25, 1862. Frank was a dear and intimate friend of the writer. Our friendship began in the halls of "Old Vic.," ripened in our close associations as fellow medical students, continued unabated in mutual correspondence while the writer was absent from the country, and subsequently as fellow-practitioners—a friendship which culminated when the writer was called to minister to him professionally on his dying bed. The writer vividly remembers the bleak January day when all that was mortal of Frank Bull was laid away in the quiet tomb. He remembers the darkened room, the solemn service, the falling tear, the military pageant, for he was an officer of the Queen's Own, the office of pall-bearer, and the last sepulchral rites, earth to earth, ashes to ashes, dust to dust. Alas, what is this life, except, as in this case, there is a certain promise of a future brighter existence.

Dr. Frank Bull stood very high in the estimation of his medical confréres, as well as of all who had the good fortune to know him. In his death it was recognized that the profession had suffered a distinct loss, and that bright promises of professional distinction had been destroyed.

DR. GEORGE BURNHAM,

Born at Cobourg, Ontario, September 4, 1814, was the son of John Burnham, one of the four brothers who emigrated from New Hampshire to Cobourg towards the close of the last century. Of these the Hon. Asa and the Hon. Zaccheus soon became prominent in Canadian public affairs. They were all Loyalists of the most ardent type. Two large books on the genealogy of the Burnham family furnish a complete and interesting account of those members of it, who, between 1635 and and 1836, had gone from Herefordshire, the manor at Norwich, Norfolk, and other places in England, to the Colonies in America.

Two of the brothers were members of the Legislative Council of Old Canada and were men of wealth and influence. During the war of 1812-15, Hon. Zaccheus Burnham, of whom Mr. Henry Morgan, in his "History of Celebrated Canadians," speaks in high praise, had the command of a fleet of bateaux on Lake Ontario, and was able to do considerable service to his country. In the "Life of Colonel Talbot," he is spoken of in terms of admiration.

The subject of this sketch at first engaged in the study of law, and had nearly completed the course for the bar, when he decided to adopt medicine as a profession. He commenced his studies with Dr. McSpadden, of Port Hope; then studied at Toronto, and afterwards in New York, at Bellevue Hospital.

Having obtained his degree in 1839, he and his brother, a barrister, went into the backwoods, as it was then considered, in the County of Peterborough, to seek their fortunes. Dr. Burnham proved to be the man for the times and place, and took an active part in public matters. Dr. Burnham took an especial interest in educational affairs, as Chairman of the Board of School Trustees, for many years—at a time when the head master and chairman were largely responsible for the success of the school. His duties called for the exercise of qualifications of no common kind. To his exertions and ability may be largely attributed the excellent advantages the youth of that county enjoyed. His zeal was manifested by giving public lectures and private discourses on educational matters yet new to the country, and thus educating the public mind.

Dr. Burnham, in the practice of his profession, was remarkably successful. His skill, combined with his high character and many amiable qualities, commanded the respect of the public, and his professional services were much sought after, not only in Peterborough, but in the surrounding districts. This large practice he continued to enjoy until a few years before his death, when failing health compelled him, gradually, to relinquish his work to his partner and son-in-law, Dr. Boucher. He was for many years a prominent Mason, and was the first Master of Peterborough Lodge, being a charter member. In politics he was a Baldwin Liberal; but never a partizan. In an obituary notice in the *Peterborough Review*, it is stated: "He contented himself with doing his duty as a citizen, where by his great ability he was enabled to do good service in promoting educational and Christian work." At the time of the ship fever epidemic, 1847, Dr. Burnham devoted himself as a volunteer to the stricken emigrants. He took the fever himself and nearly succumbed to it. His charitable acts were not few.

Dr. Burnham married, January 23, 1847, Adeline Humphress Spalding, youngest daughter of John Spalding, of Grafton, a U. E. Loyalist, with a family history similar to his own. They had born to them eight children, of whom four are now (1893) alive, namely, Herbert, Helen S. (wife of Dr. Boucher, of Peterborough), Hampden and Georgina. He died, June 14, 1881.

G. Herbert followed in the footsteps of his father by entering the medical profession. He became an undergraduate in Arts, of Toronto University, and then took a course of study in medicine, and received his degree of M.D., 1875. Proceeding to England he obtained the diploma of M.R.C.S. Eng., 1876, and F.R.C.S. Edin., 1882. He remained in England and on the continent for upwards of seven years in the pursuit of professional knowledge. He then established himself in Toronto, as an oculist and aurist. In that capacity he is now surgeon to the Eye Infirmary, the Toronto General Hospital, and lectures in the medical department of Toronto University.

Hampden Burnham, M.A., author of "Canadians in the Imperial Service," is a barrister.

DR. DAVID BURNS.

The name is found on the U. E. list as Surgeon of the 71st Regiment. He seems to have been a person of excellent education, and was appointed Clerk of the Crown in Chancery for the Province of Upper Canada, probably soon after the organization of the Government. He was one of the first settlers of York, and one of the patentees of the Park Lots laid out fronting on the north side of what was then called Dundas Street, afterward Lot Street, and now forming Queen Street.

The Upper Canada *Gazette* or *American Oracle* announced his death, after a painful illness, on February 6, 1806.

That Dr. Burns was held in high estimation is shown by verses written to his memory, which appeared in the *Gazette* and *Oracle*, February 15, 1806:

"Hail, gentle Shade! where'er thy aerial tread
To honor'd living, and lamented dead.
Mayhap that now, conceal'd from mortal view,
The Muse's trace thou friendly dost pursue;
Or leaving Earth, on wings celestial mount,
To join thy Essence to the parent fount.
In brighter skies might shine thy setting sun,
But Heaven's high will, and not my will be done.

"Say, power of Truth, so great, so unconfin'd,
And solve the doubt, which so distracts my mind,
Why Strength to Weakness is so near allied;
Perhaps 'tis given to humble human Pride.
At times, perchance, frail Nature held the sway,
Yet dimm'd not it the intellectual ray:
Reason and Truth triumphant held their course,
And list'ning hearers felt Conviction's force.
No precept mangled, text misunderstood,
He thought and acted but for public good;
His reasoning pure, his mind all manly light,
Made Day of that, which erst appear'd as Night.
In him Instruction, aim'd at this great end,
Our fates to soften and our lives amend.
Yet he was Man, and man's the Child of Woe,
Who seeks Perfection, seeks not here below;
And Him whose fame defies the Cynic's scan,
Indeed must be, or more or less than man.

"Hail, gentle Shade! nor from the friendly Muse
This weak memorial of his love refuse;
Add this small tribute to the tear he shed,
Who lov'd thee living, and laments thee dead."

DR. ALEXANDER BURNSIDE

Appeared before the Upper Canada Medical Board, January, 1820, for examination. The Board, consisting of Drs. Macaulay, Widmer, Lyons and Powell, found him "unfit" to practise, but "recommended further study and attendance on a course of lectures." Whether he complied with this recommendation or not is uncertain; but at all events, in April, 1822, he was "found qualified to practise," and obtained his license.

A trustworthy informant says of him: "An American by birth, of no education, and one considered by all medical men of standing as a Yankee quack. The country people seemed to think that he had a knowledge of local fevers, etc., and employed him; his practice was never large at any time, but he acquired considerable property. During the first cholera epidemic he was the standing witness for the defendants upon an indictment for nuisances, always proving to the satisfaction of the jurors that the stench complained of, whether it arose from stables, tanneries, privy vaults, or any other abomination, was conducive to health; at least, he found it so in his practice." Another says of him that he had for a time "a large practice up Yonge Street. He was capable of selling water at a penny a pail. An ignorant man, but a money-maker. Fine-looking, portly, neat, tidy, always wearing a large gold seal."

This is the estimate put upon him by another writer: "A wealthy, large-hearted, New England physician, whose benefactions are now doing good to thousands, but whose name will ever be remembered as the promoter and encourager of church music, both vocal and instrumental."

Dr. Scadding thus describes him in a more attractive form: "A New England medical man, of tall figure, upright carriage, and bluff, benevolent countenance, an early promoter of the Mechanics' Institute movement, and an encourager of church music, vocal and instrumental. Dying without a family dependent upon him, he bequeathed his property partly to charities in the town, and partly to the University of Trinity College, where two scholarships perpetuate his memory. In fact, he donated the greater portion of his property to Trinity College."

Dr. Burnside was a director and trustee of the British

American Fire and Life Assurance Company, as well as Dr. Winder, Dr. King being the medical adviser.

Notwithstanding all animadversions, this fact remains that Dr. Burnside's benevolence and charitable bequests entitle his memory to the greatest respect. The relief which has been, and will continue to be, afforded at the Burnside lying-in department of the General Hospital, is beyond human estimation, and can only be weighed by an Almighty hand. He died December 13, 1854, in his 75th year.

In the long disused graveyard surrounding St. James' Cathedral, among the few tombstones placed over the graves, is one containing this inscription: "To the memory of Harriet Throckmorton, wife of Alexander Burnside, M.D., who on the 23rd of December, 1839, died as she had lived, humbly depending on the merits of her Saviour for salvation, aged 56 years."

DR. WALTER HORATIO BURRITT.

The writer has before him an interesting memoir written by Stephen Burritt, who was postmaster at Burritt's Rapids for fourteen years, giving an account of the Burritt family in America, and of their settlement in the county north of the River Rideau, first visited by his father, Stephen, in 1793. Only a few facts relating thereto can be given in these pages. The progenitor of the family in America was William Burritt, a Welshman, who came out in 1641 and settled at Stratford on the sea coast, in the colony of Connecticut. At the breaking out of the rebellion, 1776, one branch of the family took sides with the rebels, while another adhered to the British constitution, and fought for the Crown. A distinguished descendant of the former was Elihu Burritt, "the learned blacksmith." Among the U. E. Loyalists were two brothers, Stephen and Daniel Burritt. Stephen entered the British army at the age of nineteen and served seven years. He was in many engagements, and at the surrender of Burgoyne. At the close of the war, the two brothers came with the disbanded soldiers, who settled along the St. Lawrence. Here they lived until 1793, when Stephen penetrated the forest north of the Rideau and began a settlement. Daniel followed a few years later. The now smiling and prosperous country at and around Burritt's Rapids was the theatre of their vigorous and successful pioneer life. Stephen was Lieutenant-Colonel 2nd Regiment Grenville Militia, and was called in consultation by General Brock, and was on duty at Fort Wellington during the war, taking part in all the engagements in that region. He was also member of Parliament, 1810-11-12.

The subject of our sketch was the son of Daniel Burritt, whose wife was Electa Landon, also a U. E. Loyalist. In the war of 1812, he commanded a company of volunteers, which he raised and did duty at Prescott, and was at the taking of Ogdensburg. He was afterwards a colonel of militia. Walter Horatio, born September 18, 1809, was the fourth of five children. He received his primary education in Brockville, and studied medicine with Dr. Basil P. Church, at Merrickville. He attended the Fairfield Medical College, New York State. Before the Upper Canada Medical Board, July, 1835, he was found "well qualified to practise," and received his licence. He commenced practice at Smith's Falls, where he continued for some thirty-five years. He was, besides an active practitioner, a public man of influence, and was honoured by various public offices, as Village Councillor, School Trustee, being Chairman for sixteen years, and also a Coroner.

In 1870, he removed to Peterborough. He married, September, 1837, Miss Maria, daughter of James Schofield, County Leeds. Dr. Burritt had seven children. Horatio Charles Burritt, the eldest son, was born at Smith's Falls, September 2, 1840. Was educated at the Smith's Falls Grammar School, Bishop's College, Lennoxville, and studied medicine at McGill College, Montreal, receiving the degree of M.D., C.M., 1863. Shortly after he went to Washington and was appointed Acting Assistant-Surgeon in the Northern Army, and assigned to Lincoln General Hospital, Washington, where he remained for some time. He married Maria Harriet, fourth daughter of James G. Rogers, Esq., of Grafton, Ont., and settled in Morrisburgh, where he remained three years. Was appointed surgeon to the Prescott Brigade of Garrison Artillery. He removed to Peterborough, where he did a very extensive practice for fourteen years. He removed to Toronto, 1882. He was member of the Council of the College of Physicians and Surgeons Ontario, 1880-85. Dr. Burritt is a well-known leading practitioner in Toronto.

DR. JAMES CAMPBELL

Was born in South Lincolnshire, England, in 1777, and died in Kingston, Canada, January 25th, 1842, aged 65 years.

Mr. Campbell became in early life a member of the Royal College of Surgeons, London, and practised with considerable success in Hedon, Yorkshire, between the years 1800 and 1821, as a surgeon-apothecary. He was of Scotch descent. He married in July, 1811, Lavinia Scatcherd, a daughter of Mr. Thomas Scatcherd, merchant, of Hull, Yorkshire. Her two brothers, John and Thomas Scatcherd, came to Canada in 1821, and settled in Nissouri, in the County of Middlesex, Upper Canada. John represented that county for many years in the Canadian Parliament, an honour afterwards held in succession by two o. his sons. Thomas is still alive (1889), a hale old gentleman.

In 1822, intending to come out to Canada, but resolving to take a degree of Doctor of Medicine before leaving Britain, Mr. Campbell went to Edinburgh to attend the College courses in medicine there, residing in the meantime with his family at Porto Bello, a sea-side village a few miles distant. He became in due course an M.D. of the University of Edinburgh, and in 1824, with his wife and children, sailed from Greenock for Quebec, in a brig called *The Warner*, owned by and consigned to Miller, Parlane & Co., of Montreal, the founders of the house there now known as H. & A. Allan, it is believed one of the largest steamship owners in the world. Miller, Parlane & Co. became Miller, Edmonstone & Co., then Edmonstone, Allan & Co., and then H. & A. Allan.

Dr. Campbell, as he had become, had engaged the cabin accommodation of the brig, and there were no other passengers. They were six weeks on the voyage. After spending a fortnight at Quebec, where he was hospitably received by several of the old residents there to whom he had letters, Dr. Campbell came up to Montreal in the steamer *Swiftsure*, owned by the Honourable John Molson, the second steamer on the St. Lawrence. There he remained practising his profession until 1832, when he removed to Lachine, where he had purchased a small estate; the house had then recently been erected by Mr. McDougall, a retired factor of the Hudson's Bay Company.

Whilst residing on this property, the first cholera broke out, and Dr. Campbell at once threw himself into the struggle, volunteered his services at the cholera sheds, accepted no fees, but professionally and privately exerted himself to the utmost to mitigate the evils of the plague. Amongst other good deeds, he brought to his house from the cholera hospital sheds Mrs. Cockburn, formerly of Toronto, now deceased, and her children. Mr. Cockburn, then an emigrant from Berwick-on-Tweed, had been cut off by the cholera at Lachine. She and her children received every kindness from Dr. Campbell. One of her sons, the late James Cockburn, M.P. for East Northumberland, sometime Speaker of the House of Commons of Canada, always bore the kindest recollections of these days, and maintained a close friendship to the last with the sons of Dr. Campbell.

In 1837, owing to the failure of his eldest son who had gone into business in Hamilton, and for whom Dr. Campbell had become endorser in Montreal, he became compelled to sell his property at Lachine and elsewhere in Lower Canada, and to resume the practice of his profession. After several visits to other places, as Oswego, Ogdensburg and Potsdam, he finally decided to commence practice at Kingston, where he died in 1842. He held a deservedly high position in the esteem of his brethren of the profession and amongst the community at large.

Dr. Campbell had five sons and two daughters. One of the daughters died young; the other, Charlotte Anne, married M. W. Strange, M.L.A., Frontenac. The sons were Colin, Donald, Charles James, Alexander and Alfred A. Of those, Donald was Registrar, County Peel; Charles, the only one of the family now living (1893), is Assistant Receiver-General, Toronto; Alfred was Colonel of the 15th Battalion, Belleville. It remains to speak of Alexander, whose eminent position as a public man demands more extended notice. In doing so we have availed ourselves of a sketch, being one of a number of "Prominent Canadians," which have appeared in *The Week*, written at the time our subject became Lieut.-Governor of Ontario, by "Herat."

"Sir Alex. Campbell was two years old when he came with his father to Canada, having been born in the village of Hedon, Yorkshire, England. His parents gave him the best educational advantages the country afforded, first, under the tuition of a Presbyterian clergyman, then at St. Hyacinthe College, and afterward at the Royal Grammar School at Kingston. Naturally studious, he acquired at a comparatively early period the essential elements of a liberal education. His knowledge of the French language enabled him in after days to address the Senate in that language. But it was in a knowledge of his own language, and a correct use of words that he was distinguished. His style in speaking and in writing was admirable. When only seventeen years of age he commenced the study of law. Completing his course of study and having been called to the Bar, he formed a partnership with Mr. (afterwards the Right Hon. Sir) John A. Macdonald. This partnership continued for many years; and as the senior partner became engrossed in political matters, the bulk of the work in connection with the firm, which had become very large, fell upon Mr. Campbell. Giving himself up to this work and ever increasing his knowledge by study, the experience he thus acquired amply qualified him for the career of statesman, which he was destined to follow. He was regarded as one of the soundest lawyers at the Bar of Upper Canada, and had he not changed into politics, there is little doubt he might have occupied a distinguished position on the Bench.

"Mr. Campbell's first appearance in political life was in 1858, when he was elected as member of the Legislative Council of Old Canada, for Cataraqui Division. No new member probably ever had less crudeness or inexperience to rub off, and no one seemed at all surprised when, in three or four years after his first election, the member for Cataraqui Division was placed in the Speaker's Chair. In 1864, he entered the Cabinet as Commissioner of Crown Lands. From this time forward Mr. Campbell was looked upon as one of the strong men of his party, though one whose strength was shown rather in counsel than in fight.

"When in 1867 the first Government of the Dominion was constituted, Mr. Campbell was made Postmaster-General. This position he held for six years, when the new Department of the Interior being instituted, he became its Minister. Mr. Campbell held the portfolio of this department until the fall of Sir John Macdonald's government in 1873. Until 1878, he discharged the duties of leader of the Opposition in the Senate. This he did with fairness and moderation which commanded the respect of the governmental party. On the return to power of the Conservative party, 1878, Mr. Campbell accepted the position of Receiver-General; not many months later he returned to his former position of Postmaster-General. In turn, he became Minister of Militia and Defence, in 1880. Returning after nearly a year to the Postmastership, he subsequently was the Minister of Justice. Mr. Campbell was, May 24, 1879, created a Knight Commander of the Order of St. Michael and St. George, a fitting recognition of his eminent public services. Sir Alexander remained Minister of Justice until the latter part of 1885, when he again became Postmaster-General.

"In the spring of 1887, Sir Alexander Campbell was appointed Lieutenant-Governor of Ontario, which was hailed with satisfaction by his political friends and opponents alike. Before assuming the gubernatorial duties, Sir Alexander, at the request of the Government, represented Canada in England at the Colonial Conference.

"In the sphere in which he has chiefly moved, that of the Senate, his was always the most important and imposing personality, and that not simply by virtue of his office as leader of the Government or else of the Opposition in the Upper Chamber, but in an equal degree at least by force of character and talent. To have represented the Conservative party as long as he did in that Chamber, and to have done so from first to last with distinguished success, not merely from a political point of view, but from an intellectual and moral point of view as well, constituted a record of which even a man of high ability and considerable ambition might well be proud. Sir Alexander may be said to have approached as near as it has ever been given to any Canadian statesman to approach the ideal type of a senator—a man grave and strong, moderate, dignified, firm, sagacious, candid without indiscretion, politic without craft, loyal to his party, but ever mindful of his personal honour, and ever thoughtful of the public weal."

When Sir Alexander Campbell was appointed to fill the office of Lieutenant-Governor of Ontario, he received the last worldly honour he was to obtain. The hand of death closed the door to further marks of distinction in this world. On May 24, 1892, while yet the occupant of Government House, and within a few days of the end of his five years' term of office, he quietly passed away, aged seventy-one years. To show how acceptably Sir Alexander had discharged the duties of his post, and the regard in which he was held by the public, of all grades of political opinion, we cull from several obituary notices published at the time. Says one: "The death of Sir Alexander Campbell takes from Canada's public life a man of the highest character, wide knowledge and many services. . . . There were none who gave their country the benefit of a clearer judgment or a higher purpose to do that which was right." Says another: "His whole career was marked by the utmost respectability and faithfulness to a high standard of public duty. . . . During his occupancy of the Lieutenant-Governorship of the Province he so long represented, he has discharged his duties with the utmost impartiality and courtesy, and his associations with the Government of Ontario have been the most pleasant. He had the esteem of both parties for his public services and personal character." Another says: "Since he became Lieutenant-Governor, the official conduct of Sir Alexander has been faultless. He performed his social duties with liberality and impartiality, and on no occasion did he ever falter in his fidelity to his advisers, even when they were running amuck of his old political friends." One more, the *Empire*, says: "The Lieutenant-Governor of Ontario was, indeed, one of the political landmarks of our day a man who was, above all things, an honest politician, without fear and without reproach, one who did his work in life well, and who carries to his grave the esteem and regret of a great number of people who may never have personally seen his tall, stately figure or encountered his pleasant smile and genial words." Still another, the *Globe*, says: "The office of Lieutenant-Governor of Ontario has become associated with dignity, liberal hospitality, courtesy, and unswerving impartiality, and it is the general verdict that this honourable tradition was thoroughly well maintained by Sir Alexander Campbell. . . . To say of a public man that from youth to old age he served his country diligently, honestly and honourably, was faithful to his friends and fair to his foes, is high praise, and such a man was the late Lieutenant-Governor of this Province."

DR. DUNCAN CAMPBELL

Died at Toronto, April 5, 1879. He was gazetted as a licentiate of Upper Canada, June 4, 1834. The following is taken from an obituary notice which appeared in the Canada *Lancet:*

"Dr. Campbell was born in Argyleshire, Scotland, in 1811, and was, consequently, in the sixty-eighth year of his age. His early education was obtained in Caen, France, and afterwards in Edinburgh, graduating in the University of Edinburgh in 1833. After coming out to Canada, in 1834, he served as surgeon in one of the battalions in 1837, and, at the close of the rebellion, settled in Hamilton, but soon after removed to Niagara, where he remained until 1858, at which time he removed to this city.

"His medical titles were the following: L.R.C.S. Edin.; M.D., University of Edinburgh. He was President of the Homœopathic Medical Board of Ontario from 1859 until its demise, in 1869, and a member of the Ontario Medical Council from the latter date up to the time of his death, having occupied the position of Vice-President, and, at the time of his death, President of the Council.

"He was a man of good education, great intellectual power, and his services in the Medical Council in the cause of higher education were exceedingly valuable. He joined heartily in the amalgamation of the different licensing boards into the one sole licensing body in Ontario, the wisdom of which has already borne such good results to the public and the medical profession in Canada. Although somewhat imperious and arbitrary in his manner at times, he was, nevertheless, possessed of an agreeable and genial nature, and though liable sometimes to

19

give offence, he was always ready to forgive and forget. He leaves a widow and eleven children, six daughters, two of whom are unmarried, and five sons, to mourn his loss."

Lorne Colin, son of above, entered the profession and graduated, 1872. He was Medical Officer for the Silver Islet Mining Company for five years. He died at Port Arthur, January 4, 1885, aged thirty-four.

DR. G. W. CAMPBELL

Was born in Roseneath, Dumbartonshire, Scotland, in the year 1810. He entered early upon his medical studies, which he pursued in the Universities of Glasgow and Dublin. After graduating with distinction he came to Canada in May, 1833, and settled in Montreal. His marked ability soon placed him in the front rank amongst his compeers, and gave him a large share of city practice. The success following him naturally led to his being very frequently called in consultation by his confrères; and for a great many years before his death, very few cases of any importance were treated in the city without the advice of Dr. Campbell having been obtained. His grand knowledge of pathology, naturally clear insight into the varying shades of distinction between clinical conditions apt to resemble each other, made him an expert in diagnosis. Surgery was always his forte, and his great reputation was chiefly made by many successful achievements in operative work. In 1835, Dr. Campbell was appointed to the Chair of Surgery in McGill University, which position he continued to hold with credit to himself and great advantage to the school until 1875—exactly forty years—when, owing to failing health, he resigned. He was made Dean of the Faculty in 1860, taking then the place of Dr. Holmes. The duties of this office he fulfilled even after his resignation of the Chair of Surgery.

Not only was Dr. Campbell deservedly looked up to as the leading surgeon of the city, but he was held in the warmest estimation as a citizen. He was for many years Director, and lately Vice-President of the Bank of Montreal, and also Director in the City Gas Company, the Montreal Telegraph Company, and many others.

Dr. Campbell died at Roseneath, Dumbartonshire, May 30, 1882. The obituary notices show clearly the estimation in which he was held.

"The profession has lost a member from whom it received an equivalence of honour far greater than it conferred; the public have lost an able servant, using that word in its true and most expressive sense; the society in which he moved will note his absence with extreme pain. There are thousands who will deplore his death and cherish recollections of his work and his benevolence."—*M. Herald.*

"A large-hearted, broad-minded, good man; a loyal man, loyal to country, to nationality, to city, to church, to profession, to clan; a true gentleman, kind and bluff, manly and tender, who that knew him does not feel that he has lost a friend? He was almost the last of that fine body of physicians who formed the profession in Montreal a generation ago, and whose enterprise and public spirit made Montreal celebrated for the school of medicine which they founded. He was the undisputed head of the profession in Montreal."—*M. Witness.*

He will long be remembered amongst his fellow-citizens as a clear-headed and judicious business man, possessing qualities in this respect sufficiently uncommon amongst medical men.

The example of such a man as Dr. Campbell cannot fail to be productive of great good. An accomplished physician and skilful surgeon, an upright, honourable citizen, a kind and considerate friend to the poor, a loved and honoured counsellor of the rich, zealous in business, but scrupulously honourable, a firm protector of the dignity of his profession, and, above all, a thoroughly consistent Christian gentleman.

This gentleman never lived in Ontario, but he was visited by many from the Province, and who became his patients. And, moreover, like Dr. Holmes, he was a much liked teacher of medicine and surgery to a large number of practitioners of Ontario. He is, therefore, accorded a place in these pages.

DR. JAMES CATHCART.

A nephew of Dr. Martin Cathcart, 4th Dragoon Guards, was educated at Trinity College, Dublin, and obtained M.R.C.S. in

England. He came to Canada, 1832, and was gazetted as licentiate of Upper Canada in June. Having decided to practise at York, he took lodgings with Mr. McMurray and began practice. Rev. Dr. McMurray writes the "he was most successful. During the height of the cholera he exerted himself beyond his strength, with both high and low, and was most successful in his practice." Dr. Widmer stated that "had he lived he would have taken a very high stand in his profession."

Highly educated and most gentlemanly in his bearing, he rendered himself acceptable to all with whom he was brought in contact, whether professional or otherwise. He died suddenly of inflammation of the bowels about the first of September, 1832.

DR. JAMES CATTERMOLE

Was born in Suffolk, England, October 13, 1807; was the son of James Cattermole, a landed proprietor whose family pedigree extended back to the time of Queen Elizabeth. At the age of thirteen he was placed in London to receive his education, where he remained until sixteen years of age, when he was apprenticed to a surgeon according to the customs of the day. He pursued his medical studies at Granger's School and Guy's Hospital, and passed his medical examination at Soc. Apothecaries, 1830. Two years later he came to Quebec, as surgeon to an emigrant vessel. He was at York, 1832, when he passed the Medical Board in July. Dr. Cattermole practised at Guelph for three years and then returned to England. For fifteen years he was engaged in a large practice in Surreyside, London. In 1850 he came to the United States and proceeding westward as far as the Mississippi, located himself at Fort Madison, Iowa, and continued to practise there for five years; but ill-health, with the disadvantages of a new country, caused him to again come to Canada. At this time he received the degree of M.D. from the University of St, Louis, Missouri. In 1855, he made his final choice and settled in London, Ont. When the City Hospital, of London, was established, Dr. Cattermole was appointed consulting Surgeon. But he has not accepted any office or position outside of his profession, to which he has always had a strong attachment. He kept himself abreast of the times in medical science by extensive reading. He gave special attention to surgery, especially in connection with affections incident to the females, in which he was considered an expert. In later years his practice was limited to this special practice, with office work and consultations. His standing as a practitioner was high, and his practice very successful. He has been called "the most experienced and skilful physician and surgeon in the County of Middlesex." He was a member of the Church of England, and his standing has been as high morally and religiously as professionally.

Dr. Cattermole married in May, 1850, Miss Maria Dalton, of Dover, England. They had five children, two of whom died young. The one son, James Frederick, entered the medical profession. He studied at the Toronto University, and at Edinburgh, where he obtained Lic. R. Coll. Phy. Edin., 1881. He also took Lic. Fac. Phys. and Surg., Glasgow, 1881.

This obituary notice appeared November 18, 1890:

"The death is chronicled of another old and highly esteemed citizen in the person of Dr. Cattermole, after a long and tedious illness, in his 84th year. For the past two years the doctor was a confirmed invalid, whose days were lengthened to an unusual span by the devoted ministrations of those about him. Since the establishment of the City Hospital he held the honorary post of consulting surgeon of that institution. He refrained from accepting civic offices of any kind, devoting himself entirely to his practice, hence his success and high standing. For some years he was a director in the Dominion Savings and Loan Society, and also in the City Gas Company, from both of which he resigned on account of failing eyesight. He was a member of the Church of England. He was a life-member and one of the doctors of St. George's Society. In politics he was a staunch Conservative, and to the last remained a strong admirer of Sir John Macdonald. His wife survives him with two daughters—the eldest of whom is the wife of Mr. Isaac Waterman, of this city; the second, wife of Dr. F. B. Wilkinson, of Courtright—and one son, Dr. J. F. Cattermole, of West Flamborough.

DR. WM. CASE.

In four generations of this family were members of the medical profession, and all of them had the same christian name. Of the first Dr. Wm. Case we have no knowledge, except that he lived and practised the profession in the State of New Hampshire, U.S. The second one of the name was born in New Hampshire, and studied his profession in Philadelphia. He practised his profession in his native place until 1810, when he came to Upper Canada and purchased a farm, a little more than a mile east of the present limits of Hamilton in the township of Barton. At this early period in the history of the Province, there was comparatively little practice in this sparsely settled district. He therefore devoted his time to clearing the farm, and in its cultivation, and as well in attending to the wants of the settlers as a physician. In the war of 1812 he was in sympathy with his adopted country. His house was converted into a military hospital for two years, and he was left in charge when the regimental surgeon was away. There were usually twelve or fifteen patients, and sometimes as many as thirty. His son remembers having seen him take up the radial artery in the arm of Capt. Taylor, who had been wounded at Stony Creek. Capt. Taylor, who had studied law in England, left the service and engaged in the practice of law at Hamilton, and had as a student young Macnab, afterwards Sir Allan. Mr. Taylor became the first judge appointed for the county of Wentworth.

Dr. Case had six sons and six daughters. He died in 1854. Throughout his life, as a pioneer settler and practitioner, he never took a holiday. "Died at Barton, April 19, 1874, Ruth, relict of Dr. Wm. Case, and mother of Dr. Case, sen., of Hamilton, aged 94 years 8 months."

DR. WM. I. A. CASE,

Son of Dr. Wm. Case, the second, was born in Pennsylvania, 1805. The family came to Upper Canada in 1810, when the subject of our sketch was but four years old. As he grew up he took his part of the work on the farm, and at an early age assisted his father in connection with his practice, and acquired by degrees much knowledge of the profession. Opportunity for obtaining an education at this time was very limited ; but for a while he had the advantage of instruction from the Rev. Ralph Leeming, Episcopalian clergyman, of Hamilton. In 1829 he went to the Medical College at Fairfield, and graduated there, and obtained license at Montreal Medical Board, 1843. Dr. Case remembers the events in connection with the war of 1812, especially the battle of Stony Creek. Although a boy he helped his father in dressing the wounds of the patients who occupied the beds in the temporary hospital in his father's house. He also remembers well Dr. Widmer, who came there toward the close of the war as surgeon to a detachment of Wellington's soldiers. He visited the hospital. At an early period in his life he was entrusted by his father to visit and prescribe for patients, and before he attended medical lectures he had done not a little as a practitioner. After leaving Fairfield, the Doctor commenced practice at Hamilton, and in 1834 married Margaret, the only daughter of Dr. Hermanus Smith, who died, 1841, aged 22. For upwards of sixty years he continued his work, living in the same house and responding to the calls of the afflicted. The writer enjoyed an hour's intercourse with the genial old man (December, 1889), old in years but young in manner and quick of perception. He had just attended to two patients who had called. The old frame house in which he lives bears more marks of age than the Doctor. It was curious to note the door of his office. Upon its panels are three well-marked spots in an upright line, where, through the long years, the impatient callers have knocked for admission. The uppermost spot indicates where grown persons have used their knuckles, the next those of medium height, and the lowest the young child. If this door could reveal the sad messages conveyed through this portal to the Doctor by the long roll of visitors, during the more than half century, or portray their agony of speech and countenance, it would give ample verification of the words, " Man that is born of woman hath but a short time to live, and is full of misery." Dr. I. A. Case is now (1894) eighty-nine years of age. He has two children—a son and a daughter. His son is Dr. W. H. Case, who is a graduate of McGill College. He was a student one year in Toronto. Unfortunately poor health prevents his engaging in active practice.

DR. ASHERN AUGUSTUS CHAMBERLAIN

Was born of English ancestry at Peacham, Vermont, U.S., February 12, 1810. He came to Upper Canada, in 1815, with his mother and stepfather, Timothy Smith, who pitched their tent in what was at that time a comparative wilderness, about four miles from Rideau Lake in the township of Bastard, on the bank of a small stream. They built a log shanty, covering the roof with wooden troughs made by scooping out basswood trees, cut of sufficient length and split in halves. After a little time Mr. Smith built a rude grist-mill on this stream and named the place "Smith's Mills," which name it continued to bear up to about the year 1848, when it was given the name of "Harlam," at the suggestion of Dr. Chamberlain. His stepfather died about the year 1830, leaving a large family of sons and daughters, all of whom being young, their care and support devolved upon the subject of this sketch. In order to meet the necessities of the family and to pay his board while attending school in the winter, he was obliged to leave home and seek employment during the summer months, leaving the children who were old enough to assist his mother about the place and mill. His education was procured at Potsdam, N.Y., to which place he would travel each fall on foot to the St. Lawrence at Brockville, and cross the river in a canoe, and then on to Potsdam. Returning in May, he would look after the family and prepare the means for the next winter's schooling. In this way he obtained sufficient education to enable him to lay the foundation for his subsequent professional studies. During this time settlers had gradually found their way into the back townships. The bridle-paths marked by blazed trees gradually became enlarged to public highways. Small clearings dotted the woods at intervals of half a mile or more, and that kind of prosperity which after a time rewards the early settler for his suffering and deprivation, began to be realized by the inhabitants of that section. Soon the necessity for medical assistance became so great, and the number of medical men so few, young Chamberlain decided to prepare himself for that profession, and he bent all his energies in that direction. The other children had now become sufficiently large to look after the farm and mill. He arranged matters for their comfort during the approaching winter, and left home for Fairfield Medical College, N.Y., where he attended the lectures and completed his medical course. He commenced the practice of his profession at Smith's Mills, where he continued up to 1858, when he removed to Farmersville (now Athens), and continued practising until he died, 1883, having steadily followed his practice for upwards of fifty years.

His life was a busy one; in addition to his professional duties he was for many years an officer in the 8th Battalion of the Leeds Militia, holding the rank of Major. In 1837, he was ordered to Prescott with his battalion, to assist in repelling invaders from the United States. At the time of the Trent difficulty between the United States and England, he was on the alert. He was for many years Justice of the Peace.

He took a lively interest in political matters, being a Reformer of the old school. He took an active part in the Masonic Order, belonging to one of the oldest, if not the oldest, lodges in Upper Canada, known as Harmony Lodge, Johnstown District. He was postmaster from the first establishment of the office at Smith's Mills and after it was changed to Harlam, up to 1858. He received the degree of M.D. of the Philadelphia Medical College. Dr. Chamberlain was a member of the Methodist Church, and an ardent advocate of temperance, for many years being head of the order of the Sons of Temperance and Good Templars. He died at Farmersville, county of Leeds, February 20, 1883.

Dr. Chamberlain married Eliza Ann, daughter of Hulit Toffey, of Pauling, Quaker Hill, N.Y., 1835. Her mother was Martha Schofield, sister of Dr. Peter Schofield, of Brockville. She still lives at the old place, being ninety years of age, but enjoying the best of health, and able to read or write without the use of glasses.

They had two children: Adelaide A., born on August 2, 1836,

now the widow of the late J. C. Miller, of the Parry Sound Lumber Co., and member of the Local Legislature for Parry Sound District; and Dr. Theodore F. Chamberlain, late of Morrisburg, county of Dundas, where he practised for twenty-nine years. He is now living in Toronto, and holds the office of Inspector of Asylums and Prisons for the Province of Ontario.

Dr. T. F. Chamberlain was born, July 6, 1837. He studied medicine at Queen's College, Kingston, and graduated, 1862. Married Annettie Jane, daughter of Arza and Eliza Parish, of Farmersville (now Athens), County of Leeds, July 3, 1862. They have two children—Dr. Watson Parish Chamberlain, who graduated at Queen's College, Kingston, 1888, and is practising medicine at Morrisburg; and Lyeria, who is living with her parents.

DR. JACOB B. CHAMBERLAIN

Was a practitioner in Fredericksburg at an early date, before 1792, and there is testimony that he was among the first, if not the first, to practise in the townships around the Bay of Quinte. After the war of 1812, he became a licensed practitioner, as "having practised before and during the war." The following notice appeared:

"DIED.—October 6, 1841. At Fredericksburg, Doctor Jacob B. Chamberlain, aged 78. Dr. C. was one of the oldest U. E. Loyalists in the Midland District, and was one of the oldest Magistrates."

DR. THOMAS CHAMBERLAIN,

Of Bath, not unlikely a son of the preceding. Before the Medical Board, April, 1837. Had tickets from Fairfield College for one course, and for attendance at Pennsylvania Hospital. He passed in Physic and Surgery, practised at Napanee for many years, was Surgeon to the 4th Hastings Regimental Militia; and Coroner. Died, September 14, 1872.

"Charles Chamberlain, son of Dr. Chamberlain, of Fredericksburg, died on his way to San Francisco, April 25, 1862, the result of an accident on board ship."

DR. STEWART CHISHOLM,

Of Charlotteburgh, was gazetted licentiate of Upper Canada, June 20, 1831, under 8th Geo. IV., Chap. 3. He was a M.R.C.S. Eng. The *Patriot,* April 26, 1831, contains the following:

"At a meeting of the Medical Practitioners of the Eastern District of Upper Canada held lately at Cornwall, it was unanimously resolved to form themselves into a society of East. District, to be called the 'Medical Society of East. District,' and the following gentlemen were chosen President, Vice-President and office-bearers for the year: Dr. Stewart Chisholm, of the Royal Artillery, and Member of the Royal College of Surgeons, London, President; Dr. A. McNougton, Surgeon, Royal Navy, Vice-President; Dr. Dickenson, of Cornwall, Secretary, and Dr. Wylie, of Matilda, Treasurer. The principal object of the meeting was to take into consideration the present rapid increase of Empiricism in the Province, and to draw up a petition to the Legislature regarding it. The President was requested to communicate with the other Medical Societies of both Provinces on the subject."

There was, prior to 1840, a Dr. Chisholm, an Army Surgeon, living at Kingston for several years. He was an intimate friend of Bishop MacDonell, the first Roman Catholic Bishop of Upper Canada. Whether this was Dr. Stewart Chisholm is doubtful, yet possible.

DR. WM. C. CHEWETT.

The name of Chewett is intimately associated with the history of Upper Canada from the time of Col. Simcoe's advent as Lieutenant-Governor to Canada at the close of 1791; and in the records of Toronto the name is found among the original patentees of the town of York, and is conspicuous in the growth and prosperity of Toronto.

The progenitor of the Chewett family in Canada was William, commonly spoken of as Col. Chewett, who was a native of London, England, born, December 21, 1753. He was educated as an Engineer for the East India Company's Service, and received an appointment to an East India vessel, 1770. Having been seized with small-pox, he was unable to join the ship; and on his recovery he decided to come to Canada, and arrived at Quebec, 1771. He at once commenced practice as a Land Surveyor, and, in 1774, became attached to the office of Surveyor-General Holland. In 1775 and '76, he served in the Quebec militia. When Quebec was besieged by the American rebels under Gen. Montgomery, Mr. Chewett was engaged in surveying the fortifications, and in determining the distance of each rebel battery as it was erected. Subsequently he was Paymaster of Works at and in the neighbourhood of Lake Champlain. In 1786, he was surveyor in charge of the Lunenburg District, now the eastern part of Ontario, and continued for several years surveying the land for the disbanded troops and U. E. Loyalists. Here Mr. Chewett met his fate in the daughter of Major Arch. McDonell, a name famous in Scottish and Canadian history. This attachment of Mr. Chewett gave rise to a letter somewhat unique, and so interesting that it is given a place in these pages:

"CORNWALL, 22nd *April*, 1791.

"DEAR SIR,—Having found out a girl whom I mean to make a partner for life, and without which it is impossible to exist in this settlement; having no settled place to retire after the fatigues of a survey, or take care of the little property I have (this, I hope, you will not think unreasonable at the time of life I am come to, as it does not proceed from motives of folly, but of a mature and deliberate consideration), I, therefore, must pray you, as my friend, to obtain a license, for me and Isabella McDonell (she is of the family of Major Archibald McDonell, of the Long Sault), to be sent by the first opportunity, and by doing so you will oblige an old servant, who is, with the greatest respect, dear sir,

"Your most obedient, humble servant,

"W. CHEWETT.

"THE HONOURABLE JOHN COLLINS, ESQ."

In the autumn of that year, 1791, Col. Simcoe arrived at Quebec, and Mr. Chewett was recommended to him by Surveyor-General Holland to take charge of the surveys in the newly created Province of Upper Canada. Simcoe accepted the recommendation, and Mr. Chewett was instructed to report at Quebec. But he did not then receive the appointment of Surveyor-General. It would seem that Capt. Smith of the 5th Regiment, then stationed at Fort Niagara, had a friend at court. Although Mr. Chewett had, during the summer, discharged the duties of Surveyor-General, he was informed, on the 30th of September, by Gov. Simcoe, that Mr. David Smith was appointed to the office. Mr. Chewett was made Deputy Surveyor-General.

Interesting journals of Surveyor Chewett's work as surveyor in different parts of the Province, and recording many interesting events, are deposited in the Crown Lands Department. One or two may be given:

"*May* 31st, 1793.—Both Houses being assembled at one o'clock p.m., and on the appearance of the Governor the garrison of Niagara fired a royal salute, a compliment to him as the representative of the Crown. The Governor being seated, an order was sent to the Commons for their attendance. The passage to the bar was so crowded they could hardly come up to it, owing to the Sergeant-at-arms being out of the way. Methinks there should be a pole to the bar for the Commons to enter, in order to be separated from the populace. The Governor was then pleased to make a most noble and gracious speech from the throne, which made the heart of every true Briton jump for joy."

"*June* 4th, 1793.—Being the anniversary of His Majesty's birthday, attended the levee, but, being dressed in boots, was told by the sentries that none but military men were thus admitted. Returned in order to dress myself accordingly, but was too late. In the evening, an elegant ball and supper was given for all His Majesty's loyal subjects, and the ladies made a splendid appearance, though not very numerous. After supper a number of loyal toasts went round, suitable to the occasion. The company went to their homes about 2 a.m., in great good humour, and a few of the gentlemen spent the evening all night."

When the Government removed to York, the new capital, Mr. Chewett became a settler there, and his first home was in a log house on the north-east corner of York and Wellington Streets. He was appointed Registrar of the Surrogate Court for the Home District, 1800. In 1802 he became Joint Surveyor-General with Mr. Ridout.

In the war of 1812, Mr. Chewett was the Colonel in Command of the 3rd Regiment West York Militia. When the United States forces took possession of York, April 27, 1813, General Sheaffe withdrew with the regular force towards Kingston, and entrusted Col. Chewett with Major Allan to treat with the foe. In the explosion of the magazine, when a number of Canadians as well as invaders were killed, Col. Chewett received severe injuries from the falling material. Col. Chewett remained in the militia service until 1832, when he retired on full pay, having served the Government upwards of fifty years. The balance of his days was passed in the quietness of home—a well-earned repose. He died September 24, 1849, near the close of his 96th year.

James Grant, the eldest son of Col. Chewett, was born at Cornwall, November 9, 1793. He was educated at the famous school founded by Mr., afterward Bishop, Strachan, and followed his father's profession. He was connected with the Surveyor-General's Department for thirty years, and was Deputy Surveyor-General of Upper Canada. He retired on a pension. In the war of 1812 he was in his father's regiment. He married Miss Martha Smith, a daughter of Richard Robison who was in partnership with Mr. Cartwright, of Napanee.

In 1832, Mr. Chewett erected in York a block of buildings at the corner of King and York Streets, in which was established a commodious hotel, known as the British Coffee House, kept by a Mr. Keating. The present Rossin House occupies the same spot. This valuable piece of land was patented to Isabella, wife of Col. Chewett, and Dr. W. C. Chewett is the present owner. Mr. J. G. Chewett filled the position of Alderman, 1835. He took an active part in the management of the Bank of Upper Canada, and was Vice-President for many years, and afterwards was President of the Bank of Toronto. He died, December 7, 1862. Mr James Grant Chewett was much esteemed for his active co-operation in everything which tended to advance the interests of his native land. He had two sons and one daughter.

The eldest son, Wm. C., was born in Toronto, August 16, 1828, and is a Canadian of Canadians, and one of the oldest Upper Canada College boys now living. He was a medical student at King's College, and when that institution was merged into the University of Toronto, 1850, he continued to attend medical lectures, and was the first to receive a degree in medicine from the University, 1851. Dr. Chewett never entered upon the active practice of his profession, finding more congenial occupation, and he has led and still leads a busy life.

Dr. Chewett married, 1857, Miss Maria Susan, daughter of Henry Ranney, Esq., an English gentleman. Dr. Chewett has five children, living.

BASIL R. CHURCH,

Of the District of Johnston. Before the Medical Board, July, 1828. "The Board perfectly satisfied by his examination." Was a popular practitioner at Merrickville, with a good practice. Married a lady from the States, who acquired considerable fame as a Universalist preacher. He was member of Parliament in 1852. His son, C. R. Church, is the well-known practitioner at Ottawa.

PETER H. CHURCH,

Of Merrickville, Johnston District. Before the Medical Board, October, 1831. He "produced testimonials of having attended two courses of medical lectures, as also a diploma from Fairfield" Medical College. Failed in Latin.

A Dr. Church practised on the Bay of Quinte, probably the same. He studied at Fairfield. He was a remarkably strong and muscular man. It is related that when he took laughing gas at the Fairfield College, with others, it was expected he would give an exhibition of his strength, but he surprised them by taking a few steps, then giving a salute and exclaiming, "God save the King," which was, no doubt, astonishing to the Yankees.

DR. WILLIAM CLARKE

Was a native of Maryborough, Queen's Co., Ireland, and became a member of the Royal College of Surgeons, Ireland, 1836. Coming to Canada, he passed the Upper Canada Medical Board, 1839. He also became a member of the College of Physicians and Surgeons of Upper Canada, 1840 (see correspondence in Appendix). Dr. Clarke settled at Guelph when it was but a village. During a residence there of many years he was not only first in his profession, but also one of the leading citizens, taking part in almost every public affair of any importance, and filling many public offices. He was a Commissioner of the Court of Requests, was a Justice of the Peace, Reeve of Guelph, and Warden of the County, 1852; elected a member of the Legislative Assembly, 1853, and for North Wellington, 1861; was Mayor of Guelph, 1864-65, being elected on both occasions by acclamation. He was also a director of the Galt and Guelph Railway. Dr. Clarke took an active and leading part in procuring the Act to establish the College of Physicians and Surgeons for Ontario, and was elected as a representative to the Council at its organization, 1866. He continued a member for many years, and occupied the President's chair, 1869, '70, '71. '72, '73, and '74. In appreciation of his services, he was presented by his *confreres* with a silver inkstand.

Dr. Clarke was twice married, first, to the widow of Captain John Poore, who was a daughter of the famous Laura Secord. She died leaving one daughter. He then married the widow of Judge Powell, by whom he had two sons, of whom only the elder, Lionel H. Clarke, of Toronto, survived him. He had one daughter, Mrs. Power Palmer. Dr. Clarke died at Guelph, October, 7th, 1887, aged seventy-four.

DR. ROBERT WHICHELO CLARK

Was the son of John Cleland Clark, surgeon in His Majesty's Royal Navy, and was born at Leith, Scotland, in 1811. His mother was the daughter of Dr. Whichelo, a native of Germany. Studied in Edinburgh and Glasgow. Passed as Licentiate of the College of Physicians and Surgeons of Glasgow, in 1833, and came to Canada at once (same spring). Settled in the township of Percy, and practised there till the rebellion broke out in 1837. Removed to Whitby, and was appointed Surgeon to Militia (*vice* Dr. Boys). Practised there until 1858, when he moved to Ottawa, and was one of the surgeons to the Protestant Hospital there for three years. On account of ill-health of his wife he had to leave Ottawa. He returned to Whitby, and took up his old practice again. Business matters connected with the death of his father, called him to England in 1866, and he went into practice in London for four years. But it was not to his liking, from having acquired Canadian ways, and he could not conform to the preciseness of medical decorum observed there. He consequently returned to Canada in 1870, and commenced practice in Hastings, where he has continued ever since (1890). He married in 1835, and has had ten children. One of them studied in Toronto for the medical profession two years. He then went to London and finished his studies at St. Thomas' Hospital. He is now practising there with Drs. Sewell & Cosby, 13 Fenchurch Street.

The following interesting reminiscences supplied by Dr. Clark, give a glimpse of the life followed by the doctors in the early days of the Province, which the reader will be glad to see. Dr. Clark writes:

"Regarding incidents of my career in those by-gone days, I could cite many, but I fear I might be set down as another 'Munchausen' by doctors just come into the profession. At the risk of being accused of a little romance, though, I shall give a few incidents of those early days. One I still vividly remember. I had been all night at a confinement near 'The Plains,' ———, and coming home at daylight through the pine woods, I was astonished at hearing strange noises, that at first I took to be the yelling of tipsy men coming from a carousal. I was on horseback, but my horse seemed to be aware of impending danger, for I could scarcely urge her to proceed, but by dint of spur and a stout oak cudgel I had with me, I prevented her from turning tail to the coming foe. As we drew closer to the noises, the mare grew more and more frightened, till at length, on turning a sharp curve of the road, I beheld eight large wolves drawn up in file right across the road. My mare was at this sight all but unmanageable, and it was all I could do with spur and club to prevent her turning and running back. Aided by my spurs and club, and yelling with all the power of my lungs, I urged her to within about twenty paces of the brutes, who were snarling and showing their lovely white teeth to perfection. At last, I suppose, my voice, raised to its utmost pressure, prevailed, and one of them who seemed to be the leader of the gang, from his size, looked over his shoulder and trotted off into the forest again. He was followed by the whole pack, and as soon as the coast was clear, I made a bee-line for the nearest settlement as tight as a hard gallop would allow of, the mare seemingly as willing as myself to part with bad company. This was in 1834. That same winter I was called on one night by an Indian, to visit his wigwam, some ten or eleven miles through the bush, and pretty dark it was. After prescribing for my patient (a child), I was expected to remain and administer the doses, and had hard work to make them understand that it was their province to nurse and attend to the directions given. I always found the Indians as honest as in their power lay, venison and such like being good pay from them. I remember once I took about fifty skins of the musk-rat as pay, dressed them myself, and made a nice boa for my wife's adornation and comfort, and I often now think of a mighty comfortable warm cap I made for myself out of the skin of a fox I killed and dressed. I kept myself well supplied in venison and salmon by hunting in my leisure hours, spearing salmon by torchlight in a birch canoe, with another young man. But this sort of life was all very well till novelty wore off, and a family in perspective. I had two children, boys. I began to reflect that it would be better to return to civilized life, so, when the rebellion of 1837 broke out, I took a couple of months' hunting, killing twenty-five deer and any number of salmon, and bade adieu to my Robinson Crusoe life, and went to Whitby."

DR. JAMES COBBAN

Was born in Aberdeen, Scotland, September 27, 1802, and commenced his primary as well as his professional studies at an early age. He was admitted to the degree of Master of Arts at Mareschal University, Aberdeen, April 3, 1818, being then only sixteen years of age, and was apprenticed pupil of Alexander Irvine, M.D., from the year 1816 to 1820; and attended lectures in Anatomy and Surgery. He then went to London to complete his medical studies, and became an M.R.C.S. London, October 5, 1821. He was three years in Greenland; then went to the West Indies and practised at Jamaica for nine years, and finally settled in Canada, 1832. He was gazetted a licentiate of Upper Canada, October 31, 1832. "Mr. James Cobban, member of the Royal College of Surgeons, London, respectfully acquaints the inhabitants of Trafalgar and adjacent townships that he has taken up his residence at Sixteen Mile Creek, with the aim to practise the different branches of his profession. TRAFALGAR, 28th *Nov.*, 1832."

On January 9, 1836, Dr. Cobban was married to "Miss Catherine Ann, youngest daughter of the late Capt. Jarmy of the 4th Dragoons of the East Indies."

He was the third pioneer doctor between the city of Hamilton and Toronto, the two others being Dr. Bell, St. Ann, and Dr. Adamson, near Port Credit. Subsequently he removed to his farm near the town of Milton, where he soon stood high in public esteem, and few succeeded better in the laborious duties of the profession to which he belonged. His memory will long be cherished by all who knew him and experienced his kindness and generosity. Dr. Cobban was considered one of the most noted and skilful practitioners in county of Halton. He was gazetted Surgeon to 5th Regiment of Militia of Gore, November, 1838. He displayed extraordinary fortitude and resignation during his lengthy and severe illness, "valvular disease of the heart," which terminated in his death on February 21, 1857. His widow survived him only six weeks. His family consisted of two sons and three daughters. One son engaged in the study of medicine, but died while a student. One daughter married Dr. Clarkson Freeman, who was in partnership with him before his death, and succeeded to his extensive and lucrative practice. Another daughter became the wife of his brother, Dr. Wm. Freeman.

DR. GEORGE COLLS

Came to Upper Canada as Surgeon to a detachment of the Royal Navy in 1816. He was stationed most of the time at Kingston, doing duty at the dock-yard until its reduction in 1834. In 1830 he is mentioned as a supernumerary, with James Taylor, Assistant-Surgeon, Royal Navy, stationed at Grand River. On June 4, 1834, he was gazetted as having obtained the provincial license to practise in Upper Canada, and denominated Surgeon on half pay of the Royal Navy. Under date, July 22, 1834, the following advertisement appeared in the Kingston and Toronto papers:

"KINGSTON, UPPER CANADA, MEDICAL ACADEMY.

"*Under the Auspices and Patronage of the Lieutenant-Governor, Sir John Colborne.*

"Mr. Colls, Surgeon, Royal Navy, will open an establishment on August 1. His terms are as follows: With board and lodging, washing, etc., £100 per year; without board, etc., £50.

"The gentlemen will be taught with great care the duties incumbent upon them as professors of the general science, in every branch, theoretically and practically. Their morals will be carefully watched, and their religious duties will be impressively enforced upon them according to their tenets. They will be taught Anatomy, Surgery, Medicine, Midwifery, etc. Lectures will be given weekly; clinical lectures will be daily given.

"Mr. Colls will teach the following languages, with which he is well acquainted: French, Spanish, Portuguese, Italian and Dutch. These will be gratuitous. £25 will be required in advance as an entrance fee, part of annual payment. July 22, 1834."

There is no record found of the result of this venture by Dr. Colls. The only additional information available relates to his death:

"DIED.—At Fort Erie, in the forty-fifth year of his age, Dr. George Colls, Royal Navy. Mr. Colls came to Canada with a detachment of the Royal Navy in the year 1816, and served at

Kingston dock-yards as Surgeon until the reduction of the yard in 1834, since which he had been residing in the country. He was a gentleman of very high attainments as a scholar, he also ranked high in his profession, and from his social qualities he will be long remembered and much regretted by his numerous friends."—*The Royal Standard*, Dec. 22, 1836.

DR. FRANCIS CONNIN.

In 1825, the Hon. Peter Robinson, brother of Sir John B. Robinson, under the auspices of the British Government, brought a number of settlers from Ireland to the wilderness where Peterborough now stands. There were 415 families, comprising 2,024 persons altogether. In their passage each ship carried a Surgeon of the Royal Navy, who accompanied the emigrants to their destination. Among them were Drs. Connin and Reed.

Dr. Connin seems to have lived a useful life among the settlers, and was a Justice of the Peace for the County of Peterborough. In June, 1831, he was gazetted Surgeon to the 4th Northumberland Infantry. The only other information concerning him is found in a local history by Thomas W. Poole, M.D., page 70: "In March, 1857, died Dr. Connin, a veteran Surgeon of the British Navy (forty years), who had been in many notable engagements, and for the services he rendered, received a medal and two clasps. He was acting Surgeon to one of those transport vessels which brought to these shores the immigrants of 1825, under the late Hon. Peter Robinson."

"MARRIED.—June 1, 1842, at St. Catharines, near Peterborough, Colborne District, Wm. Taylor to Mary Helena, third daughter of F. Connin, Esq., Surgeon, Royal Navy."

DR. JAMES CONNOR.

The first record found of Dr. Connor is a letter (now in the Archives Department, at Ottawa), dated 1783, from the Adjutant-General to the commandant of the garrison, which says that

"Dr. Connor may be reinstated." The following gives further information about him :

"KINGSTON, *October* 14, 1789.

"In consequence of a requisition I have had from Mr. Connor, Mate of the General Hospital, attending the sick belonging to Marine and Army Departments, I have the honour of sending you the enclosed list of medicines, and request you will take the trouble of having them sent immediately.

"(Signed) JOSEPH BUNBURY,
"*Capt. 5th Regt., Comm'r., Kingston.*

"*To* CAPT. LE MATRE, *Quebec.*"

The next record is a "Memorial of James Connor, Mate of the General Hospital." It states that he has been "in the service since the year 1776, when appointed by Your Lordship at Chambly. Was on the expedition against Fort Stanwix with Colonel St. Leger, whose thanks he received for his activity and attention to numbers of wounded, both soldiers and savages. The same fall he was with the army under Gen. Burgoyne as far as Fort George. Was upon different dangerous and hazardous scouts with Sir John Johnson. That attention to his duty in the General Hospital was his study, and manifest to his superior officers of the hospital, whose general approbation was testified by a joint certificate which is enclosed. After the reduction in 1784, he went to England, where, after suffering infinite distress for want of friends or interest, he was at last appointed on the peace establishment. That ever since his station never has been changed, but continually kept at the back-posts, by which he lost the benefit that other mates enjoy of agreeable, populous and cheap stations. That from the scarcity and dearness of provisions, a long and severe illness (a certificate of which I beg leave to enclose), and having a family to support, was involved in debt. That execution was ordered against him, signed by Mr. McLean, with whom at that time he was upon the most unreserved intimacy, and whose family negroes he was a slave to for above two years. He was taken by the sheriff, and in the anguish and distress both of heart and mind and jealousy to Mr. McLean for signing the execution against him without any previous notice, that he made the charge to Mr. McLean now complained of. That never before this distress befell him, received a shilling from mankind, though it has ever been the custom in the General Hospital; further, he could not think himself wrong in charging Mr. McLean, as he had purchased medicines for the use of him and his people, and was sued at Court for part of them, to a greater amount than Mr. McLean paid him, which Mr. McLean is witness to, he being one of the judges. That independent to his trouble and attendance which was incessant, he did not charge him more than the expenses he had been at for him, which plainly appeared by Dr. Gill's charge for medicines for about six weeks for them the sum of £21, and if he had even laid out no money for Mr. McLean, could not think himself in any error in recovering money from him for his attendance, as it ever has been and and is at this moment, the custom with gentlemen of the General Hospital to recover money for their attendance and from some people from their commissions much more intimately connected with the service than Judge McLean. And from some of their present local stations never being changed, are not only practising in the line of their profession, but some of them supporting their families and making fortunes by it, which your memorialist though the oldest mate in the Province, remained with his family in the dearest and most unhealthy part of the Province, where there was no money to be had for practice, and barely the necessaries of life at the dearest rate. That he cannot defend himself from the malicious reports of individuals whom he does not know, and from whose malice few can screen themselves, but will bring vouchers from every and all of the commanding officers of the posts where he was stationed, of having done his duty and never being absent a single hour, and that the operations and cures he has performed will show that he never has neglected his duty nor lost a patient, neither army nor navy, since he has been stationed at the back-posts. That he reported the situation of the place, the disorders prevalent, the remedies they yielded to, and his opinion of the cause to Dr. Nooth, and solicited his further information and advice on the subject, and also solicited from Dr. Nooth his interference for proper accommodations for the sick and wounded which was a grievance much to be complained of, by which he humbly hopes Your Lordship will see he ever was attentive to the health of the troops committed to his care.

"He is now in the most distressing and trying situation ever a man was in, after such a length of service, and the distress and hardships that attended his getting into bread at home, which is now the support for a family and the payment of debts, for which his pay is mortgaged, being referred to the War Office, where he has neither friend nor interest, for a crime which ever was, and is the practice of the General Hospital, not having a guinea to bear his expense, nor to leave his family for their support in his absence, humbly implores Your Lordship's humanity in not ordering him home or separating him from his family, but in Your Lordship's goodness you will be pleased to order him to Oswego, where there is no hospital mate, or to any other post in the Province—he solemnly declares it will be the last cause of complaint he shall ever give while in the service.

"Quebec, August 17th, 1790."

It would seem that Dr. Connor had proceeded to Quebec to urge his request.

Reference is made to Dr. Connor in a letter from Sir John Johnson to Gen. Haldimand about an expedition on Lake Ontario and a vessel driven into Niagara by a gale, which speaks of "a quarrel between Capt. Duncan and Dr. Connor, since made up."

The next record found is this: "David Fleming—Appointed surgeon's mate in Canada, *vice* Connor, removed to Dominica. War Office, March 3rd, 1794." It is most probable that Dr. Connor, instead of going to this distant station, resigned his position and commenced private practice, being one of the first to do so in New Canada. His field of practice included all the region around the Bay of Quinte at that time settled. After living at Kingston for a time, he made his home in Ernesttown. He was well remembered by the past generation of the inhabitants of the Bay. A letter, dated Fredericksburg, June 21st, 1789, from John Furguson to Wm. Bell, Kingston, was conveyed by Dr. Connor, as is shown by the words on the cover,

"Hon'd by Doctor Connor," which seems to show, that he engaged in private practice before he left the service.

He had the reputation of being somewhat unsteady in his habits. His name is associated with a somewhat thrilling incident in connection with the judicial functions of Judge Cartwright. In 1788, Upper Canada was divided in four districts, to each of which a Judge was appointed. To the second district, Mecklenburgh, Richard Cartwright was appointed. From a letter in the writer's possession, it is learned that the court was opened in December, 1788. It probably sat at Finkle's Tavern, Ernesttown. Among the cases Judge Cartwright was called upon to deal with, was that of a man charged with stealing a watch. The article was found upon the man, and although he declared he had bought it of a pedlar, yet, as he could not prove such to be the case, the pedlar not being at hand, he was adjudged guilty of the crime, and, according to the code at that time, was sentenced to be hanged. Dr. Connor, who was present at the trial, stood up in court and appealed against the decision of the Judge, but those present hissed him down. The unfortunate man was duly executed, and was the first person in Upper Canada to be hanged. Subsequently the pedlar returned and corroborated the dying words of the unfortunate man.

The first surgical operation in the Province of which there is any record was performed by Dr. Connor, who removed a large tumour from the neck of one of the family of Roblins, from the Fourth Town, now Adolphustown. After practising for a number of years along the Bay, Dr. Connor returned to Ireland, his native place. He had married a Miss Howard, of "Isle Tanti," now Amherst Isle. A son in after years filled the post of purser on one of the Bay of Quinte steamboats.

DR. EPHRAIM COOK

Was born at Hadley, Mass., June 14, 1797, being the son of John Cook, a native of the same place. As a farmer's son he did his share of farm work. His education was acquired at the district school and Hopkins Academy in Hadley. Here he also commenced the study of medicine, and afterwards attended lectures at Boston. He came to St. Thomas, Upper Canada, 1830, and there pursued his medical studies until April, 1831, when he appeared before the Medical Board. His examination was "perfectly satisfactory." He then established himself in practice in Oxford County, near the site of the Village of Norwich. At that time there was no sign of a village, and there was no other physician within twenty and thirty miles of his place. Dr. Cook soon had a large practice, which he successfully conducted for upwards of forty years, when failing health from excessive labours compelled him to restrict his labours to office work, or at most, to visits in the village. The doctor was rewarded for his hard work by acquiring considerable wealth.

Dr. Cook's attention to his profession did not prevent him from attending to other matters. He was for a time at an early date, postmaster of Norwich, when there was a weekly mail. It arrived on Saturday and the mail was delivered on Sunday. He occupied many positions of trust and honour in the township and county, and in 1854-58, he represented the South Riding of Oxford in Parliament. He was manager of a local bank, and a director of the Port Dover and Lake Huron Railroad, the building of which he materially aided.

Dr. Cook married Phœbe, daughter of John English, from Ireland, January, 1834. She died, July, 1879, aged ninety-six. They had three sons; the eldest, George A., and the youngest, John H., entered the legal profession. The other, Ephraim C., entered the medical profession.

Dr. Ephraim Cook died, Dec. 28, 1881.

DR. GEORGE COOPER,

Was born at Strathavon, Lanarkshire, Scotland, 1794. He entered upon the study of medicine with the view of going to the West Indies. He received his diploma from the University of Glasgow, 1817. He shortly after accepted an appointment at a place called Dollar in Fifeshire. He was principal surgeon to the parish, and was also physician to a large academy at that place. He continued in practice here until 1819, when he was induced by an old friend and school-fellow, Dr. Hugh Caldwell, of Quebec, to come to Canada. Having arrived, he proceeded westward until he reached Belleville, where he took up his residence. In 1822, he married, at Montreal, Miss Hannah, daughter of James Clarke, of Scotland. Dr. Cooper did not engage in very active practice. He, however, conducted a very successful business as chemist and druggist, until his death, which took place in 1836, at the comparatively early age of forty-two, after being an invalid for nine years. Only one child was born to them in 1823, a daughter who became the wife of Dr. James Lister, of Belleville.

DR. BENJAMIN SAYRE CORY

Was born in Milton, Saratoga County, New York, August 13, 1805, and came to Canada when a boy, with his parents, who settled at Pleasant Bay, in the Township of Hillier, Prince Edward County, about the year 1820. He was educated at the College of Physicians and Surgeons, then located at Fairfield, Herkimer County, New York, where he attended his first course of lectures in 1825-26 ; after which he commenced the practice of his profession at Wellington, Prince Edward County, then a primitive frontier village. Subsequently he attended his second course of lectures, in 1829-30, at the above institution, from which he graduated in the latter year. He returned to Canada, and having passed the Upper Canada Medical Board, July, 1830, he resumed his practice, which he continued uninterruptedly during the ensuing twenty-eight years, forming many warm attachments among the people in that section of Prince Edward, by his genial, courteous manners and kindly disposition, and was highly esteemed, as his large and lucrative practice testified.

In the summer of 1854, his brother David, who had passed the Upper Canada Medical Board, July, 1833, and located at Waukegan, Ill., died from cholera, leaving a large practice ; when the subject of our sketch having visited Waukegan to look after his brother's affairs, was induced to remove there with his family, and assume the practice his brother had left, as well as to afford a wider field for his large family of boys. This he did in the autumn of that year, greatly to the regret of his numerous friends and patrons in Wellington and vicinity.

He remained in the practice of his profession at Waukegan, until the winter of 1880, when, at the age of seventy-five years he retired, and with his wife, returned to Canada, living with their daughters in Hamilton, until his death in December, 1885.

Dr. Cory was married, January 16, 1828, to Fanny Young, daughter of the Hon. James Young, of the Carrying Place, Prince Edward County, and thirteen children were born to them. Mrs. Cory and eleven of the children are still living (1889). The eldest daughter married, October 1, 1851, George William Baker, of Hamilton, son of Captain George W. Baker, formerly of the Royal Artillery.

One of the daughters married Thos. C. Mewburn, son of Dr. Mewburn, of the Customs, Hamilton.

"DIED.—At the residence of her daughter, Mrs. J. R. Thomson, Herkimer Street, Hamilton, on Friday, 17th April, 1891. Fanny, widow of the late Benjamin Sayre Cory, M.D., in the 84th year of her age.

DR. CHARLES WILLIAM COVERNTON

Was the second son of James Covernton, of Seven Oaks, Kent, England, and of Antigua, West Indies, by Elizabeth Grace Baisley, of Wormleighton, Warwickshire, England. He was born at Penton Place, Walworth, 1813. His education was received first at the Academy of Mons. Duhamel, Kent Road, and subsequently at the Episcopal College of the Abbé Haffrangue, Boulogne-sur-mer, France. At the age of fifteen he was placed as a private pupil with Dr. Dugald McKellar, practising at Battersea, a suburb of London, fellow-townsman and intimate friend of John Galt, the novelist, at one time Commissioner for the Upper Canada Land Company. After two years of pupilage, he became a student at the Windmill Street School of Medicine, Piccadilly, and attended St. George's Hospital in the immediate neighbourhood. After four years of pupilage and attendance at the above institutions, he proceeded to the

University of Edinburgh, where for two years he attended the course of lectures there given, as also at the Extra Mural School, at which Doctors Gregory, Macintosh, John Lizars, Alexander Lizars, Liston, Robertson, Kemp, Read and Fletcher formed the teaching staff, and from whom certificates of attendance were obtained. Early in 1835, the University of St. Andrews nominated the above gentlemen their examining body for the degree of Doctor of Medicine of their ancient University. The requirements to be admitted for examination were two years at the London and two at this Extra Mural School of Edinburgh. The first examination under these new regulations took place early in March, 1835. At this date Dr. Covernton, with many others whose course of study complied with the University requirements, repaired to the old town of St. Andrews, and obtained the M.D. degree.

After an extended tour through Scotland, Dr. Covernton returned to England, and in August of the same year obtained the diploma of the London College of Surgeons. The examiners were Sir Astley Cooper, Sir Benjamin Brodie, Guthrie, White, Keats, Vincent, Sir William Blizzard, and Sir Anthony Carlisle, the two last at that time being over eighty years of age. The field for practice at that time in view was in the army, and consequently the diploma still required for a general practitioner in England, namely, that of the Apothecaries' Hall, was not deemed necessary. Subsequently, owing to parental objection to the long banishment in foreign countries that service might involve, the diploma of the Hall was obtained. In consequence of a long and severe illness, a sea voyage was deemed requisite; and being offered by a friend who owned a large East India ship, the *Tulloch Castle*, chartered for a voyage to Quebec, the position of surgeon, Dr. Covernton accepted, and in the early days of March, 1836, left from Gravesend for the ancient city of Quebec. The voyage of nearly nine weeks was attended with so much discomfort that on landing, June 1, he resolved not to return with the ship, but to remain for some months in Canada and to visit some old West India friends who had for some time been settled in Kingston, as also one of his youthful friends at that time in the Upper Canada Land Office, in Toronto, subsequently a prominent barrister, and now

Chief Justice Sir Thomas Galt. A letter of introduction to Mr. Henry Atkinson, at that time the owner of "Spencer Wood," Quebec, was the occasion of a delightful visit at that charming abode, and resulted in his forming very roseate views of Canada, not exactly confirmed by the tedium of travel in those days from Quebec to Toronto. At Kingston, six weeks were pleasurably spent, the population of the Granite City then being about 12,000, the same as that of Toronto, including two regiments of the line, a battery of artillery, and a company of engineers. Dr. Covernton arrived in Toronto in July, and through his friend, Mr. T. Galt, had soon a pleasant circle of acquaintances, among them Mr. Hitchings, the nephew of an old acquaintance, the Rev. Mr. Hitchings, of Wargrave, Berkshire; I. Lee, or Shakespeare Lee, as he was familiarly known; W. M. Street, subsequently manager of a bank in London the less; Walter Mackenzie, then a law student residing at Osgoode Hall, and the gifted John Kent in the same quarters. The medical men of Toronto, whose acquaintance was made during his six weeks' visit, were Doctors Widmer, King, Hornby, Nicol and Turquand, the two latter admitted to practice shortly after. Stopping at the hotel with Dr. Covernton was a young law student, now Sir Adam Wilson. Finding that in proportion to population, the aspirants for success in the practice of medicine were as numerous if not more so than in the Old Country, he retraced his steps to Kingston with the purpose of returning to England, *via* New York. Shortly after arriving at Kingston he received a letter from his brother who had with his wife reached Toronto from England, *via* New York, requesting him to return to Toronto. He consequently abandoned for the time this idea of returning to England. He accompanied his brother and his wife on a visit to Col. Delatre, of Drummondville. From thence he went to Hamilton and finally to Simcoe. He visited the Rev. Mr. Evans, Rector of St. John's, Woodhouse, near by, to whom, as well as to many others, Mr. Covernton had letters of introduction. The Doctor's brother purchased land in this neighbourhood and settled upon it, where he continued to live until his death, in 1885. This section was formerly Long Point District, then it was given the name of Talbot District, and subsequently the appellation of Norfolk County. At the date of 1836 there were only of regular and irregular practitioners, Doctors Charles, David, and Elias Duncombe, who were brothers, and Dr. Crouse. The two chief unlicensed practitioners were the so-called Doctors Bostock and Nash ; but of herb-doctors and eclectic doctors there were not a few. At this time Dr. John Mackelcan removed from Guelph to Simcoe. Dr. Covernton and he conferred together, and decided that with such a great extent of country professionally served by so few regularly educated practitioners, there was a good opening for both of them. Dr. Covernton selected the neighbourhood of Vittoria, where his brother had purchased a farm, and Dr. Mackelcan, Simcoe. The following year the rebellion broke out. Dr. Covernton had been appointed some time before surgeon to Colonel Rapelje's regiment of militia, but an opportunity was afforded him of joining Colonel Macnab's men of Gore, and with his friend Dr. Hamilton, of Dundas, he went with them through North and South Norwich, then rejoicing in the name given presumably by the Loyalists in consequence of the two townships being the hot-bed of disaffection, " Sodom and Gomorrah," but a few days sufficed for the entire clearance of the malcontents, a large number of whom sacrificed their farms and crossed over to the United States. Thus ended his short and bloodless military career, the position of surgeon to the regiment only involving for some years the attendance at the muster of the regiment on the Queen's Birthday, when it went through the farce of a two hours' drill. The militia regiments some years after were disbanded, and a volunteer force substituted, which has since developed into a well-trained and uniformed force. In 1847, Dr. Mackelcan removed to Hamilton, and Dr. Covernton purchased his property, succeeding to his clientele, retaining a good deal of his own in the Township of Woodhouse.

In 1853, Dr. Covernton, with his wife and the widow of Dr. O'Reilly, as also with a sister-in-law of the latter, the mother of the Rev. H. Waters, at one time one of the assistant clergymen at St. James' Cathedral in Toronto, made a four months' visit to Europe. Among their fellow-passengers on their return was Professor Wilson, of Toronto University, afterwards Sir Daniel, who had been a student in the Art classes in the University of

Edinburgh, whilst Dr. Covernton was attending the Medical. Dr. George Wilson, his brother, subsequently elected first Professor of Technology in the same university, was at the same time an attendant of the classes in medicine.

In 1869, Dr. Covernton was elected the territorial representative of the Gore and Thames Division of the Council of College of Physicians and Surgeons of Ontario. He was Vice-President of the same, 1870-71, and President from June, 1871, to December of same year, when he resigned in consequence of having been appointed to a Chair in the Medical Branch of Trinity University, as the by-laws of the Medical Council prohibited teachers at medical schools from holding office. In 1871, he became Chairman of Board of Examiners, holding that position for two years. He was also an Examiner in Toronto University. Re-appointed for 1884, '85, '86, Examiner in Sanitary Science and Psychology in same university. In 1871, he was appointed one of the Professors of the remodelled Medical Branch of Trinity University. In the spring of 1882 he was appointed by the Government a member of the Provincial Board of Health. In 1882, he was appointed the delegate of the Provincial Board of Health to the Fourth International Convention of Hygiene, assembled at Geneva, Switzerland, at which were assembled delegates from all parts of Europe, America (North and South). In 1885, as delegate of the same Board, he attended the annual meeting of the British Medical Association that year convened at Brighton, England. On the expiration of the term of office of the first President of the Provincial Board of Health, Dr. Oldright, he was succeeded by Dr. Covernton. In 1890, he was appointed delegate of the Provincial Board of Health to the Ninth International Congress assembled at Berlin; and in 1891, conjointly with Dr. Cassidy, delegate to the Tenth International Congress, assembled in London, England. During the session he was one of the forty-five delegates to the Congress invited to Osborne who were received by the Prince of Wales, and subsequently presented to Her Majesty. Dr. C. W. Covernton married, in 1840, Frances Elizabeth, daughter of Hutchins W. Williams, Marian Square, Dublin, a banker. Had nine children, one died an infant.

Wm. Hutchins Covernton, the eldest, was born, 1841. Educated at Guelph by Arthur Farmer. Student at the Toronto University in Arts. Took the degree of M.B., in 1861, or '62, shortly after became surgeon in the American army during the war for two years; then visited England. Returned as ship-surgeon, when cholera broke out on vessel. His management of the sanitary matters of ship disinfection was so satisfactory that the owners presented him with $100. Shortly after this he went to South America, and married a native lady of high standing.

Charles McKenzie Covernton, born in 1850, educated in medicine at McGill and Harvard, passed his final examination at the age of twenty, but could not receive his diploma. Before he attained the age of twenty-one, died suddenly of hæmorrhage of the lungs, October 22, 1870.

Theodore Selby Covernton, the fourth son, born, February 21, 1854, matriculated at Toronto University in Arts, 1869, and after passing the first year's examination, commenced the study of medicine as Clinical-Assistant under Dr. Joseph Workman at the Asylum for the Insane, Toronto, where he remained till a short time after graduation, when he was appointed Assistant-Superintendent of the Hamilton Asylum. After twelve years' asylum experience, Dr. Covernton went out to China as surgeon of a steamship, and on his return to England held the position of Resident Physician to the Cumberland Infirmary, Carlisle.

Whilst in London he studied sanitary science under Professors Corfield and Cassal of University College, spending a period of six months in the Hygienic Laboratory of the International Health Exhibition; then passed the examination for the diploma in Public Health at Cambridge University, November, 1884. Returning to Canada, he was shortly afterwards appointed chief of a staff of medical inspectors sent by the Ontario Government during the epidemic of small-pox at Montreal, to prevent its spread to this Province. Dr. Covernton discharged his duties so satisfactorily that he received a flattering testimonial, and a purse of $500 from the leading merchants and manufacturers of Montreal.

In 1885, he was appointed Lecturer in Sanitary Science at

the Woman's Medical College, Toronto, and in the following year Lecturer on the same subject in Trinity Medical College.

Carlton Covernton is a druggist in large business at Montreal. He married a niece of Sir George Stephen.

One daughter is the wife of P. H. Drayton, barrister, who was formerly an officer in the 16th Regiment, then exchanged to the Canadian Rifles, and afterwards in the 76th Regiment. He sold out to study law, and distinguished himself by taking the four scholarships of the Law Society. Called to the Bar, 1881. Is now (1893) Lecturer and Examiner at Osgoode Hall. Has been Alderman of Toronto, and for three years filled the office of Chairman of the Local Board of Health.

Dr. Charles James Covernton, eldest son of James Covernton, brother of Dr. C. W. Covernton, was born in England, 1832, and came with his parents to Canada, in June, 1836. Educated first at the Grammar School in Simcoe, County of Norfolk, subsequently at Upper Canada College, where he took high honours. Commenced the study of medicine with his uncle, Dr. C. W. Covernton, in 1848; in 1850, entered the medical branch of Trinity College, and passed the Medical Board, May, 1853. Returning to Simcoe, he took charge of his uncle's practice during his four months' absence in England. He then proceeded to England, where, shortly after, he obtained the Membership of the Royal College of Surgeons, and subsequently became a Licentiate of the College of Physicians of Edinburgh; was offered an appointment in the navy, but preferred another offer for the West India Mail Service, in which he was engaged for several years. At the time of the Crimean War, he became Surgeon on the Peninsular and Oriental Line of steamers. During that time the steamer was chartered by the Government as a troop-ship, and he had extended opportunities of witnessing the long engagements of our forces in the Crimea; and he was with the Guards when they entered Sebastopol. Subsequently he was in India during the Mutiny, and towards the close was the surgeon of the troop-ship that conveyed Lord Elgin to China.

He married a lady whose acquaintance he made on shipboard returning from India; and, within a couple of years of his marriage, bought a practice in Knighton, Radnorshire, where he continued to reside until his death, which occurred in 1890. He was unanimously elected a member of County Municipal Council, which superseded the old Magistrates Court of Quarter Sessions.

DR. WM. CRAIGIE,

From Ancaster, appeared before the Medical Board, April, 1835. Was a member of the Royal College of Surgeons of Edinburgh. He was "found fully qualified, and received the certificate of the Board." The subjoined account of Dr. Craigie, with list of his publications, is taken from "Morgan's Bib. Canaden.":

"Craigie, William, M.D. A Canadian medical practitioner. Born in Aberdeenshire, 1790. Died at Hamilton, Upper Canada, 1863. Studied for medical profession at Mareschal College, Aberdeen, and at the Universities of Edinburgh and Dublin. Contributed monthly meteorological reports to *Spectator* (Hamilton) for a number of years, and also reports on same subject to the Smithsonian.

"Miscellaneous Collections:

"I. Mean results for each month for eleven years (1835 to 1845 inclusive), of a Register of the Thermometer and Barometer, kept at Ancaster, C. W.—*B. A. Journ.*, 1846.

"II. List of indigenous plants found in the neighbourhood of Hamilton, with the dates of their being found in flower and examined.—*Can. Journ.*, 1854.

"III. Mean results of the meteorological observations at Hamilton.—*Ibid.*, 1857-8-9-60-61."

DR. GEORGE GILLESPIE CRAWFORD

Was born, August 10, 1809, at St. Joseph's Island, Lake Huron. He was the son of Col. Louis Crawford, a U. E. Loyalist from the State of New York, who was in command at the time at St. Joseph's Island, and who had a brother, also a Colonel in the British Army. Dr. Crawford's mother was the daughter of

Dr. David Mitchell, of the 8th Regiment. Col. L. Crawford was connected with a land company for a time. We learn from Mr. George Mathewson, who often heard Dr. Crawford relate the early events of his life to his father, that immediately after Napoleon's escape from Elba, Col. Crawford's regiment (89th?) was ordered to England. George was then six or seven years old, and remembered the regiment staying at York a day or two, which was impressed upon his mind by his personal attempt to capture some apples in an orchard at the present corner of King and Frederick Streets, by creeping under the gate, in which raid he was caught and got a good shaking instead of the apples. The first brick house built in Toronto, long known as the Canada Company Building, was erected there. Col. Crawford took his son to Glasgow, and soon after died. Young Crawford found a home with George Gillespie, after whom he seems to have been named. Mr. Gillespie had him educated, and he afterward studied medicine with Dr. Alexander Gillespie, to whom he was apprenticed. He took a medical course at Edinburgh University and graduated as F.R.C.S. Edin., with honours, 1828. He received the appointment of Assistant-Surgeon to the 71st Regiment, and had charge of some companies at Liverpool for a time, when he accompanied the regiment to Canada, 1829, and was quartered at Penetanguishene, where he assumed the office which his uncle, Dr. Mitchell, had held. The following year he retired from the service, and engaged in business in the firm of Newbigin & Co., in York. In 1832, he was gazetted a licentiate of Upper Canada, being designated as an A.M., M.D. But Dr. Crawford did not engage in practice. He at this time possessed considerable wealth. His father had acquired large tracts of land in different parts of the Province, all of which was inherited by the doctor. We learn on good authority that Dr. Crawford at this time was second to none among the first families of York. He lived in his own substantial white brick mansion on one of the Park lots on Queen Street, about where is now Manning Avenue, and here dispensed lavish hospitality to society people. We are told that "when he gave a dinner party it was generally of the most select in both viands and guests," while the doctor was the best of table talkers. Of carriage and horses, "his turn-out was the smartest in the place." Unfortunately Dr. Crawford's venture in business was followed by great financial loss, and afterwards, bank failure swept away much of his patrimony. Dr. Crawford in his later years lived a retired life; but he had a number of chosen friends, and with these he often referred to his early days when at school and college in Edinburgh.

Dr. Crawford was twice married. A son by his first wife went to Australia, where it is supposed he died; a daughter also by the first wife, married Mr. Dickson, barrister, of Belleville, now dead, where she still resides. A son by his second wife, lives in Buffalo, and his widow and a daughter live in Toronto.

He was a charter member of St. Andrew's Lodge of Freemasons, Toronto. In some way Dr. Crawford was concerned, by accusation, in the affair in which one Morgan published an alleged expose of the secrets of Freemasonry, in 1831, which caused no little excitement at the time. Morgan disappeared, and it was charged that the Freemasons were at the bottom of it. Dr. Crawford died at Toronto, 1893, and was accorded a Masonic funeral.

DR. LUTHER CROSS

Is mentioned as one of the early residents of Pelham Township, Niagara District. Dr. Luther Cross (probably the same), of York, appeared before the Upper Canada Medical Board, April, 1831; but in consequence of an attack of fever, his examination was postponed. In October, he appeared again. He produced testimonials of having attended two courses of lectures at Baudain and Berkshire; also a diploma from Baudain College. The Board is (was) perfectly satisfied by his examination. He was a native of the United States.

In 1842, he was practising in Hamilton. Soon after he removed to St. Catharines, and was registered as living there in 1866 and 1887.

DR. JOHN CRUMBIE

Was born, 1794, and died, 1874. The following sketch of his life appeared shortly after his death: "Another pioneer has passed away. One by one the first settlers of the County of

Peel are disappearing from amongst us. In the death of the late Dr. Crumbie, the County of Peel has lost a good citizen, and the inhabitants of Streetsville and neighbourhood a true and faithful friend, whose place will be hard to fill. Dr. Crumbie was born in Scotland, where he received part of his education and taught for a time in the parish school. In the year 1819, he emigrated to Canada with his father's family. His father settled in Chinguacousy, where he lived for many years and died at the ripe age of eighty-six years, highly respected by all who knew him. Dr. Crumbie commenced his life in Canada by teaching school in the Niagara District, having obtained a certificate from the late Bishop Strachan. After teaching a private school for a short time with success, he was engaged by the late Colonel Street to teach his family, in whose employ he remained four and a half years, having, during this time, for his pupils some who afterwards held very prominent places in Canada, among whom we mention the late T. C. Street, Bishop Fuller, Walter Dixon and the late Judge Burns. He then went to study medicine at Fairfield College, New York (there being no medical college in Canada at that time), where he graduated in 1827. He then returned to Canada, obtained his license the same year, and commenced to practise his profession in Streetsville, where he remained until his death. At the time of his settlement in this place, the surrounding country was almost a wilderness, with few roads, and very many of them only sleigh paths through the bush. At that time the inhabitants were nearly all very poor, and many a time has the familiar form of the 'Old Doctor' been seen on horse-back, with a basket of provisions on his arm and saddle-bags behind him, wending his way through the woods to the relief of some poor family in distress by sickness and poverty, where, instead of claiming a fee, he left them the wherewith, not only to relieve their suffering, but to supply the want of necessaries of life. Being blessed with a sound and vigorous constitution, which he husbanded by a life of constant activity and very temperate habits, he was enabled to endure an amount of hardship which few now-a-days have any idea of, often being called thirty or forty miles away through a comparative wilderness; when he would be several days away at a time, going from house to house, relieving suffering wherever he found it. Having, by constant and persevering exertion, accumulated a considerable amount of wealth, he was enabled to assist many of his neighbours, and was never known to send the needy away empty. By his frank, noble and generous disposition, he has endeared himself to all who knew him, and by whom he will long be remembered with the kindest feelings of friendship, reverence and esteem. As an example, we may here be allowed to quote the expression of an eminent scholar in his letter of sympathy, which has just been received. He says: 'Though his life is lost, his lifetime has not been lost. A more prolonged career of usefulness, uprightness and honour it would be difficult to find. His walk through life is a noble example to young men. His courageous frankness is as rare as the diamond, and shone from his cheerful face with a brilliancy which smote all dissemblers. I never knew so noble a specimen of moral fearlessness as the "Old Doctor." I doubt if from his cradle he ever told a lie.'

"In addition to his professional duties, being a thorough scholar himself, he always took an active interest in the educational interests of the county. He was for many years one of the county examiners, and used all his influence in supporting the schools of the neighbourhood. He was also one of the oldest magistrates in the county, for which position his sterling honesty well qualified him.

"In 1831, he married Miss Waite, who was born in Fairfield, N.Y., April 24, 1815, with whom he had become acquainted during his college course. Although they had a number of children, they all died in infancy. Dr. Crumbie, having no children of his own, adopted his niece, Mary Crumbie, who was married to J. G. Cooper, Esq., formerly of Nelson, in 1870. They now live in the family mansion at Streetsville."

DR. W. R. CUBITT,

Born in the county of Norfolk, England, was educated by a private tutor, and when a young man farmed his own estate, "Erpingham." Subsequently he studied medicine, and took his degree of M.D., at Glasgow, 1823. He commenced practice at

Ashby de la Zouch, in the county of Leicester, a town then known for its chalybeate springs and baths. He published a treatise on the medicinal qualities of these springs, which was well received by the profession. He also wrote a work upon "Angina Pectoris," and kindred complaints, many of which, he contended, arose from or were similated by indigestion. This work received a very complimentary notice in the *Medico-Chirurgical Review* of that date. In 1833, Dr. Cubitt came to Canada and settled in what is now the town of Bowmanville, with his three sons, one of whom, Colonel Cubitt, alone survives, and resides at Bowmanville (1893). Dr. Cubitt was licensed under 8th Geo. IV., Chap. 3.

In early life, Dr. Cubitt married Mary, eldest daughter of the Rev. Mr. Churchill, rector of Blickling and Espingham. The Cubitts are of an old Norfolk family, many of whose members have attained high military rank. Among them was the late Colonel Cubitt of the Royal Engineers, well known at Kingston, Ont., in years gone by. Lady Emily Cubitt, the wife of the British ambassador at Washington, is of this family. The Churchills are strangely connected, being lineal descendants of Oliver Cromwell and the celebrated Duke of Marlborough. Dr. Cubitt died in his sixty-fifth year, in 1844.

DR. WILLIAM HENRY DALTON

Was the son of Thomas Dalton, who was a well-known person in Upper Canada, being the publisher of the *Patriot* for a number of years. He was an Englishman from Birmingham, who had come to Newfoundland, where he lived during the war of 1812-14, and where William Henry was born. One effect of the war in Newfoundland is remembered. The young son was at that time very delicate, and it was necessary to have eggs for his diet, for which nine shillings a dozen was paid. Thomas Dalton came to Upper Canada in 1814, when William Henry was three years old. Kingston was selected as a home. It was there he began the publication of the *Patriot*, 1828, which was done with considerable ability. Young Dalton entered the office and learned the printing business with his brother, Robert Gladstone, and generally assisted his father. In 1832, the family moved to York and transferred the paper as well. This was a matter of regret to his patrons at Kingston, and seems to have been also a cause of regret to Mr. Dalton. However, as the organ of the Government, it was much to Mr. Dalton's advantage to publish the paper at headquarters. During the latter part of the time Mr. Dalton conducted the *Patriot*, political feeling ran very high, and he gave and received many a trenchant blow with his opponents. On a tombstone resting upon his grave in the old graveyard of St. James, on the east side of the cathedral, are these words to the memory of Thomas Dalton: "Born in Birmingham, England, April, 1792. Died, October 26, 1840." His widow died, June 14, 1859.

When William Henry was twenty years of age, he forsook printing and began the study of medicine. He became a student of Dr. King's, with whom he remained five years, until he procured his license to practise. He had as fellow-students H. H. Wright and James Mitchell, of London. Dalton had not only the benefit of Dr. King's private practice, but that of the General Hospital, and he seems to have received much of the attention of the hospital physicians, who gave him instruction. It speaks well for the course of instruction he received from Dr. King and others, and the ability and attention of himself, that he was able to pass his examination with no other facilities for learning. His whole medical education was obtained in Toronto, while his general education was principally acquired at the printer's desk.

The short-lived College of Physicians and Surgeons of Upper Canada had just taken the place of the old Upper Canada Med. Board, as an examining body, and it was from this institution that Mr. Dalton received his diploma and acquired the right to practise medicine. He was the seventh person to become a licentiate of the College, which was on November 1, 1839. (See proceedings of the College.)

Dr. Dalton opened an office in Toronto, and remained there for a year or more. He then removed to Ancaster, taking the place of Dr. Thomas Rolph, who had just left the place. Here he continued for many years. He also practised at Dundas,

Hamilton, and Wellington Square (Burlington), but notwithstanding these removals, retaining much of the same practice. Altogether he remained in this district about twenty years. During this time he was a prominent actor in a highly sensational trial of another medical man, who was tried and convicted for outrage upon one of his patients. It was his evidence which caused the conviction.

In the winter of 1859-60, Dr. Dalton took up his abode in Bolton village, where he practised until 1875. During this time he was appointed a coroner, and had a reputation as a medical jurist. Dr. Dalton practised near Toronto, on the Davenport Road, for twelve years, when he came into the city, where he lived until his death, January, 1890.

He married, 1842, Susan, daughter of James Warbrink, who, before he came to Canada, was an extensive manufacturer at Bradford, England, where he was the first to introduce machinery operated by steam. The issue of this union was ten children, five sons and five daughters. Seven children are still living (1889). One, John J., lives in Toronto, with whom his father lived at the time of his death. Mrs. Dalton died, 1888.

The Doctor's brother, Robert G. Dalton, was well known as the Master in Chambers at Osgoode Hall for many years. A sister, Emma, married, May 1, 1841, Adam Wilson, barrister, afterwards Sir Adam, who adorned the Bench for many years. Another sister, Mary, married Dr. McMichael, the well-known barrister, of Toronto. Sophia married Wm. Bartlett, for some time connected with the Indian Department. One sister remained unmarried.

A daughter of Dr. Dalton married Rev. Mr. Parker; another, Rev. Mr. Mills, both of the Church of England. Another daughter makes her home with her uncle, Robert G. Dalton.

Respecting Dr. Dalton's father, it is deemed proper, in the interest of Canadian history, to supplement the notice given with the following, taken from Morgan's "Bib. Canaden.":

"Thomas Dalton, a Canadian journalist, was for many years prior and up to his death, editor and proprietor of the *Patriot* (Toronto), then the leading Conservative journal in Upper Canada. Of a strong and fervid mind, he displayed indefatigable zeal as a public writer in strengthening the tie between Canada and the mother country; his efforts were unflinching to crush every measure calculated to disturb the harmony that should always exist between the parent state and her dependencies. Mr. D. was considered the most vigorous public writer of his day in the Upper Province. He was one of the first to advocate a confederation of all the British American colonies, and his political foresight has been strikingly evinced in the fulfilment of many of his predictions. We close this brief and imperfect notice of this distinguished writer, with the following tribute to his worth, taken from a Toronto journal:

"'In the cause of his country, he was sometimes ardent to a degree which all his friends could not approve. But those who knew him best were the most convinced of the sincerity with which he declared his opinions upon the public questions of the day. He was an Englishman in heart and mind, as well as by birth; was proud of his Saxon lineage, was proud of British freedom, which he considered the light of the world, and the best adapted to carry forward the human family from improvement to improvement in all time to come. In private life he was friendly, amiable and cheerful.'"

DR. JOHN PORTER DALY,

Of York. Before the Medical Board, April, 1828. The Board was "perfectly satisfied with his examination." He was a native of Montreal, and had just come to York, where he engaged in practice. In 1831, he married Eliza Ann, eldest daughter of Samuel Ridout, and about the same time disposed of his practice to Dr. Rees, removing up Yonge Street to where is now Thornhill. Remained there two years, and returned to York, and resumed practice. In 1835 or '36, he went to Natchez on the Mississippi. Subsequently he removed to Havana; here he lost his wife by death, 1842. His subsequent life is unknown. He was a clever practitioner, and had a large practice while in York.

DR. JAMES ACLAND DE LA HOOKE

Was born at Plymouth, England, November, 1814. His father, James Hooke (properly and anciently De La Hooke), was an attorney, and was married to Augusta Dillon, of Cornwall, England. Some years afterwards he went to Cambridge, and was ordained a minister of the Church of England, and became the Rector of Upper and Lower Gravenhurst, Bedfordshire. It may be mentioned that one of his ancestors, whose name was James De La Hooke, took a fancy to have his name on the dial of his watch; but the "De La" was omitted, leaving only "James Hooke." For a long time after, the family went by the name of Hooke, until the doctor's father, in 1825, restored the original name, and since then the family has been known both in England and Canada as "De La Hooke."

In 1830, young De La Hooke became an articled student of William Wooton, M.R.C.S., at Harold, County Bedford, and his indentures were transferred to W. M. Tracey, M.R.C.S., St. James' Square, London, with whom he remained until the expiration of his indentures. During that time he attended lectures on chemistry at the Royal Institution, delivered by Brande and Faraday; Anatomy at the Hunterian Theatre, Windmill Street; Practice of Medicine, Midwifery and Hospital Practice at St. George's Hospital; Surgery, Forensic Medicine, Materia Medica and Botany at King's College; and Surgical Practice at University College Hospital under Robert Liston. In 1836 he obtained his license from Apothecaries' Hall. In 1837 he was admitted a member of the Royal College of Surgeons, England. On his arrival in Toronto, 1839, he applied to the Governor for a provincial license, and was told by the Secretary to make application to the College of Physicians and Surgeons of Upper Canada, and undergo an examination before he could practise, which, with reluctance and a natural feeling of injured pride at such an ordeal, possessing as he did diplomas from England, he submitted to, and was granted a license. It will be seen in the proceedings of the College of Physicians and Surgeons of Upper Canada, that Dr. De La Hooke was the first person to receive its Diploma.

On June 1, 1839, Dr. De La Hooke landed at Toronto, where

he remained a week, and then located at Weston, Ontario, and commenced practice. The following spring he removed to Goderich and practised for three years, when he took up his residence on the London Road, near the Bayfield River, a mile from the now village of Clinton, formerly called Reid's Corners, a tavern being, at that time, the only building there. In 1844, he married Miss Sarah England, a native of Canterbury, England, who had been on a visit to her brother-in-law, James Gordon. Dr. De La Hooke, after marriage, went to Ohio and commenced practice at Cumminsville, on the Miami Canal. Owing to bad health he soon returned to Weston, where his wife died, January, 1845. In 1847, he married Maria Louisa Denison, daughter of Captain Thomas John Denison, of Retirement Vale. In 1870, he removed to Toronto, where he now (1894) resides. His wife died, July 1, 1887. They lived together forty years, and had six sons and one daughter. Three of the sons are now alive, James Acland, Edwin Dillon Alexander, and Thomas Denison Auley.

Dr. De La Hooke relates some of his experiences as a practitioner which will be read with interest, and which shows the contrast between the present and the past:

No one who has not had the experience of professional life in Canada fifty years ago, in the early settlement of the west and north-western portion, can have any idea of the fatigue and hardships endured by medical men. In very many instances they received no pay for their onerous services, for in those days the settlers were very poor and were struggling very hard to meet instalments on the land they had settled on. If the Doctor got a bag of oats, a small quantity of flour, a few pounds of bacon, part of a quarter of beef, or even a bunch of shingles, he did not repine. Fees were very low and money very rarely seen. Long rides through the bush, only a road cut through where sawlogs were drawn to the mills, made the Doctor's life one of toil, as well as tedious, arduous and irksome in the extreme.

Dr. De La Hooke, in a memoir, says: "He was once called to see a little boy who had accidentally swallowed a fish-hook to which a piece of line was attached. He was found in great pain, and the Doctor feared to draw on the string to dislodge the hook, lest he should cause injury to the pharynx; so he took a good-sized bullet, drilled a hole through its centre, and passed the string through it, and pushed the bullet into the pharynx, thereby dislodging the hook from its attachment. On withdrawal, the point of the hook was found imbedded in the bullet so as to be easily extracted. The injury to the soft parts was comparatively trivial, and complete recovery the result."

During the year 1847, the emigrant fever was raging amongst the newly arrived emigrants in Toronto. The hospital being overcrowded, a number of them were removed to Weston and located in a barn. Dr. De La Hooke was the only medical man in the village, and it fell to his lot to attend them, and endeavour to keep the disease confined to one place. He supplied them with medicine, wine when required, as well as other necessaries, and paid part of the funeral expenses of the only one who died. The patients and their families were between twenty and thirty in number. By isolation and care the spread of the disease was prevented; but during his attendance his private patients would not permit him to enter their houses. Dr. De La Hooke records that he neither got credit for what he had done, nor even thanks, nor any recognition, pecuniary or otherwise, from the municipality or the inhabitants of Weston. He considered this a public calamity, affecting the health and welfare of every resident in the vicinity, and that his services were worthy of some reward, or at least acknowledgment of diligent and faithful service rendered to the community. He had one consolation: he had fearlessly and honestly, as well as conscientiously, done his duty to the sick and to the inhabitants of the village. (If these patients were removed to Weston from an overcrowded hospital in Toronto, the village could hardly be expected to pay the expenses.)

On one occasion during his residence in Weston, he says: "I was called to attend a man named James Smisson, who had both his legs crushed and mangled in a threshing machine, to such an extent as to necessitate immediate amputation. I removed both legs below the knees, and was ably assisted by Dr. Reardon, an old naval surgeon, and Dr. Thistle. I operated on the 8th of August, after dark, and on the 8th of the following month both stumps were healed, and no unpleasant symptoms occurred. I may here mention the only light I had were two home-made tallow candles. After his recovery, I made application to the municipality for some remuneration, as the patient was very poor; and one of the councilmen, a man who had plenty of means, told me I should have made some party responsible for my account before I touched the patient, who, at the time, was suffering pain and bleeding profusely. In 1866, I was walking up Main Street, Buffalo, and recognized my old patient, who had a fruit stall, or table, on which were a few peaches and other fruit, and in acknowledgment of my services he gave me two peaches. This was all I ever got for what I had done for him. He was poor, but I believe his intention was honest, if he had the means to pay me."

The Doctor continues:

"During my residence on the London Road, I was summoned by the pathmaster to do statute labour, and bring a spade with me, as they intended to take out stumps. I informed him I had a machine for that purpose, and he requested me to bring it with me, for it was just the thing required. I started next morning, taking my tooth instruments with me, stump forceps, etc. The pathmaster was surprised (I had not brought either spade or stumping machine), and still more so when I produced the tooth instruments. I told him the understanding was to bring my stump machine, as he intended to have stumps taken out. I offered, if any of the men had decayed teeth, to extract them, and that they should do my statute labour, and in that way pay me, which was at once agreed to. I operated on several men, put up my instruments and went home, all parties being satisfied with the exchange of work, and I was perfectly contented that my statute labour was to be done without any outlay of money, which was a very scarce commodity in those days.

"On one occasion when visiting a patient, I got a couple pairs of live ducks as part payment of my fees. I put them in my buggy, and on my way home met a gentleman. While we were conversing, the ducks began to quack, and he remarked that this was a novel way of advertising, and he had no doubt it would prove a very successful one. I felt very much chagrined and left him, reflecting that should the ducks continue quacking, it would not redound to my credit in the minds of those I might meet. I never put live ducks in my buggy afterwards.

"A certain doctor always carried an ivory tube, and attached a bladder to it when he administered an enema. On one occasion he had left it at home, and it was too far to go back for it; but an old woman who was present went out to the bush and procured a piece of elder, trimmed it up, and attached a bladder, which worked very satisfactorily. Shortly after, he was similarly placed—his ivory tube was left at home. He at once remembered the old woman's substitute, and got a piece of elder, trimmed it up, and affixed a bladder to it and proceeded to use it, but found that he could not empty the bladder. On withdrawing the elder from the rectum, he found he had neglected to take the pith out of the piece of elder.

"During my residence in Goderich, one winter's night I was summoned to go to the Big Sable River to attend Petit Caselet, who had been severely injured, and was in the employ of Brewster & Smart, who owned the mills at that place. I hired a man and double horse-sleigh, and started on my journey at 11 p.m., of thirty miles down the London Road. The snow was deep, the track nearly filled up, for it was snowing very fast and drifting, accompanied by a very cold and strong wind. At 7 a.m. the following morning, I reached the half-way house between Goderich and London, where I got my breakfast, the fare in those days being bacon and eggs; also fed the horse, and rested for two hours. I had now the worst part of the journey to go, about sixteen miles through the bush, the road only having been blazed; no beaten track, for the snow had filled it up. Late in the evening I reached my destination, very cold, tired and weary. I at once proceeded to examine the patient, and found he had a compound fracture of the thigh, the bone protruding through the soft parts about three inches. There was also a compound fracture of the tibia and fibula at the upper third of the leg, the bones protruding through the soft parts, the integument and subjacent tissues covering the knee-joint being very much contused. These injuries were confined to one extremity. I sawed off the ends of the bones, and reduced the fractures, carefully avoiding any undue pressure from splints or bandages. The following morning I left the patient, who had passed a comparatively comfortable night. Two days after, I visited the patient again, and his condition was more satisfactory than I had anticipated. After this I saw the patient twice a week for nearly three months. At the expiration of that time, he had so far recovered as to leave his bed. About three months afterwards, I saw my patient, Petit Caselet, who was moving about on crutches, and the only deformity observed was that he was unable to bring his heel to the ground by about an inch, evidently due to the injury sustained by the soft parts in the vicinity of the knee, and permanent contraction of the flexor tendons. The result, however, was so far satisfactory; he had the use of the limb and the power of locomotion, which was more than ever I expected he would regain. When I first saw the patient, the party in charge of the mills requested me to give the man every attention, and he would pay me. On presenting my account, he ignored my claim and his responsibility. I sued him, and got judgment, and when the sheriff went to make a seizure, this man told him he had no share or interest in the business but to do his work and get his wages, and that he was employed by the firm who owned the mills and lived in Detroit; and in this way I was defrauded of the amount of my bill, and superadded was an outlay of ten dollars for the hire of the man and sleigh."

Dr. De La Hooke's connection with the Canadian Militia and Volunteer force was as follows:

July, 1842, was gazetted surgeon 1st Battalion Huron Militia;

June, 1853, transferred to 2nd Battalion York Militia;

September, 1854, surgeon to York Light Dragoons;

June, 1856, surgeon to Squadron of York Cavalry;

1866, surgeon to the Governor-General's Body Guard at Fort Erie during the Fenian Raid;

July 11, 1879, promoted to the rank of Surgeon-Major.

In 1881, he sent in his resignation, after a period of forty-six years in the Militia and Volunteer Force. During the Fenian Raid, from the inadequate and deficient supply of blankets and other necessaries, as well as from exposure, he, as well as many others, contracted rheumatism, a disease he has more or less suffered from ever since. After his resignation in 1888, he made application to the Militia Department for a gratuity or compensation for long and faithful service, and for disease contracted during the performance of duty to Qûeen and country. His application was ignored by the Minister of Militia, on the grounds that he had neglected to put in a claim on his return from the frontier, and that there was no provision for contingencies such as his case. His reason for omitting to make a claim at that time was that he only suffered from occasional attacks, and did not desire to be a burden on the Government.

He was medical officer of the day to the Ontario Rifle Association, from the time it was inaugurated until 1888, when he resigned his commission in the Volùnteer Force. He was on duty always one day at the annual rifle matches; on several occasions, two days, and one year, for four days.

Dr. De La Hooke, in his memo., says: "In concluding this record of my professional life during a period of fifty years, dating from 1839, when I arrived in Toronto, all the incidents I have portrayed are positive and reliable facts, and related without fiction or romantic exaggeration, and I do not take any undue or particular credit to myself for my share in the services it was my lot to perform. As many other professional men in those days have experienced similar trials and hardships, I would here remark that medical men, with very, very few exceptions, are at all times ready to render assistance to the sick and needy at all hours and under any circumstance, and that no other class of men perform so many unrecognized and unrequited acts of kindness as they do. In the foregoing recital I have been very careful to relate the incidents as accurately as they occurred. I could mention many more, but enough has been told to show the hardships and privations others as well as myself endured in the early settlement of the country. When I landed in Toronto I was the possessor of $200, and if I had only been so fortunate as to get only two-thirds of my lawful earnings, I should at this period of my life be comparatively well off, and able to retire from active practice. However, I brought nothing into this world, and my only ambition through life was to be able to lay by enough to support me in my declining years; but I cannot take anything out of this world or leave anything behind but a reputation, I trust, of having been an honest and conscientious practitioner."

DR. PETER DEIHL

Was a son of John Justice Deihl, a native of Germany, who, in his will, speaks of his father's estate in Darmstadt, in Hesse. He was a merchant at Montreal, and was married to a sister of Dr. Daniel Arnoldi. Dr. Arnoldi was of German extraction. The family had passed into Italy, where the original name Arnold was changed to Arnoldi. Dr. Daniel Arnoldi was an eminent physician of Montreal, and his fourth son, Francis Cornelius, was likewise an eminent physician in Toronto, from 1855 till 1862, when, on New Year's day, he died, very much respected, and his death very much regretted. Dr. Deihl was born in Quebec, May 22, 1787. His father's intention was that he should enter into some business pursuit. He died while his son was yet young. Two of the executors of his will were Charles Blake, surgeon, and Henry Loedel, the latter of whom had been surgeon to the Hessian troops, and who had been employed by the British Government in the American Rebellion of 1776.

Not unlikely it was by the advice of these two doctors that Peter decided to study medicine, or perhaps the fact of his mother's father being a doctor had its influence. He studied medicine with Dr. Blake, of Montreal, and afterwards went to Edinburgh, 1807, and attended medical lectures at the University and Royal Infirmary. Dr. Blake was a particular friend, and seems to have been like a father to him, as the following letter shows. It is given in full as it throws light on the events of that time. It is now in the possession of Mrs. E. H. Van Koughnet, of Toronto, to whom the writer is indebted for valuable information respecting both Dr. Deihl and Dr. Macaulay. The letter is addressed to Mr. Peter Deihl, student at Edinburgh; dated Montreal, Sept. 7, 1808, and was received Nov. 24, bearing the mark, "Port Glasgow, ship letter":

"DEAR PETER,—I have seen Mr. Labrie who has given me good accounts in regard to the progress you are making in your profession, which gives me infinite satisfaction. He says the Students have been at a loss for Subjects; this is a loss, indeed, for without plenty of Subjects, Anatomy is not to be learnt. It is probable your Lectures might have begun ere this Reaches you; if so, you must not throw away your Money for nothing; but if your Lectures are not begun, or you think proper, after the first Course is ended, it is my Wish you set off for London, and attend at e/y Dissections at St. Thomas's, or any other place you may think better. Anatomy is the Basis of Surgery, and if you are not Minute in it, you never will get on. Your Midwifery Lectures I suppose you are Competent to, and your Operations in Surgery I hope you have tried; if not, when you are in London be particular in it. I desired Mr. Gerrard to send an Order for you to receive £30. I ordered Mr. Gerrard since to give you £50 more. I have established a Correspondence with Mr. Gerrard here, that you are to be supplied occasionally by their House in London, viz., McKenzie, Parker & Co. I have that good opinion of your conduct and situation that you I'm sure will enter into no extravagence except such as must support your Education; this is at present necessary, if lost, it can never be regained; at the same time if a play or any novelty you would wish to see, don't deny yourself. I am very much Obliged to Mr. McKendley for his attention and kindness to you; and if you have Received the £50 pay off all your Debts; and never leave a place behind with one Shili'g Debtor. Let me hear from you immediately upon receipt of this, that I may know how to Direct to you; and desire some Friend at Edinbourgh to forward Your Letters to London after you leave it. Your Uncle is well and doing well.

"I am, Dear Peter,

"Your Sincere Friend,

"CHAS. BLAKE.

"P.S.—Mrs. Blake sends her best Wishes, and little Harriet says she sends you a kiss."

The uncle here referred to was Dr. Daniel Arnoldi. Dr. Blake was a prominent surgeon in the military service during the American Rebellion of 1776-83. His name is found in connection with several medical men, sketches of whom are found in these pages. In the Haldimand Collection, in the archives at Ottawa, are numerous official communications from or to him, or in which reference is made to him.

A communication from Gen. Haldimand to Dr. Blake, Dec. 7, 1778, speaks of his resignation of the surgeoncy of the 34th Regiment.

Dr. Deihl having completed a course of studies there, returned to Canada in the summer of 1809, and entered upon the practice of his profession in the Lower Province. In 1813, he was appointed to the medical staff, and shortly after attached to the Canadian Regiment, with which he served during the war. In the spring of 1814, being in garrison at Fort Henry, opposite Kingston, he accompanied a detachment of his own and of the Nova Scotia Regiment, under Colonel Darling, in twenty-six boats, to convey ammunition and provisions to the army, then in great straits, on the Niagara frontier. The following letters show that he was on duty at Fort George in 1814; consequently, he was an eye-witness of the stirring scenes enacted on the Niagara frontier during the closing period of the war:

"KINGSTON, *July* 14th, 1815.

"SIR,—I am surprised that the receipt sent from the Commissariat Department, for the purpose of enabling you to draw your pay from December to April, hadn't been received so late as the 11th inst. They were sent by Mr. Greene to the Commissary at Fort George.

"Your name was down on the pay list at York, from April to June, and I have desired S. S. Thom (surgeon) to inform you and Mr. Athenach how the pay is to be drawn.

"As the return for the Batt. and Forage is made out at Quebec, I cannot say whether your name was on it or not.

"If the regiment remains at Fort George, will it be attended with any inconvenience to draw your pay from York? If it is not, a return shall be made out for that station.

"Procure a bill on the Commissary-General for the surplusses of the hospital due, and endorse it to me.

"In the event of medicines or comforts being wanted for the

sick in hospital, you will apply for them to Staff-Surgeon Thom.

"I hope you have got the Purveyor's stores sent to York.

"I have the honour to be, Sir,

"Your most Obedient, Humble Servant,

"JAS. MACAULAY,

"*D.I.H.*

"MR. DEIHL, *H.A.*"

"KINGSTON, *July* 28th, 1815.

"DEAR SIR,—When I last wrote to you I forgot to send the certificate you requested and which is now enclosed; I can get a copy of it from you at any time when convenient to yourself.

"I had a letter from Mr. Thom mentioning that he was to visit the frontier, and if the consumable stores left with you were not sent to York, he will arrange the business with you; let the utmost care be taken of every article, and the wine kept in a cool place, otherwise it may be damaged.

"I wrote you respecting the supplies of the hospital, which should be settled without delay.

"I expect to leave this in a day or two and proceed to the Lower Province. Any letters for me you may put under cover to Mr. Geddes.

"I am, yours truly,

"JAS. MACAULAY."

From a letter addressed to Dr. Deihl, by Dr. Macaulay, it appears that he was attached for a time to the staff at York:

"[Private.]

"KINGSTON, *April* 16th, 1816.

"DEAR SIR,—You will observe by the General Orders from Quebec that you are to proceed without delay to that place. You must not lose any time unnecessarily as if in time you will go in the same ship with Sir Gordon Drummond; but before you leave York deliver all the forms of Returns and any official papers which may be necessary for the guidance of your successor.

"The bay is full of ice which prevents the vessels from leaving this; but I trust it will not remain much longer.

"I am, yours truly,

"JAS. MACAULAY.

"*To* MR. DEIHL."

He was sent to England in a transport with a detachment of artillery, under Sir Gordon Drummond. When in London he applied to be confirmed in his appointment to the Medical Department, and having undergone an examination by a Medical Board, he was pronounced qualified; but, after some correspondence, was informed that he could not get a commission as reductions were taking place to a large extent. He then continued in London attending the hospitals and lectures, and took his diploma as a member of the Royal College of Surgeons. Before returning to Canada he went on a tour on the continent, spending some time in visiting hospitals and other public institutions, where he might increase his stock of learning; and (contrasting the slow mode of travelling with the quick movements of modern days) he travelled, on one occasion, in a *diligence,* 400 miles direct to Paris. Having returned to Canada in 1818, he commenced practice with Dr. Arnoldi, of Montreal, where he remained till 1828.

He was connected with the Montreal General Hospital, as the yearly reports of that institution for 1827 and '28 show, being signed by Peter Deihl and W. Caldwell, M.D., as attending physicians.

In 1828, Dr. Deihl removed to York. He was gazetted as a Licentiate of the Medical Board, October 14, 1828, and November 27 following, he was gazetted as a member of the Medical Board, the commission being dated October 24. At the following meeting of the Board, in January, 1829, he took his seat. In November, 1828, he formed a partnership with Dr. Widmer, and for a number of years they had almost the whole practice of York and its vicinity. The contrast between these two was very marked. While Dr. Widmer was stern and bluff with the manner of a martinet, Dr. Deihl had a quiet, pleasant manner and a gentle disposition. The former was heroic in treatment of disease, as well as in manner. Of their skill many instances are remembered. One may be mentioned, taken from the *Christian Guardian*, March 20, 1830:

"A person about ten miles from York met with a severe accident, by which the hip was put out of joint. Many unsuccessful efforts had been made to reduce it. After the lapse of some days he was brought in to the York Hospital, where in about an hour Drs. Widmer and Deihl effected a reduction, and restored one who expected to be a cripple for life to his family and occupation."

The partnership continued until 1835, when, on account of ill-health, Dr. Deihl gave up practice and took an extensive tour in the United States as far as the Rocky Mountains. He then lived for a time at Kingston. His stay there, however, was short. The following card, dated June 27, 1836, appeared in the *Patriot*, of Toronto: "Dr. Deihl informs his friends and the public that he has returned to the city of Toronto, and intends to practise his profession. Residence, 57 Lot Street." He built for a residence and office on Richmond Street, near the present Canadian Institute, the framed building well known to the older citizens of Toronto, as it was afterward the home of Dr. King, and it remained the residence of his widow up to the time of her death.

In 1837, when the rebellion took place, Dr. Deihl was appointed surgeon to the 4th Battalion of Militia under Col. Hill, and in 1838, Deputy Inspector of Militia Hospitals. He went with the battalion to Kingston, Prescott and Cornwall. On March 19, he advertised his house to let and the sale of his furniture. When the battalion was disbanded, 1843, he again made Kingston his home until 1853, when he, with his wife, went to Europe. He returned to Toronto in 1855. It does not appear that he again engaged in practice, but passed the evening of his life in quietness at his residence on John Street. An obituary notice says that he was, at the time of his death, the oldest man in the city, and that "he was very active, mentally and physically, until a few weeks previous to his death, when he received some internal injury by a fall, which eventually caused his death." This took place, March 5, 1868, at nearly the age of 82.

It was said of him in the notice, that he was "faithful and

indefatigable in all he undertook, upright, and of the strictest integrity, an humble and sincere Christian ; he passed through life in an unobtrusive way, leaving behind him the stamp of a good and honest man."

Dr. Deihl married in 1829, Anne, daughter of Dr. Macaulay, who died, October 5, 1877, aged 71.

A portrait of Dr. Deihl in the possession of Mrs. E. H. Van Koughnet, shows a striking face and good head, with features strongly Teutonic. She also has his picture on ivory taken in the uniform of a militia surgeon, and another taken when he was old.

DR. ROBERT DENMARK

Was born at Titchfield, Hampshire, England, about 1809. His father, Alexander Denmark, was also a physician connected with the fleet at Portsmouth, in the Royal Navy. Dr. Robert Denmark was also a surgeon in the Royal Navy, and on his father's death, about 1839 or '40, resigned his commission, then being on the coast of Africa at Madagascar. He then came to Canada, and settled in the township of Seymour, county of Northumberland. He married Rosalind, daughter of Captain Rowed, also of the Navy, whose family came to this country in 1835, and also settled in Seymour. Captain Rowed died in France. Dr. Denmark resided in Seymour till his death in 1852, his wife having died in 1847. He never actively practised his profession, but as there was only Dr. Ponton in the township at the time, he usually responded to calls whenever wanted. Dr. Denmark's only son, George, is a well-known barrister of Belleville.

ALFRED H. DEWSON,

Son of a British officer, served five years' apprenticeship to the army surgeon at Kingston (Dr. Barclay of the 15th). Was with him during the cholera invasion of 1832. He failed in his application to the Medical Board, October, 1833. Before the Board again, July, 1835. "Possessed a degree of Doctor of Medicine from the University of New York." Obtained certificate for license. This card appeared in the *Correspondent and Advocate:* "Dr. Dewson begs leave to inform the inhabitants of Toronto that he has commenced the practice of Physic, etc. 62 Yonge Street, August, 1835." He married a Miss Baby. The Quebec *Mercury,* July, 1837, says: "It is announced in General Orders that Dr. Dewson, of Toronto (son of Lieut. Dewson of the 15th), has been appointed to assist Dr. Shortt of the 24th, until further instructions."

Dr. Dewson practised at Windsor for many years. He was surgeon to the 2nd Battalion Incorporated Militia, 1837 (Queen's Light Infantry).

DR. NOAH DICKENSON

Was one of the band of U. E. Loyalists. He was gazetted surgeon to the 2nd Stormont Regiment of Militia, May 1, 1828. He died at Cornwall, February 28, 1840, " in the 63rd year of his age, after a residence in Cornwall of upwards of forty years, during which he possessed the confidence and esteem of all who knew him."

DR. JAMES JOHN DICKENSON

Was born at Cornwall, Upper Canada, 1819. He entered McGill College, 1842, and took the degree of M.D. in 1846. He at once proceeded to the Quarantine Hospital at Grosse Isle as a volunteer to assist in attending to immigrants affected with ship-fever. He commenced practice at Cornwall in 1847, where he continued until 1879. He died, May 10, 1884. He stood high as a practitioner, and was regarded as a leader in the profession.

Dr. Dickenson had great taste in military matters, and was conspicuous in local regiments. Prior to studying medicine, he was an ensign for seven years, and took part in the affair at the Windmill, in 1837. After commencing practice, he was for a good many years in command of a troop of yeoman cavalry.

A Dr. Dickenson was practising in Hamilton in 1842. Came there from London, England. Was known as an intelligent, gentlemanly person, and had a large practice. Married, but no children. Died about 1846.

DR. JOHN ROBINSON DICKSON,

Son of David and Isabella (Robinson) Dickson, was born at Dungannon, County of Tyrone, Ireland, on November 15, 1819. He studied medicine with Dr. W. McLean, of Dungannon; was educated at Belfast and Glasgow colleges, and in the latter he obtained a license to practise midwifery. He arrived in Canada with the family, 1838. Was in partnership with Dr. Hutchison at Peterborough for two years; then went to New York, where he spent nearly a year to familiarize himself with the treatment of squint, club-foot, and other deformities. He attended medical lectures at the University of New York, receiving in 1842 the degree of M.D., the first granted by that institution; thus he was senior alumnus. In the same year, returning to Canada by the solicitation of friends, he passed his examination as Licentiate of the Medical Board of Upper Canada. It seems that he thought of practising in Niagara District, as that is given as his place of residence in the minutes of the Upper Canada Medical Board when he passed. He, however, settled in Kingston, where preseverance, steady habits, and marked ability, especially as a surgeon, brought him rapidly to the fore. From 1846 to 1854, he was a visiting physician at the Kingston General Hospital; from 1854 to 1856, a visiting surgeon; in 1856 was appointed a Clinical Lecturer, which position he resigned in 1860, to be reappointed Clinical Lecturer on Surgery in 1861. In 1854, chiefly through his exertions, aided afterward by Hon. Sir John A. Macdonald, the Medical Department of the University of Queen's College was founded. The minutes of the first meeting are as follows: "At a meeting, held August, 1854, at the residence of the Hon. Attorney-General Macdonald, Brock Street, Kingston, which meeting had been convened (at the suggestion of Dr. Dickson) by circulars addressed by Mr. Macdonald to every member of the medical profession resident in this city. Dr. Sampson being called to the chair, Dr. Stewart was appointed secretary to the meeting on the motion of Dr. Dickson. After discussing very fully the expediency of attempting to establish a medical school in connection with Queen's College, it was decided to adjourn the meeting for a fortnight in order to allow time for more mature deliberation. At the adjourned meeting, at which all the members of the profession in the city were in attendance, Dr. Sampson in the chair, and Dr. Stewart acting as secretary, after a very full expression of opinion, it was resolved that it is desirable to make an effort to establish a medical school here, to which resolution the only dissentient voice was that of Dr. Stewart. The chairman then stated that he was too old to write lectures, but would lend every assistance in his power to the school, and proposed that Dr. Dickson should be appointed Professor of Surgery, which motion being seconded by Dr. Baker, was carried unanimously. Dr. Yates was then proposed as Professor of Medicine, which was also carried unanimously. Dr. John Stewart, on motion of Dr. Dickson, was then named to the chair of Anatomy; motion carried. Dr. Harvey was proposed as Demonstrator of Anatomy, but at the request of Dr. Stewart, this motion was withdrawn. The nomination of Dr. Meagher to the chair of Midwifery was then carried. It was finally resolved, that Dr. Harvey should be recommended for the chair of Materia Medica. Somewhere about this time, or perhaps previously, Mr. Ireland called on Dr. Stewart and ascertained his views relative to the prospects of establishing a medical school here. Dr. Stewart ridiculed the idea of such an undertaking, and said he would have nothing to do with a scheme of that kind, unless he would be granted a salary of about (£600) six hundred pounds per annum."

During this and the two succeeding years, Dr. Dickson was a city alderman, and at this time, in connection with the late James Morton, built a branch line of the Grand Trunk Railway from Kingston Junction to the city, which, though only about three miles long, added greatly to the prosperity of the place. He took a great interest in railroad matters. In 1858, under the auspices of Queen's College, he delivered a very able public lecture on "The Evidences of Design from the Structure of the Human Body," and in 1860, another on "Comparative Physiology." In 1860, while on a trip for health, he visited the various London (England) colleges, and succeeded in obtaining for Queen's University recognition of her medical degrees. During 1861, he contributed three articles to the *British American Medical Journal*, viz., "Removal of the Inferior Maxilla," "Vaginal Hysterotomy" and "Resection of the Elbow-joint"; and since then, a number of communications on other subjects, including "Electricity," have appeared in different journals from his pen. In 1862, he was appointed Surgeon to the Provincial Penitentiary at Kingston, which position he held for about eight years. His "Prison Reports" were very ably and carefully gotten up. In 1863, he obtained the following degrees: M.D., Queen's University, Kingston; Membership of the Royal College of Physicians, London; Membership of the Royal College of Surgeons, England. From 1866 to '69, he was a member of the General Council of Medical Education and Registration of Upper Canada, and at its formation in 1866, he was unanimously elected its President for the year. This body is now known as the Council of the College of Physicians and Surgeons of Ontario, and without its license no one is allowed to practise medicine in the Province. In 1866, the Medical Department of Queen's became the Royal College of Physicians and Surgeons in affiliation with Queen's University, for which he obtained the necessary charter, and of which he was appointed President and Professor of Surgery, positions which he held through his lifetime. The new college at its first convocation conferred upon him the degree of Fellow Royal College of Physicians and Surgeons, Kingston. The greater number of his large collection of anatomical casts he presented to the College. In 1867, he obtained the degree of Fellow of the Royal College of Surgeons, Edinburgh. In 1869, he received the appointment of Medical Superintendent of Rockwood Lunatic Asylum, Kingston, and devoted himself with great zeal to the study of mental disease, hygiene and ventilation. Electricity was also a favourite study, particularly during the last ten years of his life. He devoted a great amount of care to the preparation of his "Asylum Reports." One of his first acts was to introduce the system of purely voluntary labour among the inmates, with most beneficial results to mental and bodily health, and a very marked lowering of the running expenses. No accidents resulted to patients from this change, the women making articles of dress, knitting socks, washing, etc., while the men engaged in boot-making, tailoring, carpentering, blacksmith and tinsmith work, baking, cooking and laundry work, quarrying, farming, and gardening, the latter three occupations transforming the barren "*rock*" and scraggy "WOOD" into beautiful lawns, terraces, gardens, orchards, etc. One spot was left in its original condition as a sample of former times and appropriately named "The Wilderness." At 3 p.m., coffee and bread was served out to all hands at work, and plenty of time given to enjoy it, and a happier and jollier set of mortals could scarcely be found than those who were fortunate enough to be able to work. Another and bolder reform was to abolish the use of alcohol and beer at the Institution, and substitute coffee and other drinks. He was the first in Canada to take this step purely on the grounds of health, and had to appear before the Parliamentary Committee in Toronto as a result. He began his speech of one hour and a half's duration with no one on his side, but when he sat down all had been won over by his clear and masterly argument, and since then more than one asylum has tried successfully the same principle. He was a member of the Association of Superintendents of Hospitals for the Insane of North America, and at one time Vice-President of the Canada Medical Association. A life of constant toil and unceasing study with too few holidays told on his strength, and in 1879, in opposition to the wishes of all friends of the Institution, but for the sake of what health remained, he resigned his position.

Holding marked temperance views from his youth, he lost no opportunity of impressing them upon his students; his connection with public institutions confirming and strengthening these views, he was ever ready for temperance work. For the last thirty-seven years of his life, he was an elder of the Presbyterian Church of Canada.

In 1839, he married Anne, only daughter of James Benson, of Kingston, formerly of Fintona, County Tyrone, who survives him. Two of his sons died before him, one at the age of fifteen during his second year of college life, the other being

Staff Assistant-Surgeon of Her Majesty's Forces, at Allahabad, India, at the time of his death.

His widow and two daughters reside in Kingston—one an M.D. of the Woman's Medical College, Kingston, 1886. The youngest daughter is wife of the Rev. George Bruce, of St. John, New Brunswick. The eldest son, William King, is an accountant in Toronto; Edwin Hamilton is an attorney-at-law, etc., at Waco, Texas; the youngest, Charles Rea, an M.D. of Queen's, 1880, and of the University of New York, 1881, is practising in Toronto, the fortunate inheritor of his father's large and very valuable collection of surgical and electrical instruments and books.

About three miles from Kingston, beautifully situated at the foot of Lake Ontario and head of River St. Lawrence, lies Wolfe Island, one of the largest and best settled of the famed Thousand Isles. Here, at the residence of his youngest son, who was at that time practising there, the subject of our sketch passed peacefully and happily away on November 23, 1882. Two days later his remains were followed to their last resting place in Cataraqui cemetery (Kingston) by the professors and students of Queen's and the Royal Colleges, and a large circle of relatives and friends.

DR. ALFRED DIGBY

Was a native of County Meath, Ireland, and a member of the Royal College of Surgeons, Ireland. Soon after obtaining his diploma he came to Canada, and first engaged in practice in Montreal. He then removed to Hamilton, where he pursued his practice with success. Finally he settled at Brantford, about 1835. Dr. Digby was looked upon as a man of great ability, not only as a physician, but as a politician in the various walks of life. Dr. Digby married Miss Catherine Busby, of Montreal, by whom he had four sons and two daughters. He died, 1866, and his widow, 1878. His son, James W., entered the medical profession. He was born in Brantford, 1842, became a matriculant at Toronto University, studied medicine at McGill College, Montreal, and graduated as

M.D., C.M., 1862. He afterward studied in New York, and obtained an appointment in the United States army, in which he served during the war. In 1866, he succeeded to his father's practice at Brantford, where he has continued to enjoy a large practice and the reputation of being skilful in his profession. His standing as a public man is shown by the positions of trust and honour bestowed upon him by his fellow-citizens, having been deputy reeve, town councillor, mayor for three years, and also a trustee of the College Board.

Much of the above information has been obtained from "Cyclopædia of Canadian Biography."

DR. WILLIAM DOUGALL

Was one of the first physicians to practise in Upper Canada. Shortly after the conquest of Canada, having left his home in Ireland and proceeded to England, he obtained an appointment as surgeon to a surveying party under Joseph Frederick Dunbar (De Bar) who was about to survey the coast around the Bay of Fundy. He was thus employed for three years, and then engaged in mercantile business at Halifax. During the rebellion of 1776-83, he was privateering, and at the close of the war he proceeded to New Hampshire and practised his profession for ten years. Coming to Upper Canada, he practised at Ernesttown, on the Bay of Quinte, for two years, at Fredericksburg one year, and two years at Adolphustown. Finally, in 1799, he settled at Hallowell, where he practised for six years, when he retired.

Dr. Dougall had an extensive practice, and was long remembered for his trim attire in "tights" and his silver buckles. During the war of 1812, he was surgeon to the militia. The Doctor had suffered some loss during the war of 1776, and he drew considerable land, 600 acres, in Rawdon, besides 200 acres each in several other places.

His son William, aged 77 (1864), informed the writer that he, William, was present at the surrender of Detroit to General Brock in 1812, and showed a medal of which he was the recipient. On it is: "Fort Detroit, Victoria Regina, 1848, To the British Army, 1793-1814."

His youngest daughter married James Rogers Armstrong, a brother of Dr. Armstrong, formerly of Picton.

DR. JOHN DORMER,

Born in Ireland, was gazetted Licentiate of Upper Canada, October 20, 1829. He settled at Kingston, and thus announced himself to the public: "Surgery and the Practice of Physic.—Dr. Dormer will give attendance to those who may require him professionally in front of the house belonging to Mrs. Reid, in Market Street, within one door of Mr. J. W. Armstrong. Dr. Dormer begs to remark that having pursued his studies in some of the principal medical schools of England, and that having had extern practice in that country and in the Colonies (three years of which he has been at the head of an Infirmary), he will be found, on trial, a safe and efficient practitioner. Advice to the poor gratis. December, 1829."

His position among his compatriots is indicated by the fact that at a public dinner on St. Patrick's Day, 1830, he occupied the position of vice-president.

Among the births announced in the paper of 1836, is "the Lady of Dr. Dormer, of a daughter." He was still practising at Kingston in 1838, but his appearance then did not indicate great prosperity.

DR. JOHN DOWDING,

The son of a British officer, was an M.R.C.S. Eng., and was gazetted under 8th Geo. IV., Chap. 3. Practised at Ancaster and Dundas, and subsequently at Brantford. The following interesting historical incident, taken from the Dundas *Weekly Post*, of March 8, 1836, cannot be overlooked: "About the 20th of last month, Dr. Dowding, one of our medical practitioners, was called to attend a lady of this town in her confinement; he did so, and before the matter could be brought to a successful issue, thought it advisable to call in Dr. ———, another gentleman of the same profession, to consult upon the exigency of the case. Some difference of opinion arose, it appeared, as to the treatment of the patient, and from that a demand for satisfaction was made on the part of the former to the latter. After some epistolatory correspondence between them, the challenge was accepted by Dr. ———, and the parties accordingly met on the morning of 27th ult. After exchanging two shots without effect, the seconds interfered. The affair terminated by a retraction on the part of both, as will be found on a perusal of the report below. Thus the whole affair ended in smoke; and we hope the past case will be the last of a similar kind to raise the excitement in our community:

"BRANTFORD, *February* 27th, 1836.

"*Dundas 'Weekly Post.'*

"A meeting having taken place this morning between Dr. Dowding and Dr. ———, after an exchange of two shots each between the parties, the seconds interfered, and although a reconciliation was not effected between them, it was agreed that Dr. Dowding should retract the words, 'liar, scoundrel and coward,' applied to Dr. ———, and that the latter should in like manner retract the words, 'liar, villain, scoundrel and fool,' applied to Dr. Dowding, and that all reflections upon the character of either party as a gentleman, now published or in the press, should be considered as retracted.

"(Signed) LLOYD RICHARDSON,
(In behalf of Dr. Dowding).
E. SAUNDERS,
(In behalf of Dr. ———).

DR. CHARLES DUNCOMBE.

Among the early physicians of the western part of Upper Canada, Drs. Charles, David and Elijah Duncombe were conspicuous, the first two of whom became members of parliament. They were natives of the United States, and settled in Burford, a few years after the war of 1812. That they were considered loyal is manifest from the various appointments they received, especially Charles, who was the most clever of the three.

Dr. Charles was a well-known personage in his time among Upper Canadians, not so much, perhaps, as a physician, as a politician, member of parliament, and a participator in the rebellion of 1837. The first record we have of him is in the minutes of the proceedings of the Upper Canada Medical Board, which states that "Chas. Duncombe, of Delaware Town, London District, passed his examination before the Medical Board, October 5, 1819." That Dr. Duncombe was of more than ordinary standing in his profession is attested by his being appointed by the Lieut.-Governor to be a member of the Upper Canada Medical Board. We find that at the January meeting of the Board, 1832, commissions were read appointing additional members upon the Board, and Dr. C. Duncombe appeared at the meeting as one of them. In 1825, he was made Surgeon to the 2nd Middlesex Militia.

Dr. Chas. Duncombe lived at the Village of Bishop-gate, on the side town-line between Burford and Brantford townships, in the County of Brant, and his field of practice radiated for many miles in every direction, over five or six counties. He was a man of good information, well read, and is described as a many-sided man. In his profession he was not without considerable skill. He did not confine his professional labours to the well-to-do, although he acquired considerable wealth, but would ride mile after mile, through swamp and forest, to visit patients too poor to give a fee. Naturally he acquired personal influence in the community. His manner was attractive, and very soon his popularity caused him to be sought out as a fitting person for parliamentary honours.

His political career began in 1834, when he was returned as a member for Oxford. On February 8, 1836, the "Speaker reported that he had received from the commission appointed by a resolution of the House at the last session for collecting certain information, two letters." One of them reads thus:

"TORONTO, *February* 24th, 1836.

"SIR,—Drs. Duncombe, Morrison and Bruce being by a resolution of the Honourable the House of Assembly appointed a commission to enquire into the system and management of schools and colleges, in order to report fully upon the systems of education pursued in the United States, one of the commissioners, Dr. Chas. Duncombe, was requested and authorized to visit that country, acquire a knowledge of the subject, and report thereon. That gentleman has done so to our most entire satisfaction.

"(Signed) T. D. MORRISON,
WM. BRUCE.

"*To* THE HON. M. S. BIDWELL."

The same year Dr. Duncombe visited England and presented a petition to the Imperial Parliament, reflecting on Sir Francis Bond Head, and this procedure was not without fruit. The charges were so supported by proof that ultimately the Lieut.-Governor was retired of his post, somewhat under a cloud. At this time the political sky in Canada was overcast, which ended in rebellion the following year. In the petition presented were strong protests against the dominant party of the country, and Sir Francis Bond Head was violently assailed. It was alleged that Dr. Duncombe was not authorized by anyone to speak on behalf of Canadians. At that time there was an association in Toronto called the "City of Toronto Political Union Society." On December 14, 1836, probably when the Doctor had returned, a meeting was held at which Dr. W. W. Baldwin, the president, was in the chair. Resolutions were adopted endorsing the action of Dr. Duncombe. The Society also endorsed the proceedings of the "Constitutional Reform Society," which had prevailed upon him to repair to England. One of the resolutions was moved by Dr. Tims, and another by the Rev. Dr. O'Grady. We thus get glimpses of the fact that prominent persons were engaged in the agitation which culminated in rebellion, but wisely stopped short before committing acts of a treasonable character. But Dr. Duncombe did not stop short of this. Indeed, he was the leader of the rebels in the western part of the Province. But the small band collected by him soon dispersed, whilst he had to flee the country; and we read in the *Patriot*, of December, 1837, a notice offering £500 for his apprehension as a traitor.

The following account of his escape, taken from the "History of Brant County," is interesting: " For a month, Duncombe lay concealed at the house of his sister, Mrs. Shennick, a few miles from London. Charles Tilden was, with several of the Hagel family, among the Scotland insurgents. Living near Amherstburgh, he happened to be specially well acquainted with the entire western frontier, and noticed that, although Sir Francis Head's agents had placed guards all along the line, to prevent the escape of 'rebels,' now that a month had passed from the first excitement, the vigilance was much relaxed. Tilden went to see Duncombe, who, in the depth of winter (January, 1838, was a specially cold season) was kept hid in a hay-loft, and supplied with food by stealth, by those who left the house as if to feed the cattle. Tilden urged him to attempt escape disguised as a woman, which Duncombe's smooth, round face rendered possible enough. The attempt was dangerous. A reward had been offered for his head, and all over the country the noble savages of the Grand River Reserve were on the lookout for his scalp and the blood-money it would bring. They left the house next day in an old-fashioned farmer's box-sleigh. Tilden drove; Mrs. Shennick and Duncombe sat side by side, the latter disguised as an elderly farmer's wife. Mrs. Shennick's little girl, a child of nine, was taught to address him as 'Auntie.' All day they drove along without molestation. At night they stopped at a country hotel, where, there not being sufficient accommodation, Charles Tilden had to sleep with one of the hotel-keeper's boys, while the three 'womankind' had a room to themselves. Unable to sleep from the excitement of his position, Dr. Duncombe sat up all night. At early dawn they drove away breakfastless, and arrived, after several hours' drive, at the crossing place, which was at a village opposite what is now Marine City, Michigan. They drove into the yard of a tavern where were the soldiers of a party in command of a sergeant, posted there to watch the crossing place, and, if possible, arrest the 'rebel' chief. Very calmly Tilden watered his horses, and then addressing the sergeant in command as 'Captain,' asked if the ice was safe, and if he would kindly send one of his men to guide them to the right track. The sergeant asked whence he came. Tilden replied, truly enough, that he came from London, and was going with his aunt and mother, to visit some friends, whose names he mentioned, on the opposite coast of Michigan. The sergeant ordered one of his men to accompany them across the ice. When they had got half way across the river, the young soldier said that they could easily find their way for the rest of the track, and was about to leave them. Dr. Duncombe handed Charles Tilden fifty cents for the soldier, and while the latter was thanking them, felt very much inclined to send Dr. Duncombe's compliments to the sergeant who had furnished them with a guide, but refrained, lest he should spoil the chance of some other unfortunate, who might try the same stratagem for evading the blood-hounds of the Family Compact government. In a few minutes he stood 'a free man on a free soil.' They entered a store to buy some food for Mrs. Shennick's little girl, and Duncombe, now careless of preserving his feminine demeanour, soon attracted attention. When it became known that this was the Canadian Republican, Dr. Duncombe, a crowd gathered, and with characteristic American humour, insisted on Dr. Duncombe making a speech in his woman's dress. Thus he escaped capture, which, in those days, would have been certain death. A long and prosperous career in the States lay before him. Charles Tilden's son lives in possession of a farm of two hundred acres, which Dr. Dun combe deeded to him as an acknowledgment of his father's generous friendship."

Dr. Duncombe was pardoned in 1843, but he had made arrangements to permanently live in the States; he, however, made a visit to his friends in Canada.

The following tribute to Dr. Duncombe, with two others of the profession, is given by Dr. Hodgins in an article on the "Educational System of Ontario": "The year 1836 is noted in our educational history for the efforts put forth, under the direction of the Legislature, by a memorable trio of doctors (Dr. Duncombe, Dr. Morrison and Dr. Bruce) to extend and improve our common school system. These commoners brought in an elaborate report and appended to it a voluminous bill, in which it was proposed to grant $60,000 per annum for the support of these schools."

DR. DAVID DUNCOMBE, from London District, appeared before

Medical Board, January, 1828, and obtained a certificate for a license. He engaged in practice in County of Norfolk. June, 1834, was elected to represent that county in parliament; continued in practice for many years. *Req.* Waterford, 1887. One of his daughters married Wm. Bowlby, of Waterford.

ELIJAH E. DUNCOMBE, from St. Thomas, before Medical Board, April, 1830, and "recommended to attend a course of lectures." April, 1831, obtained certificate from the Board for license. He spent his life in practice at St. Thomas, where he died of old age.

CHAS. S. DUNCOMBE, of St. Thomas, before Medical Board, October, 1849, had diploma from Geneva College.

DR. THOMAS DUGGAN

Was the eldest son of Col. George Duggan, of Toronto, who for many years held the position of coroner. Thomas studied medicine with Drs. Widmer and Deihl, also Dr. King. It does not appear that he studied anywhere else. He passed the Upper Canada Medical Board, July, 1833. This card appeared in the *Patriot,* York, August 6, 1833: "Dr. Thomas Duggan, having obtained the necessary license to practise Physic, Surgery and Midwifery, from His Excellency the Lieut.-Governor, will in future reside in York, corner King and George Streets. N.B.—Advice to the poor gratis." The York Directory for 1834 gives Dr. Duggan as at corner King and George Streets. He was one of the Managing Committee of the Emigrant Society of Upper Canada, 1835. During the rebellion, 1837, he was Assistant-Surgeon to the Queen's Light Infantry.

Dr. Duggan made this announcement, March, 1839: "Dr. Thomas Duggan, in consequence of the lamented death of Dr. McCague, and by the desire of every person of Thornhill and its vicinity, has been induced to take up his residence at Mr. Joseph Miller's Inn on Yonge Street, for the purpose of practising his profession in all its branches."

Some time before 1846, Dr. Duggan removed to Hamilton, where he acquired a good practice, and ended his days. He died, March 4, 1874, aged sixty. He left several children, one of whom is a lawyer in Buffalo, N.Y.

DR. WILLIAM DUNLOP.

The following is taken from a review in *Fraser's Magazine*, July, 1832, of "Statistical Sketches of Upper Canada, for the use of Emigrants," by a Backwoodsman. "The Canadas as they at present commend themselves to the enterprise of emigrants, colonists and capitalists."

The reviewer says: "A pleasanter little book never came out of the press—full of information of all kinds, full of reading, full of sagacity, full of humour. It is a voice speaking to us from the forests of Canada—from the centre of woods that have seen generation after generation of men pass away into the ocean of eternity, as Niagara dashes into the gulf below; and pleasant does that voice burst upon our ears, even as the voice of a friend whom we thought we had lost for ever. We may say with Solomon, 'As cold waters to a thirsty soul, so is good news from a far country.'

"In short, our Backwoodsman is he whom men and long-robed women called the 'Tiger'—a title by which he was most beloved. His own name is William Dunlop, or, as he chose to call it, 'Wull.' Of Dunlops the best, extensively rivalling even the cheeses of that honoured appellation, he can trace his family to Ragman's Roll, and his father is the laird of Kippoch, and therefore Kippoch is he called in the western wilds of Scotland. But leaving questions of pedigree to heralds, we find Dunlop a surgeon in the Connaught Rangers in early life, and as he mentions in this little book, actively engaged in the campaigns of 1813, '14 and '15, against the Yankees in what was then generally known by the name of Mr. Madison's war. Forgotten out of America, as the battles of that war are nowadays, there was some hard partisan fighting, in which the Doctor, laying down the lancet for the bayonet, and inflicting wounds instead of curing them, played no unconspicuous part."

The following account of Dr. Dunlop during the war is taken from "Twenty-seven Years in Canada West," by Major

Strickland. He says: "For the following characteristic traits I am indebted to my friend, Colonel Fitzgibbon. Dr. Dunlop, in his youth, was assistant-surgeon in the 89th Regiment on the Niagara frontier during the campaign of 1814. He was at that time a young man who appeared to have outgrown his clothes; at least, the sleeves of his coat reached but a short way below his elbows, and his trousers did not nearly reach his ankles. He was careless, if not slovenly, in his dress, and he seldom applied a razor to his chin. His proportions were almost Herculean, and his movements and gait were awkward and ungainly.

"When our army attacked Fort Erie by assault, we were beaten back with much slaughter, great numbers of our men falling killed or wounded under the fire of the enemy. As daylight appeared, Dunlop, whose vocation, be it remembered, was that of man-curer, not of man-killer, ran through the firing to witness the scene, when, seeing that some of the wounded could not get to the rear beyond the range of the enemy's fire, he gallantly caught up a poor fellow and carried him to a place of safety, immediately returning to take up another, and so on until he had thus taken bodily possession of ten or twelve of his patients.

"One man, wounded in the knee, he heaved upon his back and bore to the rear, but on laying down his burden the Doctor found that the soldier had received in transit a mortal wound in the back, and so intercepted the shot which otherwise would have taken effect on Dunlop himself. It should be stated that he brought with him, slung over his shoulders, six of the soldiers' wooden canteens filled with wine intended for the wounded, with which he refreshed them, and attended professionally to their hurts under a noble tree out of the reach of the shot he had so bravely encountered for their benefit.

"Those who enjoyed the friendship of this warm-hearted man had frequent opportunities of knowing his kind and feeling disposition, for there never was a finer jewel, though roughly set, than poor Dunlop. His cheerful and undaunted spirit formed him for an efficient leader of British emigration.

"The 89th was chiefly composed of Irishmen, and among them he learned the management of those refractory subjects better than any one of their own officers. His influence over them was very great, and during his long residence in Canada, after he left the army, he exerted his influence over the Irish emigrants and settlers, to the great benefit of the poor people themselves and to the advantage of the public. In a violent party riot in the city of Toronto, about the year 1830, he did more than any other Justice of the Peace then present in quelling the disturbance."

He was a humorous, witty man, and never regarded time or place when any opportunity occurred for displaying his facetious propensities. Upon one particular occasion I remember, he amused the House of Assembly by his comical questions and witty rejoinders. I think it was seven or eight years ago, when Montreal was the seat of Government, that a bill was brought before the House to tax dogs and whiskey. The Doctor, who spoke on this occasion, asked if any member present could inform him how many quarts of whiskey were usually made from a bushel of wheat, Indian corn or rye?

The member for the Second Riding of Northumberland replied: "He believed sixteen quarts."

"I believe," rejoined the Doctor, "the young gentleman is right, but Heaven defend me from your sixteen-quart whiskey! I like a stiff horn. I have read of the beast with two horns, and of the beast with ten horns, but I am a beast of many horns."

We now return to the article in *Fraser's Magazine:*

"Peace being proclaimed, and the Treaty of Ghent (which, as he observed, 'came upon them suddenly,' and, we may add, much to their grief) having put an end to American campaigning, he went with his regiment to Calcutta, exchanging the blanket coat for the muslin jacket, and using brandy and water to keep out the intense heat of India with as much activity as he had formerly employed it to keep off the intense cold of Canada. Manifold were his occupations in the land of the Moguls. In addition to his medical and military duties—his convivial and charioteering occupations—he edited a newspaper and contracted to clear the island of Saugur, falling with equal fury upon Silk Buckingham and the tigers. After having killed some incredible number of the latter nuisances (whence, and not from any resemblance of that king of cats, he has the name of 'Tiger'), the jungle fever subdued him, and he was obliged to come home on half pay. He fixed first in Edinburgh, where he gave a course of lectures on Medical Jurisprudence, the mixture in which of fun and learning, of law and science, blended with rough jokes and anecdotes not always of the most prudish nature, will make them live long in the memory of his hearers. He also wrote sketches of Indian life and other papers for Blackwood, under the signature of Colin Ballantyne, R.N., a *nom de guerre* under which, we believe, he figured in India during his controversies with Buckingham, whom he ever and anon delighted in calling the 'Cobbler.' Tired of Edinburgh, he came to London, where he lived a most miscellaneous life, turning his hand to everything. He edited, for a short while, the *British Press*, a journal now gone to sleep; but could not like the business of a morning paper, as it interfered too much with other occupations of a more agreeable kind.

"He then published an edition of Beck's 'Medical Jurisprudence,' an American work, to which he wrote a preface and appended many curious notes; and started a Sunday newspaper for the India interests, entitled the *Telescope*, the history of which would be a comedy of the drollest kind. It did not succeed badly, but at the end of a year he was tired of it; and having become connected with the joint stocks of those days—our history has now reached the famous year 1825—he figured in brick, iron, salt and other companies, as secretary or director. He personally superintended the salt works of this last-named company somewhere in Cheshire; but as 'Tiger' is an honest fellow—a strictly honest fellow, in every sense of the word—it is perfectly unnecessary for us to add that he made nothing of the bubbles, except what salary he may have received. The future biographer of Dunlop will have to recount that at this time he founded a club of a most peculiar description, which he called by the picturesque title of 'The Pig and Whistle'; but the time is not yet ripe for the history of that celebrated association. John Galt had, about this time, succeeded in organizing the Canada Company, which has since treated him with such signal ingratitude; and Dunlop accepted office under it in the year 1826, with the sounding title of 'Warden of the Black

Forest,' and immediately started for Canada, where he has ever since remained, teaching to hew the beech the hand that held the glaive, and performing all the duties of his laborious office with vast benefit to the country and the Company. He is, at this present writing, one of the most popular men in Upper Canada, and, of course, universally consulted by emigrants of all classes on their affairs. This brings us to the consideration of the little book before us:

"Some authors," he says, "write for fame, some for money, some to propagate particular doctrines and opinions, some from spite, some at the instigation of their friends, and not a few at the instigation of the devil. I have no one of these excuses to plead in apology for intruding myself on the public; for my motive, which has at least the merit of novelty to recommend it, is sheer laziness. To explain this, it is necessary to state that, for some years past, I have been receiving letters from intending emigrants containing innumerable queries respecting Upper Canada; also from the friends of such children of the forest—*in posse*—who seasoned the unpalatable task of writing on other people's business with the assurance so consolatory to my vanity, that I was, of all men in the Province, the one they considered best qualified to give such information, etc. These letters, always couched in the most polite terms, commencing with the writer's 'sincere sorrow for taking up so much of my valuable time,' and ending with 'the most perfect reliance on my knowledge and candour,' required to be answered; and so long as they came 'like angel visits, few and far between,' it was no great grievance to do so. But, after having written some reams in answer to them, and when every other packet brought one—and no later ago than last week I had two to answer—things began to look serious, and so did I; for I found that, if they went on at this rate, I should have no 'valuable time' to devote to my own proper affairs. And, therefore, it being now mid-winter, and seeing no prospect of my being able to follow my out-of-door avocations for some weeks, I set myself down, in something like a pet, to throw together and put in form the more prominent parts of the information I had been collecting, to the end that I might be enabled in the future to answer my voluminous correspondents after the manner of the late worthy Mr. Abernethy, by referring them to certain pages of 'My Book.'"

The Doctor in his concluding paragraph says: "Now, gentle reader, that you have got this length, permit me to compliment you on your patience; a virtue which I shall no longer call upon you to exercise, than by requesting you, in the diplomatic phrase, to accept the assurances of my highest consideration until we meet, as I hope we shall do next summer, on the banks of Lake Huron."

The reviewer then adds: "Meet him wherever we may, we shall meet a good fellow, whose various wanderings over the world have filled him with shrewd, good sense, and stored him with wealth of tale and anecdote beyond that of any other man now living. It is recorded of him that, on his return from India he entertained the company after dinner every day with stories, and that he never repeated one a second time during the voyage. What an immense and multifarious stock he must have laid in since!

"Farewell, then, dear 'Tiger,' and whether we meet you on the banks of the Huron, over the hind-quarter of a bear, clad in the skin of the same animal, and talking much in his tone and accent, or on the banks of your native Clyde, predominating over a bowl of that cold punch manufactured by you in a manner surpassing that of all other sons of men, or in your favourite region of the Strand, chasing away the midnight hours with fluid suitable to the time—wheresoever, whensoever, and howsoever the meeting may be—warm shall be the greeting and cordial the welcome,

> "'And we'll go nae mair a-roving,
> A-roving in the night;
> And we'll go nae mair a-roving,
> Let the moon shine ne'er sae bright.'"

Dr. Maginn, the editor of *Fraser's Magazine*, who produced a portrait of Dr. Dunlop, taken from Maclise's "Gallery of Illustrious Characters," described the Doctor as "six feet three inches, and measures two feet eight across the shoulders."

Dr. Dunlop was born about 1795, Greenock, Scotland, and came, as we have learned, to Canada, in 1826, with Mr. John

Galt, in the service of the Canada Company. John Galt, in writing about him, said that he "held a roving commission in the Company." For a time subsequently, his connection with the Company was discontinued. But in December, 1829, he was restored by the Canada Company to his office of "Warden of the Woods and Ranger of the Forests," for which he received £400 per year. Dr. Dunlop was for a long time a contributor to *Blackwood's Magazine*. Among other things he wrote "The Autobiography of a Rat," contributed to the *Canadian Literary Magazine*. He founded, in 1836, the City of Toronto Literary Club, before which he lectured on various subjects of interest. He was the first representative for the Huron District in the Provincial Parliament for the County of Huron in 1841, and continued dnring the first and second Parliament after the union of Upper and Lower Canada, but resigned in 1846. He was, 1841, Chairman of a Select Committee of the Legislative Assembly, to report on the petition of Mr. Robert Gourlay.

Dr. Dunlop was well acquainted with the conditions of Upper Canada. He says in the preface of his little book:

"Since the year 1826, my principal employment has been to traverse the country in every direction, and visit nearly every township in it, for the express purpose of obtaining statistical information." He had much to do with the settling of Guelph. It is recorded that he "took part in cutting down the first tree, a large maple, to found the town of Guelph. After the tree fell, the Doctor pulled a flask of whiskey from his bosom, and we drank prosperity to the city of Guelph."

Dr. Dunlop, among his numerous and varied ventures, was on the lookout for the acquisition of property and other investments. We find in the Upper Canada *Gazette*, May 24, 1832, a notice of a meeting of stockholders of the Grand River Navigation Company, recently held at Brantford. He was elected one of the directors. In a communication to the *Correspondence and Advocate* it is charged, "In the Home District a few officers of the Government, with Dr. Dunlop, are officers of a company of speculators."

The Doctor made his influence felt in the capital of York. "At a meeting of the adherents of the Church of Scotland in the town of York, held on the 3rd March, 1830, John Ewart,

Esq., in the chair, it was, on motion of Dr. Dunlop, seconded by Mr. H. Carfrae, unanimously resolved to take immediate steps for the erection of a place of worship in connection with the Church of Scotland, and for the calling of a clergyman of that Church to officiate therein as their minister." Among other noticeable projects, Dr. Scadding records that he, with Dr. Rees and Mr. Chas. Fothergill, at one time intended to establish in Toronto a museum of natural and civil history, with a botanical and zoological garden attached. For this purpose a grant of land from the Government was received.

He was one of the pioneers on Lake Huron, and lived at Goderich for some time, where he was a person of note. In Mackenzie's rebellion, 1837, he was colonel of the Huron Invincibles.

The will of Dr. Dunlop is of such an extraordinary character that it is given here in its entirety:

"In the name of God. Amen. I, William Dunlop, of Fairbraid in the Township of Colborne, County and District of Huron, Western Canada, Esquire, being in sound health of body, and my mind just as usual, which my friends who flatter me say is no great shakes at the best of times, do make this my last will and testament as follows—revoking of course all former wills:

"I leave the property of Fairbraid and all other landed property I may die possessed of, to my sisters, Ellen Boyle Story, and Elizabeth Boyle Dunlop, the former because she is married to a minister whom (God help him!) she henpecks: the latter, because she is married to nobody, nor is she likely to be, for she is an old maid and not market-rife; and also I leave to them and their heirs my share of the stock and implements on the farm, provided always that the enclosure round my brother's grave be reserved, and if either should die without issue then the other to inherit the whole.

"I leave to my sister-in-law, Louisa Dunlop, all my share of the household furniture and such traps with the exceptions hereinafter mentioned.

"I leave my silver tankard to the oldest son of old John, as the representative of the family; I would have left it to old John himself, but he would melt it down to make temperance medals, and that would be a sacrilege—however, I leave my big horn snuff-box to him, he can only make temperance horn-spoons of that.

"I leave my sister Jenny my Bible, the property formerly of my great-great-grandmother, Bethia Hamilton, of Woodhall, and when she knows as much of the spirit of it as she does of the letter, she will be another guise-Christian than she is.

"I also leave my late brother's watch to my brother Sandy, exhorting him at the same time to give up wiggery, radicalism, and all other sins that do most easily beset him.

"I leave my brother Alan, my big silver snuff-box, as I am informed he is rather a decent Christian, with a swag belly and a jolly face.

"I leave parson Chevasse (Maggie's husband) the snuff-box I got from the Sarnia Militia, as a small token of my gratitude for the service he has done the family in taking a sister that no man of taste would have taken.

"I leave John Caddle a silver tea-pot, to the end that he may drink tea therefrom to comfort him under the affliction of a slatternly wife.

"I leave my books to my brother Andrew, because he has been so long a jungley-wallah, that he may learn to read with them.

"I give my silver cup with a sovereign in it to my sister, Janet Graham Dunlop, because she is an old maid and pious, and therefore will necessarily take to horning, and also my granma's snuff-mull, as it looks decent to see an old woman taking snuff.

"I do hereby constitute and appoint John Dunlop, Esquire, of Fairbraid; Alexander Dunlop, Esquire, Advocate, Edinburgh; Alan C. Dunlop, Esquire, and William Chalk, of Tuckersmith; William Stewart and William Gooding, Esquires, Goderich, to be the executors of this my last will and testament.

"In witness whereof I have hereunto set my hand and seal the thirty-first day of August, in the year of our Lord one thousand eight hundred and forty-two.

[L.S.] "(Signed) W. DUNLOP."

"The above instrument, of one sheet, was, at the date thereof, declared to us by the testator, William Dunlop, Esquire, to be his last will and testament, and he then acknowledged to each of us, that he had subscribed the same, and we at his request signed our names hereunto as attesting witnesses.

"(Signed) JAMES CLOWTING.
PATRICK MCNAUGHTON.
[L.S.] ELIZABETH STEWARD."

"I, Daniel McDonald, Registrar of the Surrogate Court of the County of Huron, hereby certify that the within is a true and correct copy of the original last will and testament of the said William Dunlop, Esquire, deceased.

"Given under my hand and seal at Goderich, in the said county, this eighteenth day of April, in the year A.D. 1881.

[L.S.] "D. MCDONALD, *Registrar.*"

"Died, June 29th, 1848, at Cote St. Paul, Dr. Wm. Dunlop, aged 57."

"Dr. Dunlop had a brother (Capt. Sandy) almost as eccentric as himself, residing with him, and they kept a housekeeper possessed of means, from whom they had been compelled either to borrow money, or, what was much the same thing, to go in arrears in the payment of her wages, in order to tide them over an emergency. It was found, on an examination of the accounts, that they were hopelessly in her debt; the Doctor, therefore, startled his brother by stating that the only way out of the difficulty was for one or other of them to marry Betty. This was agreed upon at last, and the Doctor gave his brother a penny with which to toss up for the wife. It is said that the coin had two heads so that there was after all no element of chance in the matter. The coin went up, the Doctor cried 'heads,' and of course head it was. The housekeeper was nothing loth, and the brother was married to her without unnecessary delay."—*Rattray.*

"Died, at Fairbraid, near Goderich, February 28th, 1841, Robert Graham Dunlop, Esquire, M.P.P., Commander, Royal Navy, in his 51st year."

DR. DARIUS DUNHAM

Came into Upper Canada as a Methodist preacher, in 1792, being one of the first two Methodist ministers sent to Upper Canada by the Methodist Episcopal Church of the United States. Prior to that, he had been a minister for four years in New York State. He had previously studied for the medical profession, but where, or to what extent, is not recorded. In 1800, he ceased to labour as a preacher, and settled down on a farm in the neighbourhood of Napanee, and resumed the practice of medicine. No doubt he had, during his twelve years of itinerancy, found occasion to treat the body as well as attend to the wants of the soul, and subsequently while practising, he continued to exercise the function of preacher on Sundays. Many amusing stories are related of him while a preacher; and he was known as "Scolding Dunham." He was a fine-looking man, and secured as a wife one of the most comely of the daughters of the settlement of Napanee, a Miss Detlor; and in so doing, broke the heart and upset the mental balance of the first pioneer Methodist minister to Upper Canada.

His son, E. A. Dunham, born, July, 1814, although unostentatious, was highly esteemed in the Methodist Church, being for a long time a class-leader and acceptable local preacher. He published for some years a most valuable work on holiness, "The Christian Casket," at Napanee. He removed to Port Burwell, 1861, and thence to St. Thomas about 1880, where he died, February 27, 1891. "He was a man of strong conceptions of duty, a devout student of the Word of God, an honest, upright, consistent Christian, whose memory will be cherished most by those who knew him best."

DR. WILLIAM DURIE

Was born in the Metherton of Dunfermline in Fife, Scotland, October 4, 1779. He belonged to a very old Scottish family, of which there is a record from the year 1200.

This interesting document, which, through the courtesy of Mrs. Durie, we have been permitted to read, commences thus:

"History of the present family of Craigluscar; drawn by Charles Durie, Esquire, the present laird, 1768 (A.C., 1200). This family came first to Britain with William the Conqueror, who settled upon them an English barony, where they lived a considerable time. At length, Joan, sister to Henry, King of England, being matched with Alexander II., King of Scotland, a gentleman of this family came under the Queen's patronage, and procured from her husband, the King, a pretty considerable estate hard by Leven, to which he gave his own name."

The record drawn by Charles Durie had been continued, and although intended only for a family history, is not without considerable general interest. The impartial manner in which events are recorded is very praiseworthy. This quotation is not without interest: "One of the line in the sixteenth century, Henry by name, had the good fortune to marry one Margaret McBeath, a Highland gentleman's daughter. This lady was an excellent botanist, very conversant in medicine, and knew particularly the nature of children's diseases. Her merit shined as much at Court as in her own family. She became a great favourite of James VI.'s queen, who resided in the Abbey of Dunfermline, where she brought forth several children. There were but few complaints amongst the royal offspring in which Margaret McBeath's advice was not taken as the safest and best. Her profound knowledge particularly distinguished itself in the recovery of Charles I., after the best physician in the kingdom had despaired of his life."

Without attempting to outline the course of events in the successive generations of the family, it may be stated that they acted a conspicuous part in the various passing events, some of a most important character. We read that a daughter was married to Sir Robert Bruce, of Clackmannan. Then we read of Robert, "who commanded a company in Flanders, under King William, after serving the three kings immediately preceding, in the rank of Lieutenant; James, Thomas and Henry, who served as volunteers in the Dutch service, where they died of a flux, after eating too much fruit. One daughter by the name of Janet, who was married in the year 1665, to Alexander Campbell, of Persio, in the shire of Perth; whose estate was ruined supporting the Duke of Argyle, for which he afterwards got no thanks." Another has a company in a Regiment of Scots Infantry, then in the French service. Now we read of one who was "a good scholar, very conversant in the Latin and Greek authors." Another "was conversant in the history of all nations, but more particularly those of the sacred writings. No one could pretend to a more distinct conception of the situation and extent of all countries on the globe." Again, one is in the army and passes many years in the East Indies to return with an impaired constitution, and to retire on half pay. A number of others also entered the army; one is in service in New South Wales, and on returning is wrecked in the South Seas. And now we have come to facts collected by the subject of this sketch, and written by Major Robert Durie.

He says: "Before I close the account of my, and Charles', family, I cannot forego the pleasure I have in handing down to the family the following honourable and handsome tribute paid to my Uncle Robert who was retired in the East Indies. My brother of that name was there for twenty-three years, and had many an opportunity of hearing how deservedly beloved he was by all ranks, both European officers and native soldiers. The latter, though against their religion, buried him, and while the army lay at Cuddalore showed every respect to his tomb, by burning a lamp every night upon it. My brother mentions that he only remembers another instance in the funeral of an officer by the men of his battalion, as when an officer dies, or is retired in India, he is carried to his grave by European soldiers."

The following extract is from a letter of a Capt. Taylor of the Bombay Army, dated Bombay, November 10, 1784: "I must now lament the fate of poor Durie, a man esteemed by all as a gentleman and an officer. What instance can be given more pleasing than the tribute paid him by the gallant corps which he commanded. He fell amongst numbers at the attack of Cuddalore. He was buried during the action, but the esteem of his people would not permit him to be undistinguished. In the evening of the day he was taken up; they washed his body, clothed it in fine linen, and conducted him to his grave in the style of the country, while each shed a generous tear for the man they respected, rendered yet more respectable for his soldier-like fortune, leading his men to victory and to honour."

Dr. Durie was educated at Kinross, and began the study of medicine at Edinburgh, October, 1793, with Mr. Moncrief. While yet with him in 1797, he was offered a commission in the Royal Artillery, and being released from his engagement with Mr. Moncrief, he accepted the offer. His commission on parchment, now before the writer, is as follows:

"*George R.*

"George the Third by the Grace of God, King of Great Britain, France and Ireland, Defender of the Faith, etc. To our Trusty and Well-beloved William Durie, Gentleman. GREETING.—We do by these Presents, Constitute and Appoint you to be Assistant-Surgeon to a Corps of Artificers and Drivers to be attached to the Artillery serving in our Kingdom of Ireland, whereof Charles Combers, Esquire, is Captain Commandant.

"You are therefore carefully and diligently to discharge the Duty of Assistant-Surgeon by doing and performing all and all manner of Things thereunto belonging; And you are to observe and follow such Orders and Directions from Time to Time, as you shall receive from the Master General of our ordnance in our said Kingdom for the Time being, or any other superior Officer, according to the Rules and Discipline of War. Given at Our Court at Saint James the Twentieth Day of November, 1797, in the Thirty-eighth Year of Our Reign. By His Majesty's Command.

"(Signed) PORTLAND."

It will be seen from the date of the commission that he was only eighteen years of age when he entered the Royal Artillery service. He served in the south of Ireland at Cork and Clonmell, and at Dublin. While stationed at Clonmell, he married Miss Helena, daughter of Arthur Lee, Esq., of Coppa, and sister of Sir Francis S. S. Lee, A.D.C. to the King.

A second commission on parchment, before us, says: "To our trusty and well-beloved William Durie, etc., etc. We appoint you to be an Assistant-Surgeon on the Medical Establishment for the Military Department of the Ordnance, etc., etc. Given at our Court at St. James, the first day of January, 1804."

A third parchment informs us that on November 18, 1805, he was commissioned to be Surgeon in the Royal Artillery. It is probable that between the two periods last mentioned, he was on duty at Woolwich or Chatham. At all events he was at the former place in 1805. After his appointment as Surgeon, he served in the Mediterranean, and was at Malta and Gibraltar, 1808. Here he remained until 1813, or later, and so efficiently discharged his duties that he received the thanks of the Board of Ordnance, and also this letter:

"WOOLWICH, *June* 22nd, 1813.

"SIR,—I have just read with very great pleasure your interesting account of the Case of Aneurism, which, in my opinion, does honour to your skill and perseverance; that the termination of it has hitherto been successful, must be highly satisfactory; but if even the event had been otherwise, that so much had been done for the preservation of the patient must have been fully appreciated by everyone who could judge of the delicacy and difficulty of the task you had to perform.

"I have also been favoured with your letter of the 18th ultimo, and the accompanying Returns, which are correct and satisfactory. I wish, however, that the particulars of men who die may be inserted, agreeably to the inclosed Form.

"Mr. Dymoke has reported that he arrived at Messina on the 31st of March.

"I have the honour to be, Sir,
"Your Obedient, Humble Servant,

"(Signed) JOHN WEBB,
"*Insp.-Gen., Ord. Hosp.*

"WILLIAM DURIE, ESQ.,
"*Surgeon, Royal Artillery, Gibraltar.*"

A fourth commission appointed him "to be a Resident Surgeon" in the Ordnance Department, dated September 26, 1814. He continued on duty on the staff at Woolwich and Chatham until some time before 1823. He was then stationed at Island Bridge, near Dublin, until 1826. Returned to Woolwich and became "Assistant Inspector-General Ordnance Medical Department." With this rank he retired from the Royal Artillery, 1836, on half pay, when he received the Order of Knight of Hanover.

Dr. Durie arrived in Canada, September, 1836, and resided in Toronto about a year, when he took up his residence on Yonge Street, near Thornhill. After his arrival he was offered a professorship in the University of King's College, by Bishop Strachan, which he declined. A new commission appoihting members of the Medical Board, September 25, 1838, contains the name of Dr. Durie. By virtue of being a member of the Medical Board, he became a Fellow of the College of Physicians and Surgeons, Upper Canada, 1839, and was present at the first meeting. When the Medical Board was revived, he was again one of its members, July 28, 1841, and in 1845. But Dr. Durie very rarely attended the meetings. He lived in comparative retirement, doing a little practice principally as a consultant. At Craigluscar, about half a mile this side of Thornhill, and named after a family residence in Scotland, he passed the autumn of his life. He had received as half pay a guinea per day and allowance for three servants. He returned to Toronto a few years before his death, where he died, June 14, 1871, aged 92. His body was buried at Thornhill.

Dr. Durie had ten children, five of whom, we believe, were sons—Arthur Lee, Wm. S., George, John and C. H. Durie. One daughter married Charles Carbruld, Esq., of Orillia; another, Walter McKenzie, Toronto, Clerk of the County Court, recently deceased (1890); another married the Rev. S. B. Ardagh, rector of Barrie; and another, Hon. Justice Gwynne, Supreme Court, Ottawa. Two died unmarried. Arthur Lee, after passing through the Royal Military College, Sandhurst, went to India 1820, as lieutenant and adjutant in the 31st Native Bengal Infantry. He died in India, August, 1829.

The third son, Wm. S. Durie, was born at Gibraltar, and became a prominent personage in Canadian military matters. In November, 1828, he entered the Royal Military College at Sandhurst. From the several commissions now before the writer, it is learned that his first was to be Ensign in the 6th, or 1st Warwickshire Regiment of Foot, from January 20, 1832, dated May 4, 1832, and signed "Goderich." The second commission appoints him to be Lieutenant in the 94th Regiment of Foot, from May 8th, 1835, dated August 27, 1835, signed "Russell." This certificate shows the high standing attained by him:

"ROYAL MILITARY COLLEGE.—At a Collegiate Board, held for the Half-yearly Public Examinations, on the 8th and 9th of December, 1834,

Gentleman Cadet William S. Durie being qualified, according to the prescribed Rules of the Royal Military College, to hold a Commission in His Majesty's Service, and having accordingly, on passing five Public Examinations, been recommended for the same, and having, over and above the required qualifications, made such further progress in his studies as, by the rules of the Establishment, entitles him to a certificate recording the special approbation of the Commissioners, we, the Commissioners and Members of the Board, are of opinion that Gentleman Cadet William S. Durie is worthy of this honourable distinction and do grant him our Certificate accordingly.

"(Signed) EDWARD PAGOT, *Gen.*
MONNASEL DOUGLAS, *Maj.-Gen.*
J. GARDINER, *Maj.*
G. SINCH, *Adjt.*"

The third commission appoints him to be Lieutenant in the 83rd Regiment of Foot from August 11, 1837, dated November 24, 1838, signed "Russell." The next commission is "To Lieut Wm. S. Durie, late of Her Majesty's 83rd Regiment. To be Adjutant, with the rank of Captain in the Militia (of Canada), from November 28, 1838, signed 'George Arthur' (Sir George Arthur, Lieut.-Governor Upper Canada, Major Commanding Her Majesty's Forces), dated April 10, 1839." In December, 1855, he was appointed Captain in the Volunteer Militia Rifle Company, Barrie. April, 1857, he was commissioned to be Lieut.-Colonel in the Militia Force of Canada, signed by Edmund Head and de Sallebury, Col. Adjt.-General, Militia. Another commission, dated October, 1860, appointed him Lieut.-Colonel in the 2nd Batt. Volunteer Rifles of Canada, from April 27, 1860.

The origin of the title of the Queen's Own Regiment is referred to in a communication to the authorities, dated March 3, 1863. Col. Durie wrote: "I have now the honour to state that I have been requested to convey to His Excellency the Commander-in-Chief, the warm acknowledgments and sincere thanks, I may safely say of every officer, non-commissioned officer and man belonging to the battalion under my command (in which I need scarcely say, I cordially participate), for His Excellency's kindness in so effectually promoting our wishes in having obtained Her Majesty's gracious permission that the 2nd Battalion of Volunteer Militia Rifles shall be designated 'The Queen's Own Rifles of Toronto,' and I may safely add that it will be the sincere and earnest desire of every officer, non-commissioned officer and man belonging to the battalion to render themselves worthy in every respect of so high and honourable a distinction."

The production of the following document will be acceptable to many:

"BRIGADE OFFICE, TORONTO, CANADA WEST,
"*February* 2, 1865.

"SIR,—I am directed by Major-General Napier, C.B., Commanding the District, to express to you the great gratification he experienced at his recent inspection of the 2nd Administrative Battalion of Volunteer Militia under your command.

"The Major-General was pleased with all he saw, but his particular attention was attracted by the following points which show the high state of efficiency that the battalion has arrived at under such a short period of your command. The physique of the men is excellent. They stand steadily under their arms, and are well set up, particularly considering the short time that they have been at drill. The few movements the Major-General was enabled, owing to the contracted nature of the ground, to witness were steadily performed, and showed attention was paid by all ranks. The cleanliness and order of the barrack-rooms would be a credit to any regular regiment. The discipline of the battalion appears to be of the first order, amongst all ranks. The arms and accoutrements were remarkably clean and in good order.

"Your having established in such a short time, an officers' mess, a canteen, a library and recreation room, and all these working so well and so ably managed, meets with the Major-General's highest approval.

"Not a man of the battalion having to make a complaint is always a matter of congratulation to a commanding officer, as there can be no stronger proof to the General Officer inspecting that the interests of all ranks have been carefully looked after.

"The Major-General was much gratified at the verbal report he received from you of the support you have invariably received from the officers under your command; and you will be pleased to convey to these officers the Major-General's appreciation of their zeal and conduct in general.

"In conclusion I am directed to inform you that the Major-General has had great pleasure in reporting to the Lieut.-General Commanding, with a view to his report being forwarded to His Excellency the Governor-General, of the very high state of efficiency that the battalion has arrived at under your command, at the same time drawing attention to his high appreciation of the able manner in which you have exercised command, and your well-directed zeal, which has resulted in such a satisfactory manner.

"I have the honour to be, Sir,
"Your Obedient Servant,

"HALL,
"*Major of Brigade.*

"*To* LIEUT.-COL. DURIE, etc., etc.,
"*Commanding 2nd Administrative Battalion*
"*Volunteer Militia, Niagara, C. W.*"

Colonel Durie was retired in 1881. He died at his residence, Spadina Road, Toronto, June 3, 1885.

"Died at Thornhill, May 29, 1843, John Durie, Esq., eldest surviving son of Dr. Durie."

DR. HERBERT MELCHOIR VON EBERTS

Was a surgeon in a Hessian regiment with the British army in the rebellion of 1776-83. After the war, he lived in Montreal till 1794, when he was appointed governor of the district around Detroit, comprising the present State of Michigan, which was still in the possession of the British. Two years later when the territory passed to the United States, Dr. Eberts settled at Sandwich. He was engaged in storekeeping on the Detroit River until the war of 1812-14, when his place was sacked by the American invaders. He finally settled in the township of Chatham, the place being still known as the Eberts' farm. He recommenced business. His sons William and Walter succeeded him in the trade, and in time the business was transferred to the town of Chatham.

DR. ROBERT EDMONSON

Was born at Ballymena, Ireland, September 22, 1802. He attended the University of Glasgow, and took the degree of C.M., 1827. He was in practice in County Down, Ireland, until 1829, when he emigrated to Canada, and was gazetted as a practitioner, October, 1829. He settled at Brockville, then but a small village, and for forty years pursued his noble calling, enduring all the hardships incident to the pioneer physicians. He was greatly esteemed by all classes, for he was attentive to the poor as well as the rich. He was very skilful in his profession.

The writer is informed by one who lived in Brockville in 1831, that he was then noted as a surgeon. At that period the line between physician and surgeon was well marked. Dr. Hubbell, who called himself a physician, feigned to look down upon Dr. Edmonson because he was "only a surgeon." Dr. Edmonson was, apart from his medical attainments, a good scholar, and it is recorded that he translated the Old Testament out of the Hebrew text as a pastime, while the rest of the family were asleep. He was actively associated with the incorporated militia; was captain during the Mackenzie rebellion, and was present at the battle of the Windmill, at Prescott, 1838. He attained the rank of lieutenant-colonel. At the time of the Trent affair, he was on the alert, ready to take up arms for his country. Dr. Edmonson identified himself with every movement for the welfare of the public, and held many offices of trust: he was mayor of Brockville. He was an elder for a long time in the Presbyterian Church; was for a time President of the Bible Society, and was a sympathizing friend of the young men beginning life. In 1866, Dr. Edmonson received the honorary degree of M.D., from the University of Victoria College, and afterwards was elected President of the Medical Alumni Association of that college. Dr. Edmonson married, 1828, Miss Eliza Sarah Cumming, of Antrim, Ireland. He had one son and four daughters. The son died while young. The eldest daughter, Emily, married Charles Turnbull, of Belleville, who died at an early date. Annie married Dr. H. A. Gordon, of Leicester, England. Catharine Louisa married Colby W. Foster, of Brockville, who died early, and Helen married H. Drummond, of Winnipeg. Dr. Edmonson died, May 7, 1871. A local paper said, in an obituary notice: "At the time of his death he held a prominent position in many organizations having for their object the progress of the town and the good of the people. He was also a very skilful physician and an accomplished scholar, a man of enlarged and liberal mind, honest intentions and irreproachable personal character. Many of the inhabitants of the town and country around will feel very much the loss of one who was so universally beloved and respected as Dr. Edmonson."

The writer has a most pleasant recollection of Dr. Edmonson, who was extremely affable and a noble-looking and behaving person.

DR. JAMES FAIRFIELD.

Among the names of the first settlers on the Bay of Quinte, in the township of Ernesttown, is that of Fairfield. On lot 37, where is now the village of Bath, Wm. Fairfield pitched his tent while the country was yet an unbroken wilderness. His name is on the U. E. Loyalist list, and he ranked among the officers in drawing land. It is recorded that he had twelve children, all of whom lived to marry. Four sons, Benjamin, Jonathan, Stephen and William, are also on the U. E. list, and drew land in Ernesttown. In the early history of this district, the Fairfields hold an important place. We find that the first person to engage in the trading business at Bath was Benj. Fairfield. All of the name seem to have trod in the higher walks of life. Their descendants may be found in many parts of Canada. Several daughters of the family married well-known public men, some being physicians.

Wm. Fairfield the younger had five sons; one studied law and practised at Kingston; one was a farmer, and two sons, James and John K., both born at Bath, entered the medical profession. It is not known to what extent they were able to qualify themselves for medical practice. It is most probable they studied with some of the army surgeons stationed at Kingston. John, at least, studied for a time in the States, "went there to finish." Probably James also completed his studies in the States.

James, the eldest, passed the Medical Board in April, 1827. The Board "were well satisfied and find him duly qualified." He married an English woman and settled in Prince Edward District, at a place long known as Sodom, now possessing the name of Demorestville. Here he practised until his death, which took place at a comparatively early period. He was surgeon to the 3rd Prince Edward Regiment of Militia. He left, to be cared for by his widow, one son and seven daughters. The son engaged in the legal profession, but died young. Of the daughters, one became the wife of Dr. Pruyn.

DR. JOHN K. FAIRFIELD,

From Kingston, appeared before the Medical Board in October, 1835. Had been a pupil of Dr. Baker, and had tickets of two courses of lectures at Fairfield Medical College, and passed a satisfactory examination. He practised north of Belleville. Further information is wanting, except that he had two sons. Sisters of Drs. James and John K. Fairfield married medical men—Joanna to Dr. Forward; another to Dr. Taylor, of Philadelphia. Dr. George Baker married their cousin, as also did Dr. Ashton, of Bath.

Before this work appears, another Dr. Fairfield will be enrolled on the list of practitioners of this Province. Chas. A. D. Fairfield is now (1889) attending his last course of medical lectures at Trinity Medical College, having previously been a student at McGill.

DR. JONATHAN FOOT

Was the son of Dr. Solomon Foot, of Vermont, and brother of Senator Foot, United States. He was born, October 31, 1804, and graduated at the Vermont Medical College, at Castleton, 1829. The following year he proceeded from Rutland, Vermont, westward to Buffalo and thence to "Little York." He had letters of introduction to Dr. Burnside and others, who advised him to locate in Whitby township. The first thing was to obtain his license to practise, which he did in October following. But he had previously been at Whitby, having arrived at Oshawa on September 4, 1830. His examiners were Drs. Widmer, Powell and Deihl. His commission is dated November 9, 1830.

In February, 1835, he was married to Robina, daughter of W. Dow, Glen Dhu, Whitby. In the early years of his practice it extended to Scarboro' on the west, and the township of Hope on the east, and north to the limit of the settlement. This was done on horseback. Fortunately he was a man of iron frame and great endurance, and he spared neither himself nor horse when the welfare of his patients required it. Rich and poor alike were promptly attended to with sympathetic kindness. In this path of duty, with "unsullied honour" he trod through his long life, and died, January 2, 1885, in his eighty-first year, leaving an "untarnished reputation." He was a member of the Presbyterian Church, and had "an unfaltering trust in God." The pall-bearers were Judge Burnham, Sheriff Paxton, Elder Smith, Samuel Beall, James Thompson and George McGillivray.

Two sons and three daughters survived him. We are indebted to his daughter, Mrs. Henry Warren, of Orillia, for obituary notices by local papers.

DR. WILLIAM FORD

Was born, July 13, 1807, at Broomly, near Montrose, Scotland. When eight years old he was sent to England to a boarding-school. He acquired his profession in London, and became a member of the Royal College of Surgeons, England. He practised in London for two years, when his brother Charles having given him a sugar plantation in the West Indies, he went there to reside, but finding the climate did not agree with him, he came to Canada, and was received as a guest by Col. Delator. He invested his money in the lumbering business in York, Grand River, which failed. He then took up the practice of his profession in York, where he remained a few years. He then, 1848, removed to Simcoe, Norfolk County, and succeeded Dr. Park in practice there. Here he remained four years, but finding his health failing, he accepted a government situation. This was in 1852, when he was appointed accountant in the Crown Lands Department, Dr. Rolph being the Commissioner and the Government being at Quebec. He continued to hold this position until June 10, 1880, when he was superannuated. He then bought a place at Lambton Mills. Dr. Ford married, shortly after coming to Canada, Mary, daughter of Capt. Park, who took an active part in the war of 1812, and sister of Dr. Park. After taking up his abode at Lambton Mills, his wife died. He then lived with his eldest son William, for a time, and then with his eldest daughter, Mrs. F. A. Howland, until his death, at Toronto, March 23, 1891, being eighty-three years old. Dr. Ford left two sons and three daughters.

DR. JOHN FRASER,

Born, Ayrshire, Scotland, March 14, 1806, the twenty-first and youngest child of William Fraser. He graduated at College of Physicians and Surgeons, Glasgow, 1825, when nineteen years of age. Had a large practice in Ayr and Doune, where he continued for twelve years. Came to Canada in 1837, and at first settled on the town-line between Pelham and Thorold, Niagara District. He finally settled at Fonthill. He passed the Medical Board, October, 1843. Beside his diploma from the Royal College of Physicians and Surgeons, Glasgow, he had numerous tickets of attendance on lectures and hospital practice. In 1854, he was elected Member of Parliament for Welland County. He refused to be a candidate a second time. "Professionally, Dr. Fraser's services were in request for fifty miles around. In both his profession and politics, he was a close student and observer of every new development, as well as benefiting by the experience of the past, the result being that he attained an enviable professional prominence. He held many positions of honour and trust." He was district surgeon of the sedentary militia. He was warden of the county in 1856, when the county buildings were erected. He took an active part in securing the location of the county town at Welland, and in the purchase of the marsh lands tract by the county, the wisdom of which has been shown by the subsequent course of events. He was an adherent of the Presbyterian Church and a member of the Masonic fraternity. Socially he was a great favourite, being warm-hearted and gifted with a true Scotch love of congenial company; nor was his the less valued by reason of his well-known eccentricities, one of which was his indisposition even to allude to his own affairs. Another strange trait of his character was that although reasonably careful in entering all charges for his services, he seemed to have a chronic disregard of having his accounts collected, so that although he left a comfortable property, it is estimated that he lost five times as much by outlawed accounts during his nearly sixty years of practice. He was possessed of a strong mind, hard, good sense, and never spared in expressing his opinion, yet his very frankness, sterling integrity and absolute dislike of sham in every form, made him respected and liked by even his opponents.

Dr. Fraser never married. He died at Fonthill, October, 1882.

One of this name is mentioned in connection with the Hospital Department at the Garrison Hospital, Oswego, 1783, and in October same year, at Garrison Hospital, Carlton Island. Dr. John Fraser, probably the same, was at Niagara as surgeon to the 68th Regiment. He was in civil practice about 1828 or '29. Was a Scotchman, fond of sport and a good shot, and is still remembered by Capt. Geale, of Niagara, as having taught him to shoot pigeons.

DR. JOHN GAMBLE.

The "Family Record of the Gambles of Toronto," by John William Gamble, published in 1872, for distribution among the family, gives an interesting genealogical account of the family for nearly two hundred years. By the kindness of Clarke Gamble, Q.C., of Toronto, the writer has had the privilege of perusing this volume and extracting much valuable information.

Dr. John Gamble was the eldest son of William Gamble, of Dunross, near Enniskillen, Ireland, whose wife was Leah Tyrer. He was born, 1755; studied his profession at Edinburgh; and emigrated to America in 1779, landing in New York in September. He at once entered the King's service (the rebellion being then in progress) as Assistant-Surgeon to the General Hospital. Subsequently he was attached to the "Old Queen's Rangers," and for some time did duty as surgeon with this famous regiment. At the peace of 1783 he went to New Brunswick. On May 18, 1784, he married Miss Isabella Elizabeth, daughter of Dr. Joseph Clarke, who was a Loyalist refugee from Connecticut, and who had served in the British army at New York. Dr. Gamble practised his profession at St. John, N. B., until 1793, when, having been appointed Assistant-Surgeon to the Queen's Rangers by Lieut.-Governor Simcoe, he joined the regiment at Niagara, leaving his wife and five daughters with Dr. Clarke. The family continued here until 1798. Mrs. Gamble, then, with her five daughters, the eldest but thirteen, accompanied by her father, and a sister, afterwards the wife of Hon. Samuel Smith, set out to join her husband, who was with his regiment at York. The journey must have been a trying and a perilous one. They ascended in a bark canoe the River St. John, portaged to River

Du Loup, "sheltered only by the heavens and the primeval forest," and so on up the St. Lawrence and across Lake Ontario. In 1802, the Queen's Rangers were disbanded, and Dr. Gamble removed with his family to Kingston, where he commenced the practice of his profession, in which he held the first place. He continued to enjoy a large practice until his death, which took place September 1, 1811, at the age of 56.

Miss Isabella Elizabeth Clarke was in her seventeenth year when she became the wife of Dr. Gamble, and her long life was devoted to her husband while he lived, and her large family. She remained in Kingston until 1820, when, with the portion of her family then at home, she removed to York, and there continued to reside, surrounded by her offspring until her death, March 9, 1859. Her eldest son, J. W. Gamble, in his "Family Records," says that she "trained up her children in the fear of God, and fitted to discharge the duties of their station, who lived a widow nearly half a century, and died in her ninety-second year,—to the memory of such a mother, truly a mother in Israel, are the following pages affectionately dedicated."

Dr. Gamble had thirteen children, four sons and nine daughters. Of these latter, the eldest, Isabella, was married to Dr. Robert Charles Horne, Assistant-Surgeon Glengarry Light Infantry; Mary Ann, to Col. Sinclair, R.A.; Sarah Hannah Boies, to Dr. James Geddes, Assistant-Surgeon Medical Staff; Leah Tyrer, to Hon. William Allan, father of Hon. G. W. Allan. Catherine died in Kingston about 1816, aged fifteen years. Jane was married to Benjamin Whitney, of Kingston; Rachel Crookshank, to Sir James Buchanan Macaulay, C.B., Chief Justice; she died at Sparkford Hall, Somerset, England, July 17, 1883. Magdeline was married to Thomas William Birchall. Mary Ann died unmarried in 1883.

Dr. Gamble left three sons. The eldest, John William, who was born at York Garrison, 1798, passed a large portion of his life in the discharge of public duties. He was appointed a Justice of the Peace in the Commission of 1827; Chairman of the Quarter Sessions, in 1836; District Councillor for Etobicoke, in 1842; County Councillor, 1850, and served eight years; elected M.P. for South Riding of York, in the early "forties;"

was a Member of the Provincial Legislature many years; was a Justice of the Peace forty-six years, Warden of the County two years, Chairman of the Quarter Sessions six years, County Councillor fourteen years. Besides he held a number of responsible positions. He was also Colonel of the 2nd Battalion Reserve Militia, County of York. His first wife was Mary Macaulay, daughter of Dr. James Macaulay.

Dr. Gamble's second son William engaged in mercantile pursuits, and was one of the first wholesale merchants in York; his firm was Gamble & Birchall. He subsequently established one of the largest flour mills in the then Province of Upper Canada—the brand, "Milton Mills, Etobicoke," being one of the best and most widely known. He subsequently moved to Toronto, where he died about the year 1882.

Clarke Gamble, Q.C., the fourth son, so well known in Toronto, entered the legal profession. He studied under Sir James B. Macaulay and Judge Hagerman, and was called to the bar in 1832, and at once commenced the practice of the law in York, now Toronto; was appointed a Bencher of the Law Society at Michaelmas Term, 1840. He was made Queen's Council, May 26, 1867, and has followed the practice of the law in Toronto continuously "from his call to the bar until the present time." He is the senior member of the firm of C. & H. D. Gamble & Dunn, and is the oldest practising barrister and attorney in the profession in Canada.

Clarke Gamble's eldest son John Henry was born in Toronto, 1844, and after being educated at Upper Canada College and Cheltenham, England, entered, by examination, the Military Academy at Sandhurst, 1860; was gazetted sub-altern in the 17th Regiment, 1862, then stationed at Quebec; was promoted to lieutenant, 1865; became captain, 1877, when his regiment was in India. His battalion was one of the first to cross the Afghan frontier when the war broke out there, 1878. In the campaign that followed, the 17th had its full share of danger and hardship, and was specially complimented by the Brigadier-General. On the way back, after the war ended, the 17th suffered greatly by cholera and dysentery, and many died, among whom was Capt. Gamble, who died in the Kyber Pass, July 14, 1879. Capt. Gamble's worth is attested in the following extract from the Regimental Orders, by Lieut.-Col. A. B. Utterson : "It is with the deepest sorrow and regret that the commanding officer has to announce . . . the death of Capt. Gamble. He was a most able officer, zealous and conscientious in the performance of his duties, and a good friend to all. . . . In the death of Capt. Gamble, the 17th loses an officer whom it will be hard to replace." And the following, the voluntary testimony of Col. (Brigadier-General) Cobbe, under whose command the 17th Regiment was placed for a time, but who was not personally interested in or attached to that regiment: "It is with feelings of the deepest sorrow that Col. (Brigadier-General) Cobbe has heard of the death of Capt. Gamble, at Lundi, Kotal. Although this officer had only served for some few months under Col. Cobbe's immediate command, the period was quite sufficient to enable him to form a most high estimate of his character and capability, and to appreciate his value as a most useful and excellent officer, and for whom he had contracted a very strong personal friendship. Col. Cobbe requests the officer commanding the battalion to allow this memorandum to be published in Regimental Orders as a record of his personal feeling, as well as of his sympathy with the officers and soldiers of the Battalion of 17th Regiment at the loss sustained by them in the death of Captain Gamble."

DR. JAMES GEDDES

Was born at Halifax, N.S., 1780, and received his early education at King's College, Windsor. His medical education was acquired in the University of Aberdeen, and in the hospitals of London and Edinburgh, after the completion of which he received his appointment as Army Hospital Assistant. The dates of his subsequent promotions are not known. He accompanied the British forces to Holland, under the Duke of York, and here, while encamped on the sands at Walehesen, he contracted rheumatism, to which he was a martyr for the rest of his life. In the returns from the War Office, 1803, giving the Hospital Staff to be employed in Canada, as a peace establishment, James Geddes' name is given as a hospital mate.

On April 17, 1804, he was married to Sarah Hannah Boies Gamble, daughter of Dr. Gamble of the Queen's Rangers. He was stationed at Amherstburgh and afterwards at the Island of St. Joseph, near the Sault Ste. Marie, the remotest military hospital at that time. From 1807 to 1834 he lived at Kingston; part of the time, at least, he was on duty at the military hospital —his name is found mentioned in that connection in 1810. During the American war of 1812-14, he accompanied a naval expedition to Sackett's Harbour, under Sir James Yeo. In 1822, he was on the "Military Staff of Upper Canada Medical Department, as Hospital Assistant." But he also engaged in private practice, being contemporary with Dr. Sampson.

Dr. Geddes had sixteen children, eleven daughters and five sons. Of the former, two died in early age; the other nine were all married—four to medical men (Drs. Henry, Hallowell, C. S. Sewell and D'Evelyn, of Woodbridge), two to military men (Generals Gold and Munn), one to Judge Armstrong, one to Mr. Leaycroft, a merchant; one to Rev. Wm. Macaulay, Picton; and one to Rev. John Grier, of Belleville. Of the sons, two followed mercantile pursuits, one was a barrister, one engaged in railroad service, and another, James Gamble Geddes, became a clergyman. He was born at Kingston, and was educated primarily in Kingston High School, after which for six years he studied theology in Chambly College. He took orders in 1834, when twenty-three years of age, and was curate in St. George's Church, Kingston, for three years. After that he was curate in Three Rivers. In March, 1835, over fifty-six years ago, he went to Hamilton and organized the first Episcopal parish there. For forty-five years he was rector of Christ Church cathedral, and during that time held many public offices as well. When the diocese of Niagara was formed he was made dean. In 1879, he retired from the parish of Christ Church cathedral, and went to England as rector of Tatsfield, Surrey. He returned to Hamilton, and after being rector of Chippawa for two years, returned to Hamilton to pass the rest of his days. He died, November 16, 1891. His children are: John Gamble and Geo. W. Allen Geddes, Mrs. C. Brough, Mrs. (Major) Phipp, and Mrs. (Dr.) Walters. The dean was of a remarkably long-lived family.

In August, 1834, Dr. Geddes died of Asiatic cholera, which he contracted in the faithful discharge of his duties as Physician to the Gaol. He was a man of gentle and amiable disposition, very sympathizing with the sick and suffering by whom he was greatly beloved, and his early death (at the age of fifty-four) much regretted.

In the Midland District accounts from 1827 to 1841, among the items of expenditure is: "Dr. Geddes, Surgeon attending Gaol, £25."

The widow of Dr. Geddes lived to the age of ninety-two.

DR. JOHN GILCHRIST,

Son of Samuel Gilchrist, a farmer and mill-owner living at Bedford, New Hampshire, was born, February 5, 1792. He studied medicine at New Haven, Conn., and obtained his diploma. He practised a short time at Goffstown, and then, 1818, came to Canada and took up his residence a short distance from Cobourg. Dr. John Gilchrist was the first candidate to present himself to, and the first to secure a certificate, for a license to practise in Upper Canada, from the newly organized Medical Board. This is the entry in the minutes:

"*January* 5, 1819.—Board met. Present: Drs. Macaulay, Widmer, Lyons and Powell. Dr. John Gilchrist, of the Township of Hamilton, in the District of Newcastle, appeared, and being examined and found duly qualified to practise Physic, Midwifery and Surgery, he received a certificate to that effect accordingly."

Dr. Gilchrist was the eldest of four brothers who engaged in the practice of medicine. They all settled in the central part of Upper Canada. A peculiarity is mentioned that each had erected a similar place of residence, in which taste and utility were combined. The pattern of these houses was taken from the dwelling of a favourite teacher at the medical college where they studied.

In 1822, he was gazetted surgeon to the 1st Northumberland Regiment of Militia. A few years later Dr. Gilchrist removed to Otonabee and became an enterprising farmer, and in 1825, erected, in the township of Otonabee, a grist-mill and saw-mill. The village was named Keene, after a place in his native state. In the winter of 1829-30, he opened the first store in Keene. About this time a school-teacher, David Housteon, suffered from a severe illness. Being in a precarious state, Dr. Gilchrist was sent for to visit him, which he did more than once. On his recovery, his gratitude to the Doctor expressed itself in a letter of thanks, in which he lamented that "he had no money, but promised to pay him as soon as he could." In reply he received the following letter, replete with the spirit of true Christian charity, which we present to the reader, all the more readily from the fact that we have but few written memorials of the kind physician or the enterprising citizen from whom it emanated:

"*Reply to the Moneyless Patient:*

"SIR,—When you see a fellow-creature in distress, relieve him as far as your abilities will allow; and in so doing, you will discharge the debt you owe to

"JOHN GILCHRIST, *Otonabee*."

Dr. Gilchrist was appointed a justice of the peace for Otonabee.

In 1831, this card appeared: "Dr. John Gilchrist informs his friends that he has rented his property in Otonabee, and shall in future give his undivided attention to the medical profession. He presumes that experience of nearly fourteen years in the most successful mode of treatment, etc., etc., will secure him patronage."

This also appeared: "The undersigned experiencing much inconvenience from the long and, in many instances, endless credit which he has given in his professional business, will in future conduct his accounts in a very different way. To all such as pay him down or within a month after his discontinuing to attend them as patients, a deduction of 25 per cent. will be made on his usual charges. And such as allow their accounts to run over a year are informed that not only a doctor's, but a lawyer's, *bill* will be to be paid.

"JOHN GILCHRIST.

"Cobourg, January 11, 1831."

He was an unsuccessful candidate for the Legislative Assembly in 1834, and again in 1836. But the election of 1841 resulted in the selection, by a considerable majority, of Dr. Gilchrist as member of parliament for the new Colborne District, which position he continued to fill during the next four years. In 1842 he was elected Treasurer of the District, and continued in office until 1846. Dr. Gilchrist had taken up his abode in Peterboro'.

In the Mackenzie Rebellion, twelve persons were arrested in the Newcastle District on a charge of sympathizing with the rebels. Of these, Dr. John Gilchrist was one.

In 1849, he removed to Port Hope, where he continued to practise until near the time of his death, which took place in September, 1859.

Dr. John Gilchrist married a daughter of Dr. Jonathan Gore, a prominent physician of Goffstown, N.H., by whom he had nine children, some of whom are still living (1890).

DR. SAMUEL GILCHRIST

Studied medicine with his brother John, and attended Dartmouth College, N.H., from which he obtained a diploma. He was before U. C. Med. Board, April, 1823, but failed to pass. He, however, succeeded in obtaining a certificate to practise, January, 1824, and settled at Port Hope, where he continued to practise until his death, August 20, 1849. Dr. S. Gilchrist was commissioned surgeon to the 1st Durham Regiment of Militia, Nov. 26, 1827. He had the reputation of being an able man and sound practitioner, and was much respected.

JAMES EIKIN GILCHRIST, another brother, also studied medicine with his brother John, and at Dartmouth College, and received his diploma. Appeared before Med. Board, January, 1832. "The Board was perfectly satisfied by his examination." He settled at Cobourg, where he practised until his death, 1871. Dr. "Jam," as he was familiarly called, was very much respected and fully trusted by his patrons, who were very numerous.

DR. HIRAM GILCHRIST, the youngest of the four brothers,

studied with his brother Samuel, and took his degree of M.D. at Dartmouth. Before Med. Board, April, 1834, but failed in his Latin. He took up his residence at Port Hope, where he practised probably with his brother Samuel. He died, April, 1852. Like his brother, he had a high reputation as a practitioner.

MATHEW GILCHRIST, from Cramahe, Newcastle District, was probably related to the four brothers. Before Med. Board, April, 1823. Failed to pass. "Admonished and recommended further study." But appearing again, January, 1824, "the Board was perfectly satisfied, and granted certificate to that effect." Dr. M. Gilchrist was elected to represent Northumberland in the Provincial Parliament. Married a daughter of Joseph Keeler, of Colborne. Was a good practitioner and had a good practice.

DR. GEORGE E. GIVINS

Was the son of Colonel James Givins, who was intimately associated with Governor Simcoe in founding the capital of the Province. We learn from Dr. Scadding's "Toronto of Old," that Colonel James Givins was one of the companions of Governor Simcoe in the first exploration of Upper Canada. Before obtaining a commission in the army, he had been as a youth employed in the North-West, and had acquired a familiar acquaintance with the Otchibway and Huron dialects. This acquisition rendered his services of especial value to the Government in its dealings with the native tribes, among whom also the mettle, and ardour, and energy of his own natural character gave him a powerful influence. At the express desire of Governor Simcoe he studied and mastered the dialects of the Six Nations, as well as those of the Otchibways and their Mississaga allies. The writer remembers seeing a considerable body of Indian chiefs kept in order and good humour mainly through the tact exercised by Colonel Givins. This was at a council held in the garden at Government House some forty years since (1837), and presided over by the then Lieut.-Governor, Sir John Colborne. Colonel Givins was Superintendent of Indian Affairs down to the year 1842. Dr. Scadding again says, speaking of "Goodwin's Creek," the stream which enters the bay by the cut-stone gaol (foot of Berkeley Street, Toronto): Lieutenant Givins (afterwards Colonel Givins), on the occasion of his first visit to Toronto in 1793, forced his way in a canoe with a friend up several of the meanderings of this stream, under the impression that he was exploring the Don. He had heard that a river leading to the North-West entered the Bay of Toronto, somewhere near its head, and he mistook the lesser for the greater stream, thus on a small scale performing the exploit accomplished by several of the explorers of the North American coast, who, under the firm persuasion that a water highway to Japan and China existed somewhere across this continent, lighted upon Baffin's Bay, Davis Strait, the Hudson River, and the St. Lawrence itself, in the course of their investigations. At that time the ground on which Toronto stands was covered by the primeval forest, except around the "old French fort." Doubtless, Colonel Givins came to York to reside at the same time as Governor Simcoe (1794). He was quartered for a time at the Old Fort, where two children were born, Henry Hamilton and a daughter, who married Colonel Hillier, aide-de-camp to Sir P. Maitland, and who is still living in England (1890).

In the register of St. James' Cathedral, Toronto, is recorded that James Givins, late Chief Superintendent of Indian Affairs, died, March 7, 1846, aged 87.

The framed house which Lieut. Givins some time after erected north of the asylum grounds, has only recently (1890) disappeared, the last of his children but one, who lives in England, having passed away from earth (1890). In this house at "Pine Grove," were born to Colonel Givins, James Givins, who became a judge; Cecil Hamilton Givins, Rev. Canon (Saltern) Givins, Halton Givins, Adolphus Givins, Elizabeth Givins and George E. Givins, the subject of this sketch. George seems to have obtained his general and medical education in Toronto, but he also pursued his studies in England. He was in Toronto in 1841, and at the first meeting of the Medical Board, after the collapse of the College of Physicians and Surgeons, Upper Canada, July 5, after the commission had been read, was appointed secretary to that body. Three days later he "appeared before the Board for examination, and gave such answers as were satisfactory, therefore received the certificate of the Board." At the October meeting, when a fresh commission appointing the Board was received, it was resolved, "That Mr. George Givins be continued as secretary." In the minutes of July 4, 1842, is found this entry: "The secretary, Mr. George E. Givins, having this day tendered his resignation of the office of secretary, which being accepted, Edwin Henwood was appointed in his place." It is probable that Dr. Givins soon after took leave of his native place to join the British army in the East India Company's service. Mr. R. C. Givins, son of the Rev. Saltern Givins, now living in Chicago, says: "The Duke of Wellington gave my grandfather, Colonel James Givins, three commissions in the British army; one was used by Dr. George Givins, and that was how he became a medical officer in the British army. The other two commissions were given to his nephews, sons of Judge Givins, of London. I believe Dr. George Givins occupied quite a prominent position on the medical staff of the British army in India, and in his best days was quite a noted physician. He died a widower without children, at the age of 67—I think, about 1883." He became Surgeon-Major, and was on the medical staff in India for twenty years.

DR. JOHN DE COURCY GILL.

In 1780, Dr. Gill was stationed at Carlton Island, which had been known as Deer Island prior to its becoming a military post (1778). He was here also in 1784. He retired from the service, as is shown by the following:

"Memorial to Lord Dorchester, dated at Fredericksburgh, Bay of Quinte, 28th May, 1791.

"John De Courcy Gill, who has been a Mate in the General Hospital in Canada, and since the Reduction has been in this District following his profession as a medical man, has lost all that he had in the world by fire, his house having caught fire (owing to the bad construction of the chimney) on night of 28th April last, and burnt with such violence that Mrs. Gill miraculously escaped burning in the flames. The loss of the furniture, etc., we consider (although of considerable value), was trifling when compared to the loss of his medicine, which was really valuable, and must be deemed not only a private but public loss. We, therefore, hope your Lordship would take his case into consideration, etc., and afford him such assistance as may be deemed meet. (Signed), P. Van Alstine, Nicholas Hagerman, John Ferguson, and fifteen others."

The three persons named, Major Van Alstine, Nicholas Hagerman and John Ferguson, were all prominent men in the Bay of Quinte region. The first was the leader of a band of Loyalists, who settled Adolphustown; Hagerman was the father of Judge Hagerman, and Ferguson was one of the first settlers of Kingston.

"Memorial of John De Courcy Gill, Surgeon's Mate to the late General Hospital, and late Acting Surgeon to the Office of Ordnance, in Province of Quebec:

"Served as Mate in the War Establishment of the General Hospital in this Province, from the year 1776 to its dissolution in 1783, and was continued as Garrison Surgeon to Carlton Island until 1784; the year following he was appointed Acting Surgeon to the Office of Ordnance at this place. In that service he continued three years, when he was superseded by the Master-General's appointment of a Surgeon to that Establishment. That he is the only Mate of the late General Hospital left unprovided." The petitioner sets forth the manner of his loss by fire, and that he and his wife were left perfectly naked as they burst through the flames from their bed. That they lost everything, and asks for an appointment in the Physical Department or in any other. Dated at Quebec, 15th July, 1791.

The foregoing is all the information available respecting this pioneer doctor.

DR. JAMES GLENNON.

The York *Gazette* of June 20, 1807, has the following editorial notice:

"Sanctioned by the authority of the respected names of Lewis Farquharson, Esq., of Schenectady, and James McCabe, of

Albany, the editors feel themselves not only justified but called upon to introduce Doctor Glennon to the inhabitants of this country. Animated with the pleasing hope that his professional abilities and character are such as render anything further unnecessary on their part, they are the public's humble servants."

The Doctor's card appeared as follows:

" *Dr. Glennon* (*Late from Europe*)

" Respectfully begs leave to inform the Public and the Inhabitants of York in particular, that he has commenced business at the house of Mr. Paul Marian. He flatters himself that the opportunity he has had of acquiring a knowledge of his profession, at one of the first colleges in Europe, will enable him to permit the approbation of those who may be pleased to favour him with their commands.

" N.B.—He has on hand an assorted stock of genuine medicines carefully chosen under his immediate inspection. July, 1807."

In February, 1808, Dr. Glennon advertised for a " young man who will be instructed in Greek and Latin, and the practice of Physic and Surgery."

Dr. Glennon most probably was the only practitioner in York at that time who gave the whole of his time to practice. Dr. Baldwin was engaged with law, and others were connected with some branch of the public service.

Dr. Glennon seems to have remained in York until at least 1811, as we find in an " accompt " of Rev. Mr. Stuart, who was in control of the church at York, and was also district school teacher from 1807 to 1811, " to Dr. Glennon for tuition of his sons Barney, Harry and Marshall." No further information of Dr. Glennon has been obtained.

DR. GEORGE GOLDSTONE,

The son of Dr. George Goldstone, was born at Bath, England, January 25, 1806. He studied medicine at Edinburgh, and took the degrees M.D., M.R.C.S. Eng., and was Secretary of Apothecaries' Hall. For some years he was surgeon on board an East Indian merchantman. He came to Canada about 1835, and was licensed under 8th George IV., Chap. 3. He practised in Cobourg and the surrounding country until 1862, when he retired and removed to Quebec.

"The record of Dr. Goldstone's professional life in Canada," says one well acquainted with him, "was that of a pioneer doctor. He oftentimes was called at midnight in winter to visit patients many miles away, whose homes lay in the midst of forests far from neighbours or help of any kind, and far even from a beaten road. He frequently rode on horseback sixty miles a day, it being impossible to drive a carriage through the uncultivated country. He was on duty with the militia in the rebellion of 1837 as surgeon to the Northumberland militia. His work during the cholera of 1840 was of a most difficult and painful nature. He was a noted and very successful surgeon." The following extracts from letters of a few yet living who were his contemporaries, afford ample evidence of Dr. Goldstone's worth: "All classes loved and respected him, the poor remembering him as a kind friend. He was an especially clever surgeon." Dr. Laing, of Dundas, whose parents and whose own family Dr. Goldstone attended for many years, writes: "By his skill, careful attention and sympathy he gained a high place in the esteem of his fellow-citizens, and by his liberal and generous treatment of the poor, as well as by his gentlemanly bearing, irreproachable morals and kindly manners in the society with which he mingled, he endeared himself to all. He was a useful member of society and an ornament to his profession." Mr. A. R. Boswell, Barrister, and ex-Mayor of Toronto, informs us that Dr. Goldstone attended his father's family for many years. Mr. Boswell also speaks of the many excellent qualities of head and heart which characterized Dr. Goldstone's life, and of the premature death of Dr. Goldstone's son, a boyhood and college friend.

Dr. Goldstone married Sarah Eleanor Racey, eldest daughter of John Racey, Esq., of Quebec, January 23, 1837. They had eight children, five of whom are still living—two, Mrs. Susan Hamilton and Miss Goldstone, now (1893) residing in Toronto.

Dr. Goldstone died at Quebec, December 30, 1872. He was buried in the Church of England cemetery in Cobourg.

DR. JAMES GRAHAM

Was born in Wyoming, in the valley of the Susquehanna, Pennsylvania, U.S., October 29, 1782. His parents, who were Scotch, emigrated to America and located in Wyoming shortly after the war of 1776 commenced. The terrible massacre of the settlers by the Iroquois Indians, which occurred at that place on July 3, 1778, obliged them to flee, and they escaped on horseback with their son, then four years of age, and came to Canada, and afterwards located on wild land in the County of Oxford, where they had born to them seven sons and two daughters.

James Graham, the eldest son, the subject of this notice, pursued the study of medicine under Dr. Sumner, then an eminent physician of Grimsby, whose practice extended throughout the whole Niagara District. It was under his tuition that young Graham completed his professional studies, when he was appointed a surgeon on the staff of General Sir Isaac Brock, and served in that capacity during the continuance of the war of 1812, having been present at the battles of Queenston Heights and Lundy's Lane.

It was during this war that Dr. Graham was united in marriage, August 22, 1813, to Elizabeth Sutherland, daughter of Col. Sutherland of the Glengarry Highlanders, then stationed on active duty in Lower Canada. On the close of the war and the proclamation of peace, he, with his wife, settled on a farm in the Township of Woodhouse, in the County of Norfolk, Upper Canada, where he successfully cultivated the farm and acquired an extensive medical practice. The farm purchased had belonged to Dr. Rolph, father of the Hon. Dr. Rolph, and was near where Joseph Van Norman had, for a great number of years, the first large iron foundry in Ontario. His visiting circuits extended from Walsingham to Waterford, and from Port Dover to Walpole, travelling long distances over bad roads, through woods and sparsely settled districts, sometimes on horseback or in a sulky with his well-trained favourite pony. His patients hailed his arrival on his visits, not only as a skilful physician, but as a friend and adviser ever ready to assist and sympathize with them in their struggles, as fellow-settlers in a new country. Fees for his professional services was a secondary consideration with Dr. Graham, and in those times when money as a circulating medium was scarce, payments were generally in kind, and having a large farm himself, he would accept manual labour in time of harvest and seeding, or any article of farm produce they might give as an equivalent offer in payment.

Dr. Graham continued the practice of his profession in the same county until enfeebled by advancing years and their concomitant infirmity. He was active as a politician, and ever exerted his influence in the advancement of the best interests of his adopted country. He was also an ardent adherent of the Church of England, and gave liberally of his substance in support of the religious principles he professed. His hospitality was unbounded. The judges on their circuits, and the clergy on the occasion of their annual convocations in Woodhouse, ever found a pleasant, genial and hearty welcome to his house. Nor was he ever known to neglect cases of poverty, sickness or distress brought under his notice. As an instance: At one time a family of emigrants from Ireland arrived in his neighbourhood. They were without means, and father, mother and children were struck down by typhus, or ship-fever. Dr. Graham was appealed to, and attended them during their sickness. There was no hospital to send them to, and he caused an unoccupied log-house on his own farm to be fitted up for their accommodation, had the sick family removed into it, supplied from his own house necessary clothing, fuel and food, visiting them daily, and by careful medical treatment and nursing, subdued the disease and restored the sick ones to health, gave them temporarily work on his own farm, and ultimately secured places in the neighbourhood, where they were able to support themselves in comparative comfort and independence. He was appointed Surgeon to the 1st Norfolk Regiment of Militia, June, 1822.

Dr. James Graham died at Woodhouse, July 24, 1854, aged 72 years. His remains were interred in the family plot in the burial ground attached to the Rectory of Woodhouse, the late Rev. Francis Evans being the incumbent. Being one of the old respected inhabitants and early settlers in the county, the whole population mourned his loss.

Dr. Graham's family consisted of four sons and two daughters. Two of his sons adopted the profession of medicine. The second, Thomas Rolph Graham, commenced his studies with his father, and having a natural aptitude for surgery, performed some operations successfully while yet a student. He completed his studies in the United States, practised in Buffalo, N.Y., Cleveland, O., and also at Pittsburg, Pa., where he died.

The fourth son, John Rolph Graham, studied at the Rolph School of Medicine, shortly after its establishment in Toronto. On obtaining his M.D., he commenced practice in Tilsonburg, Township of Durham, County of Oxford, where he died.

His second daughter, Sarah Elizabeth, married Mr. Joseph Lesslie. Two sons of Mr. Lesslie entered the medical profession. Joseph Walter Lesslie, M.D., Toronto University, is a well-known practitioner in Toronto.

ROLPH B. LESSLIE, M.A. and M.D., Toronto University, has more than a local reputation. He is one of the number of Canadians who have distinguished themselves in the Old World, as is shown by this abstract from the *London Medical Directory*, 1890:

Rolph Lesslie, M.A., M.D., University of Toronto, Canada, L.R.C.P. England; Fellow of the Royal Geographical Society, London; Chevalier of the Order of Leopold; Chevalier of the Order of the Congo Star instituted for the reward of distinguished service in Africa; Order of the Medjidie 4th class; Turco-Servian, Turco-Russian and Zulu war medals; educated at University of Toronto, St. Thomas' Hospital, London, Vienna and Berlin; served as Surgeon-Major with the Turkish army during the Servian war, and was present at the siege and capture of Alexinatz; accompanied the victorious army on its march from Alexinatz to the Danube across the Balkan Mountains, and continued his active and adventurous carėer until the time of his lamented death, which occurred at Dominica, September 20, 1893.

DR. HENRY GRASETT,

Born, September 9, 1774, in County Longford, Ireland; was the son of Dr. James Grasett, of Dublin and Barbadoes. Educated at Mercer's Hospital and Westmoreland Lock Hospital in Dublin, where he attended from 1790 to 1794. He entered the army as hospital mate by commission, dated December 27, 1794; appointed surgeon 48th Regiment, March, 1797. Whilst hospital mate, served in Martinique, St. Vincent, and as a prisoner of war at Guadaloupe in charge of the British sick and wounded. Having joined the 48th Regiment in St. Lucie, he was at the capture of Trinidad, January, 1797. The regiment returned to England in 1797; September, 1798, he embarked with the 48th for Gibraltar, and there remained until May, 1800, when the regiment went to Minorca, and same year to Malta, and was at the capture of that island, where the regiment was stationed for three years. Returned to England, August, 1803, and remained on home duty until March, 1805. Ordered to Gibraltar, and was at that garrison until May, 1809. From thence the regiment went to Lisbon, and joined the army under command of Sir A. Wellesley. Was actively employed in the field until 1811, when he was appointed surgeon to the forces (staff-surgeon). In that capacity he served at different hospital stations in Spain and Portugal, to February, 1813, when, in consequence of severe illness, he was, at the recommendation of a medical board, ordered to England. In August, 1813, he embarked for North America, at which station he was, in 1814, appointed surgeon-in-chief, and so continued until after the General Peace. He was in charge at Montreal until May, 1819.

"Died, January 19th, 1843, Henry Grasett, Esq., M.D., aged sixty-eight, Deputy Inspector-General Army Hospital, father of the Rev. H. J. Grasett."

"Married, September, 1843, John H. Hagarty, Esq., barrister-at-law, to Anne Elizabeth, eldest daughter of the late Henry Grasett, Esq., M.D., Deputy Inspector-General of Army Hospital."

DR. GEORGE ROBERT GRASETT,

Born, August 3, 1811, at Lisbon, Portugal, his father being with the forces of Sir A. Wellesley. in Spain and Portugal.

He came with his father, Dr. Henry Grasett, to Quebec, 1813, and was educated there and at Montreal. He studied medicine with his father, and became a Licentiate of Lower Canada. Passed the Medical Board of Upper Canada, July, 1838. He had ample certificates of a regular course of education. His place of residence was Amherstburgh, where he practised until 1840. He was appointed assistant-surgeon 2nd Battalion Incorporated Militia, August, 1839. Through Sir George Arthur he applied for a commission as assistant-surgeon in the Regular Service, and, May 9, 1840, was ordered by the Director-General of the Medical Department of the army to proceed to Chatham (England) Military Hospital to be attached there until eligible for a commission in the service. He went to England, but for some reason refused the appointment and returned to Canada, and practised for some years in Amherstburgh, County of Essex. Ill-health caused him to come to Toronto, and with rest and the comparative ease of a town practice, he was restored to health. In 1844, he was secretary and librarian of the Medico-Chirurgical Society, Toronto. He had taken the practice of Dr. Rees, who was devoting his time to the matter of a lunatic asylum. He was appointed, June 19, 1847, Health Officer and Medical Superintendent of the Emigrant Hospital, Toronto, at the time the ship-fever was raging. "In this capacity," says Dr. Joseph Workman, "he was more than diligent in taking clinical notes, studying the disease and in endeavouring to arrest the progress of the fearful pest." The result was that he himself contracted the disease and died, July 17, 1847, at the house of his brother, the Rev. Mr. Grasett. He had almost reached the age of thirty-six, and never married. Dr. Grasett contributed an article "On the Diarrhœa of Infants," also "On Poisoning by Opium." Dr. G. R. Grasett was the brother of the Rev. Dean Grasett.

This tribute to Dr. Grasett appeared in the *Patriot*, July 20, 1847:

"It is with the most heartfelt regret that we record the death of one of the most estimable men that has ever adorned our little circle. Doctor George R. Grasett was taken from us on 16th inst. by an attack of typhus fever, contracted in the discharge of his duties as Medical Superintendent of the Emigrant Hospital. Sought and cherished as he deservedly was by the higher classes of society, he was *beloved* among the poor. In him they always found one ready to listen and prompt to assuage their distresses. His medical knowledge was always at their command. His quiet, unobtrusive, gentle manner was in striking contrast with the genuine vigour of his mind; his perception was clear, his deductions satisfactory. But his highest praise is that which belongs to the humble followers of Christ. Earnestness and humility marked his Christian character, and we have to wonder how one so few years among us, and over whose head so few years have passed, should have become so dear to us. Love to God was the key to his whole character, and this, with his other endearing qualities, will cause his memory to be long cherished by all who knew him."

Dr. Fred. Le Maitre Grasett is the son of the much revered Dean Grasett, brother of Dr. Geo. R. Grasett, and grandson of Dr. Henry Grasett. He studied his profession in Toronto, and afterwards at London, Edinburgh and Dublin, staying about seven years in Edinburgh, during which time he was House Physician and Surgeon to the Edinburgh Infirmary. He won the right to wear these letters: B.M., C.M. Univ. Edin., 1873; M.R.C.S. Eng., and L.R.C.S. Edin., 1875; F.R.C.S. Edin., 1877. Dr. Grasett worthily fills the Chair of Surgery at Trinity Medical School, Toronto.

DR. PITKIN GROSS

Was born at Burlington, and graduated at Hanover, before coming to Canada. He passed his examination before Drs. Macaulay, Widmer and Lyons.

Dr. Gross settled in Murray, now Brighton. The country was sparsely settled. He was called upon to perform surgical operations when he had not the necessary instruments. In fact, the only instrument he had was the inevitable lancet. But his skilful ingenuity enabled him to form implements by which to perform amputations with great success. On one occasion a lumberman, at the Carrying Place, met with an accident and gangrene resulted within the abdomen. He made an incision and removed a portion of the omentum, washed out the cavity and the patient got well. Finally, the patient ran away to escape paying his bill. On another occasion he had been called some distance to see a patient, and while absent a messenger overtook him to secure his services to see a man still further away, who had met with an accident. Dr. Gross proceeded on his way with as much speed as the path through the woods and a jaded horse would allow. Having reached the log-house of his patient, he found the nature of the injury to the man was such that, to save his life, amputation of the thigh was immediately necessary. He had positively nothing with him either to amputate, to arrest the hæmorrhage, or unite the flaps. But his skill, courage and ingenuity were equal to the occasion, and the man's life was saved. He obtained a portion of a scythe or sickle, to which, by the aid of a blacksmith, he attached a handle. He then, by means of a thumbscrew—however he got it—manufactured a tourniquet, and made a hook to take up the arteries; finally, with a darning needle and linen thread he prepared to stitch the flaps. Having completed his arrangements—which took some twenty-four hours—he, with scarcely any assistance, accomplished the operation. The instruments made to meet a pressing emergency, were afterwards repeatedly employed to perform surgical operations. For many years the doctor's practice extended east, west, and north some forty and fifty miles, and over most of Prince Edward District; and he found it necessary to keep six horses to visit all his patients. Probably, indeed there is hardly a doubt, Dr. Gross did more hard work, as a practitioner, than any other person in the country, and yet he reached the mature age of eighty-two.

The writer had the pleasure of being a confrere of Dr. Gross for a few months. He was a genial, kind-hearted man, and showed no little ability. He was evidently a bold surgeon. One case we had in consultation, where a large tumour existed in the abdomen, and which a *post mortem* proved to be cancerous disease of the kidney; yet he had strongly advised to make an incision.

The Doctor was very popular and had a deservedly high reputation as a medical man. He was appointed surgeon to the 2nd Regiment Prince Edward Militia, January 18th, 1822. He died in September, 1873, aged 82.

DR. JAMES GRANT

Was born in Invernesshire, Scotland, 1801. He acquired the degree of L.R.C.S., Edinburgh. In 1832, he came to Upper Canada and settled at Martintown, Glengarry. Here he soon obtained a large practice which he pursued for twenty-five years, when he removed to Ottawa. He was surgeon to the Dundas 1st Regiment of Militia, during the rebellion, 1837. Dr. Grant found time to take part in other than professional pursuits. He was a conspicuous public man, taking an active part in the affairs of the country. He contested on one occasion, Glengarry County, against the Hon. John Sandfield Macdonald. He was a most vigorous and very able speaker. He was much beloved and respected by the people of old Glengarry. Dr. Grant had four sons and nine daughters, most of whom are still living. His eldest son deserves some mention in these pages.

DR. JAMES ALEXANDER GRANT, K.C.M.G.—The following sketch is derived from Rose's "Cyclopædia of Canadian Biography," and the Ottawa *Citizen:*

"He comes of a distinguished and able family. His father was Dr. James Grant, of Edinburgh, and for many years a prominent surgeon in Glengarry, Ont.; and his paternal grandfather was the learned James Grant, author of 'Essays on the Origin of Society,' and 'Thoughts on the Origin and Descent of the Gael.' A little while after the publication of the latter work, the author was presented with a large silver vase bearing the following inscription: Presented by the Highland Society of Scotland to James Grant, Esq., of Corrimony, advocate, as a testimony of his treatise on 'The Origin and Descent of the Gael,' 1819. This was a prize essay in which many of the most noted scholars in Scotland competed. The vase is in possession of Dr. Grant, in Ottawa. It may be interesting to note, as we pass, that Dr. Grant's correct appellation is Chief Grant, as he is the present chief of the Grants of Corrimony. His mother was Jane, *nee* Ord, and she brought her son to this country in her arms. Young Grant received his education in Arts at Queen's College, Kingston, and took his medical degree, 1854, at McGill, Montreal. Having obtained his diploma, he settled at Ottawa. His great skill and noteworthy success in his profession soon attracted attention, and very speedily began the first of what afterwards became a magnificent practice. He has been successively physician to the Governors-General of the Dominion from Lord Monck to the present occupant of Rideau Hall. Honours have fallen fast upon Dr. Grant, but well have they been earned. He has been president of the Mechanics' Institute and the St. Andrew's Society of Ottawa; has been president of the College of Surgeons of Ontario; was a member of the International Medical Congress held at Philadelphia in 1876, and was created one of its two vice-presidents. He is a Fellow of the Royal College of Physicians and a member of the Royal College of Surgeons, London, a member of the Royal College of Surgeons, Edinburgh, and of the Geological Society of England. Dr. Grant is likewise a member of the Royal Society of Canada, and is ex-president of the Dominion Medical Association and representative of the University of Ottawa in the Medical Council of Ontario. In the literature of his profession, Dr. Grant is a gentleman of distinguished repute. He has published, in British and Canadian periodicals, a large number of able, lucid and comprehensive essays on medical and scientific subjects. In addition to his contributions to his own professed science, he is a geologist of high standing, and has made most valuable contributions to the literature of that important science. His style is clear, forcible and cultured, and his work has attracted very wide attention. Dr. Grant has likewise taken a share in public life. He sat for eight years in the Dominion Parliament for the County of Russell, and is at present the representative of the Capital in the Dominion House. Dr. Grant introduced the original Pacific Railway Bill. He likewise advocated the admission of the North-West Territories into the Dominion of Canada at a time when some men regarded the proposal with hostility, and others deemed the territories to be an illimitable and dismal stretch of frosty plain, whereon little grew but lichens. Dr. Grant married, January 22, 1856, Maria, daughter of Edward Malloch, who sat for Carleton in the Legislative Assembly of Upper Canada. The fruit of this union was twelve children, four of whom are dead."

It may be added that Sir James Grant is one of twenty-five

honorary members of the British Medical Association, and is a corresponding member of the *Associazione de Benemeriti Italiani*, Palermo, Sicily, and was awarded the gold medal of the association for high standing in medical science.

Dr. Grant was created a Knight Commander of the Most Distinguished Order of St. Michael and St. George, 1887, an Order originally called into existence in the year 1818. He is the only Canadian outside of politics upon whom the honour of a K.C.M.G. has been conferred. His selection for it was a fitting recognition of his eminence in his profession.

Dr. James A. Grant, son of Sir James, was educated in Arts at University of Queen's College, 1878; M.D., C.M., McGill College, 1882; L.R.C.P. London, 1883, and is now (1894) practising at Ottawa.

DR. JOHN GRANT.

Born in Scotland, 1804. After a course of medical study at Glasgow, he took the degree of M.D., and became a Licentiate of the Faculty of Physicians and Surgeons, Glasgow, when but twenty years of age. Among the books left by Dr. Grant was a copy of "A Dictionary of Chemistry. By Andrew Ure, M.D., F.R.S. Published, 1824." At the front part of the book is written as follows: "This premium, a mark of pre-eminence in the study of Materia Medica and Pharmacy, was presented to Mr. John Grant by the votes of his fellow-students, and is bestowed with much satisfaction by Andrew Ure, M.D., F.R.S."

Dr. Grant came to Canada the same year, 1824, as surgeon to a ship sailing from Glasgow to Quebec. On board the vessel was Peter Shaver, M.P., of Upper Canada, a wealthy lumber merchant, and on his advice Dr. Grant came to the County of Dundas, and commenced the practice of his profession. Among the papers left by Dr. Grant is a document which says: "John Grant, of Matilda, in the Eastern District, surgeon, makes oath and saith, that he is the person named in the annexed diploma. (Signed), John Grant. Sworn before me at Augusta, in the District of Johnston, the 15th day of February, 1828. (Signed), — Walker, J.C.D." This was doubtless the occasion of his obtaining his license to practise. At the time of the rebellion,

1837, Dr. Grant was commissioned surgeon-major to Colonel Chrysler's Battalion from Dundas County, and was at the storming of the Windmill. After the rebellion he practised at Williamsburg, and in 1847, when the emigrant fever prevailed, he was appointed surgeon to a temporary hospital, and received instructions from Government to act as surgeon on the steamer *Gilderslieve*, Captain Maxwell, which conveyed the emigrants from Montreal to Kingston. For a number of years Dr. Grant was coroner for the united counties of Stormont, Dundas and Glengarry.

Dr. Grant removed to Toronto, 1853, and soon formed a friendship with Drs. King, Telfer, Primrose, Bethune, and other leading physicians. He was appointed by Lieutenant-Governor Sir Edmund Head, physician to his household, and to the family of his aide-de-camp, Captain Utalic, and continued to discharge these duties until Sir Edmund was recalled from Canada. Dr. Grant was also surgeon to No. 1 Co. of the Volunteer Rifle Corps which became the Queen's Own Rifles. For a time he practised at Brampton, and was physician to the gaol there, and coroner for the counties of York and Peel. Returning to Toronto, he continued to practise until his death. In 1885, Dr. Grant formed a class of ladies for instruction in the management of wounded and sick persons in cases of emergency, when his instructions were much appreciated, and he was presented by the ladies with a gold-headed cane.

Dr. Grant married Miss Shaver, a neice of Peter Shaver, M.P., and by this happy union he had eight children. All of them predeceased him but John, who is engaged in the drug business, Helen, and Marion, who is the wife of Dr. Malcolm Ranney, of Georgetown. Dr. Ranney took his degree of M.D. at the University of Glasgow, 1855, and obtained the license to practise in Upper Canada the same year. Dr. Grant died at Toronto, March 3, 1893.

DR. ROBERT J. GUNN,

Born at Caithness, Scotland, February 14, 1815, was the son of Rev. Alex. Gunn, of the Kirk of Scotland. He was educated at a private school and at the University of Edinburgh. He studied his profession also at Edinburgh and became Lic. R.C.S. Edin. He then practised at Thurso for two years, and, in 1842, emigrated to Canada and settled at Whitby, then consisting of only a few houses, where he continued to practise, which became very extensive; and in the first years of his work he encountered much hardship in his rides of thirty or more miles over half-made roads. But he never refused to attend the calls of the sick, rich or poor, whatever might be the state of the weather, by night or day. Dr. Gunn did not appear before the Medical Board until April, 1846, when he obtained his license to practise.

Dr. Gunn enjoyed the confidence of the public, which he served as school trustee and chairman of the Board for many years, as a justice of the peace, town councillor, and mayor for two terms. He was appointed surgeon to the gaol when Ontario became a county, 1853. He was also an elder of the Presbyterian Church.

Dr. Gunn married, October 24, 1849, Miss Agnes Pringle, of Whitby, a native of Edinburgh. Two daughters grew up, one of whom became the wife of Angus McKay, farmer, of Pickering; the other, the wife of John Ball Dow, barrister, of Whitby.

DR. WM. CHARLES GWYNNE.

His father was Rev. Wm. Gwynne, D.D., of Castle Knock, near Dublin. His mother was the daughter of Rev. N. Nelson, Dunshaughlin, County of Meath, Ireland. Fourteen children were born to them, a number of whom died while young. Six sons grew to manhood, five of whom came to Canada, viz., George, Hugh Nelson, Wm. Charles, John Wellington, and James. John Wellington was the first to come to Canada; while yet young, Wm. Charles came in 1832, as a ship-surgeon to Quebec. George and Hugh came the following year, and James some years later. George, a clergyman, lived in York for a time, and officiated at St. James' Church, prior to the time of Rev. Mr. Grasett. The incumbency was offered to him, but not satisfied to remain in the country, he returned, after a year, to Ireland. Hugh Nelson, who was, as well as his bro-

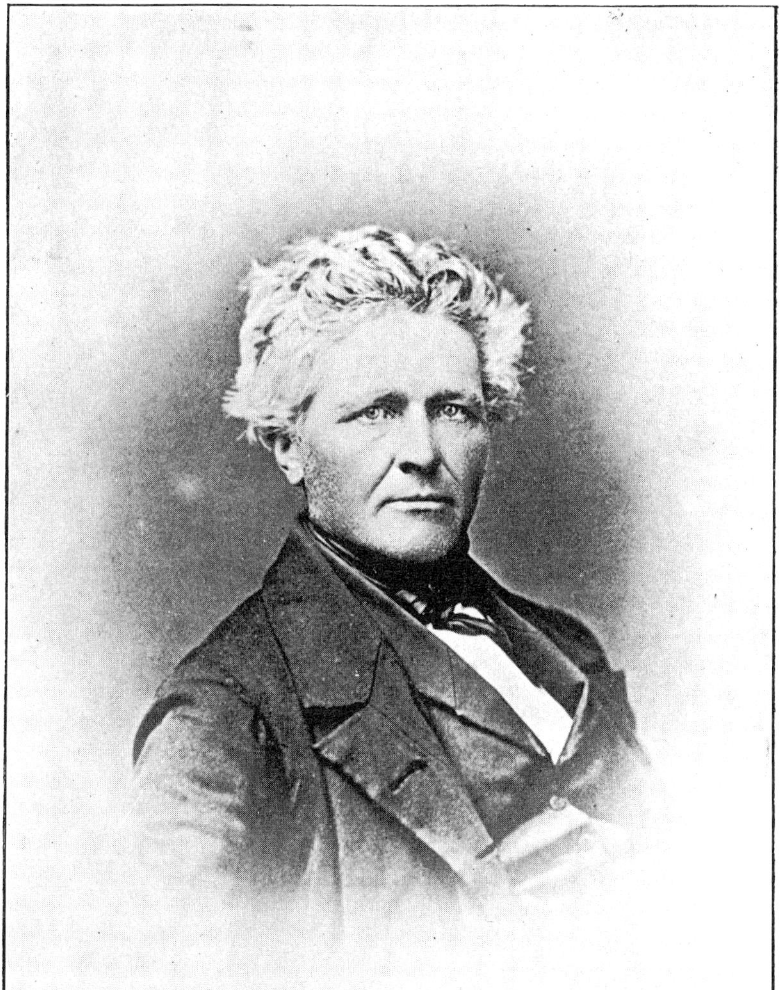

DR. WM. CHARLES GWYNNE.

ther, a scholar of Trinity College, had been offered a fellowship, but wishing to see Canada, he declined the offer, and was for a time a master in Upper Canada College. He then removed to the country, where he lived until 1840, when he became Secretary-Treasurer of the Law Society. This position he retained until a short time before his death, December, 1872.

John Wellington, who had been a student of Trinity College, Dublin, for four years, on his arrival in Canada, commenced the study of law in the office of Thomas Kirkpatrick, Kingston, who was an old friend of the family. He was called to the bar in 1837. He married Julia, youngest daughter of Dr. Durie. He was appointed Judge, Common Pleas, 1868, and in 1879, Judge of the Supreme Court of Canada, a position he yet adorns (1891).

James became a barrister, and was in practice at Berlin and Galt until his death.

A sister, Elenor, came to Canada in 1876. She became the wife of Rev. Thos. Green. Mrs. Green, now a widow, is still living in Toronto (1890).

Wm. Charles was born, April, 1806. He received his general and medical education at Trinity College, being a private pupil of Surgeon Adams, of Stephens' Green. Eight years were devoted to medical study, and he took the degree of M.B. at Trinity College. The following certificates signed by two distinguished surgeons of that day, tell of the high estimation in which he was held :

"DUBLIN, *July* 23rd, 1831.

"I have been intimately acquainted with Mr. William Charles Gwynne for several years past and know him to be very highly qualified in all the departments of medical science. He is well calculated in every respect to faithfully discharge the duties of any medical or surgical situation to which he may be appointed, both from his high professional qualifications and his most excellent moral character.

"EPHRAIM McDOWEL, M.D.
"*One of the Surgeons to the Richmond Hospital.*"

"DUBLIN, *July* 25th, 1831.

"I have had the pleasure of knowing Mr. Gwynne during the last four years, and observing the close attention he paid to professional pursuits while a pupil of the Richmond Surgical Hospital. I have, therefore, no hesitation in stating that he is in every respect, particularly well qualified to act as physician and surgeon to any dispensary or hospital, and that he will be found a great acquisition to any institution of the kind.

"RICHARD CARMICHAEL.
"*One of the Senior Surgeons of the Richmond Hospital.*"

He further pursued his studies at Edinburgh for a year, and was a favourite pupil of the famous Lizars. He then engaged as surgeon to a vessel sailing to Quebec, and came on to Kingston. His friend, Mr. Kirkpatrick, introduced him to Dr. Sampson, who proved a kind friend, and who took an interest in starting him in practice. The cholera was then raging, and Dr. Gwynne found plenty to do. But the disease was more alarming at York, and thither, on the advice of Dr. Sampson, Dr. Gwynne proceeded, and entered with enthusiasm into the work of controlling the dread malady, and his management of cholera cases was attended with remarkable success. He then permanently settled in York, and was gazetted a licentiate of Upper Canada, July 9, 1832.

This marriage notice appeared in the paper, May 4, 1835:

"By the Honourable and Venerable Archdeacon of York, Wm. Charles Gwynne, M.B., to Ann Murray Powell, youngest daughter of the late Wm. Dummer Powell, Esq., and granddaughter of the late Hon. W. D. Powell, formerly Chief Justice of the Province."

Dr. Gwynne seems to have given his undivided attention to practice, and endeavoured to secure the advancement of the profession and education generally.

In the rebellion of 1837, Dr. Gwynne was surgeon to the Queen's Rangers.

Dr. Gwynne seems to have had his opponents in high quarters, but his ability and skill was recognized by the public. (See pages 88, 89.)

Dr. Gwynne took his seat as a member of the Upper Canada Medical Board, October, 1838, and thenceforth took an active part in its proceedings, being very rarely absent. When the College of Physicians and Surgeons of Upper Canada took the place of the Board, he contributed his part in its management; and when the Upper Canada Medical Board came again into operation, he was commissioned, May 31, 1841, one of the members.

During these years of practice, Dr. Gwynne seems to have incurred the disfavour of some of his fellow-practitioners. Fresh from his studies, he had learned that the practice of blood-letting, then greatly in vogue, was often unnecessary and harmful, and strongly urged the new doctrine. He held very decided opinions and had unlimited faith in his own judgment and powers of diagnosis particularly.

One instance of many is remembered even yet, of his correct diagnosis—that of a case where the son of a distinguished citizen, in a wild frolic one night, undertook to climb a lamp-post to extinguish the light. The unfortunate young man fell to the ground and sustained fatal internal injury. In the consultation of medical men who met around the patient, Dr. Gwynne alone concluded that the liver was ruptured and that death would ensue. A *post mortem* examination verified this opinion, and Dr. Gwynne's friends ever after referred to it as a triumph of expert skill.

It is not for us to-day to adjudge the matter nor to decide who was the most blameworthy for the frequent misunderstandings which arose between him and his confreres. We are more interested to know that Dr. Gwynne was essentially a reformer, as well in medicine as in politics, in educational matters as in every other relation of life.

N. F. Davin, in *The Irishman in Canada*, remarks: "The ideas of Dr. Gwynne with regard to education were advanced, and he petitioned the Legislature with regard to the constitution of the Council (of King's College). This was regarded by Bishop Strachan as "a contoomaashus sleight of our authority," and he tried to have Dr. Gwynne and his friends dismissed. But liberal ideas were then coming to the front, and the efforts of Dr. Strachan failed. Dr. Gwynne next devoted himself specially, and not without success, to reforming the financial affairs of King's College. As to the general principles of foundation and management, he advocated every reform which was ultimately made. He denounced class distinctions such as can hardly be conceived at the present time. His skill in physiology, comparative anatomy, and cognate subjects, combined with happiness of expression, made him a lecturer to whom the student listened with rapt attention."

In January, 1842, Sir Charles Bagot became Governor-General. He was a fair-minded man, and did not commit himself to either of the political parties. He took into his confidence the leading men of both parties. On account of illness, he filled this responsible position less than a year and a half, and in consequence of failing health, he solicited his recall. He resided at Kingston, then the capital, and during his illness his medical attendant was Dr. Gwynne, whom he had summoned from Toronto. He enjoyed the confidence of His Excellency to a large extent, and remained with him during the winter and until his death, May, 1843. It had been hoped that he might be able to proceed to England, and Dr. Gwynne was to accompany him.

As the friend of Baldwin and Hincks, to whom the Governor showed marked attention, Dr. Gwynne, being a clever man, would, with some advantage, have the ear of the Governor; and there is reason to believe he in some measure guided the Governor in matters relating to King's College, which at this time was receiving a good deal of attention from His Excellency. The proceedings of the Medical Board show that strenuous efforts were being made to have established a medical faculty of the University of King's College, by corresponding with Sir Charles Bagot, who was chancellor. It is somewhat remarkable that before Sir George relinquished the reins of power, Dr. Gwynne was appointed by a commission a member of the Council of King's College. It is more remarkable that in the commission he was designated Professor of Anatomy and Physiology. This was September, 1843, before the medical faculty was established. At the next meeting of the Council after this, September 25, when Dr. Gwynne first took his seat, the first step was taken to form a medical department. The proceedings of the Council given elsewhere show the successive steps taken to accomplish this end, and at every move, the guiding hand of Dr. Gwynne may be seen. It was he who drafted the report, in 1843, of the "Medical Committee," which the Council adopted. It was he who designed the building for anatomical study in which the lectures were at first delivered. This building is yet to be seen to the west of, and adjacent to, the old Parliament buildings on Front Street (see illustration), the west wing of which was occupied by King's College. Here Dr. Gwynne was wont to spend much of his time, even extending into the night, after the medical school was established, giving instructions to his pupils, especially his favourite one, Mr. Small, who for many years practised in Toronto. The merging of King's College into Toronto University, January, 1850, only made Dr. Gwynne the more enthusiastic in his labours. No wonder he was a favourite with his students. But when, in 1854, the medical department was swept away by the action of the Legislature, Dr. Gwynne, with some others of the professors, felt that the end had come for all aspirations in the pursuit of medical science. He lost all interest in medicine and even cared not to remain in the country. He consequently arranged to return to the Old Country, and in the summer of 1854, departed, with the intention of remaining away if he could find a suitable home, his family having preceded him. He devoted some time to travel—one winter was passed in Paris, and a second, in the north of France. But after being away for two years, Dr. Gwynne was persuaded that only in Canada would he be satisfied to live, and so he returned. Thereafter he devoted his time to farming and the study of insect life, of which he was very fond. He possessed a good deal of landed property, but which was encumbered by mortgage, and which he was unable to discharge in his lifetime, and the property he left has become very valuable by the growth of Toronto.

He had four children, three of whom were sons, who died in infancy. His daughter still (1894) lives in Toronto, cherishing the memory of a loving father.

Dr. Gwynne died, September, 1875, aged 69, on board the steamer *Miramichi*, while on a trip to the lower provinces, where he had gone to recruit his health, which had been impaired by worry and disappointment.

His widow died, May, 1883.

DR. CYRENUS BENJAMIN HALL

Resided at Fort Erie. He received his medical education at Fairfield Medical College, where he attended two courses of lectures. He passed the Upper Canada Medical Board, April, 1836, and commenced practice at Fort Erie. Subsequently he practised at St. Thomas, and had a large amount of professional work. He held the position of Coroner for the Niagara District, and was Assistant-Surgeon to the Queen's Light Infantry during the rebellion of 1837. Dr. Hall settled in Toronto in the latter part of the sixties. The following (date lost) is taken from the London *Free Press*: "We notice in the advertisements in our columns this morning, the appointment of C. B. Hall, M.D., late of the county of Elgin, as Associate Lecturer in the chair of Surgery in the Medical Department of Victoria College, Toronto. It will, no doubt, give sincere pleasure to his numerous friends in this section of the country, and his services cannot fail to add to the reputation of the College, after an ample experience of nearly twenty years."

He received the degree of M.D., Geneva University, Switzerland, 1846. Dr. Hall was a very active member of various medical associations, and a well-known practitioner in Toronto. He died, April 1, 1880.

DR. WILLIAM HALLOWELL,

Was born at Quebec, April 9, 1814. At the age of seven he was sent to Scotland to be educated. Pursued his medical studies in Edinburgh, France and Germany, and received the degree of L.R.C.S. Edinburgh, 1834, and M.D. from the University, Giesen, Germany, 1836. At the age of twenty-four he returned to Canada, and obtained the provincial license of Lower Canada. He then received a commission to the 83rd Regiment of the line, as assistant-surgeon, and was in several engagements during the rebellion in Lower Canada, in 1837. He afterwards retired from the service, and for many years practised his profession successfully in Kingston, Canada. He then removed to Toronto, where he practised till the time of his death. He was one of the promoters of Trinity Medical School,

Toronto, in which he occupied the chair of Materia Medica and Therapeutics. In 1858, he received the degree of M.D. from Toronto University. He was a Master Mason of Lodge Canongate Kilwinning, No. 2, Edinburgh, his certificate of membership being dated May 10, 1836. He was also a member of St. George's Society, and was one of the first who applied for the establishment of a branch in Kingston, Canada, to which he was appointed physician, his certificate of membership being dated April 23, 1846. He was at one time surgeon to the Field Battery, Toronto.

Dr. Hallowell was married at Kingston, July 25, 1839, to Sarah Hannah Boies, daughter of Dr. Geddes, of Kingston, by whom he had eleven children—six daughters and five sons. Chas. Geddes Hallowell, of the Canada Company, is the only male representative of the family now (1891) living in Toronto. Dr. Hallowell had been in bad health for many years, suffering from asthma and disease of the heart, an attack of the latter causing his death, October 20, 1873, in his sixtieth year. His widow still (1891) resides in Toronto.

DR. ROBERT DOUGLAS HAMILTON.

The following is taken from Morgan's "Bibliotheca Canadensis":

"Born at Muirhead, Lanarkshire, Scotland, January 16, 1783. Died at Scarborough, near Toronto, April 2, 1857. His father had been a stonemason but gave up that trade and leased a farm, upon which the subject of this notice was born. After receiving his elementary education at the Grammar School of Stonehouse, in his native county, he studied the classics and natural philosophy at the Universities of Glasgow and Edinburgh, at the latter of which he also studied and completed his medical education. From April, 1808, till November, 1809, he was Assistant-Surgeon to Her Majesty's hospital ship *Tromp*. He practised for a short time at Cornwall, England; and during the Peninsular war, having volunteered his services as a surgeon, served with the British army in Spain and Portugal. In 1827, he emigrated to the United States, and in

1830, he removed to York, Upper Canada, and settled at Scarborough, where he continued to reside until his death. Throughout life, he devoted a large portion of his time to literature and literary pursuits. He early cultivated the muses, and was a frequent contributor to the newspaper press in whatever place he resided. He was the author of several works, a list of which we give below. In Canada he contributed several series of letters on literary, political and other subjects to the newspaper and periodical press, under the *nom de plume* of 'Guy Pollock,' commencing first, we believe, in the *Canada Literary Magazine* (York), in 1833, and subsequently in the *Courier* of Upper Canada, the *Herald*, the *Palladium* and the *British Colonist*, all, at one time or another, published in Toronto. He left a large number of manuscript writings, written in both Britain and America; poems, novels, dramas, essays on politics, agriculture, etc. These, we understand, are soon to be published, together with a memoir of the author, written by his kinsman, Dr. J. R. Dickson (Glasgow). Dr. Hamilton was a man of large mental endowments and great cultivation. In politics, we believe, he was a Tory, or at any rate a Conservative in his leanings, and at one time was a candidate for a seat in the Canadian Parliament."

Among other works, Dr. Hamilton published the following: "Essays," in 1812; "Craignethan Castle," a poem, in 1817; "The Principles of Medicine on the Plan of the Baconian Philosophy," in 1822; "Dr. Shaddon of Goslington," by Mungo Coulter Goggle.

Dr. Hamilton was commissioned a member of the Upper Canada Medical Board, September, 1838, and was a Fellow of the College of Physicians and Surgeons of Upper Canada, 1839.

DR. JAMES HAMILTON.

The following well-written sketch, which appeared in the *Canada Medical and Surgical Journal*, embraces almost all that needs to be said in giving the subject a place in this work:

"We regret to have to record the death, on the first of March, 1877, of one of the oldest and one of the best-known medical men in the Dominion, Dr. James Hamilton, of West Flamboro', Ont. He was born at the village of Douglass, in Lanarkshire, in 1797. Receiving a preliminary education at the parish school, he proceeded to Edinburgh as a medical student, and after four years' study obtained, at the early age of 19, the diploma of the College of Surgeons, the date of which is 1816. Thus qualified, and being anxious to see something of the world, he came to Canada as surgeon on a vessel, and was induced by friends to begin practice in Montreal. After enjoying himself for four months, and doing, as he told the writer, very little practice, he returned to Scotland. In 1818, he again visited Canada with the intention of permanently settling, and after visiting many localities, began practice in Ancaster, a small village about five miles from the head of Lake Ontario, and at that time the chief place of business between York (Toronto) and Niagara. Here, as the only medical man at the head of the lake, he quickly obtained an extensive practice, so extensive, indeed, that the greater part of the day was spent in the saddle. His district at that time lay between the Grand River and twenty miles down the lake on either side, an area about sixty miles by twenty. In 1820, he moved across the valley to West Flamboro', about two miles from Ancaster, having purchased one of the most beautiful sites in Western Canada, immediately above the town of Dundas, and overlooking Burlington Bay and Lake Ontario. Here he continued to live until the time of his death. Dr. Hamilton possessed qualities of mind and body which fitted him in the highest degree for his profession, while the strict and conscientious attention which he paid to all cases, early secured for him a lucrative practice. In all public matters Dr. Hamilton took a deep interest, but had no great desire for parliamentary honours. He was one of the original promoters of the Great Western Railway, of which he was for many years a director, latterly holding the position of consulting surgeon. At the time of the rebellion he held a commission as colonel of militia, and took an active part in its suppression. By his professional brethren Dr. Hamilton was held in the highest esteem, and most deservedly so, for one by one he had welcomed them heartily into his district, holding out to each the hand of good-fellowship. He took a deep interest in the Ontario Medical Council, and represented the Burlington and Home District from 1869 to 1872. It is much to be regretted that Dr. Hamilton has left us no record of his medical experiences, which, extending as they did over a period of sixty years, would have formed a most valuable contribution to Canadian medicine. To the end he maintained an interest in the progress of the art, and frequently in conversation would refer to the great improvements in medicine and surgery. Possessed of an accurate memory stored with interesting incidents both medical and social, he was a most delightful companion, and will greatly be missed at friendly gatherings in Wentworth. To within a year ago Dr. Hamilton enjoyed an unusual measure of health; indeed, in his long career he was only once laid up by illness. For nearly a year before his death symptoms of declining vigour were apparent to his friends, and signs of grave disease of the heart were discovered. The death last year of his son, Dr. Andrew Hamilton, of Melbourne, Que., was felt very keenly by him, and he never fully recovered from the fatigue of a hurried railway journey undertaken at the time. To the end, however, he was cheerful and resigned, though loath to depart, and on Christmas day, when the writer of the present sketch saw him for the last time, and on leaving spoke of his long and honourable career, he replied that nothing would please him better than to exchange his rusty old body for a young and active one, and work on for another eighty years."

It may be added that Dr. Hamilton was appointed Surgeon to the 1st Gore Regiment of Militia, April, 1823, and what was of more importance, he was appointed by the Lieut.-Governor a member of the Upper Canada Medical Board, in 1838.

Dr. Hamilton married Miss Hatt, of Dundas, who was related by marriage to Sir Allan Macnab.

DR. JOSEPH HAMILTON,

Son of Robert Hamilton, who was a pioneer merchant in Upper Canada, even before 1783. He removed from Lower Canada to Deer Island, known afterwards as Carlton Island, a military station during the rebellion of the thirteen colonies. He settled at Fort Niagara, and afterwards at Queenston, which village he founded and named Queen's Town about the close of the war, 1783. He was extensively engaged in supplying goods to the western military posts as far as Detroit. His name is intimately associated with the early history of the Upper Districts. When Lord Dorchester, in 1788, divided the territory now comprising Upper Canada into the four Districts of Lunenburgh, Mecklenburgh, Nassau and Hesse, Robert Hamilton was appointed Judge of Nassau, which extended from the River Trent to Long Point on Lake Erie. When General Simcoe organized the Government of Upper Canada, July, 1792, Robert Hamilton was summoned to become a member of the Legislative Council, a position he continued to fill while he lived. Robert Hamilton acquired great wealth, and it is recorded that he died worth £200,000. He died, March 8, 1811. Upon Queenston Heights is the old Hamilton homestead. Ascending the heights from Queenston and proceeding southward towards the Falls, the traveller passes through the Hamilton estate. On either side of the road for miles are stately maples. These trees, we are informed, were planted by Dr. Joseph Hamilton.

In the register at St. Mark's Church, Niagara, it is recorded: "July 22, 1792, James, son of the Hon. Robert Hamilton, was baptized at St. Mark's." "December 15, 1796, Catherine, wife of Hon. Robert Hamilton, was buried at St. Mark's." "August 9, 1798, Joseph, son of Hon. Robert Hamilton, was baptized at St. Mark's." "February 29, 1800, Peter Hunter, son of Hon. Robert Hamilton, was baptized." "April 11, 1802, John, son of Hon. R. Hamilton, was baptized." It has been stated that the Hon. Robert Hamilton had seven sons; of these, John, the youngest, became most distinguished. Educated at Edinburgh, trained to business in a wholesale house in Montreal, he settled at Queenston, and entered on the business of boat-building, and became the owner of a large number of the first steamboats which plied on Lake Ontario. It is recorded that "his energy and enterprise was remarkable, and he continued in this business until 1862." In 1831, he was called to the Legislative Council of Upper Canada, and for over half a century he took part continuously and carefully in the upper branch of each successive Legislature, wearing the title of "Nestor of the Senate." So much it is deemed proper to say about Dr. Joseph Hamilton's brother John in this connection; but it comes far short of giving a full account of this pioneer steamboat builder and proprietor and distinguished legislator. The Hon. John Hamilton died, October 10, 1882.

Of the history of Dr. Joseph Hamilton, but few facts are available. It is most probable that he, like his brother John, received his general education in Edinburgh, and likewise his medical. He took the degree of M.R.C.S. Edinburgh. Dr. F. C. Mewburn says he practised for a time in London, England, and returned to Canada, 1835. He took up his abode at the homestead, Queenston Heights. Here he devoted his time to farming and beautifying his place, and his handiwork may be seen in the solid stone fence and majestic maples along both sides of the road. He did not altogether neglect his profession; but the most he did in it was in the way of consultation, in which his opinion had great weight. While living here, November, 1840, Dr. Hamilton was engaged in "an affair of honour." The principals were Dr. Hamilton, attended by W. H. Dickson, Esq., and James Boulton, Esq., attended by Lieut. Power, K.D.G. The parties crossed the river, where two shots were exchanged, without damage to either party, and the affair ended. The *casus belli* is understood to have originated in some matter of business.

After some years, date uncertain, but probably 1844 or 1845, he removed to Toronto and engaged in active practice. He had been appointed a member of the Upper Canada Medical Board, 1838, but his name does not appear in the minutes as present at any of the meetings. In 1845, Dr. Hamilton was again commissioned a member of the Board, and thereafter he was almost invariably present at its meetings up to July 6, 1847, when his name appears for the last time. The end of his earthly career had come. It is stated that Dr. Hamilton was in partnership with Dr. Hodder. In 1846, we find him Treasurer of the Medico-Chirurgical Society.

Dr. F. C. Mewburn says of Dr. Joseph Hamilton: "The Doctor was a man of high attainments, most gentlemanly in manner and appearance; he had practised in London, England, as a physician; but came back to Canada, 1835, and commenced farming at Queenston. His only connection with the profession was in consultation, and his opinion was highly valued. He removed to Toronto; died in the discharge of his duty there, having contracted typhus at the Emigrant Fever Hospital." Dr. Mewburn then touchingly refers to acts of kindness he had shown to himself by Dr. Hamilton.

The year 1847 was made terrible in Upper Canada by the scourge of typhus or ship-fever, which was brought in by Irish emigrants. A large number of them had come out and found their way to different parts of the Province, carrying with them the elements of the fatal disease. The writer remembers a family who took up their abode near his father's house, and every one of them was swept away. It was the same all along the way from Quebec upward. A large number came to Toronto. Emigrant sheds were prepared as hospitals, and the Board of Health took active steps to give proper attention to those smitten with the malady. Physicians were appointed to attend them, but some declined. Among those who accepted the post and incurred the risk, was Dr. Joseph Hamilton, also Dr. Grasett. Both of these died of the fever, and both died as gallant and heroic a death as if on the field of battle.

HENRY HANSON

Passed the Upper Canada Medical Board, April, 1846. The following obituary notice is taken from the London *Free Press*, after his death, in 1885:

"The Doctor was born in Cheltenham, England, in 1823. His father, who was a captain in the army, died young. In early life the Doctor was apprenticed to a celebrated surgeon, Dr. Fricker, of his native town, for five years. The young man proved to be an apt student, and was now far advanced in the elements of a medical education. In 1844, being then twenty-one years of age, he came to Canada and settled in the London District on a farm near the present village of Hyde Park. For a time he taught school in the township of

Southwold, after which he attended lectures in the Rolph School, Toronto, at which institution he graduated with honours in 1846. In the meantime, however, he studied with and assisted the late Dr. Salter in the drug store. In the year 1846, he commenced his practice on the farm he had taken up when he first came to London. The country was sparsely settled then, and a country surgeon had necessarily a long distance to go in order to see many patients. Doctors, too, were scarce, and their practice extended over a large area of country. Dr. Hanson's practice for a number of years extended all over the west, there being no regularly qualified physicians nearer than London, Sarnia and Goderich. Along with the distance travelled there were either no roads at all, or such as were part of the year almost impassable. Then the early settlers were comparatively poor and the money scarce, and if a doctor had a large field for his operations, he accumulated wealth very slowly. His bills were often settled in trade, as the commerce of the country was principally carried on by barter. The hardships of a pioneer physician like Dr. Hanson can hardly be realized by professional men now, whose practice only extends to the suburbs of the city, or at the most of a radius seven or eight miles in the country. In the old times it was quite common for the subject of this sketch to be called up in the middle of the night, in all kinds of weather, and ride twenty or thirty miles on horseback, on roads and through woods where no vehicle could travel. Whether sick or poor, the Doctor was always prompt and earnest in his endeavour to alleviate suffering. Bad roads, stormy weather or poverty never prevented him from being at his post. He has befriended many a poor man—never making a charge, but leaving it to their own honour to pay him what they liked when they got in better circumstances. His skill as a surgeon, his urbanity of manner, and his strong social qualities soon gained for him a large practice, extending over the western part of this peninsula, especially in the townships of London, Lobo, East and West Williams and Bosanquet. He was thus widely known all over. Four years ago, after an active practice of thirty-four years in the same place, he sold his farm at Hyde Park and removed to the city, so as to be relieved from the arduous duty of so large a country practice. . . . . He leaves a family of ten children, of whom eight were sons, amongst them being Dr. Hanson, of Rat Portage. After an illness of several weeks he died at his residence, Mill Street, aged 61."

His son, Dr. Hanson, continues (1894) in practice at Rat Portage.

DR. ALEXANDER HARVEY

Was born near the town of Peterborough, 1821. His father, John Harvey, came to Canada, 1817, and was a pioneer settler in the township of Smith. Here he died much respected, 1865. Dr. Harvey, the second son, commenced his medical studies, 1846, and pursued them in New York and at King's College, Toronto. He passed in a "highly satisfactory" manner the Upper Canada Medical Board, April, 1849. In 1861, he took the degree of M.D. at the New York University. He practised in the county of Peel for five years. In 1855, he took up his residence in Peterborough, was appointed Coroner, 1858, and was commissioned Surgeon to the 5th Batt. of the Peterborough militia. He married (1852) Eliza, daughter of W. McCormick, from Ireland. Registered, Peterborough, 1887.

DR. THOMAS HAY

Was the third son of Lt.-Col. James Hay, of Seggieden, Perthshire, Scotland, and was born, June 4, 1804. The following list of documents, now in possession of his son, T. A. S. Hay, C.E., of Peterborough, gives information as to his course of study and its successful completion: Indenture and certificate of five years' apprenticeship, June 16, 1820, to May 6, 1826; Edinburgh University tickets for attendance on different subjects, from 1821 to 1825; certificates for two years' attendance at Edinburgh Infirmary, 1822-23; five certificates from different professors of Universities, from 1822 to 1829; eight certificates of private course of lectures, from 1821 to 1827; diploma as Dresser at Edinburgh Infirmary, November 4, 1824; diploma R.C.S. Edinburgh, March 27, 1825; diploma in Midwifery, University Edinburgh, March 6, 1826; degree of M.D., University Edinburgh, 1826; certificate from Apothecaries' Company, London, May 31, 1827; diploma R.C.S. England, January 4, 1828; certificates of pupilage at Queen Charlotte's Lying-in Hospital, July 10, 1829. It will be seen that Dr. Hay omitted no means of thoroughly qualifying himself for the practice of his profession.

In 1840, Dr. Hay came to Canada and settled at Peterborough, where he continued to practise during his life. He married (November 20, 1842) Anna M., eldest daughter of Hon. Thomas A. Stewart, Legislative Council, Upper Canada. Mrs. Stewart has left an interesting leaf of Canadian history in her "Experience as a Pioneer," so well related by her daughter, E. S. Dunlop, under the title of "Our Forest Home," published for distribution among the members of the family. In this record Dr. Hay is incidentally described as a "kind-hearted, amiable, sensible man, highly educated, . . . an excellent, clever man, and most kind and attentive." Dr. Hay had charge of Dr. Huchison's practice while that gentleman was visiting Europe; and the same writer says again, 1844, "the more we know of Dr. Hay the more we see to admire in his character. He is a blessing to us. He is in good practice, but it is a life of hardship and trial—far-off calls and wretched roads, often bad pay. Doctors are exposed to dangers both by land and water. One awful night the trees were falling on all sides for ten miles on his road."

Dr. Hay died, March 9, 1857, and his widow, January 16, 1889. One son—an eminent C.E., of Peterboro'—and one daughter survive.

DR. WALTER HENRY

Was born at Donegal, Ireland, January 1, 1791; educated at Trinity College, Dublin; studied for the medical profession under Sir Everard Home. Dr. Henry says, respecting his pupilage with Sir Everard: "I spent a year in London where I was a pupil of Sir E. H., a great geni of his day, though by no means the best man or the best surgeon in the world. I owe him little, but I owe a cleverer man, at that period young, much. Even then, green and inexperienced as I was, I had a presentiment that Sir Benjamin Brodie would attain to the distinguished eminence which he has since reached." During the period of his studies he attended St. George's, Guy's and St. Thomas' Hospitals, and was a member of the Medical Society of Guy's Hospital. After becoming an M.R.C.S. England, he entered the army as hospital mate, equivalent to assistant-surgeon, and rose through the various grades of the service until he was appointed Staff-Surgeon in 1839, and Deputy Inspector-General of Hospitals in 1845. We learn that he served with the 66th Regiment from May, 1811, to the close of the Peninsular War, at Toulouse; including the siege of Badajos, battle of Vittoria and the action in the Pyrenees; battles of Nivelle and Nive; engagements at Garris; battle of Orthes and the action at Acre. He also served with the same corps in the Nepaulese War in India, in 1816-17, and in the Canadian rebellion, 1837-38. He was with his regiment in St. Helena during the last four years of the life of Napoleon, and at his death, was charged with the duty of preparing the bulletin of the *post mortem* appearance of the body, which was published by the British Government. He was stationed in Canada from 1827 to 1841. From Quebec he removed to Halifax, N.S. Dr. Henry was in Toronto in 1834, and seems to have engaged in practice, at least we find that he attended, in his last illness, Chief Justice Sir Wm. Campbell. Dr. Henry writes: "My worthy patient became very weak towards the end of the year, his nights were restless, his appetite began to fail, and he could only relish tid-bits; medicine was tried fruitlessly. At the point of the sandy peninsula opposite the barracks are a number of little pools and marshes, frequented by these delectable little birds (snipes), and here I used to cross over in my skiff and pick up the Chief Justice's panacea. On this delicate food the poor old gentleman was supported for a couple of months; but the frost set in, the snipes flew away, and Sir William died." Whilst at Quebec he wrote a considerable portion of the work, "Trifles from my Portfolio,"* and had the book

* "Trifles from my Portfolio; or recollections of scenes and small adventures during twenty-nine years' military service in the Peninsular

printed there. Of his other writings, only those published in the *Albion* (N.Y.), from 1837 to 1845, over the signatures of "Miles," "Piscator," and "Scrutator," have come to the writer's knowledge. The two letters signed "Miles," are succinct and trustworthy contemporary accounts of the rebellion in Canada in 1837-38. "Scrutator's" letters were on the politics of Nova Scotia, and were dated from Halifax in 1843-44. In one of these a paragraph indicates an early intention of the Doctor, subsequently carried out, to settle somewhere under the British flag on this side of the Atlantic. In a few remarks, Dr. Bartlett, the then editor of the *Albion*, truly characterized them as "those admirable letters." The letters of "Piscator," two in number, are on "Salmon Fishing in Canada," and evince an intimate and thorough acquaintance with the subject. Dr. Henry was also the author of a paper, "Observations on the Habits of the Salmon Family, in the Trans. of the Lit. and His. Soc. (Quebec)," 1837. In 1852, he was appointed Inspector-General of Hospitals in Canada, where he remained during the remainder of his life, retiring upon half pay in 1856, and dying at Belleville, June 27, 1860, where he had carried out his intention of "settling under the British flag."

For some of the foregoing we are indebted to Morgan's "Bib. Canadensis."

The writer can testify to the absorbing interest which a perusal of Dr. Henry's writings creates. The graphic description of the events he witnessed in Wellington's peninsular campaign, and during the two years of his service in India; the story he relates of the last days of Napoleon, his death and the *post mortem* examination, are all intensely interesting. Also, his description of events in which he took part, or of which he spoke as an onlooker, in England and Ireland, read like a

---

War and invasion of France, the East Indies, campaign in Nepaul, St. Helena during the detention and until the death of Napoleon, and Upper and Lower Canada." By a Staff-Surgeon. Quebec, 1839, 2 vols.

Second edition published under the title of "Henry's Military Life." London, 1843 ; 2 vols., pp. 300-384.

"The style of the work throughout is masculine, correct and classical, and such as to reflect honour on the author as an officer and a scholar."—*Montreal Gazette.*

romance. His account of the Canadian rebellion in 1837-38, is likewise full of interest to Canadians. It may be mentioned that Dr. Henry is by no means complimentary to certain doctors, members of parliament, who were conspicuous at that time.

Dr. Henry married Leah Allan Geddes, daughter of Dr. Geddes, and granddaughter of Dr. Gamble, of whom sketches are given elsewhere. Dr. Henry had at least three sons and two daughters, whom the writer had the pleasure of knowing while practising in Belleville, 1864-69. The eldest son, Walter James, was then practising medicine also in Belleville, in partnership with Dr. Lister. He was a graduate of McGill College. He removed to Ottawa, where he practised until his death, September 2, 1874, while yet only thirty-seven years of age. The writer found in Dr. Walter James Henry something more than a clever practitioner. He possessed as well all the qualities of a high-bred gentleman, a kind and sympathizing friend, and an unostentatious Christian.

DR. EDWIN HENWOOD

Was the second son of Dr. James Dimble Henwood, of Helston and Penzance, Cornwall, Eng., where he was born, December 23, 1819. Three brothers, James Dimble, Edwin and Reginald were all physicians, as well as the father. James D. practised in Penzance for a time, and then in London, England, until his death. Edwin studied medicine for some time with his father, but from the glowing description of the future of Upper Canada given him by his father's friend, the late Governor, Sir Francis Bond Head, he determined to set sail for Canada, and gave up his medical studies. He, with his younger brother Reginald, came to Canada in the summer of 1842, and after having stayed in Quebec and Montreal for some time, came to Upper Canada, and shortly after settled in Toronto. By the advice of Dr. Gwynne, who had known his family in England, Edwin resumed the study of medicine, and whilst doing so filled the position of apothecary to the Toronto General Hospital, then situated at the corner of King and John Streets.

It is recorded in the minutes of the Upper Canada Medical Board, July 4, 1842, "The Secretary, Mr. George Givins, having this day tendered his resignation of the office of Secretary, which being accepted, it was proposed by the President, and seconded by Dr. Gwynne, that Mr. Edwin Henwood, the resident Apothecary of the Hospital, be appointed his successor, which was carried unanimously."

In January, 1845, Dr. E. Henwood passed his examination before the Medical Board, and almost immediately after was appointed House Surgeon to the Hospital, which appointment he held until 1848, when he resigned to engage in practice at Hamilton. Soon after he was appointed Surgeon to the Hamilton Hospital, and continued to hold that position till 1868, when he became consulting surgeon, and remained so for a number of years.

Dr. Henwood held a number of public positions, among which were that of Coroner for the city of Hamilton and that of Gaol Physician. He continued in active practice till within a year of his death, which took place October 31, 1882, in the sixty-third year of his age. He was twice married, his first wife being the daughter of Dr. William Case; the second a daughter of Angus Murray, Esq., of Aberdeen, Scotland. He left six children, four daughters and two sons. One son, Dr. J. M. Henwood, studied medicine at Trinity College, Toronto, and graduated at that university, 1889. After spending some time in the hospitals of Europe, he commenced practice in Toronto.

DR. REGINALD HENWOOD

Was the youngest son of Dr. J. D. Henwood, and was born, 1827, at Helston, Cornwall, Eng., where he received his early education at the Grammar School under the headmastership of Rev. Derwent Coleridge. He came with his brother Edwin to Canada, 1842. Both became residents in the Toronto General Hospital. Reginald remained here for several years, availing himself of the clinical advantages offered in the hospital, at the same time attending the medical lectures of Professors King, Gwynne, Beaumont, Sullivan, Nicol and others,at King's College. Having passed the Upper Canada Medical Board, April, 1846, he was shortly after engaged by the Toronto Board of Health to take charge of the fever hospital which had been opened for the care of emigrants during the terrible epidemic of typhoid, or emigrant fever, then prevailing. He remained in charge of this institution until its close. He then took up his residence at Brantford, where he has remained in the active practice of his profession, excepting a short time he sojourned in Toronto. At the solicitation of the civic authorities, he returned to Toronto during a severe epidemic of cholera, and took charge of the cholera hospital which had been established near the River Don, about where the General Hospital now stands. When the disease subsided, Dr. Henwood returned to Brantford and resumed his practice, which he still pursues (1894) in conjunction with his son, with his usual activity. Besides attending to his large practice, Dr. Reginald Henwood has found time to respond to the calls of public duty which his fellow-citizens have made upon him from time to time. He has been President of the County of Brant Medical Association on several occasions. He is a member of the medical staff of the John H. Stratford Hospital at Brantford, and is President of its Medical Board. He has also been the representative at the Ontario Medical Council for the Erie Division. He has served several years as an alderman at the Council Board, and was twice elected mayor of the city. In 1852, he married Annie (who still survives), the youngest daughter of the late Dr. Alfred Digby, Brantford, and by her had four sons and a daughter, three of whom are living, his second son, Reginald, having died of typhoid fever, and his daughter Caroline of scarlet fever. In religion, Dr. Henwood is a Churchman; in politics, always a consistent Conservative.

His son, Alfred James, entered the profession, and after laying a good foundation in medical study, attended McGill College, and took his M.D., C.M. from that university in 1879, also becoming member Coll. Phys. Surg., Quebec. In 1882, he likewise became a member of Coll. Phys. and Surg., Ontario.

DR. GEORGE SAMUEL HEROD

Was born in Lancashire, England, May 26, 1827. Received his general education in private and boarding schools at Edinburgh, Queen Elizabeth's School, Mansfield, and at Birmingham. He left England, August, 1840, and arrived at Guelph the following November. Studied medicine with Drs. Orton and Clark until November, 1843, and then attended lectures at the Medical Department, King's College, Toronto. Continued at the College until 1847, when he passed the Upper Canada Medical Board in July. He took charge of the Emigrant Hospital at Hamilton, with Dr. Dickinson, and was in charge until June, 1848. He then commenced practice at Georgetown, Halton County, and remained there until April, 1854, when he removed to Guelph and entered into partnership with Dr. Wm. Clark, M.P. In the early years of Dr. Herod's professional life, he had many hard rides over rough, primitive roads. The country was thinly settled, there were few villages and towns and they wide apart. Physicians and surgeons were scarce, and at one time his circuit extended over a radius of thirty miles. Dr. Herod has always been in active general practice and has had a liberal share, being the leading physician in Guelph for a quarter of a century. He is now the oldest doctor in the county of Wellington. He has been county coroner and gaol surgeon since 1854; was appointed surgeon of the Wellington Battalion on its organization, and held the position until his resignation. He was member of the town council for several years, a member of the school board for some time, and mayor of Guelph for two years. These various appointments are ample evidence of the Doctor's high standing as a physician and as a citizen.

Dr. Herod married Margaret, daughter of Thomas Sandiland, for many years manager of the Gore Bank, Guelph. He has two children living and has buried two. Still in possession of vigorous health, his many friends look forward with the expectation of having Dr. Herod a long time to administer to their wants and cheer them by his presence.

DR GEORGE HERRICK

Was born at Cork, Ireland, 1789. He acquired the standing of B.A. at the University of Dublin. He studied for the medical profession in Edinburgh as well as Dublin, and took the degree of M.D. at Edinburgh. Coming to Toronto, Dr. Herrick issued the following in the public press :

"GOVERNMENT HOUSE,
"*September* 26, 1838.

"His Excellency the Lieutenant-Governor has been pleased to grant a license to practise Physic, Surgery and Midwifery within this Province, to George Herrick, Bachelor of Arts of the University of Dublin, and Doctor of Medicine of the University of Edinburgh.

"George Herrick, M.D., and Surgeon A.B.T.C.D., and late of the city of Cork, respectfully informs the citizens of Toronto that he has opened an office for the practice of Physic and Surgery at No. 42 Lot Street, adjoining the house lately occupied by Dr. Rolph, where he will give his undivided attention to the practice of the profession in its various branches. Dr. H. having brought from England a supply of the most genuine medicines, which will be compounded by an experienced assistant, he trusts that the confidence which a generous public may repose in him will not be misplaced.

"Dr. H. will give gratuitous attendance to the poor afflicted with eye diseases, from 8 to 9 every morning.

"Toronto, October 3rd, 1838."

"*South Charitable Infirmary.*

"At a meeting of the Trustees of the South Charitable Infirmary, held on Wednesday, June 6, 1838, Sir James Pitcairn, M.D., in the chair, the resignation of Dr. Herrick having been received, it was unanimously

"*Resolved,*—That while we accept the resignation of Dr. Herrick as Senior Physician to the South Infirmary, we cannot help expressing our regret that this Institution should be deprived of the valuable services of a physician whose energies have been so long devoted to its best interests, and that at a period when his extensive and enlightened experience is capable of affording such great advantages to the poor; it was also

"*Resolved*,—That the above resolution be communicated to Dr. Herrick through the Secretary, accompanied by an assurance of the high esteem of this Board, and of their warm thanks for his long continued and valuable services to the Infirmary, and that it likewise be published in all the Cork newspapers.

"J. PITCAIRN, M.D."

"At a meeting of the Physicians to the Cork Lying-in Hospital, held June 19, 1838, Dr. Herrick's resignation having been received, it was unanimously

"*Resolved*,—That we cannot record the retirement of our respected colleague, Dr. Herrick, without sincerely and deeply lamenting the loss which this hospital sustains, in being thus deprived of the benefit of his valuable services—services which have been at all times, for a period of more than twelve years, afforded to the patients with benefit to them and honour to himself.

"(Signed) JOHN COPINGER, M.D., *Chairman*."

A new commission was read at the meeting of the Upper Canada Medical Board, July, 1845, and among the new members was "George Herrick, Doctor of Medicine, Professor of Midwifery, University of King's College." Dr. Herrick was almost always present at the Board meetings.

Dr. H. was a favourite with those who enjoyed his friendship. His eccentricities did not lessen their esteem. He remained a bachelor, and almost every night he had a half dozen around his hospitable board. They were sure of a pleasant time. He would neither have carpet nor gas in his house. His custom was to give two special dinners each year, one on Christmas day, the other on his father's birthday. His choice of guests was generally among the younger men. The Doctor was always fresh and cheerful at dinner, as he usually took a sleep between four and six. Yet he retired early, generally at nine, and would in his own way tell his guests to move off.—*N. F. Davin.*

As Professor of Midwifery and Diseases of Women and

Children at King's College, he was liked by the students. His lectures were considered to be concise and thoroughly practical. Among other amusing things he would say in his lectures was, pointing with his thumb over his shoulder, "You must not take the advice of those people over there," meaning the medical teachers of the United States; "because if you do you may as well leave the place at once." It is related that on the occasion of delivering his introductory lecture, he had forgotten that the public were invited to attend, and the presence of ladies was a cause of embarrassment. At the hospital he would not say to a patient, "Put out your tongue;" but would indicate what he wanted by putting out his own.

Dr. H. enjoyed deservedly a high reputation in the practice of midwifery. This the writer—who followed him around the wards of the old hospital—well remembers. He was on familiar terms with his confreres, and always called Dr. King "Rex." As Mr. Davin says, he was of the old school of Irish gentlemen. In appearance he was tall and stout.

Mr. Clarke Gamble says he was "a typical Irishman, clever, well educated in his native country, and London and Edinburgh. His specialties were Diseases of Women and Children. He had a very large practice, and like his fellow-countryman and most intimate friend, Dr. King, was a great favourite with all with whom he came in contact, both young and old. His well-known figure on Church and King Streets, his left arm behind his back, and the right swinging as he moved at a good pace, will not be readily forgotten."

DR. ANSON HEYDEN

Was a good type of the enterprising adventurers from the States who found their way into Upper Canada in its early days. Possessing many good qualities, he was, while he remained in the country, a useful citizen. He settled in Thurlow, back of Belleville, after staying a while at the front, some time prior to 1817. He had studied medicine in New York, but to what extent is unknown, and held a diploma, but having presented himself before the Medical Board in July, 1819, he failed to obtain a license. Nevertheless he had a good practice; in fact, was the only doctor in Thurlow when Dr. Smith came to Belleville, in 1817. He acquired some land, whether by purchase or marriage with Miss Mott, whose father was a pioneer of Thurlow, is unknown. He built a house, large for the period, on the concession corner, and a village sprung up long known as Heyden's Corner. This building was used not only as a dwelling and surgery, but as an inn. The writer well remembers the appearance of the place when attending school in the neighbourhood. Dr. Heyden found time, beside practising and conducting the inn, to look after public affairs. His enterprise and public spirit was recognized by electing him township clerk in 1837. But alas, his active sympathy with William Lyon Mackenzie in his rebellion placed him in a compromising position, and on the approach of the red-coats one day, he fled, never to return.

DR. HAMNETT HILL,

M.R.C.S. Eng., and L.S.A., third son of John Wilkes Hill, a medical practitioner in the eastern part of the city of London, Eng., very near to the "Tower" so rich in historic reminiscences, was born, December 15, 1811. At the early age of eight he was consigned to a boarding school in the village of Peckham, under the management of — Wanostrockt, LL.D., author of "Wanostrockt's Epitome of Blackstone." He remained at this celebrated academy for about eight years, and when about sixteen, he was placed to study medicine under the care of Mr. Philip Harlock, a surgeon residing in St. Paul's Churchyard, to whom he was regularly articled, as was the custom in those days, the fee paid therefor being £200 sterling. At the end of this engagement (five years), he returned to the paternal mansion, pretty well grounded in Materia Medica, Pharmacy and Practical Chemistry. Shortly after he commenced the orthodox two years' hospital course at the London Hospital, in a neighbourhood now too familiarly known as the immediate vicinity of "Jack the Ripper" outrages. During his surgical course he became the pupil of Sir Wm. Blizard and Mr. Luke in the surgical wards, and of Dr. Thos. Davis and Dr. Gordon in the medical wards.

Having finished the prescribed hospital course of two years, required before presentation for examination at Apothecaries' Hall and the College of Surgery, he successfully passed through each ordeal, and joined his uncle, Mr. Lawrence, Surgeon-Extraordinary to His Majesty William IV., and one of the surgeons to the Sussex County Hospital at Brighton, as visiting assistant, where he remained about four years, frequently acting as house surgeon *pro tem.* at the hospital.

At the time of the Canadian rebellion, in 1837, troops were sent out from England to assist in quelling the insurrection. Dr. Hill thinking the War Department might gladly avail themselves of Volunteer Medical Officers to accompany the troops, made application to Lord Hill, the commander of the forces at that time, through the Inspector-General of Hospitals, Sir James McGregor. The latter was all courtesy and kindness, producing a long list whereon were recorded three hundred names, his own nephew standing about one hundred and fifty on the list before him. "If you like," said he, "I will place your name, of course, at the bottom; but if you will take my friendly advice, I should say, turn your attention to something else, as you will be too old (over twenty-seven) by the time you can possibly arrive near the top of the list." Dr. Hill resolved to take the advice so kindly offered by the courteous old officer and made his bow. However, by this time he had a bad attack of "Canada on the brain," and made up his mind to pay a visit to his maternal uncle, the Hon. Hamnett Pinhey, then residing in the township of March, a military settlement on the Ottawa River, about twenty miles from By-town, now Ottawa. He was most hospitably received by his relative, with whom he spent a most agreeable year and a half. By this time he had become so enamoured of Canadian life, that he purchased a small farm on the river front, where he intended to out-do the illustrious Roman Consul Cincinnatus in combining medicine with agriculture, and both with pleasure; but alas, the unpromising state of the health of the sparsely settled neighbourhood, promised but a precarious subsistence, and but for this he might have remained in that locality. A better prospect seemed to be looming up at this juncture in By-town, from whence he received promises of support from influential residents, to wit, Major Boulton, R.E., Capt. Baker, R.A., and other prominent civilians. He consequently removed to that town, where he immediately found his professional abilities duly appreciated. Prior to this he had succumbed to the fickle goddess, in the person of one of the daughters of his former host, to whom he was shortly after married at the Parish Church of St. Mary's, in the township of March, May 18, 1844. The issue of this union was three sons and four daughters, of whom at the present time survive but two daughters and four grandchildren.

At this period, 1844, the practice of the medical profession was very laborious, the roads were execrable, and locomotion was on horseback, on foot or in canoe. No such thing as a railway was ever thought about, and such a thing as a wheeled carriage was not seen for some years after. Of course, in winter with plenty of snow, it was more agreeable. The Doctor can look back to a winter when he travelled three hundred miles in six days with the same horse, whilst in a day of twenty hours, ninety miles was accomplished on two horses, thirty being done before breakfast, and sixty by midnight. "On dismounting, it is almost needless to observe, he slept the sleep of the righteous." Canoeing was a most delightful means of progression if the weather was good and not too early in the spring, and not too late in the fall; and a journey of one hundred miles or so was thought nothing of. A trip of that kind is recorded, to visit a case of serious protracted disease of the knee-joint, requiring amputation. To have performed the operation and have left the patient out of reach of medical assistance, without after treatment, was almost certain death. So, after much persuasion the patient allowed himself to be placed in a large birch bark canoe, on a species of hand-barrow, and thence was lifted out at the head of each rapids, and portaged to the still water again; and in this way was brought down to the city, where his leg was safely removed the next day, and he returned home after about three weeks.

About the year 1850, an agitation arose to found a Protestant hospital in the city, which was carried out successfully on a small scale. It was named the County of Carleton Protestant

Hospital. Dr. Hill was appointed surgeon, the duties of which he fulfilled without assistance for a while; when Dr. Charles Sewell was appointed consulting surgeon. Subsequently Dr. (now Sir James) Grant was appointed on the attending staff. He subsequently became consulting surgeon. Dr. Hill is now also consulting surgeon.

After the death of Dr. Vancortlandt and of Dr. Sewell, he was appointed consulting surgeon to the Roman Catholic Hospital, which position he occupied for more than twenty years, with Dr. Beaubien as attending surgeon. Of course, the very long connection with these institutions gave him very much experience in operative surgery, so that almost every variety of that branch of the profession came under his immediate noticc; such as the many varieties of dislocations, amputations, ligatures of arteries, trephining, strangulated hernia, lithotomy, trachæotomy, ovariotomy, Cæsarian section, craniotomy, paracentesis of abdomen and chest, resection of bones, etc., etc., with an infinite variety of minor operations. Many of these cases considered of a more or less interesting nature were recorded in some of the leading medical journals of the day.

In a communication to the writer (1890), Dr. Hill in his genial manner says: "Domestic affliction and increasing age prompted the propriety of relieving himself from the more arduous duties of professional life; two or three months for summer recreation and enjoyment for his very small family broke up his professional connections, and gradually his business became small by degrees, and beautifully less. His lady friends, with ever-longing hopes of maternity, could not await his return from summer jaunts, and sought fresh fields and pastures new, and although he has never made known his retirement from business, at the age of seventy-nine he now finds that business has given him up; and now finds quite enough to occupy the balance of his days in attending to his financial affairs, and ministering to a few old friends who desire and deserve his gratuitous attendance."

It is a great gratification to the writer to be able to count Dr. Hill as a very kind friend, the remembrance of whose hospitality is a green spot on the plains of life lying behind.

DR. EDWARD MULBERRY HODDER.

Dr. Hodder was the son of Captain Hodder, R.N., and was born, December 30, 1810, England. He entered the navy in 1822 as a midshipman under his father, but only took one cruise, leaving the service at the expiration of one year, having a strong desire to study medicine, for which profession he had a preference. Educated as a boy, first at Guernsey Grammar School, afterwards at St. Servans, France, he began his medical studies in London under the late Mr. Amesbury, very celebrated as a surgeon, with whom he spent five years. At the close of his career as a student, he passed the Royal College of Surgeons of England. He afterwards went to Paris, where he spent two years more in the study of his profession, and subsequently visited Edinburgh, and there, too, passed a considerable time in seeing the practice of the then famous teachers of that city. He began practice in London, where he remained but two years, and thinking his prospects would be improved by removal to St. Servans, in France, he settled there for a time. After remaining a single year, he visited Canada, 1835, returning to France again in a few months. For the next three years he practised his profession in this French town, when he resòlved to make his home in this Province. He settled in the neighbourhood of Queenston, in the Niagara District, where he remained doing a very extensive practice for five years. In 1843, he removed to Toronto, where he continued to practise up to the time of his death.

In 1834, he married Frances Tench, daughter of Captain Tench, of the 87th Royal Irish Fusiliers. In 1854, he was elected a Fellow of the Royal College of Surgeons of England, and in 1865, a Fellow of the Obstetrical Society of London, and was, at the time of his death and for some years past, one of its honorary local secretaries. In 1845, he received the degree of C.M. from King's College, Toronto, and M.D. from Trinity College in 1853.

In 1850 he established, in concert with Dr. Bovell, the Upper Canada School of Medicine, which that year became the medical department of Trinity College. For several years Dr. Hodder was a member of the Faculty of the Toronto School of

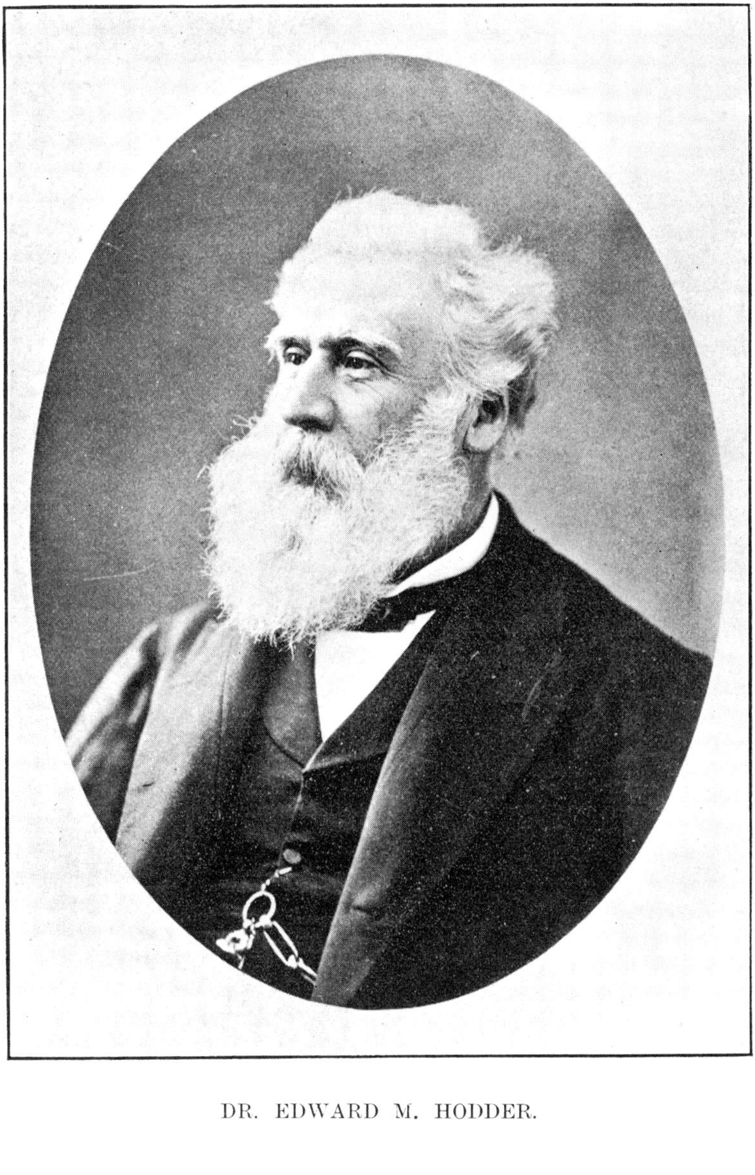

DR. EDWARD M. HODDER.

Medicine, but on the revival of his old school in 1870, he was, by the unanimous wish of his colleagues, appointed Dean of the Faculty, which position he held at the time of his death, having been reappointed in 1877, when the Act incorporating the school passed the Provincial Legislature. From 1852 to 1872, he was one of the leading members of the active staff of the Toronto General Hospital and of the Burnside Lying-in Hospital, and at his decease was senior consulting surgeon to both of these institutions, as well as to several others of like character.

Although devoted to his professional work, Dr. Hodder found time in the way of recreation to gratify his continued love for the water. He was mainly instrumental in forming the Royal Canadian Yacht Club, of which he was Commodore for many years and up to the time of his death. A local paper said of him: "In Dr. Hodder our city loses a man of no ordinary value; while to thousands over the length and breadth of the Province his death will make a blank very difficult to fill, for medical men of his long experience and great and acknowledged skill are not too numerous in any country, and the death of one such is a truly public loss."

This is the testimony of Clarke Gamble in writing about the early medical men of Toronto: "Dr. Hodder's name was a household word in Toronto. Skilful, cautious, affable and handsome, he was a universal favourite, particularly with the gentler sex." Dr. Hodder had been President of the Upper Canada Medical Board, also President of the Toronto Medico-Chirurgical Society in 1862, and President of the Canada Medical Association in 1875. He was the representative of Trinity College at the College of Physicians and Surgeons from 1872 until his death.

His death took place, February 20, 1878, aged 67.

In the *Practitioner* for July, 1873, is an article from the pen of Dr. Hodder, of Toronto, on the transfusion of warm milk into the veins of patients in the later stages of Asiatic cholera. The experiment was tried in the Hospital, Toronto, during the cholera epidemic of 1849. In the first and second cases the patients rallied immediately and ultimately recovered. In the third the patient, although *in articulo mortis*, rallied for a time after the transfusion, but the operation not being seasonably repeated, the patient succumbed.

DR. RUFUS HOLDEN,

The third of six sons of James Holden, of Augusta, U.C., was born, January 16, 1809. He received his education at Ogdensburg, and then entered the store of Billa Flint, Brockville. He then removed to Cobourg, where he remained four years. Then, removing to Belleville, he commenced business as a druggist. Soon after, Merrick Sawyer became a partner in the business, and Mr. Holden pursued the study of medicine. He attended the Pennsylvania College at Philadelphia, and received the degree of M.D., 1842. He then engaged in practice at Belleville, but subsequently took a post-graduate course at McGill College, Montreal, and in 1844 received a degree of Doctor of Medicine and Surgery at McGill University. After this he entered on a very large and successful practice in Belleville, making diseases of women and children a specialty. Here he continued to practise up to the day of his death, March 30, 1876. Dr. Holden was a member of the town council of Belleville for five years, and in 1864 was chosen mayor.

One who knew him well, says: "Dr. Holden was kind even to a fault, sincere, benevolent. Few die more universally respected, even beloved. The street through which the funeral passed was thronged by many of the poor to whom his unostentatious charities had been dispensed. On his grave may well be inscribed, with unvarnished truth, the words of the Patriarch, 'The blessing of him that was ready to perish came upon me, and I caused the widow's heart to sing for joy.'"

The following notices by the Belleville newspapers show the high estimation in which the subject of this sketch was held:

"Another of our oldest and most estimable citizens is gone. Dr. Rufus Holden, for over forty years a resident of Belleville, passed away this morning, but he was attending to his practice as usual yesterday. It appears, however, that he passed an uncomfortable night, although he was able to rise this morning, and was in the act of dressing when he fell in a swoon. An hour afterwards his spirit had taken its flight.

"When the Doctor came to Belleville it was an unpretentious town. About ten years ago, having amassed a competence, he delegated his professional duties to younger men, but his active temperament and robust health demanded employment, and some four years later he found himself as busy as he had been during any part of his life, both in town and the adjacent country. He may, therefore, be said to have literally died in active service."

Another notice says: "The Doctor possessed a most genial temperament, which, combined with large benevolence and a firmly developed Christian character, made a valuable member of society. Few men enjoyed higher distinction in connection with the Church, and he was also prominently associated with the temperance organizations of the country. He was mayor of the town for one or two terms, and in 1867 he contested the West Riding of Hastings in the interests of the Reform party, but without success. He was President of the Tract and Bible Societies for several years, and the Evangelical Alliance had no more earnest and interested co-laborer. In the John Street Presbyterian Church, he was a pillar of inestimable importance. The family and extensive connections have the sympathy of the whole community. But their loss is his gain."

His family consisted of one son and seven daughters. The son, J. C. Holden, is a member of the large manufacturing firm, Ames, Holden & Co., Montreal. One daughter is the wife of Rev. Prof. Gregg, D.D., of Knox College, Toronto; another is married to the Rev. R. F. Burns, D.D., late of Fort Massey Church, Halifax, N.S.,; another to Thomas Ritchie, Esq., dry goods merchant, Belleville; two unmarried daughters reside in Belleville, and two died in childhood.

The writer must not omit to give expression to his own feelings of high esteem for the worth of Dr. Holden. Among his earliest recollections is the occasion when he was a patient of Dr. Holden, also of seeing him pass and repass on his way in attending to country patients. While a confrere of Dr. Holden, 1864-69, the writer found him always kind, courteous, and sympathetic.

DR. WILLIAM HOPE

Was born on January 15, 1815, near Belfast, in County Antrim, Ireland, and was the son of John Hope, who was married to Ann Forsyth of the same county. In 1822, John Hope came from Ireland to Kingston, Canada, with his family. The fact that the trip from Montreal up the river occupied three weeks, gives one a glimpse of the state of things in this country in those days. Robert Hope, now of Newburgh, the eldest son of the family, went into business as a general merchant in Bath, then a place of some importance. William was clerk for him for some years, but having decided to study medicine, he went to Kingston, and for some time had the advantage of attending a school taught by Mr. Jeffers, father of the Rev. Dr. Jeffers, a man whom Dr. Hope recollects as being possessed of much of the intellectual power which has since distinguished his gifted son. He completed his general studies at the Kingston Grammar School, then taught by a Mr. Baxter, a famous teacher of those days, under whose rod most of the professional men of the time in the Midland District passed in their youth. Young Hope then went into the office of Dr. Adamson and afterwards Dr. Sampson, both of Kingston. Mr. Hope studied and saw practice with them for upwards of four years, attending two courses of lectures meanwhile at Fairfield, in the State of New York, where he graduated as M.D., in January, 1838. He took out his license under the Medical Board of Upper Canada in the same year. Dr. Hope at once settled in Belleville, where for forty-three years he devoted himself assiduously to the practice of his profession. His extensive and, in the earlier days of bad roads, very laborious practice, did not, however, engross his whole attention: everything that made for the improvement of the community, had not only his sympathy, but his active support. He was for years a member of the old board of police, and when our municipal system came into operation, he was for a long time a member of the town council; he was mayor in 1860. Dr. Hope was for many years a school trustee, and was largely instrumental in introducing the free school system into Belleville, the first municipality in which it was established in Upper Canada. Dr. Hope was appointed surgeon to the county gaol by the Quarter Sessions when the county was first established; he was also surgeon to the Deaf and Dumb Institute from its beginning; he held both these appointments until he resigned them on becoming sheriff. He was appointed surgeon in the 2nd Battalion of Hastings Militia, in 1847. He was a member of the Board of Examiners of the Medical Council for the years 1871 and 1872; and his professional brethren elected him for many years President of the Belleville Medical Society, an honour which he resigned into their hands on retiring from active practice. Dr. Hope married in 1843, Augusta, only daughter of the late Sheriff Spencer, of Northumberland. Her only brother is George B. Spencer, of Winnipeg, who organized the customs service in Manitoba and the North-West, and remained at its head until his retirement from active service a few months ago. Dr. Hope was a member of the Bible Society from its first organization in Belleville, and has been several times and is now the President of that branch. He was appointed in April, 1881, sheriff of the county in which he had lived so long and so worthily.

The foregoing is extracted from a biographical notice in the "Encyclopædia of Canadian Biography." The writer must not omit to give his personal testimony to the worth of Dr. Hope, whether as a practitioner, a Christian worker, a public man in various capacities, the chief magistrate, or as a citizen generally, also as a confrere. Among his earlier recollections is to have seen again and again, at all hours—at early dawn or at nightfall—Dr. Hope passing along the road in his vehicle, going to or returning from the bedside of a patient. Nor does he forget the first visit made by the Doctor to his father's house, where the gravity of the case made it necessary for him to remain over night, to be ready for contingencies.

DR. ROBERT HORNBY,

An Englishman by birth and education, was gazetted Licentiate Upper Canada, Dec. 9, 1833, as an M.D., University of Edinburgh, and Licentiate Royal College of Surgeons, London, and

Extraordinary Member of the Royal Medical Society of Edinburgh. He went to Cleveland, Ohio, for a time, but returned to Toronto and engaged in practice. A contemporary says: "He was an estimable man and a clever physician; but on account of deafness, he did not attain to the position nor acquire the amount of practice his abilities and acquirements entitled him to."

In April, 1836, the Medical Board was re-constructed, and Dr. Hornby was one of the new members. From this time it is seen that Dr. Hornby was a very regular attendant at the meetings of the Board. October, 1838, a new commission was issued, and Dr. Hornby was again one of the members. He continued an active member until the College of Physicians and Surgeons of Upper Canada assumed its duties, when he was likewise an active member while it lasted; and when a new Medical Board was commissioned in 1841, he was a member again, and his name is recorded as present at the meetings up to April, 1850.

Dr. Hornby was on duty in 1837 as Assistant-Surgeon to the Royal Foresters.

He died, we believe, March 4, 1869, aged 56.

DR. ROBERT CHARLES HORNE,

An Englishman by birth, was a member of the Royal College of Surgeons, England. He was Surgeon to the Glengarry Light Infantry Regiment, which was for a time stationed at Kingston prior to its being disbanded. He married, at Kingston, the eldest daughter of Dr. John Gamble. After his regiment had been disbanded, Dr. Horne removed to York. This was about 1815 or 1816. It is uncertain whether Dr. Horne engaged in practice. At all events, in 1817, we find him "Printer to His Most Excellent Majesty," and editor of the *Official Gazette*. The first newspaper published in Upper Canada was the *Upper Canada Gazette*, or *American Oracle*, commenced April 18, 1793, at Newark, now Niagara-on-the-Lake. When the seat of government was removed to York, the *Official Gazette* naturally removed also. When Dr. Horne became the publisher, the word *American* was dropped, and the title became the *Upper Canada Gazette*, or *Oracle*. It is interesting to notice that at first the term American was used in Canada, and that a monopoly of the word by the United States was not recognized. The cause of the change made by Dr. Horne may have been to strip the title of everything savouring of Yankeeism, or possibly to make the name of the paper shorter. He continued the publisher until 1821, when he resigned the position. Not long before this he became involved in a difficulty with the Parliament, on account of imperfection in the reports of Parliamentary debates, which he had allowed to appear in the columns of the *Gazette*. On being summoned to the Bar of the House, Dr. Horne stated in explanation that the notes of the debates were not taken by himself. He offered every apology, and submitted himself to the pleasure of the House.

In 1822, Charles Fothergill succeeded Dr. Horne as Printer. Dr. Horne became then the chief teller of the Bank of Upper Canada, a position he filled for many years, till his death.

In February, 1827, Dr. Horne issued a prospectus of a new religious and literary publication, to be conducted by the clergy of the Established Church, under the sanction of the Lord Bishop of the Diocese, to be entitled *The Christian Sentinel and Anglo-Canadian Churchman's Magazine*.

Although Dr. Horne did not engage in practice, he remained identified with the profession. In 1822, he was appointed Surgeon to the North York Regiment of Militia; and a more important position assigned him by the Governor, in 1823, was that of member of the Upper Canada Medical Board. His first attendance as such was at the April meeting. He continued an active member until the beginning of 1831. After that his name does not appear on the minutes until October, 1837, when it appears in connection with a resolution respecting King's College. He was one of the Fellows of the College of Physicians and Surgeons, Upper Canada, during its existence, and was elected to fill the office of Treasurer. He was a constant attendant of the meetings of the Fellows up to the last, January, 1841, having continued to be the Treasurer. This seems to have been the last of his work in connection with the profession. His name does not appear on the new U. C. Medical Board.

Dr. Horne filled other public offices, as Secretary to the Agricultural Society of York, in 1820; Commissioner for Taking Affidavits, 1823; Commissioner of the Peace, with Drs. Powell, Widmer and Lyons, in 1825.

"During the rebellion of 1837, Mackenzie, whom the Doctor in a humble way had most vigorously opposed, burned his residence over the head of his wife and children, who fled through the snow to the house of a neighbour on Bloor street. From the effects of this tramp through the snow, quite unprotected from the weather in any way, Mrs. Horne never recovered."—*C. Gamble.* Again it is recorded by a writer (Mulvaney): "That by orders received from Dr. Rolph, the insurrectionary executive fired Dr. Horne's house, which had been a rendezvous for loyalist spies."

Dr. Horne married Isabella Leah, of St. John, N.B., daughter of Dr. Gamble, who died, September 29, 1863, aged 78. They had two sons; one, John, was living in the neighbourhood of Sandwich; the other, James Macaulay, died December 26, 1857, aged 32. The daughter, unmarried, was recently (1891) living at St. Catharines. Dr. Horne died, October 26, 1845.

DR. JOHN HOWISON.

Little is known of Dr. Howison, except that he sojourned in Canada for a short time, played at the practice of his profession, and then returned to England, and wrote a book, entitled "Sketches of Upper Canada." His knowledge of the country was acquired principally in the Niagara District. His opinion, as expressed in his sketches, was not flattering to Canadians. He says: "They are still the untutored, incorrigible beings that they were, when the ruffian remnant of a disbanded regiment, or the outlawed refuse of some European nation," and so on. We have evidence that the Doctor was actuated by spite, or wished to supply a reason why his efforts to practise in Canada were a failure. Robert Gourlay, who was by no means a lover of the U. E. Loyalists, says, regarding the Doctor's diatribes: "It is not true, it is not fair, it is not discreet. The first settlers of Upper Canada, in my opinion, were wrong-headed men as to politics; but they were far from being bad-hearted men, and anything but the 'ruffian remnant of a disbanded regiment.' They were soldiers who had done their duty; who had regarded with reverence their oath of allegiance; who had risked their lives a hundred times over in support of their principles; who had sacrificed all which the world in general holds dear, to maintain their loyalty and honour. They were anything but the 'outlawed refuse of some European nation.' They adhered to the laws of Britain; and for the laws of Britain they bled. They did not 'seek refuge in the wilds of Upper Canada, aware they would neither find means of subsistence, nor be countenanced in any civilized country.' It is a libel on the British Government to say they sought refuge, and a libel on common-sense to say that men who resolved to earn their bread by labour, under the worst circumstances in the world, could not find means of subsistence anywhere else. The whole passage is untrue, is shameful, and Dr. Howison should apologize for it in the public prints of this country. The mass of first settlers in Upper Canada were true men, and to this day there is a peculiar caste of goodness in their natures, which distinguishes them from their neighbours in the United States. Dr. Howison wrote only to trifle—very readable as a romance—the tale of a weak man. . . . They refused Dr. Howison, it would seem, and because he could not appreciate the nobility of nature when crowned by the rough circumstances of pioneer life, he must needs write a libel. No doubt his mind was influenced by Yankee tales of Butler's Rangers, and perhaps his exquisite sensibility was wounded, forsooth, because a Canadian would not touch his hat to him."

In the absence of any knowledge of Dr. Howison's professional acquirements, it may be reasonable to suppose that the cause of his leaving the country was his inability to pass the required examination of the new Medical Board.

"Dr. Howison," says Mr. J. P. Merritt, in his biography of Hon. W. H. Merritt, "spent the winter of 1819-20 at St. Catharines, and had his office at Paul Shipman's hotel. He appears to have been a man of means, and practised but little at his profession, spending most of his time in visiting around the neighbourhood. . . . On returning to England, he published the result of his observations in a good-sized volume, for the information of those intending to emigrate, the substance of which was that the country was unfit for a professional man of good education, who expected to make an income by the practice of his profession."

One incident connected with the Doctor's sojourn at St. Catharines is recorded by Mr. J. P. Merritt. A party of two ladies and the Doctor set out to attend a theatrical performance at Niagara. "The turn-out was a purely rural one. Dressed in spring attire, with white pants of unexceptional blancherie, he drove up to the house. The vehicle consisted of a one-horse waggon, imported from the Eastern States, and which had probably done good service for the Fraus and Mynheers in their first emigration from the Mohawk Valley after the Revolution. Having but one seat, a chair had to be put in for the Doctor, whose first essay showed that the safety of the ladies depended more on the gentleness of the horse than the skill of the driver. Things went on smoothly until their return, where an extra 'rut' in the last mile of the swamp caused a separation of the vehicle, leaving the driver and ladies in the road, and considerably diminishing the lustre of the Doctor's snowy unmentionables, and detracting from his skill as a navigator."

DR. ELNATHAN HUBBELL

Was a native of the United States, and coming to Canada about 1808, he settled at Brockville. Dr. Hubbell was remarkable for his large size, and a face marked by numerous nodules of the skin. It is stated that his education, both general and medical, was of doubtful extent. But he was evidently a man of considerable ability and possessed of qualities which recommended him to the community. He was fortunate in becoming connected with a well-known family of the place, by marrying Lucy, daughter of Ephraim Jones. This union brought him influence and wealth. In time he commanded a large practice, principally in the town, especially in midwifery, although there were some who doubted his skill. He adopted the sensible plan of attending families by the year. It is related that Dr. Hubbell built the first brick house in the place. During the war of 1812, a raiding party of Yankees carried him away prisoner, but shortly after released him on parole. In 1819, he was appointed a member of the Land Board for Johnston District, Dr. Solomon Jones being the chairman; and in 1822, we find him trustee of the public schools, and Commissioner of the Peace. The Doctor was one of those whom the people will talk about, and among the sayings of the day which have been handed down, is, that "he was very fond of hot cakes." But a love for hot cakes, although generally regarded as a Yankee characteristic, is very general among the U. E. Loyalists.

Dr. Hubbell died about 1850. He had a large family, concerning which information is not available, except a marriage notice which records that, at Brockville, November 25th, 1841, Thomas Mair, Esq., was married to Amelia, youngest daughter of Dr. Hubbell.

DR. JAMES HUNTER

Was born in Yorkshire, England, 1790, and came to Canada in 1823, and settled in Niagara District. It is unknown whether he had studied medicine prior to leaving England, but probably not, as it seems he was a student at Fairfield. In April, 1826, he passed the Medical Board, which "was perfectly satisfied with his examination." He commenced practice at Whitby, where he remained until 1837, when he was implicated in the Mackenzie rebellion. Being arrested, he was released on bail ($16,000), and absented himself until the trial, when he returned, and was acquitted on the same day that Lount and Matthews were executed. This was in April, 1838. He was afterwards threatened with re-arrest, but managed to reach the States before he could be detained. He returned to Canada in 1841, and resided for some time in Newmarket. He died in Buffalo, in 1850.

Dr. Hunter was small in stature, but a busy, energetic man. His love of the medical profession was inherited by his descendants who are still known in the medical world.

DR. JAMES JOHN HUNTER,

A native of Yorkshire, England, was born in 1822, and was the son of Dr. James Hunter, who settled at Niagara, in 1823. He appeared before the Medical Board, October, 1843. He had a diploma from Geneva College, N.Y., and obtained a certificate to practise ; he had attended lectures at the New York Medical University. He commenced the practice of his profession at Newmarket, in which town he remained about twenty years. He was reeve of the council during six years of that period. In the year 1860, he went to New York city, where he practised three years, when he returned to Newmarket and resumed his practice. He was a Justice of the Peace for twenty-five years. He married in 1842, Rachel, daughter of Isaac Lundy.

DR. JOHN WILSON HUNTER,

From Grimsby. Before the Medical Board, April, 1839. He had tickets of attendance on three courses of lectures at Fairfield, and a diploma from the same. He obtained a certificate to practise. "Married—At Kingston, October, 1844, John Wilson Hunter, Esq., M.D., of Hamilton, to Olivia, daughter of the late Lieut. and Adjutant John Hinds, 68th Regiment Foot."

DR. ROBERT HUNTER,

From Whitby. Before the Medical Board, April, 1846. Had a diploma from University of New York. Not being able to read a Latin prescription, examination not proceeded with. (For further information, see minutes of U. C. Medical Board, October, 1847.)

Dr. Robert Hunter was the author of "Hydro-therapeutics, or A Treatise on the Water Cure ; being a digest of the opinions and experience of some of the most distinguished physicians in Europe and America on the curative virtues of water, etc. Toronto, 1848."

DR. JOHN HUTCHISON

Was born at Kircaldy, Scotland, in 1797. He received his early education at the high school of that town, and in the year 1812, commenced his studies for the medical profession with James Corkindale, physician and surgeon, Glasgow, to whom he was indentured as student for three years. During those three years he attended lectures at the University of Glasgow, and in 1815, passed the required examinations and was granted a diploma and license from the Faculty. He then spent two years or more at Edinburgh, attending the lectures of the Medical Faculty of Edinburgh University.

At that period it was regarded as a formidable undertaking to cross the Atlantic, and young Hutchison availed himself of an opportunity which offered of accompanying an intimate friend and college chum who was about to emigrate to America. Accordingly they sailed in the latter part of the year 1817, arriving at New York early in 1818. His friend, James Grant, decided to try his fortune in Mexico, but the young doctor, preferring to live under the British flag, came to Canada, and, towards the end of 1818, settled at Port Hope. On December 8, 1818, we find he took the oath of allegiance before John Small, J.P., at York, and in accordance with the requirements of the Medical Act, he passed the examination of the Board in July, 1829. For several years from 1818, Dr. Hutchison practised at Port Hope and Cobourg, and in 1822, moved to Cavan and resided for several years near where the town of Millbrook now stands. In 1830, he was induced to remove to Peterboro', at which place he resided until his death. He had a very large practice, extending over all the townships in the counties of Peterboro' and Victoria, and many of those in Northumberland.

At one time Dr. Taylor was associated in partnership with Dr. Hutchison, so also was Dr. Dickson, afterwards of Kingston, and the late Dr. Harvey, of Peterboro', was a student with him in 1846-47.

In the fall of 1842, Dr. Hutchison visited his native land, taking with him his two oldest sons, and remaining in Scotland until the following spring. On the eve of his departure from

Peterboro', a farewell public dinner was given, at which an address was presented. Whilst in Scotland the Doctor afforded much information about Canada to many inquirers, and he was the means of inducing a number of families to make their homes in this country.

The year 1847 will be remembered as the period of the famine in Ireland, in consequence of which thousands of poor Irish people were brought to Canada. Hundreds of these poor creatures, sick and destitute, were forwarded to Peterboro', and slab shanties were erected for their shelter, outside the village, and a temporary hospital near Little Lake, far enough away for isolation. A Board of Health was organized and Dr. Hutchison was commissioned by the Emigration Department to look after the sick. Unremitting in his attention to the unfortunate sufferers, many of whom were prostrated with a malignant type of fever (ship-fever or typhus), the Doctor was stricken with the same disease, and after a week's illness, died, August 1, 1847, in the prime of life.

The Peterboro' *Dispatch* contained the following brief obituary notice:

"DIED.—On Sunday, July 1st, 1847, of typhus fever, caught while in attendance at the emigrant sheds, John Hutchison, Esq., M.D., aged fifty years, formerly of Kircaldy, in Fife, North Britain, and a resident of America since 1818. This melancholy event cast a gloom over the entire community, to whose interests he, both as a friend and a physician, had long been faithfully devoted. The writer trusts that some one of his most intimate associates will pay a just and fitting tribute to the memory and merits of our departed friend, as it would be both unbecoming and ungrateful that talent and worth such as Dr. Hutchison was largely gifted with, should pass from the busy stage of life without something beyond a passing notice."

Dr. Hutchison married, at Port Hope, in the year 1826, Martha Holland, by whom he had eleven children, six sons and five daughters; three of the latter died young. His wife and eight children survived him.

The following appointments were held by Dr. Hutchison: Justice of the Peace, Coroner, Surgeon to the 2nd Regiment of

Northumberland Militia (1822), Surgeon to the 7th Provisional Battalion of Peterboro' (1838), Member of the Board of Surgeons in the Newcastle District (in conjunction with Drs. Gilchrist and Burnham) for examining claimants for pensions, and granting certificates to those found to be disabled in consequence of wounds or other injuries received while in service in the rebellion, or in the war with the United States (1840), and Medical Attendant of the Mississaga Indians at Rice Lake (1844).

Dr. Hutchison was a cousin of Sanford Fleming, the well-known civil engineer, scientist and educationist. At the time the Doctor visited Scotland, his warm recommendation of Canada as a field for enterprise and industrious pursuits, induced Mr. Fleming's family to come and settle in the country, and they arrived about the time the Doctor died.

DR. HAMILTON DIBBLE JESSUP.

The "U. E. List" contains the names of four Jessups—Edward J., father and son, Henry J. and Joseph J. The famous corps which distinguished itself during the rebellion of 1776, known as "Jessup's Rangers," was commanded by Major Edward Jessup, a son and a grandson of the same name. The following is taken from the Brockville *Recorder*, November 26th, 1892, furnished by E. Jessup, Esq., son of Dr. Jessup:

" Hamilton Dibble Jessup was born on May 2, 1806, in the township of Augusta, county of Grenville, province of Upper Canada. He was the grandson of Major Edward Jessup, who commanded a colonial corps which was known as the Loyal American Regiment, and who was born in the Parish of Stanford, in the county of Fairfield, province of Connecticut, in 1735. He was the son of Joseph Jessup, who died in Montreal, in 1779, and grandson of Edward Jessup, and great-grandson of Edward Jessup, who emigrated from England about 1640 and settled in the colony of New York. At the breaking out of the revolutionary war, Major Jessup and his family resided at the city of Albany, New York, where he was extensively engaged in business, and in the possession of a tract of 500,000 acres of land. A staunch loyalist, Major Jessup sacrificed his fortune by taking up arms for the King. In 1777, he joined the army under Burgoyne, who was then marching against Ticonderoga, and continued in the service until the close of the war, when the Major proceeded to Canada with his corps, which was then known as 'Jessup's Rangers.' They were first stationed at Isle Aux Noix, subsequently at St. Denis, St. Charles, Riviere du Chine, Vercheres and Sorel. When peace was declared in 1783, large tracts of land were granted by the Crown to the officers and men, who, accompanied by their families in the spring of 1784, proceeded up the River St. Lawrence, thus commencing the settlement of Leeds and Grenville, Addington and the Bay of Quinte. After locating his men, Major Jessup proceeded to England, where he remained for several years. When he returned, he settled in the township of Augusta, county of Grenville. In 1810, he laid out the town of Prescott, where he died, in February, 1816, at the age of eighty-one years. Lieutenant Edward Jessup, only son of Major Jessup, was born in the city of Albany, province of New York. He became a Lieutenant in the Royal Rangers, went to England with his father, and returned with him to Canada. In 1798 he was elected to represent the Eastern Division in the Legislative Assembly of the Province of Upper Canada, and in January, 1800, was appointed by Lieutenant-Governor Hunter to the Clerkship of the Peace for the district of Johnston. In 1809, he was appointed by Lieutenant-Governor Gore as Lieutenant-Colonel of the 1st Regiment of Leeds Militia. He died at Prescott in 1815, leaving a wife and seven children—five sons and two daughters, the late Dr. H. D. Jessup being the last of the seven children. He received his education at the District Grammar School in Augusta. In 1825, he was articled to Wm. Caldwell, M.D., at Montreal, as a student of medicine; in October, 1829, he received his license to practise medicine in Upper Canada, and in February, 1830, for Lower Canada. He practised his profession for about thirty years at Prescott. During the troubles of 1837-38, he was captain of a company of militia, under Col. Young, and took part in the engagement at Prescott, which occurred in November, 1838, known as the battle of the Windmill. In 1844, he was elected to parliament for the county of Grenville. He was for several years mayor of the town of Prescott, and was two or three times made warden of the united counties of Leeds and Grenville. In July, 1856, he was appointed Captain of the 1st Volunteer Rifles, of Prescott, and in November of the same year he was appointed Lieutenant-Colonel of the Militia Force of Canada. In April, 1867, he was appointed Lieutenant-Colonel of the 56th Battalion of Infantry, and in 1873, after twenty-six years of service in the active force of Canada, owing to his advanced age, he withdrew from the force. In 1867, Dr. Jessup was appointed to the Collectorship of Customs at Prescott, which office he filled for eighteen years. At his own request he was placed on the retired list in 1885. The deceased gentleman was a life-long Conservative, and an intimate colleague of the late Right Hon. Sir John A. Macdonald. Dr. Jessup married Sophia Matilda, daughter of Michel Trudeau, of Montreal. By this union he has two sons and three daughters living, Edward Jessup, his son, being our present collector."

DR. SOLOMON JONES.

Among the names found in the "Old U. E. List" is that of Solomon Jones, "E. District Surgeon's Mate, Royal Rangers." The following petition taken from the Department of Archives, Ottawa, gives an account of his connection with the military service:

"To His Excellency Robert Prescott, Esquire, Captain-General and Commander-in-Chief in and over the Province of Lower Canada, etc.:

"The Petition of Solomon Jones, Surgeon, Humbly Sheweth:

"That your petitioner begs leave to represent to your Excellency that he is by birth an American. In 1776, he with other loyalists joined the Royal Standard, and served under His Majesty until the peace of 1783, in the capacity of Surgeon's Mate, since which time he has resided upon the Crown Lands, in the Province of Upper Canada, where, for a considerable time, himself and family suffered many hardships and inconveniences such as are attendant upon the settlement of a wild and new country.

"That your petitioner also begs leave to represent to your Excellency that he has a wife and six children, with an aged mother, to provide for, who have no other means of support, but through your petitioner.

"That from the character of your petitioner and his well-known attachment to the British Government, he begs leave humbly to solicit your Excellency to appoint him to succeed the late Mr. Latham as hospital mate at Kingston, in the said Province of Upper Canada.

"May it, therefore, please your Excellency to grant such relief in his present situation as to your Excellency's humanity and wisdom he may appear to merit, and your petitioner as in duty bound shall ever pray.

"SOL. JONES."

"MONTREAL, *March* 4th, 1799.

"I do hereby certify that I am well acquainted with the allegations set forth in the foregoing petition, as also with the petitioner whom I consider as a person qualified and capable of performing the duties of the appointment which he solicits.

"CHARLES BLAKE,
"*Surgeon, Half-pay Staff.*"

Dr. Solomon Jones was a native of Connecticut, and studied his profession at Albany.

He was with Burgoyne when he surrendered, but managed to escape to Canada. He offered his services to the Commander at Three Rivers, and continued as surgeon until the end of the war. He was one of seven brothers, two of whom died fighting for their King; one found refuge in Nova Scotia; four brothers, Solomon, Daniel, John and David, settled on the banks of the St. Lawrence, 1784. It was Lieut. David Jones who was to have married the beautiful Miss Jane McCrea, of historic fame, who was killed and scalped by Indians as they were conducting her to Fort Edward, where Lieut. Jones was with the British forces. Her "silken tresses were taken to the fort, where they were immediately recognized by Lieut. Jones." Lieut. Jones was never seen to smile afterwards, and died in early life.

It is recorded that Dr. Solomon Jones "was domiciled about seven miles below Brockville; was one of the first settlers, first doctors, and first in point of education and respectability."

A writer in 1846, relating some incidents attending the advent of Simcoe as he passed up the St. Lawrence, speaks of a meeting as follows:

"The gentry of the surrounding country collected together for the occasion, and looking spruce, though weather-beaten, in their low tasselled boots, their queer old broad-skirted military coats, and looped chapeaux, with faded feathers fluttering in the wind, had retired to the inn, and were toasting in parting goblets the 'good old cause for ever' previously to betaking themselves to their woodland path homeward, or embarking in their canoes to reach their destination by water, above or below.

"'Now, I am content—content, I say, and can go home to reflect on this proud day. Our Governor—the man of all others—has come at last—mine eye hath seen it—drink to him, gentlemen—he will do the rest for us,' cried Colonel Tom Fraser, his face flushed and fiery, and his stout frame drawn up to its full height at the head of the table.

"'We do—we do!' vociferated young Kingsmill, emptying his glass and stamping to express joy. 'Bonhomme' Tom Fraser then got on his legs, and shouted a brawny young soldier's echo to the toast of his relative.

"The mild placid countenance of Dr. Solomon Jones was lighted up by the occasion, and he arose also and responded to the toast, recounting some of the services performed by the newly appointed Lieutenant-Governor in the late war."

Dr. Jones' professional services were in demand from Cornwall to Kingston. His was among the first appointments as Magistrate in the Province. He was also a member of parliament from 1796 to 1800, and was a trustee of the public school. Finally, was made Judge of the Johnston District. He died in 1822.

Dunham, a son of Dr. Jones, born, 1793, was Ensign in First Regiment Grenville Militia during the war of 1812; Captain of the same during the rebellion of 1837-38, and subsequently a Lieutenant-Colonel. Was Justice of the Peace, 1828, and for a long time Collector at the Port of Maitland.

DR. AUGUSTUS JUKES

Was the youngest son of Andrew Jukes, M.D., a superintending surgeon on the Bombay Establishment, holding the appointment, at the period of his untimely death, of political agent at Kishm, in the Persian Gulf, and employed on a special mission to the Court of Persia. He was one of the best Persian and Arabic scholars of his day, having previously served with distinction for many years, as secretary to the embassies of Mr. Manesty, Sir Harford Jones and Sir John Malcolm, at Teheran.

Dr. Augustus Jukes was born at Bombay, October 30, 1821. In 1822, after the death of his father, he returned with his mother to England, where he continued until his thirteenth year, when he emigrated to Canada with his mother and an old friend and comrade of his father, the late Col. John Johnson, C.B., of the Engineers (father of the late Rev. W. A. Johnson, of Weston, Ont., and grandfather of Dr. Arthur Jukes Johnson, Toronto). On their arrival in Canada, they took up a considerable tract of land in the unbroken wilderness on the north shore of Lake Erie, hitherto the reserve of the Six Nation Indians, from which they were then in process of removal. Here he continued leading the rough life of a pioneer until November, 1837, when he returned to England and remained there at school until April, 1840, when he came back alone to Canada, arriving here after a very severe passage of fifty days. A few days subsequently he received from the late Hon. Francis Warden, a director of the Hon. East India Company, and an old friend of his father, a direct appointment as military cadet to India, which had followed him on the *Great Western* accompanied by the most urgent solicitations from his mother and other relatives that the appointment should be declined. Had he been still in England, he would probably have overruled all objections and accepted the nomination, but under the conditions he felt compelled to decline it, a conclusion he never ceased to regret.

The first enlargement of the Welland canal being at that time undertaken as a government work, under the direction of the late Samuel Power as engineer-in-chief (who subsequently won great professional distinction both in England and India),

Mr. Jukes obtained employment on that work, first as roadman to Mr. Thomas C. Keefer, then as one of the assistant engineers, and during the next four years was employed successively in various positions upon every section of the work, being ultimately placed as assistant engineer in special charge of the construction of that section of the work (eight miles) lying between Thorold and Port Robinson; Mr. Walter Shanly, then also an assistant engineer, being engaged upon another section of the work at Port Colborne.

The only public works then in course of construction in Canada were under the control of the Government, of which department, then called the "Board of Works," the late Hon. H. H. Killaby and Mr. Dominick Daly constituted the president and secretary; but a change of government taking place about this time, the entire staff of civil engineers on the Welland canal construction works, with one or two exceptions, from the chief downwards, were summarily dismissed at one month's notice; new appointments being made by the party which then succeeded to power. Seeing no reasonable prospect, under these circumstances, of obtaining professional occupation in Canada for some years to come, Mr. Jukes changed his profession, and in 1846 entered the surgery of the late Dr. T. Mack, of St. Catharines, as a medical student. In 1847, he removed to Toronto, and during the winters of 1847-48 and 1848-49 attended medical lectures at the University of King's College, taking, at the annual examinations, five first honours and one second. In July, 1849, he passed his examination for license before the Medical Board. Dr. Widmer, the president, when the examination was completed, publicly complimented Dr. Jukes on his proficiency, and told him if he ever desired to take service under the Government, to apply to him and he would recommend him. Later on in the same year he was appointed by Dr. French, Inspector-General of Hospitals in Canada, on the recommendation of Drs. Widmer and Beaumont, surgeon to three companies of incorporated militia, originally enlisted for three years to maintain order on the Welland canal during the reconstruction work then in progress, the headquarters of which were at Port Robinson. In 1857, these companies being disbanded, Dr. Jukes removed to the town of St. Catharines, where he continued the practice of his profession. In March, 1854, he was appointed by General Rowan, surgeon of the 2nd Battalion of Lincoln.

On March 11, 1870, the 20th Lincoln having been disbanded and merged into the 19th Battalion, Dr. Jukes was gazetted surgeon of the latter corps, which position he retained until his appointment as Senior Surgeon of the North-West Mounted Police, January 1, 1882.

In November, 1865, Dr. Jukes graduated as M.B., at Trinity College, Toronto, and in 1870, was elected first president of the Medical Association of St. Catharines and the county of Lincoln, which was then first inaugurated, and delivered before them an inaugural address, which was published by the Association shortly after in the *Canada Lancet*, in which address he first introduced to the notice of the profession, not only in Canada but of the continent of America, throughout which its adoption has since become almost universal—the treatment of post-partum hæmorrhage by the intra-uterine injection of dilute alcohol.

For some years after, Dr. Jukes received many expressions of thanks from medical men throughout Canada, by whom his suggestions had been adopted, and which have ever since been increasingly taught and received everywhere.

On January 1, 1882, Dr. Jukes, then in his sixty-first year, was appointed, as already stated, Senior Surgeon of the North-West Mounted Police, and after recruiting two hundred and twelve men for that force at the New Fort in Toronto, proceeded early in April of that year in medical charge of the division for the headquarters of the force, then at old Fort Walsh, in the Cypress Hills, North-West Territories.

During the last half century, Dr. Jukes "has contributed in prose and verse," as stated in the "Bibliotheca Canadensis," "to many newspapers and periodicals" both here and in England, but always under a *nom de plume*. Among others, are the "Selections from the Odes of Hafiz," "The Lyrical Poet of Persia;" rendered into English verse, "Christmas Eve," and other papers referred to in the above work, which appeared in the *Anglo-American Magazine* in 1852-53. He has also, in former years, given various popular lectures on literary and scientific subjects, mainly for charitable purposes, several of which were published at the time in the local press.

DR. KEATING.

One of this name was practising at York for a year or two, prior to the time of Dr. Widmer, about 1816. It is said that Dr. Widmer succeeded him in his practice. A Dr. Keating, probably the same, was practising at Kingston subsequent to this, and was there in 1818. N. F. Davin speaks of him as an Irishman at Kingston. A local writer speaks of "Surgeon-General Keating, who died in 1821." Dr. T. W. Keating was practising at Port Sarnia in 1839. It was probably the same person who advertised in the *Courier*, of Upper Canada, 1835, as follows: "NOTICE—A gentleman, lately come to the country, wishes to obtain a situation as assistant or foreman in a respectable medical house. Has served apprenticeship of five years to one of the most eminent surgeons in Dublin. Has certificate from Richmond Surgical Hospital; also ——— school in Dublin; also of four winter courses (six months) on anatomy, demonstrations with dissection; and for same period, lectures on physic, pathology and surgery; also, from R.C.S.I., lectures on physiology, materia medica and chemistry. Apply to Mr. Keating. Toronto, December 19th, 1834."

DR. THOMAS KEEGAN,

A native of Ireland, was for a time at Halifax. His advent to Upper Canada was in 1833, when he took up his abode in Brockville. But the Doctor had a disposition to migrate from one place to another. He went from Brockville to Belleville, then to Hamilton, and thence to Brantford, where it is related he died. That he lived for a time in Toronto is shown by the following notices: "Married—At York, by Bishop McDonell, George Sherwood, Esq., to Miss Keegan, daughter of Dr. Keegan, all of this town. July, 1833." "Died—At Toronto, 1st February, 1835, Edward Burk Keegan, eldest son of Thomas G. Keegan, Esq., M.D., of Toronto."

Dr. Keegan had two sons and two daughters; one of the latter, who died in early womanhood, was to have been the wife of John Crawford, afterwards Lieut.-Governor of Ontario.

The Doctor was a somewhat remarkable man, inasmuch as he wore his hair long. His face was streaked by large prominent veins, and he gave little attention to his person.

Died at Brockville, December 26th, 1842, Jessy Albro, second daughter of the late Thomas Keegan, Esq., M.D., formerly of Halifax, N.S., aged 22."

DR. JABEZ KELLOG

Was a native of the United States, studied his profession there, and graduated at Dartmouth College. He came into Canada in 1822, and finished his education with Dr. Armstrong and Dr. Sampson, of Kingston, with the former of whom he practised for a short time after passing the Medical Board in January, 1825. He commenced practice in Belleville in the same year, where he remained until July, 1835, when he removed to Hamilton. He was well liked at Belleville, and enjoyed a high reputation for skill. He was also respected as a benevolent Christian gentleman, and was secretary of the Belleville Sunday School Society, 1830; also, treasurer of the Methodist Missionary Society, 1830.

In Hamilton he soon acquired a large and successful practice, which continued until failing health obliged him to retire. After a residence in that city of about twenty years, he died of pulmonary disease universally regretted.

Dr. Kellog was twice married; first, in 1830. It was announced at Belleville on October 1, 1834, that Matilda, wife of Dr. Jabez Kellog, died in the twenty-eighth year of her age.

In October, 1835, he married Miss Mary, a sister of the Rev. Dr. Macnab. His only surviving son, Stephen Benson, was educated in Hamilton; afterwards read for Holy Orders under the Rev. Dr. Macnab, Rector of Darlington; was ordained in 1860; and, after a signally useful life, died at St. Thomas, Ont., in 1874, being rector of that parish, and universally beloved wherever known.

"Died at Cobourg, September 26, 1849, Mary, wife of Dr. Jabez Kellog."

The only daughter of Dr. Kellog is Mrs. Alfred Stow, of Hamilton.

DR. ALEXANDER KENNEDY.

Through the kindness of Dr. G. M. Shaw, the following information respecting Dr. Alexander Kennedy has been obtained:

Alexander Kennedy, born, September 23, 1802, near Dumfries, Scotland, took his degree at Edinburgh. Married his cousin, Agnes McDougall, in 1836. Came to Canada in 1845. Was two months in Hamilton; thence moved to the township of Binbrook. He purchased 200 acres, intending to clear the bush and cultivate the soil, but he was not allowed to farm in peace. So he engaged in practice, and continued until his death in 1867. His services were, highly appreciated by many. He possessed abilities of a high order.

DR. ROBERT KERR.

The following testimonials give interesting information of the events at that time, apart from the particulars respecting Dr. Kerr:

"MONTREAL, *June* 3rd, 1787.

"I do certify that Mr. Kerr, Surgeon to Sir John Johnson's 2nd Battalion from the time of its being raised to that of its being disbanded, discharged his duty with the greatest zeal in the line of his profession, and that the Service is much indebted to him, not only for his care and attention to the sick of that regiment, but to those of a variety of other corps, also Loyalists and Indians, at the posts of Carlton Island, Oswego, and Cataraqui, where he served for four years under my command.

"JOHN ROSS,
"*Major 34th Regt.*"

"CARLTON ISLAND, *May* 10th, 1787.

"DEAR SIR,—Being now on the eve of quitting the charge I had over the Loyalists in this district, I cannot in justice to your merit, before that event takes place, but thank you for your great care and attention to all ranks of those people where your assistance was necessary, and I hope for the good of the settlement that Government will give you every encouragement necessary to induce you to remain with them, as the knowledge you have of the people and country renders you much fitter for that service than any other person of your profession, even of equal abilities. That prosperity may attend your endeavours and you may live long to watch over the health of your people is the warmest wish of

"Dear Sir, etc.,

"(Signed) NEIL MCLEAN,
"*D. Inspector of Loyalists.*

"*To* MR. ROBERT KERR,
"*Surgeon to the Loyalists in the District of Cataraqui.*"

[Neil McLean was the father of Archibald McLean, Chief Justice of Upper Canada. He acted a conspicuous part in repelling the invaders on the St. Lawrence in the war of 1812. He was in command of the Stormont Militia at Chrysler's Farm.]

The exact time at which Dr. Kerr came to Newark to settle is uncertain; not unlikely he obtained the appointment of Surgeon to the Indian Department soon after he ceased to be acting hospital mate at Cataraqui in 1788. It has been recorded on a previous page that he was at Newark in the beginning of 1797, practising inoculation for the small-pox, but a traveller mentions his name as living at Newark in 1792. He did not give all his time to the work of the Department, but engaged in private practice, but likely he, from time to time, visited distant Indian posts. He acquired the reputation of being an "eminent surgeon."

His connection with the Indian Department continued for many years. Gourlay speaks of him in 1817 as "Surgeon to the Indian Department of Upper Canada at Fort George." In 1823, he is mentioned as on the "Military Staff, Indian Department, Niagara," and as on the "Militia General Staff." That he took an active part in medical matters during the war of 1812 is certain. In the programme of the funeral procession of General Brock, October 16, 1812, he was allotted a conspicuous place. He became a member of the Medical Board in 1823, but his name appears but twice as present.

Dr. Kerr occupied a good many public positions. He was appointed a Public School Trustee by the Lieutenant-Governor in 1807, and again in 1822-23. He was Principal of the Surrogate Court for Niagara.

In 1806, he was one of five appointed to be magistrates at Niagara. In this judicial capacity Dr. Kerr was well known; no one found fault with his decisions; but it was thought he was too fond of sport, especially boxing, and he was familiarly called the "boxing magistrate." He was a prominent Mason, and in 1823, he is mentioned as "Past Deputy Provincial Grand Master of the United Fraternity of Free Masons." He drew a large quantity of land. Dr. Kerr married a sister of Captain Brant. Had children, three or four sons and two daughters, all remarkably handsome. We find the record, October 3, 1816, that Robert Gillespie, of Montreal, was married to Anna Agnes Kerr, at St. Mark's. The youngest (Mary Margaret) married the Hon. Thomas Clark. Simcoe Kerr became Chief of the Mohawk nation. Was a lawyer, and practised in Hamilton.

"Died, March, 1824, Robert Kerr, aged sixty years, Surgeon in the Indian Department."

DR. JOHN KING

Was a native of Tuam, county of Galway, where he was born, 1806. He was a student at Trinity College, Dublin, also Licentiate Accoucheur of the Lying-in Hospital, Dublin. Subsequently he became Doctor of Medicine of the University of Edinburgh, and Licentiate of the Royal College of Surgeons. This was in 1830, when he was about twenty-five years of age, and soon after he set out for Canada, coming to Quebec to his uncle, Dr. Wm. Lyons, Staff-Surgeon, then quartered at Quebec, who was his mother's brother. Another uncle was John Lyons, for many years Registrar of Niagara. Dr. King did not tarry long at Quebec, but came on to York, and at once commenced the practice of his profession. He was gazetted as a Licentiate of Upper Canada, July 22, 1830. His standing was soon recognized by the Governor, as we find his name mentioned as present as member of the Medical Board at the January meeting, 1832. We find him a very regular attendant at the Board meetings for many years. His name last appears at the April session, 1855, when he was in the chair. Of his success as a practitioner, Mr. Clarke Gamble writes: "The more notable practitioner after them (Widmer and Deihl) was Dr. King, a true Irishman and the most liberal of men I ever met. He was an exceedingly clever, skilful physician and surgeon, and soon built up a most successful practice. He was a great favourite with everybody with whom he came in contact." In April, 1833, Dr. King was added to the list of magistrates of the town of York. The Doctor found time to take part in most public affairs, and was an active worker at the election of the first mayor of Toronto, Wm. Lyon Mackenzie, and at a dinner that year in honour of St. Patrick, a serious misunderstanding arose between His Worship and Dr. King. Gossiping tongues told of a challenge to fight a duel, of its acceptance, and of one of the combatants notifying the authorities so that all parties would be arrested and no blood spilt. How much truth there was in all this is now unknown. One thing is certain, the Doctor, with all his kindly nature, was, like an Irishman, hot-tempered, and history tells us that W. L. Mackenzie was all that in early days. Dr. King was one of the first aldermen of the newly incorporated city, and was elected for several succeeding years. In 1833, Dr. King was married by the Right Rev. Bishop McDonnell, to Amelia, second daughter of Livius Peters Sherwood, Speaker of the House of Assembly, afterwards the Hon. Justice Sherwood. During the rebellion of 1837, Dr. King was surgeon to the Queen's Toronto Guard. Dr. King, being always conspicuous in every movement to advance the profession, worked to secure the organization of the Medical Department of King's College, of which he was the Professor of Theory and Practice of Medicine. He was appointed by the Lieut.-Governor in 1843, and held that position while the College lasted, and then in the Toronto University until the Medical Department was abolished. During the years 1848 and 1849, he received an increase of salary of £55 11 2, an allowance for clinical lectures at the Hospital. Dr. King was long a member of the hospital staff, where his skill as a physician was apparent to all, and some of his old pupils still remember his kindly interest in their welfare and sound instruction. The writer will never forget the time when he followed the Doctor through the wards of the old hospital at the corner of King and John Streets, nor his mingled feelings of alarm and admiration to see the Doctor perform one of the first surgical operations he had ever witnessed.

The welfare of the city was always a matter of great moment to Dr. King, and in the matter of public health he took a leading part, being Chairman of the Board of Health.

Dr. King died while comparatively a young man, in 1857. Again a quotation is made from a written statement by Mr. Clarke Gamble respecting him: "He was well educated and passionately fond of his profession. He had a large practice for many years, and although a Roman Catholic, was very popular with the Orange body; personally I don't think he had an enemy. For many years before he died he was a great sufferer from his liver, which interfered a good deal with his practice, and I think he was eventually carried off by an abscess or some complication of disorder in that offending organ. He told me an anecdote of his going to New York to consult the then celebrated surgeon, Dr. Mott, who coolly proposed to his brother surgeon to cut off the ends of two ribs to get a look at his liver, and actually brought his instruments, attendants, etc., into poor King's room, and began to open his cases and display his instruments to the sufferer's gaze. Whatever modern surgery may have now achieved, this was too much for Dr. King, who, sitting up in bed (which he had not done for ten days), told the New York surgeon that he seemed to forget that his patient was as good a surgeon as himself, and if he did not pack up his traps and leave the room in five minutes (with an oath), suffering as he was he would kick him out. Mott disappeared.

The excitement did King good—the next day he got up and dressed himself and returned home."

Dr. King died, January 12, 1857, aged 53.

His widow, who was quite young when she married, still mourns her husband, and is in the enjoyment of vigorous life (November, 1889). Eleven children were born to them, of which only one is now living, the eldest son, Capt. King, of the British army, who now resides in London, England. One son, John Lyons, entered the medical profession. He was a brilliant student, obtained the diploma of the Royal College of Surgeons, England, and commanded until his death a large practice in Toronto. He was for a time one of the staff of the Victoria Medical College. He married a daughter of W. A. Murray, so well known in Toronto. A daughter became the wife of Dr. Winer, who practised at Hamilton and then at Chicago, where he died. The widow was afterwards married to Dr. Norman Bethune. She died a few years ago.

"On Tuesday, the 12th of April, 1891, at 50 Mutual Street, Toronto, Amelia, widow of the late Dr. King, and daughter of the late Judge Sherwood, in the 76th year of her age."

DR. RICHARD S. KING

Was born in Wexford, Ireland, 1817. Became a member of the Royal College of Surgeons, Ireland. He was for a short time in practice at Manchester, England, and then emigrated to Canada in 1844, and lived for a time with his brother-in-law, Dr. Morris, Fort Erie. He then commenced practice at Stonebridge. In 1847, he removed to Port Robinson, and took charge of the practice of Dr. Campbell. He was appointed to the medical charge of the troops stationed along the Welland Canal. Took an active part in volunteer movement, originating in the Trent affair, and in 1861, organized the Welland Canal Field Battery, of which he became Captain, and was in command in 1866, when the Fenians, under O'Neil, invaded the frontier. Was severely wounded in the engagement by a rifle-ball, and had to have his left leg amputated. His gallantry on that occasion gained him great praise. He was presented with two swords of honour, beside innumerable complimentary addresses. For the loss of his leg he was granted a pension by the Crown. In 1870, had command of volunteers at Port Robinson. He died, August, 1885.

A son of Dr. R. S. King entered the profession, and, after practising in Buffalo for a time, settled in St. Catharines, where he is now in practice.

DR. JOHN JOHNSTON LAFFERTY.

In the old church register of St. Mark's Church, Niagara, is the record that on August 17, 1800, John Johnston Lafferty was married to Mary Johnston. This was a daughter of an Indian of some renown, of Grand River, who had a white woman for his wife, and had received the cognomen of "Cogniac" Johnston. Dr. Lafferty practised his profession, and died at Drummondville; but the date at which he took up his abode there cannot be learned. It is stated by one authority that he had been a surgeon in the British army. Another says he was a doctor of the old school, with natural abilities, but he had not had many advantages. He had a large and extensive practice, and became popular; also well known throughout the Province in his capacity as member of the Provincial Legislature, having been elected for the county of Lincoln in 1828. He was conspicuous for his vigorous action in the discharge of his parliamentary duties; and his large, portly presence, his loud, sonorous voice, and forcible language made him a conspicuous figure in society at the young capital. Dr. Scadding, whose father's house he was in the habit of visiting on Sundays while in York, informs the writer that he had a striking appearance, with a head of bushy, grey hair. In 1834, he was defeated at the polls by David Thorburn, by one vote. Although the Doctor was at times given to the use of profane language, yet he would occupy the sacred desk in a school-house near his own residence, when no clergyman was at hand to discharge the duty. He would read the service and a sermon. It is related that on one occasion, a hot Sunday, when engaged in this sacred function, he happened to look out of the window, and found that the sheep had escaped into a field, and were committing mischief. He promptly put his head out of the window, and shouted to his son to "take the d——d sheep back again."

He carried on farming and was a great admirer of good horses, and always had the best. It was said of him that during the war of 1812, when he was amputating a soldier's leg he suspended the operation to have a look at a fine horse going by. He had a family of four sons and three daughters. Bryan, the eldest, died at Chicago, August, 1836. John became a doctor, and died at Brantford, where he had gone to practise. One daughter married Dr. Blackwell, who succeeded Dr. Lafferty, at Drummondville, after his death. The youngest, Julia, married George Miller, of Nelson, June 11, 1834.

In 1818, Dr. Lafferty, with a Dr. Smith, had an apothecary shop in the village of St. Catharines. The Doctor was considered skilful in his profession. In 1824, he was appointed surgeon to the 2nd Lincoln Regiment of Militia. The Doctor was not given to new ways, and it is said that after he had seen Dr. Telfer, who had just come to Niagara, using the stethoscope, he told a friend that the sight of the Doctor using a "telescope" was enough for him. He died, October 26, 1842, in his sixty-fifth year.

His popularity was attested by the presence of an immense concourse of people at his funeral. "There are a few left who will remember the old Doctor and his brown horse, John." One personally acquainted with Dr. Lafferty says: "He was a kind-hearted, hospitable man; it may be said of him, a fine old gentleman of the old Canadian school."

The following is from "Sketches of Canada," by W. L. Mackenzie, 1833: "Dr. Lafferty, who is a native of the province (now state) of New Jersey, and the son of a former attorney-general of that colony, served as a surgeon to the forces in the time of the war (1812); had his premises destroyed, and is not yet recompensed; and had his establishment again burnt, while attending at the Legislature at York. I stopped a day or two with him at Lundy's Lane, before the sad destruction of his house, and copy from my note-book a list of the curiosities: 'Visited this eccentric legislator, and by way of whiling away the time, took a list of all the rare and curious things, animate and inanimate, about his establishment, which is a handsome one. And first, I may enumerate himself; then a part of a mammoth's tooth, taken out of a lower jaw found on the Missouri by Mr. Stewart. It is very ponderous. A piece of Indian crockery, made of a composition of shell powdered and mixed with clay; it was brought from the Arkansas territory. A wild goose tamed; this animal was very polite, indeed, and bowed to those who fed it, with dignity. A white owl measures from tip to tip of wing, across the back, five feet four inches. The great pig. The Louisiana State pig. Two thigh-bones; one of an Indian, very large, and had been in his lifetime fractured and broken, but had ossified and got firmly together again. Skulls, jaw-bones, drum-sticks, pistols, the skeleton of an American goldfinch, a noble head of deer's horns, three or four nondescripts in bottles, preserved in whiskey, for their uncommon ugliness; 3,569 doctor's phials, bottles and jars, filled with fluids, unguents and powders of various kinds, several of the labels on which it would dislocate the strongest pair of jaws that ever lodged in a human head to pronounce. Guns, powder-horns, Journals of Assembly, Pharmacopœias, Alien Question Resolutions, *Colonial Advocate*, carefully filed (a remarkable and convincing instance of this gentleman's wisdom and good sense). *Observer*. (Several numbers of this journal were wrapped round two stuffed rattlesnakes.) Joe Bofanti on the chimney-piece. Military sashes, daggers, anatomy books, skates (a pair), five cats (two of them jet black), two dogs, mortars and pestles; specimens of petrifactions of leaves, "Lucan's Pharsalia" (1636), an electrifying machine, Greek books in abundance, and a large hornet's nest in good preservation.' I was told that Derbyshire spar (lime with the fluoric acid) may be found at the whirlpool, but had not time to go to see it."

The Doctor has a standing song, "Twelve Bottles More," and an everlasting anecdote, the authenticity of which has been disputed. The last time I heard it was in the Assembly's Chamber upon the militia question: "If," said the Doctor, "it should be determined to adopt the American laws here, and to allow the men to elect their officers, and then domineer over them—the consequences would be just the same as it had been in General Hull's army, during the invasion of Canada. One evening the General heard a noise near his tent, and sent out to inquire the cause. The reply was: 'Oh, nothing at all, General, merely a company of Kentuckians who are busy riding their captain on a rail!'"

DR. JAMES LANGSTAFF,

Born at Thornhill, Yonge Street, 1825, was the son of John Langstaff, who came from New Jersey, 1808, coming the whole way, it is told, on horseback. He settled on Yonge Street, and married Lucy, daughter of Abner Miles, of Richmond Hill. He was bookkeeper in the Commissariat Department during the war of 1812-14. He died, 1863, aged 89. James, the subject of this sketch, was the youngest of eight children. He studied medicine with Dr. Rolph, as a house pupil, for two years, and proceeding to England he attended Guy's Hospital for two years. He obtained an honorary certificate for Clinical Reports from Guy's. Returning to Canada, he passed the Upper Canada Medical Board, April, 1849, and at once commenced practice at Unionville. In the following September he settled at Richmond Hill, where he continued to practise until his death. He was for a short time lecturer at Rolph's School. Was twice married: first to Mary Ann, daughter of Henry Miller, of Thornhill; secondly, to E. F. Louisa, daughter of J. W. Palmer, of Whitby. Had four children by first wife.

DR. WILLIAM LEE.

"Died at York, 1st July, 1833, Dr. William Lee, in the 70th year of his age. Dr. Lee was an old servant of the Government, having been appointed surgeon's mate to the 49th Regiment in the year 1786, and to the 24th Regiment, in 1788. On the removal of the regiment to Canada, he was stationed for some years at Quebec. He was for a considerable time attached to the Indian Department on the Island of St. Joseph, at the port of Michilimackinac, at Amherstburgh, and subsequently at York, where, on the general reduction which was made in 1815, he was placed on a retired allowance. In the following year he was appointed Gentleman Usher of the Black Rod to the Honourable the Legislative Council, and after the formation of the Medical Board of the Province, he was appointed Secretary. Dr. Lee was an inhabitant of York from 1807 for a period of twenty-six years, during which time he secured the esteem of numerous friends, and by a cheerful disposition and unassuming demeanour acquired general respect and regard."—*The Patriot.*

While stationed at York, Dr. Lee not only dealt out medicine to the Indians visiting that place, but had to make long journeys to distant Indian settlements to prescribe for and administer medicine, even as far as Penetanguishene, which he did on horseback by bridle-paths, carrying the drugs in his saddle-bag. He took part in all the events connected with early York. He was rather short in stature and stout, had a good head, but owing to some infirmity he had a halting gait. He was Coroner for the Home District, and was appointed Surgeon to the 1st West York Regiment Militia in 1822.

Of his children, Wm. Henry, who married a granddaughter of Dr. Gamble, was connected with the public service for more than half a century. Born at Three Rivers, 1799. Entered the Civil Service in 1821. He was promoted from time to time until 1867, when he was made Clerk of the Queen's Privy Council for Canada, the chief executive authority in the Dominion. In 1872, he was superannuated, at which time the members of the Privy Council testified to his long and faithful services by presenting him with a valuable silver urn.

He died at Ottawa, September, 1878, leaving a good record in every respect. A daughter of Dr. Lee, Ann Elizabeth Lavinia, married Wm. Stanton, Deputy Assistant Commissary-General.

DR. EBENEZER LEE

Was born, 1727, at Canaan or Farmington, Connecticut, and married, June 20, 1750, Abigail Bull, who was born at Canaan, in 1728. Place of medical study unknown, but believed to be Yale. Came to Canada, 1796 or 1797. Settled at Burford Gore, now known as Oakland, Upper Canada. He died, May 9, 1811, and his wife Abigail died, January 11, 1812.

DR. WILLIAM HOOKER LEE,

Sixth son of the above, born, February 10, 1761, at Old Canaan, Connecticut, married, 1787, Phœbe Davis, who was born at Reading, Connecticut, January 24, 1771. Place of medical study unknown. He came to Canada with his father, and practised at Chippawa and Niagara District, but ultimately removed to Southwold, London District (now county of Elgin), where he died, March 30, 1829. Dr. William Hooker had thirteen children; two sons followed the medical profession, viz., Hiram Davis (third son) and James Clark (ninth son).

DR. HIRAM DAVIS LEE,

Born at Clarknett, November 20, 1791, was only a few years old when brought to Canada by his father. He was an intimate friend of the late Dr. Rolph, under whom he studied medicine at York. He was appointed Government Medical Officer for London, Upper Canada, holding a license signed by Sir John Colborne, Lieutenant-Governor of Upper Canada, dated at York, 14th day of October, 1833, which states: "He, the said Hiram D. Lee, having exhibited the proof of qualification and other testimonials as required by law." While a medical student he acted as army surgeon in the Niagara District during the war of 1812-15; afterwards he practised medicine some time in Southwold, London District; afterwards at Chippawa, Niagara District, and latterly in London, Canada West. He was Government Medical Officer for London, for which appointment the above-mentioned license was given. He died at London, September 28, 1847, during an epidemic of typhus fever, his death being attributed to his indefatigable exertions to attend his patients most carefully. The following was the obituary notice contained in the *Church Newspaper*, of October, 1847, London, Upper Canada:

"DEATH OF DR. LEE.—In a succeeding column our readers will find the distressing obituary of an able and intrepid physician, Dr. Lee, whose self-sacrifice on the altar of duty well deserves to be classed in the rank of martyrdom. The bereavement which society at large suffers from the loss of men like Dr. Lee is one of the most afflicting features of the fearful disease which has been brought into the Province by our late unhealthy immigration."

Dr. Hiram Davis Lee married, 1819, Annie Terry, daughter of Parshall Terry, a U.E. Loyalist of the Erie District. They had twelve children: Elvira, married to James B. Strathy, J.P., now residing at Kingston, Ont.; Simcoe Lee, residing in Philadelphia; Annie, married to Charles B. Daly, civil engineer, of Kingston, Ont.; Louisa, married to Herbert Austin, of New York; Edmund Roscoe Lee, living at Detroit (1890).

DR. JOHN ROLPH LEE, the eldest son, was a student with Dr. John Rolph, and afterwards studied and graduated at McGill College, May, 1843. In the same month he was accidentally drowned in the Grand River, near Brantford, through the capsizing of a boat.

DR. FREDERIC ROLPH LEE STRATHY is the son of Elvira Lee, eldest child of Dr. Hiram Davis Lee and wife of James Brakenridge Strathy, formerly of the "Pines," London, Ont., but now residing in Kingston, Ont. He was born, January 25, 1849, educated at Upper Canada College and Hellmuth College, London, Ont. Entered Victoria College as a medical student in 1866, and graduated in 1870 as M.D. In 1870 he proceeded to Edinburgh, and in the following spring obtained the diplomas of the Royal College of Physicians and also of the Royal College of Surgeons. He remained in Edinburgh till 1873, holding various hospital appointments. Afterwards he spent some time in London and Paris, returning to Canada in September, 1873. After a few months he became surgeon on the Allan Line of ocean steamers. In October, 1874, he settled in Harborne, a suburb of Birmingham, and has been practising there ever since.

Dr. Strathy was the third generation who studied under Dr. Rolph. For many generations the Lees were members of the medical profession.

DR. JAMES LISTER,

Surgeon and physician, who practised in Belleville for thirty-seven years, was one of the best educated professional men in this part of the Province. He was a son of Capt. Lister, long a commander of the Coast Guards, at Cowes, in the Isle of Wight, and was born in London, Eng., June 30, 1811. When twelve years old he was placed in a large private school near Cork, where he received an English and classical education. He then went to Dublin, took a thorough course of study in surgery, and received his degree in that branch of the healing art, and thence repaired to London, where he took a hospital course and became a member of the Royal College of Surgeons, London, 1834. In 1862, he received the degree of M.D. from McGill College, Montreal. Thoroughly equipped, Dr. Lister entered upon the active and responsible duties of his profession, practising six years near Barnstable, Devonshire. In 1841, he emigrated to Upper Canada and settled at Belleville, where he continued in constant practice until his death, March 23, 1878. He had an extensive general practice, especially in surgery, for which he always had a predilection. His reputation was not limited to one locality, as he was called to distant parts, even to Montreal and New York.

He was greatly esteemed for his kindness, as well as skill, at the sick-bed, and for his generosity to the unfortunate; was constant in his attendance upon the poor, for which he received and expected no remuneration. He never thought of asking that class of patients for a penny; and if he had one fault it was carelessness in making collections of those abundantly able to compensate him for his services. It is doubtful if he received fifty per cent. of his annual charges, and yet he left his family in comfortable circumstances. He was ever a self-sacrificing man, never refusing to respond to a call while he was in good health whatever might be the state of the weather. The result was, that overwork and exposure partially undermined his constitution, and he was an invalid for some years before he died.

Dr. Lister grew up in the Church of England, and was a constant attendant on Divine worship all his days, and lived a pure, exemplary and noble life. He married, October 4, 1843, Margaret, daughter of Dr. George Cowper, of Belleville.

Much of the foregoing is taken, at the instance of Mrs. Lister, from the "Canadian Biographical Dictionary" (1880), American Biographical Publishing Co. It was the writer's privilege to have the friendship of Dr. Lister. He has a very pleasant recollection of Dr. Lister as a fellow-practitioner in Belleville. His attitude towards a junior in the profession was very kindly and considerate.

DR. DAVID LITHGOW

Was gazetted, March 5, 1834, as licensed to practise. He published this card: "D. Lithgow, M.D., F.R.S.G. & C., being obliged to remain a short time in Canada, begs leave, respectfully, to offer his professional assistance to such of the inhabitants of the city of Toronto as may require it; and from his many years' experience and extensive practice he does so with confidence.

"Dr. Lithgow is a graduate of the University of Edinburgh, has his diploma as a member of the College of Surgeons as an accoucheur, and was lately President of the Royal Physical Society of Edinburgh, etc. The necessary documents to that effect he has laid before His Excellency Sir John Colborne, and they have been honoured with his approval.

"Dr. Lithgow has lodgings at present at No. 8 Richmond Street, where he can be consulted, or any direction left for him at the *Courier* office will be immediately attended to, and he will feel pleasure in giving his gratuitous attention to the poor *at all times.*

"Toronto, March 4, 1834."

Dr. Lithgow was not only a man of ability, but of enterprise and ambition, as the following announcement shows. But his project was altogether premature and came to nothing:

"*School of Anatomy, Surgery and Medicine, Toronto, under the immediate superintendence of* D. LITHGOW, M.D., ETC., ETC., *of the University of Edinburgh.*

"Dr. Lithgow, having taken that large and central brick

building, No. 17 Newgate Street, will open it as a general School of Medical Science early in the month of November. It shall be conducted on a plan precisely similar to those institutions in the Old Country, which have acquired such deserved celebrity from the professional gentlemen educated in them. During the season lectures will be delivered upon Anatomy and Surgery, Physiology and Medical Jurisprudence, Materia Medica, Chemistry, Practice of Physic and Midwifery.

"The Anatomical Demonstrations will be under the direction of a Licentiate of the Royal College of Surgeons, Dublin; the other courses of lectures by medical practitioners in extensive practice and of acknowledged talent, particulars of which will be made known hereafter.

"The session will be opened upon Wednesday, 12th of November, by the delivery of the first of a short course of lectures upon 'The Duties and Qualifications of a Medical Practitioner,' by Dr. Lithgow.

"Further particulars may be known by application to Dr. Lithgow as to terms of indoor or outdoor pupils, terms of lectures, etc.

"Toronto, September 24, 1834."

"*Public Dispensary and School of Medicine,*
No. 17 Newgate Street.

"Dr. Lithgow will attend every morning, between the hours of 9 and 10 o'clock, at his house, No. 17 Newgate Street, to give advice *gratis* to such persons as may require his professional services.

"Poor persons, who bring a certificate from any respectable citizen of their inability to pay, shall receive medicine *gratuitously*.

"Toronto, November 24, 1834."

He seems to have settled afterwards in Hamilton as the following shows:

"MELANCHOLY DEATH.—It is with the most poignant feelings we announce the death of David Lithgow, Esq., M.D., at his lodgings in this town, which took place this morning very suddenly. An inquest held by D. C. Beard, Esq., Coroner, has just closed its sitting, and who returned the following verdict: 'That the deceased came to his death from having taken a quantity of laudanum, or some such other deleterious substance, while labouring under a state of mental derangement and not otherwise.' Dr. Lithgow was highly esteemed in this town and neighbourhood, and his decease is greatly lamented."—*Hamilton Gazette, 1836.*

DR. GEORGE HUMPHREY LOW,

Of Trinity College, Dublin, son of Captain Low, of Ireland, who served under General Wolfe at the taking of Quebec, emigrated to Canada in 1833, and settled at Whitby, where he first commenced practice in Upper Canada. During the rebellion of 1837 he was Surgeon to the East York Militia. Subsequently removing to Port Hope, he remained there several years and then settled in Darlington. Being eminent in his profession, especially as a surgeon, he had in Bowmanville and surrounding country an extensive and lucrative practice. He died in September, 1865, aged 75 years, at his residence, Rathscamoy, Bowmanville.

DR. JAMES McCAGUE,

Of York, passed Medical Board, January 2, 1828. He seems to have practised at York for a number of years before settling about ten miles up Yonge Street. His practice extended on every hand, a contemporary says perhaps sixty miles, which he attended to on horseback. A fine-looking, portly Irishman, with a frank countenance and genial manners, with a tendency to be "wild," he was a great favourite everywhere. Dr. Scadding says he practised first at Thornhill, and was an impulsive Irishman.

Dr. McCague addressed a letter to the *Patriot*, Aug. 26, 1834, urging the efficacy of a remedy he had discovered for cholera in its worst stages. A. C. Robinson, M.R.C.S. Lond., at that time practising in Toronto, testifies as to its value in one case he had seen. The medium was "plumbi supernacit," two grains in an ounce of water. An advertisement appeared, August, 1834, by Dr. James McCague, of the sale of a farm on Yonge Street, ten miles from Toronto. When Colonel Moodie was shot by the rebels at Montgomery's Tavern, 1837, Dr. McCague was called to attend him. He was Surgeon to the 4th North York Militia. This notice appeared, March, 1839: "Died, at his residence on Yonge Street, Dr. James McCague, native of Monaghan, Ireland, and particularly distinguished during the late outbreak for his unswerving attachment to the Constitution, and for his bravery and exertion on all occasions." He left a large family.

DR. WILLIAM MCCARGOW,

The youngest child of Adam McCargow, who had retired from business, was born, May, 1819, in the Abbey Parish, Paisley, Scotland. When about fourteen, he commenced his medical studies with James Paton, M.D., with whom he applied himself diligently for three years and a half. In 1836, he commenced his collegiate course at Glasgow College, attending the lectures of Dr. Jaffery on anatomy and Dr. Thos. Thompson on chemistry. The well-known Norman McLeod was at this time a student, and he took a great interest in the election of Sir Robert Peel as Lord Proctor. Dr. McCargow was present at a meeting and heard Sir Robert's eloquent speech. His subsequent studies were carried on with a view of entering the Royal Navy. He therefore attended the best of the lectures at the College and medical schools, and put in the usual attendance at the Glasgow Royal Infirmary. Having passed the Faculty of Glasgow, and a vacancy having occurred in the Paisley House of Recovery, of house-surgeon, he was appointed to that office in 1841, after a competitive examination.

In the spring of 1842, he was induced to accept an offer from his brother-in-law, William McPherson, M.D., to join him in practice at York, on the Grand River, then in Niagara District. Accordingly he shipped at Glasgow in May, and arrived at Hamilton in July. He passed the Upper Canada Medical Board, July, 1843. After three years the partnership with Dr. McPherson was dissolved.

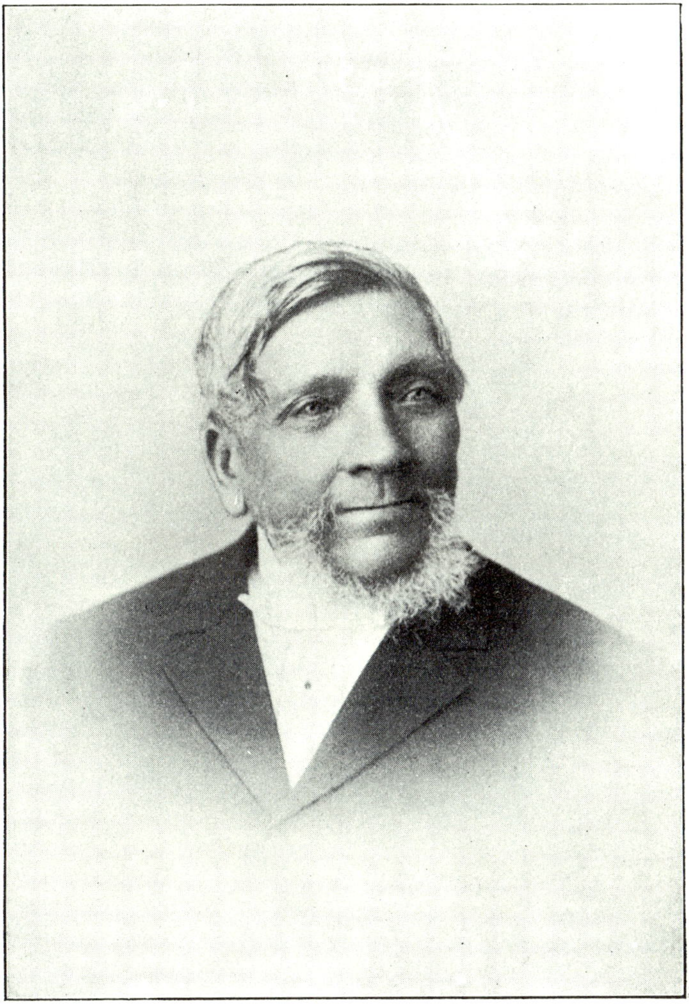

DR. WILLIAM McCARGOW.

April 24, 1846, he married Mary, second daughter of John Jackson, Civil Engineer, of Seneca. Among the first medical societies organized in this part of the Province was one by Dr. McPherson and Dr. McCargow, known as the "County of Haldimand Medical Association." He was also for a year or two a member of the first medical society in Hamilton. He was appointed to the position of medical attendant of the Six Nation Indians, 1865. This position he held until failing health compelled him to resign in 1882, when his adopted son, Dr. R. J. McKinnon, received the appointment. He held the position of a magistrate of Haldimand from 1856 until he left the country. In 1858, the office of Assistant-Surgeon of the 3rd Battalion, Haldimand, was given to him. In 1872, he held the position of corresponding member for the Gynæcological Society of Boston. He was an active member of the Canada Medical Association, and was also one of the Medical Council of the College of Physicians and Surgeons of Ontario, 1880-85. After an active practice of forty years on the Grand River, failing health compelled him to remove to Hamilton, where for some years he has been on the consulting staff of the City Hospital.

Dr. McCargow writes: "Reverting back to my forty years of practice on the Grand River, for the first fifteen or twenty years, but more particularly for the first ten years, remittents prevailed to a large extent from about the middle of July to the middle of December of each year. Then, during the remaining months, in every house there were persons suffering fom intermittents. There were occasionally severe epidemics of dysentery, which proved very fatal to the aged and children. When the potato-rot appeared in Canada, I had many cases of scurvy. Children were the greatest sufferers from it. The woodman's axe, the foundry, threshing machines and the implements of husbandry were fruitful sources of accidents to all parts of the body, particularly to the hands and limbs, so much so that amputations were frequent."

Dr. McCargow has no children, except by adoption, one of whom, the late Dr. Ranald J. McKinnon, died at Oshweken, Brant County, on March 11, 1887. An adopted daughter is the youngest daughter of the late Colonel Wallace, of Norwich.

DR. RODERICK McDONALD

Was son of John McDonald, who came from Scotland before the beginning of the present century, and settled in Cornwall. Roderick was born in Glengarry, and educated at the Cornwall Grammar School, and at Montreal. Studied medicine at McGill College, and took his M.D., 1834. He passed the Upper Canada Medical Board, October, 1835. He settled at Cornwall, and engaged in active practice until 1846, when he was elected Treasurer of the United Counties of Dundas and Glengarry. Dr. McDonald was twice elected member of parliament, serving eight years. He held commissions in the militia force, and attained to the rank of Lieut.-Colonel. He was Surgeon to the forces during the Mackenzie rebellion, and at the time of the Trent affair he was in command of the 1st Battalion of Stormont Militia. In 1862, he became Deputy Clerk of the Crown and Pleas. Dr. McDonald died, April 7, 1885.

DR. WILLIAM McGILL

Was born at Glasgow about 1814, being the son of George McGill. The family emigrated to Canada while William was yet young, and settled on a farm in the township of Whitby. William was educated at the Grammar School at Oshawa. He commenced the study of medicine with Dr. H. Low, 1835. Then attended two courses of lectures at Willoughby Medical College, Ohio, 1837-39. He commenced practice at Oshawa in 1841. In 1847, he attended McGill College, where he took the degree of M.D., 1848. By this time Dr. McGill was unusually well equipped to practise his profession; but he subsequently attended lectures at the New York University. He stood very high as a practitioner, and enjoyed the reputation of being a capital surgeon. Dr. McGill was elected a member of Ontario Medical Council for King's and Queen's Division, 1866. He was also elected a member of the first Legislature of the Province of Ontario, 1867-71. Dr. McGill was always a student, not only in medicine, but in literature, and of the Bible. As a member of the Disciples' Church, he not only acted as an elder, but frequently occupied the pulpit. He died, November 9, 1883.

He married Julia Ann, daughter of James Bates, of Darlington.

DR. JAMES MCILMURRAY,

M.R.C.S. Eng., 1833; Provincial Licentiate, 1834, under 8th George IV., chap. 3, was born in Tyrone County, Ireland, 1800, and came to Toronto, 1834. He practised in Toronto until his death, 1880. Dr. McIlmurray never married. He was very popular as a physician, to the duties of which he gave all his time. The Doctor, it is related, had a quantity of gold coins at the time of the Mackenzie rebellion. Fearing the rebels would take and pillage the city, he put the gold in a hiding-place in the stable. His servant-man happened to find it, and, being a faithful servant, he informed the Doctor of the treasure-trove, and said he would share it with the Doctor. The result is not recorded. Although Dr. McIlmurray left no relations in Toronto to mourn his loss, his removal by death was keenly felt by many friends, and those to whom he had been a faithful physician.

DR. DANIEL EUGENE MCINTYRE,

Now Sheriff of the United Counties of Stormont, Dundas and Glengarry (1893), was born in the town of Oban, Argyleshire, Scotland, 1812. He was the only son of James McIntyre, Captain in the Merchant Marine Service, who was drowned at sea while Daniel was yet a child. The mother, Mary McLaughlin McIntyre, died in 1819. Young McIntyre was educated at Oban, the parish school of Appin, and at McFarlain's Academy, Glasgow, then a noted school. He took a position in a business house, but after a short time relinquished it, having no taste for a business life. In 1829, he entered the Glasgow University as a medical student. His medical course was continued here until 1834, except one year passed at Edinburgh University. Dr. McIntyre came to Canada in the spring of 1835, and after sojourning a short time at Quebec, came to Upper Canada, and established himself at Williamstown, county of Glengarry. Being a Highlander, he was cordially received by the inhabitants of this Highland settlement, and welcomed with Gaelic words by Gaelic hearts. Dr. McIntyre not only found here congenial friends, but a few years later, 1837, a Canadian Highland wife, in the person of Ann, daughter of Colonel Alex. Fraser, M.L.A.

During the Mackenzie rebellion, Dr. McIntyre was on the staff of the 1st Glengarry Regiment of Militia, as Surgeon. He was on the steamboat *Henry Brougham* when captured at Beauharnois by the rebels, and was for several weeks a prisoner, confined at the house of the parish priest, where he was rescued by the Glengarry Regiment, which took possession of the town. He continued in the militia service as Staff-Surgeon until 1842. Having a taste for military life, he became (1854) Major of the Stormont Battalion. He subsequently retired with the rank of Lieut.-Colonel. He represented the township of Charlottenburg, in the old Eastern District Council for thirteen years, and was the first warden elected for the three united counties, 1849, and again the following year.

A staunch supporter of Baldwin and Lafontaine, he was a warm friend of that distinguished patriotic Canadian, the Hon. John Sandfield Macdonald, and took an energetic part in all the political contests in Glengarry at that period.

In May, 1850, Dr. McIntyre was made sheriff of the united counties, a position he has filled to the great satisfaction of the public. He has had seven children, of whom only two remain alive, a son and a daughter.

DR. ANDREW MCKENZIE.

"The subject of this sketch is a native of Lower Canada, a son of Daniel and Margaret (Gray) McKenzie, and was born at Terrebonne, September 15, 1810. His father was from the Highlands of Scotland, and was engaged for years with the North-West Fur Company.

"Andrew finished his education at the Grammar School of Perth, county of Lanark. At seventeen, commenced the study of medicine with Dr. Robert Gilmour, of Brockville; attended lectures at McGill College, 1829-30, and Glasgow University, 1831-32, and took M.D. at Glasgow University; practised a short time at St. Thomas, Ontario; served in the rebellion (1837-38) as surgeon to the volunteers, and in 1839 settled in London, which has since been his home. In a few years he built up a good practice. Though nearing his seventieth year, he keeps his office open, and waits upon a few families whose physician, in some cases, he has been for twenty or thirty years. Among the older class of citizens of London, few are more warmly esteemed than Dr. McKenzie.

"September 5, 1836, Dr. McKenzie married Isabella Maria, daughter of John Shore."—*Can. Bio. Dict.*, 1880.

We may add that Dr. McKenzie was gaol physician for fifteen years. Dr. Beemer, of the London Asylum, writes, January 8, 1894, respecting Dr. McKenzie, that "though at present over eighty years old, the Doctor is bright and active, and exhibits the same enthusiasm in all things pertaining to the medical science, which has characterized his long and useful professional career."

DR. ROBERT MCLEAN,

Sixth son of John McLean, was born at Martinique, West Indies, 1811, where his father was then serving in the Royal Artillery. The father served in the British army fourteen years, and retired with the rank of Sergeant-Major of the Artillery. The Doctor's mother was Isabella Graham. Both parents were born in Ireland. Two uncles also served in the army. One, Samuel, retired as Captain, after serving forty years; and William retired as Major, after serving sixty years. Both of these had risen from the ranks. Another uncle settled in Kingston. The Doctor's father held a commission as Lieutenant during the Canadian rebellion of 1837, and was present at the attack on the Windmill at Prescott.

Robert acquired his preliminary education at the Bath Academy, which had a high reputation, under the superintendence of the elder Bidwell. The following certificate indicates that he was a pupil of Dr. Sampson: "Kingston, September 16, 1836. I certify that I have known Mr. Robert McLean, student in medicine, for the last four years, and that he is a young gentleman of exemplary moral character, of good literary acquirement, and that he has, during my acquaintance with him, ever evinced a laudable desire to acquire professional knowledge. (Signed) James Sampson, Surgeon."

He also studied at Fairfield, and took a course of lectures at Jefferson College, Philadelphia, and graduated there. Returning to Canada, he passed the Upper Canada Medical Board, July, 1837, and received his license.

Dr. McLean practised at Belleville for a long time. He spent several years in Europe perfecting himself in his profession, and then returned to Kingston. His father had "left him well off in worldly goods; but the Doctor being of a generous nature, the money did not stay with him." The popularity of Dr. McLean is shown in the following extract from a communication from M. Flanagan, Esq., the much-respected City Clerk of Kingston. He says: "At a meeting of the common Council of the town of Kingston, April 7, 1846, Dr. Robert McLean was unanimously elected Mayor of Kingston, for the year ending first Monday in April, 1847; but his term of office expired with the old town on the 13th June, 1846, Kingston being then incorporated as a city. The Doctor, at this time, was one of the most popular men in Kingston, and it was considered at the time, he would, and could, contest this constituency with every prospect of success." It seems, however, that he did not seek parliamentary honours.

Dr. McLean was commissioned Surgeon of the 2nd Lennox Regiment of Militia, June, 1838. About the year 1850, he retired from practice, and passed his last days with his only surviving brother, Henry, who lived at the homestead, lot 19, concession 6, Ernesttown.

There is only one descendant of the family now living, Robt. McLean, of Harrowsmith.

DR. JAMES MACAULAY.

Dr. Macaulay's association with Upper Canada began with that of Colonel Simcoe, the first Governor of the Province, in

1792. As Simcoe was the first Chief Magistrate of the Province, so Dr. Macaulay held the chief position with respect to medical affairs, first as a member of Governor Simcoe's staff, then as Deputy Inspector-General of Hospitals, and finally as the senior member of the Upper Canada Medical Board, organized in 1819, until July, 1821, six months before his death. From the first meeting of the Board until the time mentioned, Dr. Macaulay was always present.

Dr. Macaulay was not only a prominent person in matters appertaining to medicine, but as one of the worthies who contributed to the welfare of early York, and as the founder of a distinguished family in Upper Canada, his name is conspicuous in the early history of the country.

Dr. Macaulay was a native of Scotland, born, 1759. Of his medical education and what degrees he possessed, there is no record, but we find in different notices of him both M.D. and M.R.C.S.E., attached to his name.

On November 20, 1790, he married Elizabeth Tuck Hayter, a connection of Admiral Hayter. About this time the Imperial Act of Parliament creating the Province of Upper Canada was passed, and Col. Simcoe was appointed the first Lieut.-Governor. It appears most probable that Dr. Macaulay was an intimate friend of Col. Simcoe, who induced the Doctor to join him as physician to his staff. There is evidence of this friendship in the fact that Dr. Macaulay named his eldest son, who was born in England, October, 1791, after Col. Simcoe.

Dr. Macaulay's first connection with the military service was as Surgeon to the 33rd Regiment. After his arrival at Fort Niagara, he became Surgeon to the Queen's Rangers, of which Simcoe was colonel.

When the Rangers were disbanded, it seems that Dr. Macaulay received the appointment of Deputy Inspector-General of Hospitals. Dr. Macaulay's family was living at Newark at the close of 1794, as in the register of St. Mark's Church, Niagara, is the record of the baptism of his second son, dated November 29, 1794. The third son, George, was born at York, 1796, consequently the family moved to York between these two periods. Thus Dr. Macaulay became one of the pioneers in the first settlement of York, and helped to lay the foundation of the capital. The records show that he took an active part in promoting the interests of the place. The *Upper Canada Gazette* records that a meeting was held March 9, 1801, at the Government Buildings, of the subscribers for the opening of Yonge Street. The name of James Macaulay, Esq., M.D., appears first on the list of a Commission appointed to oversee the work. Again, in 1803, the newspapers record that a meeting was held to consider steps to build a church in York, and Dr. Macaulay was one of a "Committee appointed to proceed with the work of building."

Dr. Macaulay received the patent for a park lot, where now is the heart of the city. It extended from Yonge Street westward to University Street, and from Queen Street to College Street. Near the south-east corner of this plot, some years later, a number of small lots were laid out, and upon them buildings were erected. The principal street here received the Doctor's Christian name, and the present James Street marks the spot. This village was separated by woods and fields from the young capital, the western boundary of which reached no farther westward than the present George Street. This village was known for many years as Macaulay Town. Elizabeth Street was named after Mrs. Macaulay. The Macaulay homestead was situated where is now Trinity Square, and was known as "Teraulay Cottage." This name was formed from the last syllable of the names, Hay*ter* and Mac*aulay* (Teraulay). Teraulay Street commemorates this historic and romantic name.

But the requirements of the military service in Canada made it necessary for Dr. Macaulay to leave the capital of Upper Canada for a considerable time. It is learned by a communication from the War Office to Gen. Hunter, dated Jan. 6, 1803, signed by Surgeon-General Keat, which is designated, "Returns of the Hospital Staff proposed to be employed in Upper and Lower Canada, as a peace establishment," that the army surgeons in Canada were duly graded. This document gives James Macaulay as senior hospital officer and Surgeon to the Forces.

It was necessary that the chief medical officer should reside at Quebec, where were the headquarters of the medical staff in Canada. Mr. Longmore, who had been Apothecary to the

Forces, and lived at Quebec, it appears from certain letters, expected to be the principal medical officer. The following letter, however, dispelled such hopes and anticipations:

"ARLINGTON STREET, *January* 5th, 1803.

"SIR,—I am to acquaint you that Mr. Macaulay, Surgeon to the Forces, being senior in the service to yourself, is recommended by me to His Royal Highness, the Commander-in-Chief, to remain in full pay in Nova Scotia, as senior hospital officer, and when the arrangement is approved of, you will be informed thereof and placed on half pay.

"(Signed) T. KEAT,
"*Surg.-Gen. to the Army.*

"MR. LONGMORE,
"*Apothecary to the Forces, Quebec.*"

But Dr. Longmore was unwilling to submit to this arrangement, and sought through the Lieut.-Governor of Upper Canada, Gen. Hunter, who was Commander-in-Chief of the British Forces in North America, to effect something different. And we find, in a letter from him to Major Green, Gen. Hunter's military secretary, dated March 22, 1803, certain suggestions made on the matter: "That Mr. Macaulay's appointment took place during the peace of 1783, and it was thought necessary, on the division of Canada into the Provinces of Upper and Lower Canada, that at the headquarters of each Province there ought to be a Hospital Staff Officer of some standing and responsibility in his profession, to give the principal officers and servants of Government a fair chance and every necessary assistance in cases of sickness and accident. From what I have learned in conversation with the Chief Justice, it would be a great loss to Mr. Macaulay, who has a good farm and well stocked with cattle, etc., in the neighbourhood of York, to be removed from that station, for the avenues to practice in Quebec are at present well secured. It would, therefore, be some years before he could expect to derive much advantage from this source. He would, therefore, find it difficult, with an increasing family, to support the great expense of living in this garrison on his pay and allowances. If, upon the above principles, Gen. Hunter could be induced to think it necessary for the present to continue Mr. Macaulay's residence at York, he might, for similar reasons, perhaps, be inclined to recommend a continuation of my services on the staff at Quebec."

Dr. Longmore's efforts were not without effect, as is seen in a letter from him to Major Green, Gen. Hunter's military secretary, Sept. 13th following, inclosing one from Surgeon Keat, which informs us that he had been reinstated as Apothecary to the Forces. He expresses gratitude to Gen. Hunter, to whom he gives the credit for it. He was instructed to report to the senior hospital officer (Macaulay). By this we learn that at or about this time Dr. Macaulay had removed from York to Quebec. Here he continued until the declaration of war by the United States against Great Britain, in 1812. During his sojourn at Quebec, he suffered the worst bereavement which can overtake an affectionate husband, in the death of a loving wife, March 29, 1809. We find it stated that "she was an accomplished lady, and the loss was felt by all who had enjoyed her society."

The breaking out of war summoned the Doctor to the discharge of important duties in looking after the military hospitals, and the brave militiamen whom the fate of war had brought to him for treatment of wounds or diseases. The time at which Dr. Macaulay left Quebec is shown in the following letter, the original of which is now in the possession of Mrs. E. H. Van Koughnet, of Toronto, a granddaughter:

"CHAMBLY, *August* 17th, 1812.

"MY DEAR FRIENDS,—I am now a hundred and eighty miles from Quebec, on duty, and at present uncertain where I may go to. I will not see the commander of the forces till after tomorrow. I left the children well, seven days ago, at Quebec, and James, second son, at Three Rivers, a lieutenant in the Glengarry Regiment.

"You will have heard that Upper Canada is invaded, and additional regiments are, it is said, on their march to assist General Hill. Whether I may be ordered to that Province to inspect the hospitals there when I have finished in the Lower Province, I am uncertain. I have been travelling for four days in constant rains; there will be much injury done if it continues much longer. You will conclude how very uncomfortable my situation is at present, so many little ones left with servants. I place great dependence on their own prudence, however young.

"I am to set off immediately for the next port, to inspect the hospitals of a battalion of embodied militia. The frigate was to sail on the 20th. I hope this will get to Quebec in time.

"JAS. MACAULAY."

The reference made to his children, who had been deprived of a mother's care, and that he "placed great dependence on their prudence, however young," is a touch of nature which makes us all kin. This letter was addressed to "Rear Admiral Shivers, Wickham, Hampshire, England," whose wife was a sister of Mrs. Macaulay. It is probable that Dr. Macaulay had removed his family from Quebec to Kingston during the war, where he continued to live until the early part of 1817. The Kingston *Gazette*, of May, 1817, advertises a house to let as recently occupied by Dr. Macaulay. Having returned to York, where he was to pass the remainder of his life, we find in the *Gazette*, Nov. 25, 1817, the announcement of his marriage, on the 10th of that month, to Rachel Crookshank, who was a sister of the Hon. George Crookshank, an historic name in the annals of Toronto. Wedding presents then made, exist in the family of Mrs. Stephen Heward, who is a niece of the second Mrs. Macaulay.

It is probable that the Doctor had, on leaving Kingston, ceased to be Deputy Inspector of Hospitals. When the Medical Board of Upper Canada was formed, in 1819, it was to be expected, from the position which Dr. Macaulay had held, that he should be appointed as the senior member, and as such should discharge the duties of President. This position he continued to hold until his death, which took place Jan. 1, 1822, at his homestead, "Teraulay." The esteem in which he was held is shown in the obituary notice found in the *Observer*, York, Monday, January 7, 1822:

"It becomes our painful duty to communicate to our readers the decease of Dr. Macaulay, of this town. In the death of this truly valuable member of society, charity has lost its best supporter, and the unfortunate emigrants their best friend. He was ever ready to wait upon and relieve the forlorn stranger, not only with his medicine, but with his purse; and it is to be hoped that those gentlemen who are left behind will endeavour to imitate his unbounded liberality.

"The House of Assembly, and the Honourable Legislative Council adjourned to attend the funeral."

Dr. Macaulay is described as not having a striking appearance. He was of medium height, inclined to stoutness, a good deal stooped; had a pallid face, fair hair, with spectacles on nose, which for stooping became very prominent. He lived an active life, noted for his amiable disposition, and enjoying the high respect in which he was held. He did not engage much, if any, in private practice, but his connection with the first Medical Board of the Province, as senior member, made him an important personage in the annals of the profession of Upper Canada.

The widow of Dr. Macaulay passed her peaceful days at "Teraulay" (now Trinity Square), until her death in 1840.

The children of Dr. Macaulay, by his first wife, were eight in number:

1. John Simcoe Macaulay, born in England, October 13, 1791; died, December 20, 1855; married Ann Gee Elmsley, July 2, 1825.

2. James Buchanan Macaulay, born at Newark, December 3rd, 1793; died, November 26, 1859; married Rachel Crookshank Gamble, December 1, 1821.

3. George Macaulay, born at York, November 11, 1796; died, August 7, 1828; married Jane Hagerman, October 26, 1822.

4. Elizabeth Macaulay, born at York, February 27, 1799; died, July, 1832; married Christopher A. Hagerman, March 28, 1817.

5. Mary Macaulay, born at York, February 15, 1801; died, February, 1833; married John W. Gamble, 1822.

6. Allan Macaulay, born at York, January 4, 1804; died unmarried, October 5, 1830.

7. Ann Macaulay, born at Quebec, May 3, 1806; died, October 5, 1877; married Peter Deihl, M.D., October 15, 1829.

8. Sarah Hayter Macaulay, born at Quebec, March 3, 1809; died, August 24, 1866; married John S. Cartwright, January 11, 1830.

It will be observed that the names of all who became connected with Dr. Macaulay's children are household names in the annals of Upper Canada.

The eldest, John Simcoe, was educated in England, and entered the Royal Engineers. He rose to the rank of Captain, and was a lecturer in the college at Woolwich. He was the author of a work known as "Macaulay on Field Fortification," which is still a text-book at Woolwich. A copy of the work before the writer says, on the title page: "Colonel of Upper Canada Militia, late Captain in the Corps of Royal Engineers, and Professor of Fortification in the Royal Military Academy, Woolwich, MDCCCL." In 1835, he came to Canada, and settled in Toronto. He had previously married a daughter of John Elmsley, who became Chief Justice of Upper Canada in 1796, and sister of Captain Elmsley, a name well known in the early days of York. He took part, as an engineer, in the construction of the Welland Canal. In the rebellion of 1837, he held the rank of Colonel. In 1843, he returned to England, and purchased a beautiful place in Kent, near Rochester, where he lived until his death, 1855. "He was one of the most kind-hearted and genial of men." The second son, who became Sir James Buchanan Macaulay and Chief Justice, is one of the most conspicuous figures in the history of Upper Canada. He was one of the noted band who formed the school of John (afterwards the Rev. Dr., and then Bishop) Strachan, at Cornwall.

When the war of 1812 broke out, James B. Macaulay, though then but nineteen years of age, with alacrity entered into the military service of his country. A regiment, the Glengarry Fencibles, having been raised for the special defence of the Province, young Macaulay obtained a lieutenancy in that valiant corps, and was afterwards appointed Adjutant of the regiment.

He was with the regiment on that cold winter morning in February, 1813, when, Colonel McDonald in command, they made a spirited and dashing attack on Ogdensburg, crossing the ice in deep snow, charging the batteries on the American shore with much heroism, if not complete success.

It is something to be remembered that in all these engagements—Ogdensburg, Lundy's Lane and Fort Erie—Lieutenant

Macaulay, afterwards Chief Justice, did his part well, doing his duty as a soldier, as he afterwards did in his professional career as a lawyer and judge, to the Province.

On the restoration of peace, the Glengarry Fencibles were disbanded, and Lieutenant Macaulay exchanged his sword for "Blackstone." In 1818, he became a student of law, and was called to the Bar in Hilary Term, 1822. He had not long to wait for clients.

Mr. Macaulay had been but seven years at the Bar when, in 1829, he was elevated to the Bench, as one of the Justices of the Court of King's Bench. He was associate of Chief Justice Robinson in that Court till the constitution of the Court of Common Pleas, in 1849, when he was made Chief Justice of this newly created court, and his appointment was hailed with satisfaction by the whole profession, as well as by the body of the people.

Mr. Macaulay continued to hold the place of Chief Justice of the Common Pleas till 1856, when he retired from the Bench. On his retirement, he was elected Treasurer of the Law Society; and, subsequently, a Commission having been formed for the revision of the long-accumulated Statutes of the Provinces of Upper and Lower Canada, as well as of the Statutes of Canada since the union of 1841, he was appointed Chairman of that Commission.

A few months after the completion of the revision of the Statutes, he received the honour of Knighthood, and was, July 27, 1857, appointed a Judge of the Court of Error and Appeal, a position held by him till a few months before his death. He died at Toronto, November 26, 1859.

George Macaulay became a barrister, and settled in Bath, near Kingston, on the Bay of Quinte, at one time an important place. Here he remained until his death, August, 1828.

To his daughter, Mrs. E. H. Van Koughnet, of Toronto, the writer is greatly indebted for information. She has in her possession her grandfather's (Dr. Macaulay) family Bible, in two volumes, in which are recorded the names and dates of births, marriages and deaths of the family.

Allan Macaulay was a clergyman, but died before he had filled a regular incumbency, October 5, 1830.

There are no descendants of Dr. Macaulay of that name now living; but by his daughters there are very many who are well known to Upper Canadians, especially in Toronto. Of those who married grandchildren of Dr. Macaulay may be mentioned: The Rev. K. Mitchell, B. Homer Dixon, E. Bennett, Col. Thos. Ross, M. R. Van Koughnet, J. Joseph, Hon. John Beverley Robinson, William Greey, George Boyd, Rev. J. D. Cayley, Col. Van Straubenzie, and Rev. Bedford Jones.

DR. THEOPHILUS MACK

Was the son of the Rev. Mr. Mack, an Irishman from Trinity College, Dublin, who came to Canada in 1829, expecting to be appointed a master of Upper Canada College, but, being disappointed in this, he entered the Church. He lived at Wellington Square and Amherstburgh. Theophilus was four years old when his father came to Canada. He was a pupil of Upper Canada College. During the rebellion of 1837, at Amherstburgh, being in his teens, he distinguished himself, with a number of others, equally young. He was subsequently a lieutenant in connection with the local navy, in which service he continued for eighteen months. He then commenced the study of medicine in the office of Dr. George Grasett, and at the military hospital. He received his degrees of medicine at Geneva College, U.S., 1843, and soon after his provincial license. In 1844, he commenced practice at St. Catharines. Not long after, his attention was directed to the medicinal properties of the saline waters of a well which was dug during the war of 1812, to supply salt, as none could be obtained from the States. Dr. Mack ascertained that the waters possessed medicinal qualities, and ultimately brought St. Catharines into considerable repute as a health resort. He succeeded in attracting large numbers of invalids to the place, and subsequently built an hotel and sanitarium. He was for three years Professor of Materia Medica in the University of Buffalo. By his efforts a marine and general hospital was established at St. Catharines. In 1874, he founded the first training school for nurses in Canada.

Dr. Mack died at St. Catharines, October 24, 1881, aged sixty-one.

32

DR. JOHN DUFF MACDONALD

Was born in the parish of Cromarty, Scotland, November 18, 1819, being the son of a naval officer. Dr. MacDonald may be numbered among the United Empire Loyalists. His grandfather, with several brothers, was living in North Carolina, when the rebellion of 1776 commenced. All the brothers, except Dr. MacDonald's grandfather, were the victims of rebel fury, and simultaneously lost their lives. The grandfather, being then but a youth, succeeded in making his escape, aided by sympathetic women. He then entered the army. After the war he received a grant of land, as a United Empire Loyalist, in New Brunswick; but a transition from North Carolina to that province, he felt would not conduce to his comfort, so he remained in his regiment. He finally made his home in Scotland again; and among his children were many physicians, lawyers and naval officers. The subject of this sketch received his education in Edinburgh, and became Licentiate of the Royal College of Surgeons, Edinburgh, 1839. He came to Canada in the double capacity of naval officer and surgeon; and in 1848, obtained provincial license of Upper Canada. He at first settled in Lanark, where he had to undergo all the hardships incident to pioneer life; laborious work, uncertain remuneration, with the absence of mostly all the pleasures to which he had been accustomed. So, after a time, he betook himself to Hamilton, where he has continued to practise. Soon after his advent to Hamilton, Asiatic cholera became epidemic, and Dr. MacDonald found plenty to do. When the plague disappeared, his practice did not cease. During that trying time the public had learned his worth and professional skill, and his position, as a physician, was established in Hamilton, and he has continued to enjoy a large practice. In 1867, he received the honorary degree of M.D., from Victoria University. He was a member of the Council of the College of Physicians and Surgeons, Ontario, 1872-80, and President, 1879-80. He is an ex-President of the Canadian Medical Association.

DR. JOHN MACKELCAN.

John MacKelcan was born, September 22, 1804, at Fort George, in the Island of Guernsey. He was the eldest son of General MacKelcan, R.E., Commandant of the Fort. He studied at St. Bartholomew's, and became a member of the Royal College of Surgeons, England, 1827. He practised in London, England, till 1834, when he came to Canada and obtained the provincial license. Three brothers had preceded him to Canada. He went on a bush farm at Guelph, the village consisting only of a few houses. His farm consisted of one hundred acres, and had five acres partially cleared with a log-house. He therefore took a house in the village and commenced the practice of medicine instead of farming. In his rounds of practice he rode on horseback and travelled through the bush principally by an Indian trail. He remained at Guelph only about two years. He then moved to Simcoe, County of Norfolk. Here he practised for ten years, when he made a final move to Hamilton. During the rebellion of 1837-38, he was appointed surgeon to the 85th Regulars on the death of the surgeon of the regiment.

In April, 1846, Dr. MacKelcan took up his abode in Hamilton, and he soon became known as a skilful practitioner and a worthy citizen. He was not unknown outside of Hamilton. Mr. Clarke Gamble says of him: "I first met him in the Synod of Toronto, as delegate from one of the churches in Hamilton. He appeared to me to be a man of great force of character, and was decidedly opposed to 'The Tracts for the Times,' and a most earnest opponent of the ritualistic practices of some of the clergy of the Church of England. I always heard him spoken of as an eminent physician." At the time of his death, which took place in his eighty-second year, April 15, 1886, a local paper said: "It is with the deepest regret that the *Times* is called upon to chronicle the decease of one of our oldest citizens, Dr. John MacKelcan. He was a remarkably well-informed man, and took an intelligent interest in educational and sanitary affairs, upon which subjects he wrote many letters to the press advocating his views. A few years ago the Doctor celebrated his golden wedding, and of late years had retired from active pursuits. He leaves a widow, four sons and four daughters. Dr. MacKelcan was a man who was always held in the highest respect and esteem by those who knew him, both for his ability as a medical practitioner and for his sterling integrity as a man, and now that he has passed away after a long and useful life he will be greatly missed from among us." Dr. MacKelcan was the father of twelve children, seven of whom are now living (1889), three daughters and four sons.

DR. DAVID MACKINTOSH

Was born at Inverness, Scotland, December 12, 1821. He received his earlier education at the Royal Academy of Inverness, where he was awarded the silver medal for proficiency in mathematics in the year 1839, and in the year 1841 he received the gold medal for proficiency in the same subject. From Inverness he went to the Edinburgh University, where he obtained his degree of M.D., also L.R.C.S. Edin., and in 1845 carried away with him the gold medal of the University, and the highest testimonials from each and all of the professors connected with the University.

Dr. J. Y. (afterwards Sir James) Simpson, says: "I had an opportunity of seeing much of Dr. Mackintosh at the time (referring to his connection with the Royal Maternity Hospital where he acted as House Surgeon), and of hearing still more of him, and all went to impress me with the most favourable opinion of his professional knowledge and talent and his great moral worth. I am acquainted with few or no young physicians more deserving of all possible encouragement." Dr. M.'s thesis was deemed so superior and so valuable as to have had one of the four gold medals of the University mentioned for it. Others who gave their testimonials were: James Syme, Professor of Clinical Surgery; Dr. Thompson, Dr. Martin Barry, Dr. Zeigler and Dr. John Moir, and one and all unite in speaking in the highest terms, not only of his professional ability, but also of his great moral worth, and state that his conduct was uniformly characterized by gentlemanly feeling, kindness to his patients, and zeal and diligence in the discharge of his duties.

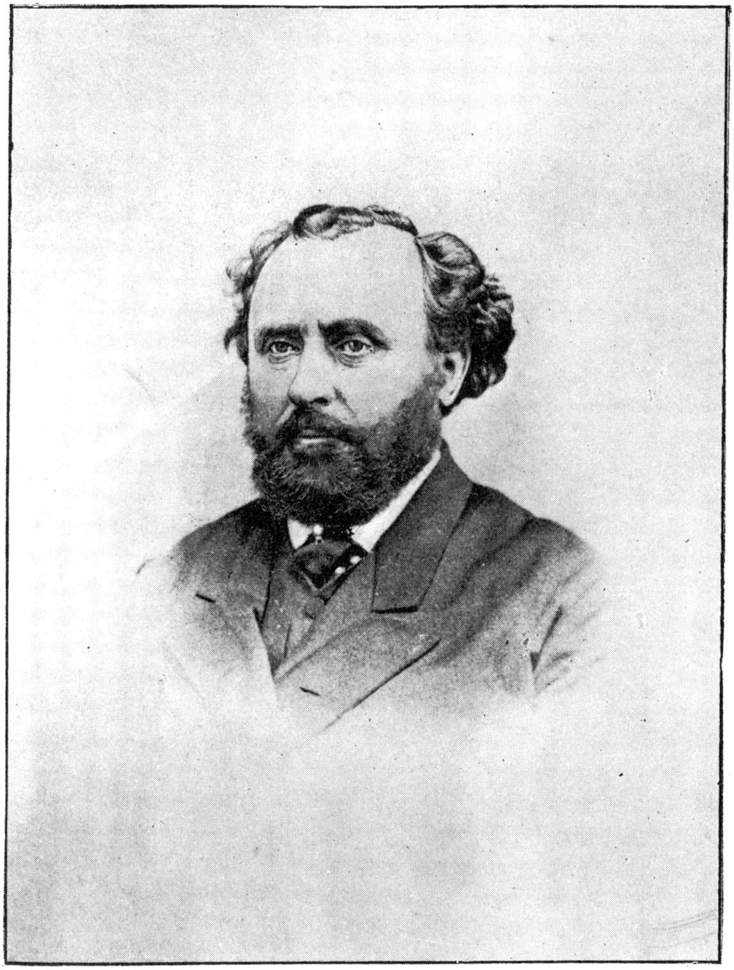

DR. DAVID MACKINTOSH.

Sir James Simpson was "Professor at Edinburgh University, Physician Accoucheur to Her Majesty of Scotland, and the discoverer of anæsthetical properties of chloroform."

Dr. Mackintosh was married, May 15, 1848, to Anne, daughter of James Ross, of Portland Place, Inverness. Shortly after, he sailed for Canada, and, having obtained his provincial license in 1855, he settled in Hamilton, where he remained up to the time of his death, March 26, 1876. In the year 1867, he was sent as a representative to the Canadian Medical Association at Quebec.

Dr. Mackintosh had a family of four sons and five daughters. He had all but lost some of them from scarlet fever, all being down with the malady at the same time; and he had to hand over his practice to Dr. MacKelcan. The eldest son was at one time considered beyond recovery. It is worth recording that his recovery was attributed to eating artificial oysters. He had been urgently asking for oysters, while unable to eat anything else; but the oysters were not in season, and none could be obtained. The eldest daughter, however, was equal to the occasion. The sick child, ignorant of the state of affairs, had brought to him what seemed to be some fried oysters, of which he partook with great satisfaction. But the dish was made up of pieces of veal, dipped in beaten eggs and powdered crackers and then fried. The subject of this piece of deception, it is related, will not to the present time believe that he did not have genuine fried oysters at that time.

At a meeting of the Hamilton Medical Association, the physicians asked the Doctor for a discourse on his treatment of scarlet fever patients, and particularly that of his son. His address was received with great enthusiasm by the members of the Society, and ordered to be printed in pamphlet form. Dr. Mackintosh was Coroner for the City of Hamilton and County of Wentworth. His death was caused by congestive apoplexy. Nine months after his death, his eldest daughter passed away, and twice since that has the angel of death entered the household; in 1881, taking the youngest daughter, a beautiful girl of sixteen years, and in 1886 the mother went to join the loved ones who were "waiting and watching."

The eldest son is accountant in the London Branch of the

Canadian Bank of Commerce; the second son is a druggist, but it is expected that some day he will take up the profession of his father, after whom he was named. The third son is in Texas, prospering as a merchant, and the youngest is in California. The three surviving daughters are also in California. One is married to James M. Wilson, of Pasadena, one of the proprietors of the "San Pasqual," one of the largest dairies on the coast of Southern California; another is in the same city doing well in her profession as a public reader and teacher of elocution.

Dr. Mackintosh was a contributor to medical literature. Especially may be noticed an admirable address to the Hamilton Medical Society on "Medical Legislation," in February, 1870. Fortunately, it is preserved in the form of a pamphlet.

The above was written in 1890. We have since learned that the eldest surviving daughter, Bella F. Mackintosh, has completed a two years' course of training at the Children's Hospital, San Francisco, and is already a successful worker in her chosen profession.

DR. THOMAS CLARK MACKLEM,

The youngest son of James and Lydia Macklem, was born at Chippawa, on the Niagara River, September 19, 1817, and was godson of the Hon. Thomas Clark, after whom he was named. The grandfather of Dr. Macklem lived in County Tyrone, Ireland. He was a member of the Church of England, as are all his descendants. His son James, the father of the subject of this sketch, came to America about 1788, and for a time lived in Northumberland County, Penn., being engaged as a school teacher. About 1781, he removed to Canada, and for a short time lived at Ancaster, County Wentworth. He finally settled with his family at Chippawa, County Welland. He engaged extensively in the milling and distillery business, and was the originator of the well-known "Chippawa Whiskey." Although Mr. Macklem had lived for a time in the States, he remained a British subject (he was a U. E. Loyalist), and in 1794 was commissioned First Lieutenant (in artillery cavalry) in the militia force of County Lincoln. This commission was signed by John Butler—"constituted and appointed (by commission from His Excellency the Lieutenant-Governor of Upper Canada) Lieutenant of the County of Lincoln." This commission shows that each of the several counties of the province had its lieutenant, as it is in England. In the war of 1812, James Macklem commanded a company in the 2nd Regiment Lincoln Militia. He had three sons and two daughters, namely: James Oliver Tiffany (named after Dr. Tiffany), Thomas Clark, Nancy and Sophia. The two elder sons, besides the business in which their father engaged, carried on an extensive foundry business, and also established a line of steamboats between Chippawa and Buffalo, and between the latter place and Detroit. The youngest son, some time after his father's death, about 1838, decided to study medicine, and accordingly proceeded to Edinburgh and entered the University. Young Macklem found friends among the university professors, but the climate of Edinburgh did not agree with him and he was obliged to return to Canada. He consequently completed his studies at McGill College, Montreal. He stayed for some time with Professor Sutherland, who was a friend so much appreciated that Dr. Macklem named after him his second son. The subject he selected for his thesis, at the time of his graduation, was consumption. The merits of this essay were such that it was suspected he had been assisted by his friend Dr. Sutherland. But the professor indignantly declared he had never seen it.

Dr. Macklem established himself in practice in his native place, and his field of labour extended over a large section of the country. He acquired a high reputation for skill in his profession, especially in the diagnosis of cases requiring the use of the stethoscope. Dr. Macklem, by his sympathetic nature, unremitting attention to his patients and kindness, endeared himself to all, and not the least to those who were poor. His professional ability was recognized by the offer of a professorship in the medical department of Trinity University, Toronto, which offer was declined in consequence of his mother's declining health.

Among those on the ill-fated train that was precipitated into the Desjardins Canal, March 12th, 1857, was Dr. Macklem.

He was recovered from the wreck in an unconscious state, in which condition he remained for many hours. He was unable to leave Hamilton for several weeks, and, although skilfully treated by the Hamilton doctors, he never entirely recovered from the effects of the shock and internal injuries he had received. In the early part of 1859 he contracted a severe cold, and, in consequence of his weakened constitution, he was unable to overcome the effects, and disease of the lungs was developed. Having hopes of recovery, he, by the advice of medical friends, proceeded to Florida with his family. The salubrious air of the pine groves allayed the difficulty of breathing and soothed his cough for a time; but the relief was very transient, and he died, December 11, 1859. His remains were brought to Canada and buried at Chippawa.

Dr. Macklem married, 1851, Caroline, third daughter of Samuel Street, Esq., of Niagara Falls, by whom he had two sons and two daughters. The eldest son, James, was drowned in childhood. The other son, Sutherland, after being educated at Trinity College, Toronto, and at the University of Oxford, was ordained priest in the Church of England, 1890. His home is at Clark's Hill, at the Falls, but he is temporarily residing in London, England (1892). The eldest daughter, Caroline, remains unmarried, and resides with her mother. The other daughter, Elizabeth, is the wife of Oliver R. Macklem, barrister, Toronto. The widow of Dr. Macklem became the wife of H. C. R. Becher, Q.C., London, Ontario.

DR. SAMUEL STREET MACKLEM, born, 1836, was the son of James and nephew of Dr. T. C. Macklem. He acquired his medical education at McGill College, being a private pupil of Dr. Sutherland, as well as of his uncle. He was engaged in practice for some years, up to 1871, at Oil Springs, County Lambton. He died at Chippawa, January 8, 1872.

DR. JAMES MACNAB.

Among the historic names connected with the history of Upper Canada, that of Macnab is equal to any in prominence, and for conspicuous service to the Crown and the Province.

As will be seen, not only Canada has been served by the Macnabs, but elsewhere the name has a place in the annals of the British realm. It is gratifying to record that one of the name was intimately associated with our Loyalist forefathers. Through the favour of the Rev. Dr. Macnab, the following interesting certificate is taken from the original:

"YORK, *February* 23rd, 1818.

"I do certify that I was acquainted with Doctor James Macnab when he acted as assistant-surgeon to the Loyalists during the first war with America; and that I attended him in his last illness, at Machiche, in Lower Canada, where he died about the beginning of the year 1780.

"ROBERT KERR,
"*Surgeon I. Department.*"

Many years after Surgeon James Macnab's death, in consideration of his distinguished services in the American revolutionary war, as the departmental records attest, his heirs received grants of land from the Crown. This gentleman was the earliest representative on Canadian soil of the ancient Clan Anaba or Macnab.

A branch of his family were Nova Scotians, who for their high character while serving under the Marquis Cornwallis, obtained the grant of their property, the Macnab Island, in the harbour at Halifax. The last head of this family in Halifax was the Hon. James Macnab, Member of the Legislative Council and Receiver-General of Nova Scotia.

Another collateral branch was that represented in the person of Allan Macnab, lieutenant in the Queen's Rangers, who accompanied his commander, General John Graves Simcoe, to Upper Canada, in 1792, to assume the office of Lieut.-Governor. During the revolutionary war he received thirteen wounds. He became sergeant-at-arms to the House of Assembly of Upper Canada, and was the father of Colonel Sir Allan Napier Macnab, who was Premier of United Canada, Speaker of the Senate, and A.D.C. to Her Majesty the Queen, "whose history," as Rev. Dr. Scadding, in his "Toronto of Old," has said, "forms part of that of Upper Canada." Sir Allan was born at the historic Navy Hall, Niagara, Feb. 19, 1796, while his father was acting as A.D.C. to Governor Simcoe, and died at "Dundurn," Hamilton, August 8, 1862, aged 66. His daughters, Mrs. Daley and the Viscountess Bury, survive him, and now reside in England. The only surviving member of this family in Canada is Miss Hannah Macnab, of Hamilton, now far advanced in years. In the early days of Upper Canada she was the reigning belle of the capital. From a letter of hers just received, it is learned that her father died on the 6th June, 1830, aged 72 years, her brother, the late David Macnab, having succeeded his father in the position of sergeant-at-arms.

A distant relative of the subject of this sketch, and, in order of time, third representative of the clan in Canada, was Archibald—"The Macnab of Macnab"—himself the noble laird, of magnificent physique, who emigrated to Canada in 1821, whither many of his clan had gone before him.

After a residence at the Chats, on the Ottawa River, for nearly forty years, he returned to Europe and died at Lannion, Cotes du Nord, France, August 12, 1860, aged 83, being the thirteenth and last of the gallant chiefs of the clan of which mention is first made in the annals during the reign of David I., in the beginning of the twelfth century. It may be regretted that the succession in this chieftainship has not been maintained, although it is now a landless, yet not an honourless, title, and the clan greatly scattered.

The only surviving daughter of the late chief, "Mrs. Macnab of Macnab," lives in Florence, Italy, where she is well known in social circles and much esteemed by all classes of people for her benevolence and good works.

Surgeon James Macnab had four sons, viz., Colin, Alexander, Simon and James, three of whom lived and died in Canada; the other, a native Canadian, was slain on the field of Waterloo. Colin, whose daughter was the wife of Col. Phillpotts, Royal Engineers, brother to the Lord Bishop of Exeter, and A.D.C. to Sir John Colborne, Lieutenant-Governor of Upper Canada, was connected with the commissariat at Niagara, and subsequently for many years held the collectorship of customs at that port. He died in 1810.

Simon was the first collector of customs, registrar, and commissioner of the "Court of Requests" at Belleville. In the war of 1812 he did duty at Kingston as Captain in command of a flank company of "Hastings Incorporated Militia," and at the time of his death, in 1821, held the rank of Lieutenant-Colonel, and was buried with military honours.

James was connected with the Commissariat Department at Belleville during the war of 1812, and for several years represented the County of Hastings in the House of Assembly, at York, where, while on duty, he died in 1820.

Alexander was sworn in as confidential clerk to the Executive Council of the Province in 1797, and entered upon his duties when Newark (now Niagara-on-the-Lake) was yet the seat of Government. In 1800, he was gazetted an ensign in the Queen's Rangers; in 1803, he joined the 26th Foot; in 1804, he became lieutenant in the 30th Regiment, and in 1809 was promoted to a captaincy. He served through the Peninsular campaign, was on the staff at the battle of Waterloo as A.D.C. to General Sir Thomas Picton, both he and his chief being killed in action at Waterloo, on the 18th of June, 1815.

A grandson of Surgeon Macnab was Captain James Macnab, of Belleville, who was accidentally killed while on duty with the volunteers in the rebellion of 1837. A son of Captain Macnab is Alexander Macnab, C.E., London, Eng., who for many years has held responsible positions under several colonial governments.

The other grandson of Surgeon Macnab was the Rev. Alexander Macnab, D.D., Rector of Darlington for nearly forty years. Two of his most important positions in former years were that of president of the University of Victoria College, and acting chief superintendent of education for Canada West. The writer cannot forego stating that he has a most pleasing recollection of the Doctor's genial kindness to him when he first entered Victoria College as a student in 1848. Dr. Macnab was constituted honorary canon of the diocesan cathedral of St. Alban the Martyr, Toronto. He died, November 15, 1891, in his 80th year.

His eldest son, Allan Napier, lost his life by accidental drowning at Montreal in 1872. He was a graduate of Trinity College, Toronto, and curate of Christ's Church Cathedral, Hamilton.

The only surviving son of the Rector of Darlington is Rev.

Alexander Wellesley Macnab, incumbent of St. Barnabas Church, St. Catharines, for fifteen years an able and successful parish priest.

DR. THOMAS MACQUEEN

Was born at Edwardsburg, Ont., January 5, 1805. He was the son of Captain MacQueen, of the Halifax Fencibles, and Grace, daughter of the Hon. Richard Fraser. He was brother to Judge MacQueen, of Woodstock, Ont. He passed the Upper Canada Medical Board, October, 1827.

He married his cousin Mary, daughter of Lieut.-Col. Fraser, who commanded the Grenville militia at the battle of the Windmill. The following is an obituary sketch in one of the local papers at the time of his death: "Dr. MacQueen graduated at Glasgow with high honours and commenced the practice of his profession at Ottawa, then By-town, where he attracted favourable notice by his first case, which was the performance of a difficult operation of tracheotomy. Called on while absent from his office, he was compelled to resort to the only means at hand, and without surgical instruments, completed the operation successfully. The characteristic boldness of his operations, united with a firm disposition and extreme kindness of manner, drew around him a numerous circle of friends including many members of his own profession. Dr. MacQueen will long be remembered among all classes and his place will not readily be supplied. His first object was, relief to the sufferer; his last, remuneration."

Dr. MacQueen removed to Brockville about 1840, where he enjoyed a very large practice, gained by skilful care in all branches of his profession, and a genial manner. He was Surgeon to the Grenville militia, and served during the rebellion of 1837 with the Brockville Rifles. He died at Brockville, June 6, 1859. His widow still (1890) survives him, living at Ottawa.

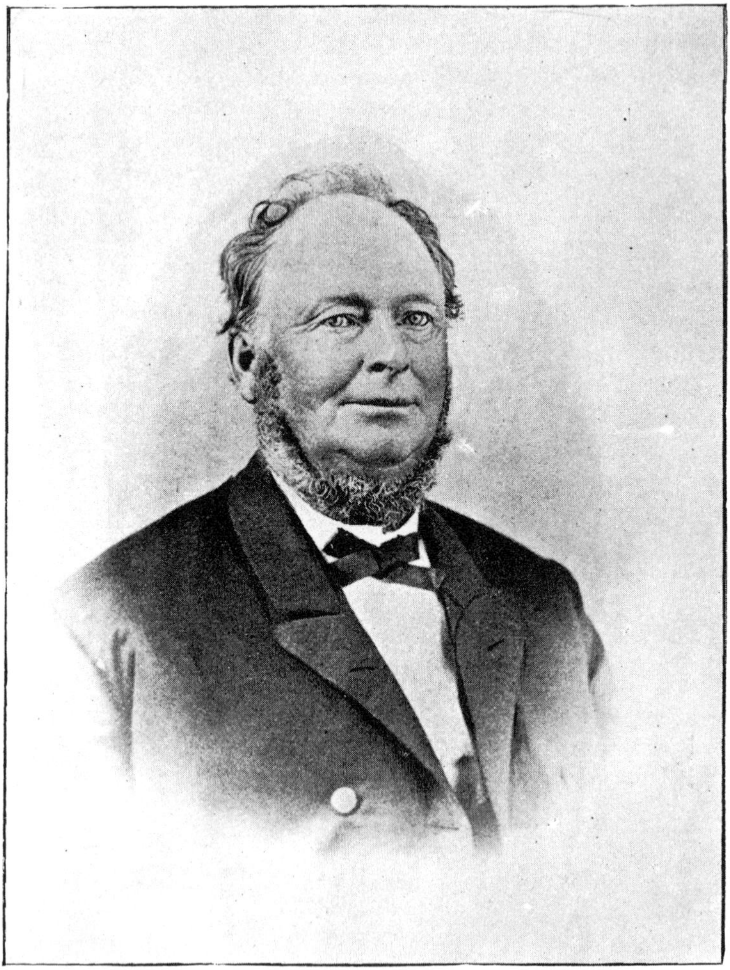

DR. NATHANIEL E. MAINWARING.

DR. NATHANIEL EZRA MAINWARING.

The subject of this sketch was of Norman origin, one of his ancestors having served as captain in the fleet which brought William the Conqueror and his army over to England, in 1066. This Captain Mesniewaring, that being the way the name was spelled in the eleventh and twelfth centuries, was rewarded for his share in the Conquest with a large grant of land in the County of Cheshire, where, for over thirty generations, the family have continuously resided.

In 1189, Sir Randolph Mainwaring was Chief Justice of Cheshire. In 1647, Sir William Mainwaring was killed in the streets of Closter while defending the city against the Parliamentary forces. In 1615, Sir Henry Mainwaring visited Newfoundland in command of five good ships, and returned to England safely, after having gained much information and rendered good service to his king and country. In 1797, Sir Henry Mainwaring, a lineal descendant of the latter, was in possession of the ancestral manor of Over Peover, in Cheshire, England.

In the parish church of Over Peover may be seen several massive sculptured tombs, upon which lie in effigy some giant warrior or sailor of this distinguished family. Amongst the numerous family monuments to be seen there, is an exceedingly beautiful altar or shrine erected to the memory of Sir Randal Mainwaring and his wife, Margery, in the year 1467, by their grateful tenantry.

The first record of the family in America that can be found bears date 1664, when William Thompson, a missionary to the Indians near New London, Connecticut, sold a section of land to Oliver Mainwaring. A portion of this land still remains in the Mainwaring family, the present (1890) owner being R. A. Mainwaring, Esq., M.D.

The late Dr. W. E. Mainwaring, of St. George, Ontario, came from this Connecticut stock. He was born in the town of Lynn, Conn., in the year 1813. When seven years old, his father moved to Canada, and bought four hundred acres of land near St. George. What is now one of the most beautiful and fertile sections of Ontario, was then a dreary wilderness. The father brought the first sheep and cattle into that section, and he also built the first saw-mill there. Public schools in those days were not known as we have them to-day, and young Mainwaring, as was customary then, acquired his knowledge of the three R's at the feet of the itinerant schoolmaster who generally gave his instruction during the long winter evenings. Notwithstanding the great difficulty in gaining book learning in those days, he succeeded in mastering sufficient of the Latin grammar and getting a firm grip of the contents of the English spelling book to qualify him for entrance into the University of New York as a medical student in the year 1836, and so well did he pursue his studies that in 1839 he graduated as an M.D. From New York he went to Dartmouth College, New Hampshire, where he spent a session in post-graduate studies. In April, 1842, he passed the examination, Medical Board, and received his license to practise. He immediately commenced practice in St. George, and in what was then called the Gore District.

In 1849, Dr. Mainwaring married Rebecca, youngest daughter of Dr. E. Stimson. For nearly forty-four years he enjoyed one of the most extensive country practices in Canada. His heart was wholly given to his profession, and no matter how cold or wet the day, or dark the night, he hastened to attend on rich and poor alike. It has been said, and truthfully, too, that he preferred to give his services to those who were unable to pay him his fee rather than to those who were wealthy. He so seldom rendered any accounts for his services, that it is not surprising to find that during the forty-four years of his practice he should have lost $75,000 from non-collection of his accounts. In the fall of 1882, he had a slight apoplectic stroke, but quickly recovered and resumed his work. In November, 1883, he was again stricken down, and died on the 18th of the same month, and was laid at rest in the St. George Cemetery. Although the day of his burial was one of the most gloomy and wet, and the roads almost impassable for mud, yet he was followed to the grave by one of the largest concourses of mourning people ever witnessed in that neighbourhood.

In politics, the Doctor was a staunch Reformer, and always took an active part in elections, but would never allow his name to be put forward as a candidate, fearing it might interfere with his professional duties. Socially, he was one of the most genial and lovable of men, and his constant urbanity and smiling face never failed to please and benefit those with whom he came in contact. He was a constant student, and kept well to the front in making use of modern ideas and theories; and, though not a public speaker, he was a veritable encyclopædia of medical, historical and biographical lore, with which he could entertain his guests by the hour.

His widow still survives him, and continues to reside in St. George (1894). His only son, R. A. Mainwaring, resides in Toronto, and is well known as an estate broker. His only daughter married Dr. Baugh, of Hamilton.

DR. JOHN MAIR,

A Master of Arts and Doctor of Medicine, a staff-surgeon (half pay) in the British army. Born at Aberdeen, Scotland, 1798, where he was educated. Studied anatomy in London under Mr. Brookes, and also attended the surgical practice at St. George's Hospital under Mr. (afterwards Sir) B. Brodie. Commenced medical studies at the University of Edinburgh, and became ordinary and subsequently extraordinary member of Royal Medical Society. In 1821, studied in Paris under Dupuytren and Broupais, and dissected with Lisfranc. Entered the army as hospital assistant in same year, having previously received certificate of qualification from Blizard and Abernethy for surgeoncy of any regiment in the service. Served in nearly all His Majesty's dependencies, attaining the rank of staff-surgeon (1st class), and retired from the army in 1852, settling at Kingston, C.W. Contributed various articles on the temperance movement to the *Gospel Tribune* (Tor.), 1851; on communion wine question, in letters addressed to the Dean of Carlisle, in the *Temperance Spectator* (Lon.), 1861; on the medical profession in relation to the temperance movement and the sacramental elements, to the *Journal of Temperance* (Can.), 1864-65; in 1849, to *Medical Times* (London), "Results of my Experience in the Treatment of Asiatic Cholera as it occurred at Kingston, C.W., in 1849.

I. "The Cup of the Lord," not "The Cup of Devils." Reprinted from *Gospel Tribune*, Toronto, 1855, pp. 21.

II. "Nephaleia, or Total Abstinence from Intoxicating Liquors in man's normal state of health, the doctrine of the Bible." In a series of letters, with addenda, to Edward C. Delavan, Esq., with coloured plates of the stomach as affected by strong drink. Albany, 1861, pp. 300.

"The entire question of 'Biblical Temperance' is discussed in Nephaleia, but particularly what is called the sacramental wine question. Dr. Mair has devoted his leisure hours for many years to a painstaking research and a careful study of most passages of Scripture bearing upon this important subject; and the result is a clear and settled conviction that total abstinence from intoxicating liquors in man's normal state, is the doctrine of the Bible."—*Temperance Spectator* (Lon.). "Bib. Canaden.," by Morgan.

DR. ANTHONY MARSHALL.

At what date Dr. Marshall came to Kingston and commenced practice, is unknown. The first notice we have concerning him is in this letter, published in a Kingston paper:

" *To the Editor:*

"SIR,—In justice to the reputation of Mr. Anthony Marshall, member of the Royal College of Surgeons, London, who contemplates making his future residence among you, I deem it my duty to give a public testimony of his professional abilities and skill, so fully evinced in the instance when I was the subject who unfortunately required his aid. Early in the month of June last, having fractured my right leg, I applied to Mr. Marshall for relief. After making use of every effort to save my limb, and finding it impossible from the extreme badness of the wound, recourse was unavoidably had to amputation, as the only means of saving my life. The operation was performed by him with consummate skill, and much to the satisfaction of myself and friends; and such was his attention during every part of my confinement, that real motives of gratitude prompt me to make this public declaration of his merits as a surgeon, and the claim he has to the patronage of the public.

"JAMES MCNOBLE.

"Thurlow, Nov. 24, 1815."

Dr. Marshall issued his card as follows:

Kingston *Gazette*, December 9, 1815: "Mr. Marshall, Surgeon, takes the liberty of announcing that he has taken Mr. Evart's house, where all calls in his line will be immediately attended to."

"Kingston, July 10, 1816: Mr. Marshall, Surgeon, has received from Montreal a fresh supply of vaccine or cow-pock matter."

"LIEUTENANT-GOVERNOR'S OFFICE,
"YORK, *Dec.* 10, 1816.

"His Excellency the Lieutenant-Governor has been pleased to appoint Surgeon Anthony Marshall, of Kingston, to examine and grant certificates of disability, to militiamen disabled from wounds received in service in defence of this Province during the late war.

"By order of His Excellency,

"EDWARD MCMAHON,
"*Assistant Secretary.*"

Dr. Marshall, after the death of Dr. Meacham, whom he attended in his last illness, removed to Belleville, being the second doctor to settle in the place. He was greatly respected as a practitioner, and as an indication of his character it may be mentioned that he, with Mr. John Turnbull and Dr. Cooper, organized a Sunday School, and was one of the teachers. Dr. Marshall was a Coroner for the Midland District. This notice appeared in the Kingston *News*, March 20, 1879: "A RIPE OLD AGE.—Mrs. Jane Marshall, whose death, at Picton, on the 10th instant, at the ripe old age of ninety-two years, was announced in the *News* of yesterday, was a former resident of this city, and sat under the ministration of the first resident Presbyterian minister, the Rev. Mr. Barclay, whose monument stands in the old Presbyterian burying ground, on Clergy

Street. Her husband, Dr. Anthony Marshall, was Secretary-Treasurer of the Building Committee for the erection of Saint Andrew's church, in the year 1820. She and the Doctor afterwards removed to Belleville, where, after his death, she taught school for many years, and was also a devoted Sabbath School teacher. She was a woman of superior attainments, and deservedly respected."

DR. PETER MARTER

Was one of the sons of Thomas Peter Marter, London, Eng. At the time of the birth of Dr. Marter, 1810, his father was Deputy Commissary-General of the British army. London was probably his birth-place. In 1815, he was in Brussels with his mother, and often said that he distinctly remembered hearing the firing at the battle of Waterloo.

In 1818, the family came to Halifax, thence to Annapolis, and afterwards to St. John, N.B.

Sir Howard Douglas, Governor of New Brunswick, and a friend of the family, became very much interested in the subject of this sketch. He gave him his entire education. He received his medical education at London, Edinburgh and Paris. At nineteen (the youngest graduate up to that date, 1829), he received his diploma from the Royal College of Physicians and Surgeons, London. He then went to Edinburgh, and thence to Paris. Among his papers are two certificates received in Paris—one dated July 24, 1830, stating that Mr. Peter Marter had attended a course in chirurgical anatomy and operative medicine, signed by Mallett, M.D., etc. The other is dated September 25, 1830, Hospital for the Poor, and is signed by Lorec. In 1831, he returned to New Brunswick, and practised for a time in St. John.

He married, in 1833, Augusta Hatch, daughter of the Hon. Harris Hatch, of St. Andrew's, and came, with his young bride, to Brantford. He was gazetted licentiate of Upper Canada, November, 1833, under 8th George IV., chap. 3. He remained in Brantford until 1858, when he took the family to Nova Scotia, where they lived but a year or two. Returning to

Brantford, he died, 1862. Dr. Marter was Surgeon to the 4th Oxford Regiment of Militia, 1837.

Mrs. Marter survived her husband fifteen years, and died in Winnipeg, 1877.

The family consisted of six children, two daughters and four sons. The eldest, Henrietta, married, 1852, Walter B. Rubridge, of Peterboro', Barrister-at-law, now Deputy Clerk of the Crown and Pleas, and Local Registrar of the High Court of Justice for the County of Brant. Jane Augusta married, April, 1855, the Hon. Edmund Burke Wood, late Chief Justice of Manitoba. The eldest son, George Frederick, is M.P.P. for the District of Muskoka, first elected, 1886, and re-elected in 1890. He married in 1862, Mary Green. The second son, Harris Hatch, married Mary O'Neil, and is reeve of the town of Gravenhurst. John Wellington married Mary Ann Harris; and Walter Peter, Minnie Findley, of Simcoe.

DR. SETH MEACHAM

Was born and educated in New Hampshire, where he also acquired his medical knowledge. It is worthy of notice that Dr. Meacham was dissatisfied with republican government, and resolved to make his home in Canada, and cast his lot among the U. E. Loyalists, who had been expatriated by the victorious rebels of 1776. In taking this step, he forsook everything in the way of riches and position. He came to Upper Canada, entirely ignorant of the country and a stranger to the people, in 1801, when about thirty years of age. His journey occupied three weeks. Crossing over at Brockville, he proceeded westward on the lookout for an eligible place at which to settle. On reaching the mouth of Myers' creek (where Belleville now stands), he found a few scattered houses and a limited population; but among them were a few who, like himself, had recently left the United States, preferring to live under the British flag. After examining the surrounding country, he resolved to make the place his home. He had not come without means, and he purchased a lot of one hundred acres in the eastern part of the township of Sidney, which is now in the western part of the city. Here, on the farm, he continued to live until his death. At this time there was no other doctor west of Kingston, as far up as Cobourg. Consequently the field of practice over which Dr. Meacham had to travel on horseback by a bridle path extended over Prince Edward District eastward to Napanee, westward to Colborne, and northward to Rawdon. It was a common thing to be absent several days, and sometimes more than a week.

At the time of the war of 1812, he was Surgeon to the Hastings Battalion of Militia, and was stationed at Kingston. At the close of the war, Dr. Meacham received very flattering testimonials from the military authorities at Kingston.

Dr. Meacham passed a brief, but very useful life. Not only was he well up in his profession, but he continued a student, and he had brought in with him a good supply of medical books and surgical instruments.

Dr. Meacham married Elizabeth Simons, daughter of Commissioner Simons, whose brother distinguished himself at Lundy's Lane. He was brother-in-law to Simon McNab, and the Rev. Dr. McNab, now Rector of Bowmanville, was his nephew.

His death took place in October, 1815, from the effects of a cold caused by exposure while visiting a patient in Rawdon. The following account of his death and funeral is taken from the Kingston *Gazette*: "Died—Universally regretted, on the morning of the 22nd inst., at his farm, in Sidney, near the River Moira, after a short and severe illness, Dr. Seth Meacham, aged forty-seven. He resided in Sidney and Thurlow for upwards of fourteen years past, during which time he exercised his profession as a physician with great success and general satisfaction to the public. He was much esteemed by all who knew him, for the strict practice of those moral and social duties which inspire respect and give true dignity to the man. His death, by the inhabitants of the adjacent townships also, will be most severely felt, having been at all times ready and willing when called upon to give medical aid to the poor, as well as to the rich. He has left a widow and four small children to mourn the loss of an affectionate husband and a most tender and benevolent parent. The remains were interred in the burying ground at Thurlow, on the afternoon of the 23rd inst., with Masonic honours, attended by a numerous train of friends and connections." It is interesting to notice by an account now before us, to William Bell, of Thurlow, that for "inoculation of six" persons, by Dr. Meacham, there was a charge of £1 10.

Dr. Meacham had two sons. The eldest, James Hubbard Meacham, now eighty-four years old, is one of the oldest inhabitants of Belleville, who has been postmaster of that city for upwards of forty years, and is known as one of the salt of the earth. Personal regard for a dear friend does not prejudice the writer in saying that a nobler, more upright man does not exist.

The second son was named Simon, who now lives at Odessa, with his son, Dr. Walter Meacham, member of the Provincial Legislature for Lennox and Addington. A daughter of Simon married a son of the Rev. Dr. Stinson.

J. H. Meacham has two sons living. The eldest, Rev. Dr. Meacham, is well known as a Methodist missionary to Japan, where he is now labouring, and whose labours have been attended with manifest success. A second son is James Bogart Meacham, druggist, of Toronto.

One of Dr. Seth Meacham's daughters remained unmarried; the other became the wife of Gilbert Bogart, of Belleville, whose daughter is the wife of Judge Dean, of Lindsay.

DR. JAMES MEAGHER

Was born at Kingston, Upper Canada, 1814. His father was in the 9th Regiment, which came to Kingston, August, 1814, after taking part in the Peninsular war. His mother was a Portuguese. He had three brothers—Jeremiah, John and Thomas. Jeremiah was a well-known personage in Kingston, and in his later years held a place in the Inspector's Department of the Post Office, Kingston. John became a druggist at Kingston. Thomas entered the legal profession, as student-at-law, in the office of Sir John Macdonald, but took an appointment as Custom House officer. A son of Jeremiah became a doctor and was attached to a company of surgeons in the North-West. He died from the effects of a fall; he had three ribs broken, but in this state and with a frozen foot he walked four hundred miles through slush and snow.

James, the subject of this sketch, was a pupil at Upper Canada College, and finished his general education there in 1832. At one of the yearly examinations he obtained the highest position, carrying away the three leading prizes of Greek, Latin and French. He then went to Montreal to study medicine in McGill College, which he did under Dr. Caldwell, the then leading medical man in that city. Dr. Caldwell died before his studies were finished, and he then studied with Dr. Racey, or "Tracey." Both of them were Professors of McGill. He remained a student at McGill until 1836, and in July of that year appeared before the Upper Canada Medical Board. The minutes of the Board say: "He had been educated in Montreal and attended the lectures at McGill College and the Montreal Hospital for two years. He passed a very creditable examination." He commenced the practice of medicine in Kingston, his native town, in 1836, "and was, as was well known to those living in his time, of high repute in his profession." He and his father were elected members of the Town Council at the same time, 1846.

At the time of the emigrant or typhus fever, 1847, in Kingston, he was one of the physicians who attended the General Hospital when that disease was so prevalent that the hospital was full of typhus patients, on account of the vessels coming with emigrants having to perform quarantine here. The disease spread to an alarming extent, filling the General Hospital to its full capacity.

When the Medical Department of Queen's College, Kingston, was created, 1854, Dr. Meagher was selected for the Chair of Midwifery.

Dr. Meagher died, December 18, 1875, aged sixty-one. The *Canada Medical Record* of that time, says: "He was a man of high attainments and of a genial disposition."

We are indebted for most of the information regarding Dr. Meagher to his brother, John Meagher, of Montreal, the head of the firm of Meagher Brothers.

DR. HENRY MELVILLE

Came from the West Indies to Niagara in the latter part of the "forties." It is said that he was the son of a British officer. He practised at Niagara for several years; came to Toronto, 1849 or 1850, and was one of the originators of the Upper Canada School of Medicine, which became the Medical Faculty of Trinity College, Toronto. He was a graduate of the University of Edinburgh and was appointed Professor of Surgery in Trinity College at the time of its organization. Dr. Melville prepared for publication, in 1852, a very interesting account of "The Rise and Progress of Trinity College, Toronto, with a Sketch of the Life of the Lord Bishop of Toronto, as connected with Church Education in Canada." This interesting volume of 258 pages contains valuable and most authentic historical information. It was published in Toronto, by Henry Rowsell, in 1852. Among the benefactors of Trinity College was Dr. Melville, who gave £20.

Dr. Melville's stay in Toronto was of short duration. He identified himself with Dr. R. Hunter, who at that time practised as a specialist, and was not regarded by the profession as a regular practitioner. He shortly after returned to England and engaged in practice. His death took place a few years later.

DR. FRANCIS MEWBURN.

The Mewburns have been in the medical profession for at least four generations. The family is entitled to a prominent place in these pages as distinguished members of the medical profession; some of its members have been equally distinguished in other professions and callings in life. The first of the name which comes under our notice is Francis Mewburn, who was born in Durham, England, 1748. He commenced the study of medicine, 1765. The indentures of apprenticeship, together with the various testimonials of attendance at lectures by some of the great men of the day, and his notes on the lectures beautifully written out, are in possession of his great-grandson, F. H. Mewburn, at Lethbridge, North-West Territories. After obtaining his diploma at R.C.S. London, he practised in Whitby for many years; also held a commission as captain in the volunteers when Napoleon threatened to invade England. He practised his profession till far advanced in years, living latterly at Danly, in the dales of Yorkshire.

He had three sons—Francis Mewburn, of Darlington (the first railway solicitor in England, of the firm of Stevenson, Pease & Mewburn, the three pioneers of the railway), John Mewburn and Boyer Mewburn, a solicitor of London.

DR. JOHN MEWBURN,

Second son of Dr. Francis Mewburn. As a student of medicine he possessed great advantages, and profited by them. He was honourably noticed by Sir Astley Cooper when he obtained his diploma as M.R.C.S. He was one of those who volunteered as assistant-surgeon to attend the sick and wounded at Haslor Hospital, after the battle of Corunna, and his account of the way they were treated was horrible. What would be said now of amputation at the shoulder-joint for wound of the circumflex artery? Yet such was done there. He was also one of those who witnessed that celebrated case of a man wounded at Corunna, who died two weeks afterwards of dysentery, and a ball was found in the heart.

Dr. John Mewburn emigrated to Upper Canada in 1832, and was gazetted as a licentiate July of that year. He resided in York for a short time, and had a very advantageous proposal to remain there, which he refused, and having purchased a farm at Stamford, settled there, where he remained all his life—a life spent in active practice—a life of usefulness, and crowned with success. "A warm-hearted, impulsive man, he had many friends, and he was always ready to assist anyone whose cause he believed to be just. From doing his duty fearlessly and honourably as a magistrate and coroner, he made many a bitter enemy." He was "a man much given to hospitality, especially to the clergy; from the Bishop to the youngest curate, from the Roman Catholic priest to the Baptist minister, all were sure of a welcome. In church matters he was always ready to give his time, and not backward in giving money likewise. Well as he treated the clergy, it must be said if he fed them well, he ruled them with not a gentle hand. . . . He was a sound churchman, and anyone staying at his house had to go to church. In all he did he aimed at being consistent." His son, in his racy way, relates this: "In explaining to his son why he had knocked a man down, for which he had to pay costs and a guinea, he said, 'Frank, you see the man called me a liar. Had he been a gentleman, I should have called him out; as he was not, I knocked him down.'" It will be seen that the Doctor had a temper. At "another time, some officers of a regiment stationed at Niagara insulted him in some way. He mounted his horse and started (using some strong language), declaring he would call out every man of them if they did not apologize. He rode fourteen miles to Niagara, and it is stated got the apology he demanded."

Dr. Mewburn was skilful in his profession, and had a high reputation. He was well known for his skill in obstetrical operations. He was the first one in Upper Canada to perform the operation whereby the offspring of a deformed woman was born alive after she had lost several children. His son, Dr. Frank C., writes: "Arriving in Canada, 1832, just as the stethoscope was introduced, there was a fortune in it. But as there was a good deal of rubbish connected with it, he threw it to one side. Some months ago a beautiful arterial preparation, arm and leg, was sent up to the American Museum. After cleaning it up, it is safe to say a finer one was never done. This was his work eighty years ago."

In the Mackenzie rebellion he volunteered for the defence of Toronto, and embarked at Niagara for Toronto.

His duties as a magistrate and coroner occupied in later years much of his time, and interfered with his practice. Moreover, his strict impartiality in dealing with evil-doers, alienated not a few.

Dr. John Mewburn was twice married. First, to a Miss Moore, afterwards to "Miss Henrietta Chilton, whose family were the real true old Tory." Mrs. Mewburn survived the Doctor many years, and died at the advanced age of ninety, well known for her kind and lovable disposition. She "read her Bible, Prayer-Book, novels and newspapers to the last." They had eleven children; of them, three sons are still living: Harrison Chilton, living on the old homestead at Stamford; Dr. Francis Clarke, living and practising in Toronto (1893); John, residing in Liverpool, England, Assistant-Manager Union Bank, Liverpool, who, in his young days, was one of the gallant fellows who sent the piratical steamer *Caroline* over Niagara Falls. Served afterwards as ensign in the Old Queen's Own under Col. Kingsmill. He joined the Volunteer Movement in England at its commencement, and is now Colonel of the finest volunteer artillery brigade in England. Thomas Chilton, the youngest son, was Inspector of Customs at Hamilton. Here it may be stated that Harrison Chilton Mewburn and Thos. Chilton Mewburn were in the cavalry troop that hunted down the American sympathizer and rebels who had successfully attacked Col. Magrath's lancers at Font Hill, and that the wounded were brought down and placed in the Queen's Own Hospital, and visited by Francis C. Mewburn under Dr. Winder, the Surgeon of the Queen's Own. Francis C. Mewburn, some years after, purchased the house.

DR. FRANCIS CLARKE MEWBURN, son of Dr. John Mewburn, was born at Whitby, Yorkshire, England, 1817. Upon his arrival with the family at York, 1832, he entered the old York Hospital. He there saw the first cholera cases that appeared in York; studied afterwards with his father, and went to Philadelphia in 1837. He passed the Medical Board in 1838, and was appointed to the Coloured Corps, with which he served two years. He practised at Weston till 1845, when he went to Niagara Falls, in which locality he resided for thirty-five years. Then he proceeded to Montreal, and afterwards to Toronto, where he has practised since. While at the Falls, the University of Buffalo conferred on him the honorary degree of M.D.

Dr. Mewburn married Henrietta Shotter, of Kent, England. He has seven children. The youngest one carried the standard in the North-West. The Doctor, unfortunately, has been somewhat deaf from his fifteenth year; but even with this great drawback, he has managed well to hold his own in the profession, and perhaps made as few mistakes as others, as he was compelled to take more time and more trouble over his cases. While at Niagara Falls, the Doctor had the pleasure of driving round the distinguished Dr. Marshall Hall. We are indebted to Dr. F. C. Mewburn for the following spirited account of his recollections and experience, which gives bright glimpses of events connected with the profession in the early days of York:

"The description of the early days of the profession in Upper Canada is taken solely from my own observation and experience; and it must be borne in mind that it is from a student's and young country doctor's standpoint. I have selected the time between 1832 and 1845, as after that the modern history may be said to commence.

"In the summer of 1832, I was attending the York Hospital in John Street. Dr. Cattermole, of London, and myself are, I believe, the only survivors (1888) who were there at that time. The staff—Drs. Widmer, Deihl, King and Rolph—have long since gone over to the great majority. One House Surgeon, Dr. Stevenson, died of cholera. Dr. Sullivan, a pupil of Dr. King's, and Dr. Woolverton, a pupil of Dr. Rolph's, are all gone. And here let me say, what a capital place this old hospital was for any young fellow who really wished to learn; many a good bedside lecture was given there. The principal figure was old Widmer—(who ever forgot him?); he was notorious for two things, his awful swearing and his good surgery. His theological views at that age were looked upon with horror. But he was an amazing favourite with the ladies, and also, I believe, with old Dr. Strachan. That only proves that both ladies and parsons rather prefer their doctor to have a certain quantity of the devil in him; and old Widmer had it fully developed. However, he was kind and attentive to the sick poor, never neglecting them; and no doubt this covered a multitude of sins. I saw him amputate a thigh for gunshot wound of the knee. There was secondary hæmorrhage and the man died. The cholera broke out after I had been there a short time. The first cases were treated with calomel and opium; they died. Then the injection of a saline solution into the veins was used on the Hospital Steward. Great things were hoped from this:

but alas, he died. After this, the General Hospital was moved into one of the new Parliament Buildings.

"Perhaps nothing can better show the difference between 1832 and 1887 than this occurrence: Dr. King and the House Surgeon went into a ward where there was only one patient, and I went with them. The two doctors looked carefully at the man, and I looked and saw that he was *well spotted.* Rather proud of my skill in diagnosis, I asked Dr. Cattermole if that was erysipelas. 'No,' he said, 'that is small-pox.' Both the doctors went their way, and young Mewburn went home and ate his dinner as usual, and I never heard there were any more cases. I heard Dr. King say, 'Cattermole, get some vaccine and vaccinate these children, as there is a case of small-pox in the house.' Can anyone imagine this in the Toronto General Hospital! These were the bleeding days; blood flowed like water. As I had learned to bleed in England, I was always ready. One day a man came in to be bled; he just wanted bleeding. He took off his coat, rolled up his shirt sleeve. Then Cattermole, pointing to me, said, 'He will bleed you.' The man took a good look at me, unrolled his sleeve, put on his coat and walked out. I was very indignant, and thought he was a fool. I think now he was a wise man. Another time I was called in to bleed a woman in York Street. Dr. Rolph had refused to do so (no doubt for good reasons). I operated at once, but to my annoyance I received no fee. Another *good* bleeding case I had in the country. It was a case of erysipelas of the leg. The man had been bled once, and I saw him the next day. The old man saw my perplexity, and so he helped me out: 'Do you think I ought to be bled again?' 'Yes,' I said. 'Then stick in your lance,' and I stuck it in, and he got well. From these cases it will be seen what recklessness there was at that time about bleeding; indeed, I was not fifteen when I first let blood (as the saying then was). May I hope that more than half a century has condoned my sins? In 1832, I remember also a most excellent address to a coroner's jury from Dr. King on peritonitis, so plain and so good that I never forgot it, and it has lasted me ever since. The man had been killed by a stab in the belly from a fish-spear. I had the Coloured Corps, two military posts, one hundred and sixty officers and men, and any number of women and children; I cannot recollect any deaths while I had charge, which ought to be to my credit; and to show the scale of pay allowed in those days to the civil medical attendants of corps, I had $500 a year and had to find medicine and my own horse. The Imperial authorities would never pay a cent for women and children.

"What a change since 1832, or since I commenced practice in 1838. In surgery, no chloroform; and no words can express the unspeakable horror of some of our cases; no pulley and weights for broken thighs; no regular wound drainage; no opening into joints; no hot water to stumps; but there was good surgery even then. I think these dreadful things were enough to make angels weep. In medicine, the furious bleedings are gone, and well would it have been had we retained the lancet, using it moderately instead of doing as we did about 1845, by taking up stimulants, and, like the bleeding, carrying it to excess. The cry was, 'Keep him up,' and very often he went up. I have lived through the era of profuse bleeding and starving, and I have also lived through the stimulants and feeding plan, and I think the last is the worst. Can we not take the good out of both? I hope so.

"Our surgical stand-bys were 'Cooper's Surgical Dictionary,' 'Astley Cooper's Lectures,' 'Charles Bell's Surgery,' and 'John Bell on Wounds.' I doubt if a better book was ever written than the last. Another was 'Lawrence on Hernia.' Not for some time did that work 'Druitt's Vade Mecum' come forth, and it was a God-send to the country doctor. In medicine we had old 'Gregory,' then the 'Cyclopædia of Practical Medicine,' and not till 1846, I think, did that priceless work of Watson's arrive.

"The stethoscope was about the year 1832 just coming into use, and those who availed themselves of its assistance had great advantage over many of the elderly men who never would learn its use. I am afraid many cases of pneumonia were not recognized till too late."

DR. FRANK HAMILTON MEWBURN,

The youngest son of Dr. F. C. Mewburn, grandson of Dr. John Mewburn, and great-grandson of Dr. Francis Mewburn, obtained his degree, M.D., C.M., at McGill College, 1880. He was first House Surgeon in Montreal General Hospital, afterwards House Surgeon in Winnipeg City Hospital for four years. The way he performed his duties was evidenced in the fact that the city physicians presented him with a handsome gold watch and chain. On leaving the hospital he obtained the position of Medical Officer to the Galt Coal Company, at Lethbridge, N.W.T. He is also acting assistant-surgeon to North-West Mounted Police, at that post (1888).

DR. ROBERT MILLER

Was gazetted to practise surgery in Upper Canada, 1832, under 8th Geo. IV., chap. 3. Dr. Robert Miller, doubtless the same, is mentioned by the Hon. James Young in his account of the settlement of Dumfries. He says: "Dr. Miller was born in the parish of Stewarton, in Ayrshire, Scotland. He was educated at Andrew's College and the University of Glasgow, where he took the degree of Master in Surgery in 1832. He arrived in Quebec on the 10th of June of the same year and came westward, looking for a suitable place to commence practice, and hearing that a physician was needed in Dumfries, he determined to have a look at the place. A letter received from the Doctor, says:

"'Between the prairie and Galt, I think there were only two houses in sight of the road. I arrived at Galt about the 18th of August, 1832. The appearance of the village was very discouraging. So far as I remember, there were only about twenty-six buildings in all, including the flour-mill, saw-mill, distillery, two stores, hotel, school-house and two blacksmith shops.'"

The Doctor came, saw, and remained. In settling in Galt, he found he had a wide field all to himself. Except Dr. Cattermole, who settled in Guelph about the same time that Dr.

Miller came to Galt, there was no medical man nearer than Dundas, Brantford, or Woodstock.

Through his skill and success, Dr. Miller became widely known as a physician, and for many years his two shaggy French ponies, one white and the other black, were among the most noted "institutions" of the village. The white one, which was universally known as Sawbones, had an unusually rough and shaggy coat, but had the merit of being able to "rack" with astonishing speed.

In 1850, Dr. Miller took the degree of M.D., at New York, and in 1860 became a Member of the Royal College of Physicians, London, England. After making a competency, he retired and took up his residence in London, England.

In 1834, Asiatic cholera was brought to Galt by a menagerie. One of the showmen was seized with the disease, and Dr. Miller, who had seen many cases at Montreal, in 1832, at once recognized the disease. He was soon overdone with work, and, at his solicitation, one Dr. McQuarrie came to Galt and rendered good service.

DR. JAMES MITCHELL,

The son of Judge Mitchell, of London, Upper Canada, studied medicine with Dr. King and Dr. Rolph, and was a fellow-pupil of Dr. H. H. Wright. The record of the Upper Canada Medical Board, of October, 1836, says: "Mr. James Mitchell, a pupil of Dr. Rolph, appeared. He had been one winter at Jefferson College, Philadelphia, and an attentive pupil of the Toronto Hospital. He underwent a severe examination with credit, and received the Certificate of the Board." Why his examination should be severe is not stated. In 1840 he was gazetted Surgeon to the 7th Regiment, Gore District.

"Married, July 16th, 1838, Dr. James Mitchell, of Dundas, to Martha, daughter of Burge McCay, of Nelson."

He died in his 68th year, at his residence, North Cayuga, 1861.

DR. JOHN W. MONTGOMERY

Was born at Newtonbrook, Upper Canada, 1827. His father, John Montgomery, was the proprietor of the tavern, "Sickle and Sheaf," on Yonge Street, where the first shot was fired in the Mackenzie rebellion. He (then ten years of age), with a cousin, were alone in the building, when a canon-ball came crashing through and knocking down the three chimneys. After a second ball entered the building, the children were taken away by friends. His father made his escape to Rochester, N.Y., and was followed by the family. Dr. Montgomery was educated here at the Collegiate Institute. In 1843, the family returned to Canada, and young Montgomery became a pupil at Dr. Rolph's school. As a senior student he acted as demonstrator of anatomy, at the invitation of the class. He qualified to practise in 1847, settled at Sutton Village, where he practised for twenty-five years. In 1872, he removed to Belle Ewart, where he practised until 1877, when he was appointed Assistant-Superintendent to the Insane Asylum at Kingston. After five years he was transferred to the Insane Asylum at Hamilton.

Dr. Montgomery was married, first, to Josephine Gorham, of New York; secondly, to Elizabeth Anderson Hawick, of Scotland; thirdly, to Charlotte, daughter of William Jones, of Kingston, Ont. He had four sons and three daughters.

DR. THOMAS MOORE,

Of the Midland District, "before Medical Board, January, 1827, was found qualified to practise." He had previously (1821) obtained Licentiate Medical Board, Lower Canada. A Dr. Moore was practising at Brockville about this time, probably the same. Appointed Surgeon to 1st Addington Regiment Militia, June 18, 1822, which indicates that he was practising some years prior to going before the Upper Canada Board. He settled at Picton, and was appointed Surgeon to 1st Prince Edward Regiment, August 11, 1828. Dr. Moore was during his lifetime highly respected as a physician and citizen. After his death (1869, aged 72), the Grand Jury at Picton, under date December 15, 1869, in a presentment, expressed "their heartfelt sympathy for the bereaved friends of the late Dr. Thomas Moore, physician to the gaol, whose loss will be greatly felt by many in this county who have availed themselves of his valuable services during the past forty-five years of his professional career among us." An obituary notice said he was "a prominent and much respected citizen of Picton." Had "practised forty-five years with much ability and success. He died, mourned by the sorrowings of hundreds who had known him and loved him for his very many commendable traits of character." Dr. Moore had two sons and several daughters.

Thomas Moore, son of above, also became a physician. He was before the Medical Board, July, 1844. "He presented a diploma from the Geneva College, State of New York." Received certificate of qualification. He practised in Demorestville until his death.

DR. WILLIAM MORRIS

Was born, County Limerick, Ireland, July 1, 1821. Educated at Ennis College; studied with Surgeon-General Sir Philip Crompton; entered Trinity College and Royal College of Surgeons, Ireland, November, 1839; continued at lectures up to 1843; attended the Dublin Lying-in Hospital; received the degree of M.D. and L.R.C.S.I., June, 1843; was Resident-Surgeon City of Dublin Hospital, 1843-44. He came to Canada, 1845; practised at Bolton's Village, Fort Erie and Buffalo. He returned to Canada at the time of the cholera and practised at Port Robinson, Delaware, five years, also at Florence. He passed the Upper Canada Medical Board 1865. Returned to the United States, and was appointed Secretary of the Board United States Examining Surgeons.

Dr. Morris was married, in Dublin, to Henrietta King, niece of A. Montgomery, Lord Mayor of Dublin, 1842. He had seven children; two are members of the profession. The Doctor writes that he had hard work when first in Canada, riding through woods sometimes fifty miles, and had to perform some of the most difficult operations, often without assistance, such as amputation of hip, resection of elbow, operation for strangulated hernia, Cæsarian section, etc.

Dr. Morris is now (1889) living in retirement at Cairo, Michigan, with his wife and daughter.

DR. THOMAS DAVID MORRISON

Was a conspicuous figure in Upper Canada, especially during the rebellion of 1836-37. He was a prominent individual of York when it was incorporated as the city of Toronto. For many years he was a leading practitioner of the Capital and the surrounding country, standing next to Drs. Widmer and Deihl. Dr. Morrison was a native of Quebec city and came to York probably about 1816. The *Christian Guardian*, of February 2, 1830, contains a letter, signed "George Ryerson," which says: "Dr. Morrison was a clerk in the Surveyor-General's office, and a nominal churchman; but from conscientious motives he joined the Methodists; for this, without a single cause of complaint alleged against him, he was dismissed from his situation and cast destitute upon the world." We give this extract to show something about his early life. The removal from the Surveyor-General's office must have been prior to his entering upon the study of medicine, and if he was left destitute, he must have been a person of industry, energy and ability to acquire a knowledge of the science of medicine to enable him to pass the Upper Canada Medical Board, which he did July 5th, 1824, and, as a result of his examination, it is recorded "the Board is perfectly satisfied by his examination." It seems that he at once commenced the practice of his profession at York, and soon found a fair patronage, especially in the country up Yonge Street. On the occasion of the arrival of Sir John Colborne at York, 1825, an address was presented to him by the citizens, and we find as the first two signatures the names of W. W. Baldwin and T. D. Morrison.

In 1831, Dr. Morrison was Vice-President of the Bible Society. At the election for the Provincial Parliament, in the Third Riding of York, 1834, he was sufficiently popular to be returned as member. He was also elected Alderman for St. Andrew's Ward, in Toronto, which had just been incorporated as a city (1834). In April, 1836, the Medical Board was reconstructed, and among the new members was Dr. Morrison, who was present at the first meeting; but his connection with the Board ceased the following year. In the same year he was elected Alderman for St. Andrew's Ward, and was chosen by the Aldermen for Mayor. During the year 1835 he had been an active member of the Toronto Board of Health, and while Mayor he was the President.

Dr. Morrison not only gave attention to the practice of medicine and civic matters, but was also an ardent politician, being in harmony with the party then designated Radicals, and was intimately associated with Wm. Lyon Mackenzie. But when that impetuous and reckless individual first submitted in secret conclave his scheme to seize Sir Francis Bond Head, take possession of Toronto and establish a new government, Dr. Morrison could restrain himself no longer, but burst forth with an impetuosity and indignation which had but seldom been observed in him. He asked if it was possible that Mackenzie could be serious in unfolding so foolhardy a design. "This," said he, "is treason; and if you think to entrap me in any such mad scheme, you will find I am not your man!" He declared that if another word were said on the subject he would forthwith leave the room.—*Dent.*

After all, however, Dr. Morrison, through the influence of Dr. Rolph, became a participant in the preliminary actions of the rebel conspirators. Although he took no active part in the rebel demonstration, he, after its collapse, was the first to be arrested. The Government believed they had sufficient evidence to secure his conviction of high treason. A committee was appointed by the Government to inquire into matters relating to the rebellion, and Dr. Morrison voluntarily appeared before it. He denied all knowledge of, or participation in, the revolt—a denial for which, under the circumstances, he ought not to be held to a severe account, as he well knew that his life hung trembling in the balance, and he could not, in strictness, be said to have had any participation in the revolt as finally consummated by Mackenzie.

The writer has read with curiosity and interest the published account of the "Trial of Thomas David Morrison, for High Treason," April 24th, 1838. It was expected that he would be convicted, and his life was trembling in the balance; however, the jury, after long deliberation, brought in a verdict of "not guilty." But, as we have seen, he had, through the influence of Dr. Rolph, really acquiesced in the armed rebellion. An interesting account of the trial may be found in Dent's "Story of the Upper Canada Rebellion."

Dr. Morrison having reason to fear a second indictment on a fresh charge, repaired to Rochester, where he remained until 1843, when he returned to Toronto.

Dr. Morrison died, March 19, 1856, aged sixty.

DR. ALFRED MORSON,

Born at Rochester, England, April, 1810, commenced the study of medicine at Aberdeen, and remained there two years; then studied at Edinburgh for a year; was a student at Paris for three years, and was under Dupuytren, Velpeau and Ricord. He also attended the Clinique of Baron Larrey, Surgeon of the great Napoleon. He then became a student at Guy's and St. Thomas' while they were one hospital, and took the degree M.R.C.S. Eng., 1834. In 1835, he held the position of dresser for the distinguished surgeon, Travers, or, as he was familiarly called, "old Ben." The writer has before him certificates to Dr. Morson from a number of famous physicians and surgeons of the day. B. Travers "certifies that Mr. Alfred Morson has been engaged as my dresser for eight months, at St. Thomas' Hospital, and that he is well qualified to perform the practical duties of his profession with ability and humanity," etc. Henry Burton, M.D., says: "I have much pleasure in offering my testimony of the diligence and assiduity displayed by Mr. A. Morson during the period of his studies at St. Thomas' Hospital, and I feel confident his ability will eventually secure him professional success." H. S. Roots, M.D., certifies the same. Robt. Williams, M.D., certifies likewise, and adds that "he leaves us with an excellent character for ability and industry." John F.

South, Assistant-Surgeon to St. Thomas' Hospital, closes a laudatory certificate, by saying: "I feel confident that in any future professional engagement into which he may enter, he will acquit himself as much to the satisfaction of those with whom he is connected as to his honour and credit." The writer cannot allow this opportunity to pass without expressing his own obligation to Mr. South for kind and effective services received from him when a student at St. Thomas' Hospital in 1855.

Dr. Morson had intended to practise his profession in England, and was preparing for an examination at the Apothecaries' Hall. But his father having removed to Canada some time previously, he was induced to follow him to By-Town (now Ottawa), where the father was living; so, towards the close of 1836, he came out in company with Dr. Durie and his family, with whom Dr. Morson was intimate.

Soon after his arrival in Canada, Dr. Morson visited Toronto, carrying the following letter from "The Macnab" to "the other Macnab." It may be here stated that "The Macnab" was the chief of the clan of that ilk. He was a man of perfect physical development, of six feet three inches. He was a polished courtier, having been at most of the courts of Europe. He came to Canada with the view of settling, and acquired a township of land in the western part of the Province, afterwards known as Macnab township. After a few years "The Macnab" returned to his native land. Allan, afterwards Sir Allan Macnab, was of the same clan. It is related that on one occasion The Macnab called on his relative Allan, and not finding him at home, left a card inscribed "The Macnab." But Allan, not to be placed in a lower position in the clan, in returning the call, gave his card with the cognomen, "The other Macnab." The letter given to Dr. Morson reads:

"BY-TOWN, *December* 26, 1836.

"DEAR KIN AND CLANSMAN,—Allow me to introduce to your particular acquaintance, Dr. Morson, who is going up to visit the Capital. I need only say he is very nearly connected with some of the clan—being uncle to a fine young family of Macnabs, his sister being married to my excellent clansman, son of the late Colonel Macnab, of the 91st Highlanders—to insure him of every attention from you. Of himself, I need say nothing, for I assure you to know him is to respect. Although this is a letter of introduction, I am going to complete it with my best wishes to your good Lady and all your family, and accept my every sentiment of esteem and regard, while ever consider me,

"Thy Leal Clansman,

"Yours most affectionately,

"MACNAB."

Soon after this, Dr. Morson received a commission from Sir John Colborne to take medical charge of the Garrison at Bytown, a position he held for fifteen years. July 14, 1847, he was appointed Surgeon to the 4th Battalion of Carleton Militia. He made application for license to practise, while Sir Francis Bond Head was Governor of Upper Canada; but there was some delay in the issuing of it. Meanwhile Dr. Morson came to Toronto with the intention of engaging in practice. After the advent of Sir George Arthur as Governor, application was made to him for license, which was issued, bearing date October 1, 1838. Subsequently, the license from Sir Francis Bond Head was received, dated March 7, 1838.

Dr. Morson practised at Montreal for two years, to which place his father had removed. From Montreal he removed to Hamilton, 1855, where he remained until 1887, and then took up his residence in Toronto, where he still lives (1893), in the enjoyment of his wonted energy and strength of mind and body. He retains in manner and conversation the *suivater in modo*, acquired by a residence at the French capital, and extensive intercourse with the educated classes.

Dr. Morson married, 1852, Mary, sister of Alexander Urquhart, a well-known citizen of Montreal, by whom he has a large family. Four sons—Alfred E., real estate agent, Toronto; William, Manager Bank of Commerce, Cayuga; George, living in Costa Rica, Central America; Walter B., in Toronto.

DR. FREDERICK MORSON.

Frederick and Alfred Morson were the sons of Thomas Morson, a lawyer of Rochester, County of Kent, England, at which place Frederick was born, 1808. He studied medicine with his brother Alfred, at Aberdeen, and at London, and obtained M.R.C.S. Eng. About 1833, through Sir George Dalbiac, of the Dutch army service, he was commissioned Staff-Surgeon in that service, and served during the trouble between Holland and Belgium. Came to Canada about 1839, and commenced practice at By-town (now Ottawa), where he continued four or five years. He then practised in Montreal several years, and at Chambly. Finally, he settled at Niagara, where he still lives (1893).

Dr. F. Morson married a daughter of Assistant Commissary-General Kupar. His only son is Judge of the County Court at Toronto. His eldest daughter is the wife of Mr. J. L. Scarth, a well-known citizen of Toronto.

DR. JAMES MUIRHEAD

Was a native of Scotland, and came to Fort Niagara with the 16th Rifles, in (or about) 1790. A traveller in Upper Canada speaks of him, 1792 : "He was a stout, fine-looking person, with a ruddy complexion." On May 19, 1795, he married Deborah, the only daughter of Colonel Butler, a lady of refinement and piety, who had been educated in England. It was probably about this time that he retired from his regiment. From this time, Dr. Muirhead was identified with the welfare of Newark (now Niagara-on-the-Lake), even before there was a village, while it was known as Niagara West, until his death. Therefore he was the pioneer doctor of the place. In every account met with of public meetings and proceedings, and by travellers, concerning the place, the name of Dr. Muirhead appears. He evidently led a busy life. Beside his practice, which was large, he attended to the duties of public offices. In 1807, he was appointed by the Lieutenant-Governor to be Public School Trustee. He was Coroner for the Niagara District, Commissioner of the Peace, and Chairman of the Quarter Sessions.

In 1812, he was engaged, probably on the staff, and was taken a prisoner of war, and retained for some time. In 1822, we find him on the militia staff as Surgeon-General. Dr. Muirhead was a Freemason, and for a time the Masonic lodge was at his house. It is not recorded that Dr. Muirhead practised to any extent through the settlements; it is most likely that he found enough to do at, and in, the neighbourhood of the town. Still, he doubtless did some riding, as the following advertisement, which appeared in *The Canadian Constellation*, in December, 1799, indicates: "A horseman's saddle, but little worn and soiled, was taken out of Dr. Muirhead's house some weeks since, by whom unknown; it has a high back and silver-plated buttons, A.H.B. in a cypher; whomsoever will return, or give information of it to the Doctor, will receive his thanks and a generous reward."

With regard to Dr. Muirhead's skill as a surgeon, there is a letter signed "Justus" in the *Upper Canada Gazette* or *American Oracle*, of December 11, 1802, which strongly eulogizes him in connection with a case of some injury to a man. He says: "When we consider the nature of the wounds, one of which was five inches deep under the arm, and the other quite through to the lungs, we must own the value and merit of the surgeon whose skilful applications and care contributed so much to this cure, much the greatest that has been effected since the Province was established."

That Dr. Muirhead took an interest in the advancement of his profession, is shown by the communication from him and Dr. Telfer in 1832 to the Attorney-General (see Proceedings of Upper Canada Medical Board), in which they speak of the prevalence of "Empirics, licensed or not," and ask for legislation.

Socially the Doctor was a favourite, and the youngsters found in him a great friend, and often a playmate. Especially he would lead them in pigeon-shooting, and there was usually a good supply for the sportsman.

Dr. Muirhead died, March 24, 1834, in the sixty-ninth year of his age, and his widow, June 29, 1844.

Dr. Muirhead had one son, John Butler, who became a lawyer, having studied with S. P. Jarvis. He married Miss Dockstater, but died before his only child, a daughter, was born. Her name was Deborah Catherine, and she became the wife of William Buell Richards, of Brockville, a barrister, who was afterwards known as Sir W. B. Richards, Chief Justice of Ontario, and then of the Supreme Court of Canada. The family of children consisted of William Muirhead, now of the Quebec Bank, Toronto; John Butler, living at Plattsburg, Pa.; Stephen O., of Vancouver, B.C.; Annie C., married to James Moore, Esq., Hartford, Conn.; and Mary L., of Vancouver, B.C.

DR. THOMAS H. MULOCK,

Son of Wm. Mulock, one of twelve children, eleven being sons, was born, 1811, at Banagher, Ireland. Three brothers and the sister are yet living (1891); the Rev. Canon Mulock, Montreal; the wife of A. G. Robinson, C.E., of Orillia, and two others living in the United States.

Canon Mulock came to Canada, 1834, and was with his father at Orillia at the time of the Mackenzie Rebellion, 1837. He joined the Royal Foresters as Lieutenant, under the command of Col. Carthew, and remained until they were disbanded, 1845. He subsequently took holy orders, and continued in the work for forty years. He now (1891) lives with his son in Montreal.

The Doctor was educated at the "Royal School of Banagher," and at the age of sixteen was bound to his uncle, Robert Mulock, apothecary and accoucheur, Dublin. With him he remained for upwards of two years, and was then indentured to a surgeon. He attended at Trinity College, Dublin, also "The Lying-in Hospital" for two terms, being a paid member thereof during the second term. He also took the degree of M.D. at Trinity College.

For a short time the Doctor practised in the town of Banagher, then on some trouble breaking out with Spain, he obtained a surgeoncy in the army. At the close of the war, which was of short duration, he returned to Banagher, where he again practised, and married Miss Smith, who died without issue. At her decease he came to Canada, 1835 or '36, and after a short sojourn in Orillia with his father, went to Newmarket, where, according to a published card, he was in 1838. He finally settled at Bond Head, where he continued to live until his death, about 1847.

In 1838, Dr. Mulock married Mary, daughter of John Cawthra, of Newmarket, who represented Simcoe County in Parliament, 1829. Mrs. Mulock survived her husband for many years, having died at Los Angeles, Cal., December 29, 1882. Mrs. Mulock founded a scholarship in connection with Toronto University.

They had five children: John, who died, aged 12; Marian, who married Wm. Boultbee, C.E., of Toronto; William, who is well known as a barrister, as the Vice-Chancellor of Toronto University, and as Member of Parliament for North York, who married Miss Sarah Crowther, of Toronto; Sarah, who married George Lount, barrister, of Barrie; and Rosamond, who married George W. Monk, the well-known and popular member of the Ontario Legislature, for many years, of Carleton County.

DR. JAMES MUTTLEBURY.

An interesting document before the writer contains the returns of the professional education and services of James Muttlebury, M.D., Inspector of Hospitals, from September 18, 1795, to June 25, 1818. By this document we learn that he saw service in many parts of the world, and was rapidly promoted, until he became Inspector of Hospitals, 1816.

Dr. Muttlebury left England for Canada in the early part of 1832, accompanied by his eldest son and a younger one. A letter written by him to his wife informs us that he reached York, May 7th, making the journey from Portsmouth to York in 67 days. He writes to his wife: "On the 8th I delivered my credentials to the Lieut.-Governor, by whom I was favourably received. Sir John introduced me to the various public officers, and when I dined with him yesterday he named me pointedly to all his guests. To-morrow we dine with Mayor Winnetts, to con over the best place for a location. On Saturday we shall take a family dinner with the Archdeacon, who has permitted me to make use of his pew on Sunday, as the military one is generally overcrowded. There appears on the part of Sir John every disposition to favour me, but I can perceive an evident wish to detain me in this place, where he says there is a good field for practice. I met the chief medical men at his table, but I do not mean to be diverted from the main object I have." This main object is revealed in a subsequent letter dated July 11, 1832. He says, it may be with a presage of his fate: "We are not without our troubles and our fears on this side the water, for the cholera has made its appearance, and has committed appalling devastation in the Lower Province, 149 deaths having taken place in one day in Montreal. It has gradually advanced with the tide of emigration to the Upper Province; Cornwall, Prescott, Kingston, Cobourg and York have severally been visited with it. We took every precaution, having previously appointed a Board of Health, and used every precaution made. We have had, on the whole, between fifty and sixty cases, of whom the major part, I believe (for I do not know), have died. It has been, and continues to be, confined to the lower orders. I have been so often absent on occasional journeys to look out for a spot on which to seat myself, that I have not seen much of the disease, but within the last three days I have made frequent visits to the Cholera Hospital, and shall continue to do so in order to study the complaint.

"20th. We are likely to be in a certain degree settled, for I have effected the purchase of an improved farm of 200 acres, fifty of which are under cultivation, at about fifteen miles from York. I pay £640 for it and half the crop—wheat, hay, corn and potatoes. . . . We took out a waggon-load of things on Wednesday, another to-day, and to-morrow we are in hopes to be able to quit York altogether for our new residence. . . . The Commissioner of the Crown Lands has given orders for a reserve in the township of Blandford to be surveyed, and has promised to give me my allotment there; it will be 650 acres."

This we glean from the worn and torn letters. It is doubtful that he again penned a line to his absent wife, as a month later he was laid in his grave, being the victim of cholera, which complaint he had been studying. He died in his house, where he had hoped to pass many a day with his family.

The circumstances of the family at this eventful period was extremely sorrowful. Dr. Muttlebury had left England with his two sons, leaving his wife and nine children behind. Two sons were immediately following. Later, his wife with one daughter also embarked, notwithstanding she had heard of the death of her husband. The following year the rest of the family also emigrated, in charge of a nurse. The family consisted of eight sons and three daughters. Although the head of the family was wanting to be a guide, the young children found a path of some distinction. Six of the sons became pupils at Upper Canada College. The eldest, Rutherford, became a barrister. He died at Toronto, 1849. His daughter became the wife of Chas. McMichael, brother of Dr. McMichael, Toronto. The second son, George, became an officer of the British army ; was wounded in action in Spain, and finally died in Africa of fever. The third, Frederick Clayton, studied law, practised as a barrister at Kingston, where he died, 1856. The fourth, Augustus, studied medicine for a time with Dr. Gwynne. He went to the West Indies, where he died, 1836. The fifth, James William, also became a barrister. In 1851, he went to Australia. Here he stayed seven years, and having acquired a fortune, he repaired to London, England, where he continued until his death, 1887. His son is at present (1889) President of the Cambridge Rowing Club, and the stroke oar of the Cambridge Rowing Crew. The sixth son, John, went to New Zealand, and was a volunteer in the war with the natives. Returning to Toronto he died, 1873. The seventh son is Francis Walter, now living in Toronto. He was in California in 1850, and remained thirteen months, when he proceeded to Australia, where he remained three years, and then returned to Toronto. The eighth son, Henry, was a student-at-law for a time, but accompanied his brother to California. He is at present in Dakota (1889). One daughter died in her teens. One became the wife of Judge McQueen, of Woodstock. Their daughter is the wife of Dr. R. A. Pyne. Another daughter, living in Toronto, is well known for her philanthropic work.

It is safe to say that in the premature death of Dr. Muttlebury, not only his family suffered an irreparable loss, but as well the young Province in which he had settled. Although he had made his home in a rural place, he would doubtless have acted a conspicuous part in the medical profession. He had been gazetted as a licentiate, June 21; and on July 23, three weeks before his death, it was announced that "The Lieutenant-Governor has been pleased to appoint James Muttlebury, Esq., M.D., and Inspector-General of Hospitals, on half pay, to be a member of the Medical Board of this Province."

The Rev. Isaac Fidler, in his "Observations" on Canadian matters, published in 1832 (he lived at Thornhill three years), draws a comparison between the medical profession of the United States and Canada, in connection with the cholera epidemic. Speaking of New York, he says it was "every man for himself. Many of the medical profession imitated the flight of their splendid neighbours, and abandoned the less fortunate of their fellow-citizens in the hour of danger. In Canadian towns, no such absence of sympathy was betrayed. In York and other places of Canada, every available assistance, pecuniary as well as medical, was rendered to the distressed; and the patients received attendance and consolation to the very last."

Reference is made to a Dr. M. (Muttlebury), who, having retired from the army, had purchased three hundred acres near Yonge Street, and had come to live there with his two eldest sons. Mr. Fidler says: "He intended to go to York, on particular days, to practise in the capacity of a consulting physician. This Dr. M. was seized with the cholera, but did not seek medical aid until he was beyond hope. A doctor was ultimately called from York." The following statement can hardly be credited. He says the doctor called from York, and thus announced to the sons the inevitable death of their father: "Your father is a dying man; there is no hope; and now where am I to obtain my fee? I must be paid immediately." The body was buried in the military burying ground at York. It was near midnight when the body reached the place of burial, and it was buried with military honours. The Archdeacon of York subsequently told Mr. Fidler that this was the only case of death among medical men by cholera.

The military burying ground, in which Dr. Muttlebury was buried, was situated at the western extremity of the broad and beautiful Wellington Place. It is now converted into a sightly public square, having been set apart for that purpose by the Dominion Government and transferred to the city of Toronto. While it was yet a burying ground, but not used as such, the writer repeatedly visited the place, looked at the graves of those taking their last rest, who were buried there in the early part of the century, and examined the head-boards, some of which had fallen from decay, and also noted the inscriptions, more or less faded, some obliterated by time. Among those yet standing was one erected to the memory of a son of Sir John Colborne, who died while Sir John was Lieutenant-Governor of the Province. The grave was within an enclosure, and beside it another grave. The plot was marked by the only tree standing in the grounds. This "other grave" was that of Dr. Muttlebury, but the head-board had crumbled away. When Sir John Colborne's child died, he decided that its body should be laid beside that of his old friend, the Doctor, for whom he had had great regard. And on this spot the remains of these two still lie. The uneven ground has been made level, all the graves have been obliterated. The remaining tablets have been placed in the western part of the square. Green grass and trim walks are daily trod by the unheeding public who come and go, while the dead sleep on beneath the sward of Victoria Square.

DR. WILLIAM BULMER NICOL,

A descendant of a Scottish family of Norman extraction, was born at Stockwell, Middlesex, England, Nov. 11, 1812, being the second son of William Nicol, Esq., one of the deputy paymasters, St. James' Palace, by Harriet, daughter of Edward Chesshyre, Esq., a landed proprietor in Cheshire. He received his education at Rev. Dr. Burney's (afterwards Archdeacon Burney) and Christ's College, Cambridge. He became a very thorough classical scholar. He arrived in Canada in 1836, and, April 7, passed the Upper Canada Medical Board. He had "tickets from the University of King's College." He at once commenced practice at Bowmanville. He was Surgeon of the Northumberland Battalion of militia during the rebellion of 1837-38, and was also Staff Surgeon to Col. Cox, commandant of that district. In 1842, he removed to Toronto, and entered upon the practice of his profession. He received commission from Sir Charles Medcalfe, Lieut.-Governor, dated December 7, 1843, as Professor of Materia Medica in the University of King's College, on the recommendation of the Home Government, which position he continued to hold when King's College was merged into the University of Toronto, and until the Medical Department was abolished. Dr. Nicol was M.D. of the University, and for many years he was Dean of the Medical Faculty and a member of the Senate. In May, 1845, he was commissioned a member of the Upper Canada Medical Board, being designated Doctor of Medicine. Dr. Nicol, it is seen by the minutes, was a very regular attendant at the Board meetings, and the writer has a very clear recollection of his kindly face on the occasion of his examination, January, 1854. He was secretary of the Chirurgical Society, composed of men much his seniors in years. During the cholera of 1849, Dr. Nicol was one of the most active in attending on the immigrants afflicted with the scourge, visiting the sheds daily. For this attention and care he received the thanks of the Government. Dr. Nicol enjoyed a very extensive practice among the oldest and best families of Toronto. He was, during their sojourn in Toronto, physician to the Governor-General and Countess of Dufferin. His death took place, December 24, 1886, having shortly before completed his seventy-fourth year.

Dr. Nicol married Maria Alves, eldest daughter of Dr. Boys, a sketch of whom is elsewhere given. His widow died, March, 1892. They had born to them three sons: William, a member of the legal profession; George, also a member of the legal profession and clerk of Assize High Court of Justice; and Henry, a graduate in medicine of Toronto University, now practising in Cookstown, South Simcoe.

It is a great satisfaction to the writer to bear testimony to the high ability of Dr. Nicol. In the diagnosis and prognosis of disease he was almost unequalled, certainly not excelled. In his bearing towards his confreres he was a model; as a professional friend he was the soul of honour.

DR. LUCIUS JAMES O'BRIEN

Was born, 1796, at Woolwich, England, where his father was then stationed. He was the eldest son of Captain Lucius O'Brien, of the Royal Artillery, and Mary Callander, daughter of Sir Frederic Callandar-Campbell, of Craigforth, head of the well-known Scotch family of that name, whose other daughters were Lady Grahame, of Netherby, and the beautiful Mrs. Richard Brindsley Sheridan. On his father's side he was a direct descendant of Brien of the tributes, first King of all Ireland, the present head of which house is Baron Inchiquin, one of the Irish representative peers in the House of Lords. Whilst Dr. O'Brien was a child, his father was appointed to an important position connected with the fortifications then being constructed at Spike Island and Cork Harbour, and at a private school in that vicinity young O'Brien received his early education. Although most of his male relatives, on both sides, were army or navy men, young Lucius had a strong predilection for the medical profession, and entered on his studies for the same at Edinburgh University in 1812, and obtained his M.D. and M.R.C.S., London, in due course. Professor Sir Robert Christison, the celebrated toxilogist, was one of his most intimate friends and classmates. His residence in Europe, after he took his degree, was not of long duration, as he accepted a very advantageous offer to go to the Island of Jamaica, where he settled at the city of Kingston as one of the firm of Spaulding, Ferguson & O'Brien. He soon had a large and lucrative practice at Kingston, Port Royal and the surrounding districts. While there the slave insurrection, which preceded the rebellion, broke out; and during the troubles which ensued he was on constant military service with Colonel Madden's Battalion of Volunteers. His practice had made him widely personally known among the plantation negroes, and the sympathetic gentleness of his manner among patients had made him many friends among these people, so that in spite of the revolting scenes daily enacted among the insurgents, he could go alone and unarmed into portions of the island where scarcely any other white man dare venture, and could leave his young wife and infant child with no other protection than that of his black servants. The Baptist missionaries among the blacks were particularly obnoxious to the slave-holders, being blamed for inciting the insurrection through their preaching. Three of these gentlemen who fell into the hands of a Kingston mob only escaped what is now called lynching, through the personal exertions of Dr. O'Brien and his brother-in-law, John Roby, Comptroller of Customs of the Port. They could not obtain the liberation of the preachers, which would have been of precarious tenure, but they managed to secure their custody in law-abiding hands until matters quieted down.

A younger brother of the Doctor, the late Col. E. G. O'Brien, who had previously settled in Canada, had frequently asked him to join him, and a growing dislike to earthquakes and hurricanes, of which he had had several unpleasant experiences, made him decide to leave Jamaica. He therefore sold out his interest in his medical partnership and made arrangement for the freedom of his slaves. He came to Canada in 1832, landing at Quebec when the cholera was at its worst. He proceeded to Toronto, then York, and after a short stay with his brother at Shanty Bay, near Barrie, he established himself at Thornhill, on Yonge Street. Here he began the combined life of country practitioner and farmer. He soon had a large, if not very remunerative practice. Here he early became impressed with the crime and misery which strong drink and gambling were causing, as those were days of cheap rum and paucity of rational amusement. In conjunction with Rev. Mr. Mortimer, the Anglican clergyman of the place, he organized a total abstinence society, which existed for several years and did a great deal of good. During this period he, for example's sake, banished all alcohol, as a beverage, from his own house—a stand which then required more moral courage than now, as, then, not to ask a visitor to partake of something of that nature was looked on as a want of hospitality and churlish. The custom prevailed among all classes alike. He was during this period an active Justice of the Peace, and noted in that capacity for his endeavours to heal old sores among neighbours, and reclaim hard cases by kindly reason rather than by severe penalties. He was at Thornhill when the rebellion of 1837 broke out, and at once volunteered on the Loyalist side. He was appointed surgeon to the York Volunteers, and moved with his family into Toronto. He remained on duty all through the rebellion, and was personally acquainted with most of the leaders. Strange to say, he and Wm. Lyon Mackenzie never met to speak afterward but once, in 1860, in the house of the latter, long after all political feeling had passed away. In his study, that evening, Mackenzie showed him a framed copy of the proclamation of £1,000 for his capture, dead or alive, saying, "There was a time you wouldn't have minded earning that, Doctor." To which the Doctor, after looking at it, said: "Yes, there *was* a time, but that has passed."

When the Medical Faculty of King's College was established, he was offered the Professorship of Medical Jurisprudence, which he accepted, and held the chair until the abolition of the Faculty with that of Divinity. In Toronto, he was for years one of the Physicians and Vice-Presidents of the St. Patrick's Society, when that organization was national and non-sectarian. He was one of the first visiting physicians of the Toronto Hospital, and always took an active interest in its welfare. His correspondence with friends in Ireland early roused him to the impending danger of typhus fever being imported from thence, and he was about the first to arouse his medical confreres and the authorities to what was likely to come. During the epidemic of the fever in '47, '48, and when the cholera came, he worked day and night among the stricken ones, and in more than one case he had to put the dead bodies in the shells, when the undertakers would not touch them. During the latter period of these epidemics, his wife was in an almost dying condition from nervous prostration; but, notwithstanding, he never relaxed his labours in the hospital, the fever sheds, and in the worst parts of the city. He was a member of the University Senate, and was strongly against the surrender of the royal charter for a provincial one. He was a steady adherent of the Church of England, and in several journals opposed the secularization of the Clergy Reserves. In politics he was a Conservative, and, notwithstanding the many other matters weighing upon him, he edited the Toronto *Patriot* in 1848-50. Much as he differed from the Radical party of the day, he bitterly condemned the violence of speech which led to the Montreal riots, and was among the most active in promoting the courteous reception of Lord Elgin in Toronto. He was for a considerable time editor of the *Churchman*, published in Toronto, and also of the *Colonist*, the Conservative organ, when under the proprietorship of Samuel Thompson. His services to that party were recognized by the late Hon. William Cayley, then Inspector-General, who in 1885 offered him the post of his private secretary. This he accepted and retained for a brief period, when Mr. Cayley, previous to retiring from the Government, tranferred the Doctor to the permanent staff of the Department. He remained afterward with the Civil Service, going with it in 1859 to Quebec, and thence to Ottawa, where he died, in 1871, aged 75.

Dr. O'Brien married twice: first, in Ireland, his cousin, Miss Devere-Hunt, by whom he had one son, Lucius, who died in Oregon, U.S., 1858; secondly, in Jamaica, Eliza Da Lindo, second daughter of Abraham Rothschild Da Lindo, one of the wealthiest planters of the Island. She survived him for some years. His children by his second wife were: Edward Roby, who died in Toronto, 1889; Richard, resident in New York State; Donough, who died unmarried, in Ottawa, 1869; George Callander; Morrough and Alfred, who both died in infancy; Godfrey Samuel, P.L.S., died in Ottawa, 1891; and Lucia, married to Thos. J. Watters, Assistant Commissioner of Customs, son of the late Hon. Judge Watters, of St. John, N.B.

In addition to the foregoing interesting sketch furnished to the writer, the following pertinent facts are given: Dr. O'Brien was gazetted as practitioner of Upper Canada, September 8, 1832, and this card appeared:

"The subscriber, in compliance with the recommendation of his friends, and the usage of the country, begs leave to intimate to the inhabitants of York and its vicinity, that he has taken up his residence at No. 239 King Street, with the intention of practising his profession.

"LUCIUS O'BRIEN,
"*M.R.C.S., London, and Member of the Royal Medical Society of Edinburgh.*

"York, 1832."

In April, 1836, the Medical Board was reconstructed, and in July following his name appears among those present at the meeting of the Board. He was present again, January, 1837, and not again till January, 1839. From this time he attended regularly, until the Board was temporarily superseded by the College of Physicians and Surgeons of Upper Canada.

Dr. O'Brien was the most prominent member of the College of Physicians and Surgeons of Upper Canada. He was present at its organization, and was unanimously elected Secretary and Registrar. He was one of the committee appointed "to draw up a code of by-laws for the government of the College." In fact, he was on all the more important committees of the College, and was the chief officer in the organization and working of the College. He also prepared all official communications to the Lieut.-Governor, and conducted an extensive correspondence. Dr. O'Brien was a member of the Upper Canada Medical Board when it was revived, July, 1841, but, as will be seen in the proceedings of the Board, some difficulty arose with regard to the position allotted him in the Commission. He did not attend the meeting, and when a new commission was issued by the Lieut.-Governor in October following, Dr. O'Brien's name did not appear. His connection with the Board had finally ceased.

Dr. O'Brien was for many years President of the Bible Society. He was a sincere Christian, an "estimable man and clever physician."—*C. Gamble.*

Col. O'Brien, M.P., and Henry O'Brien, barrister, are nephews of Dr. Lucius O'Brien.

DR. GERALD O'REILLY.

This sketch of Dr. O'Reilly is so full of interest that no excuse is necessary for giving it in full.

Gerald O'Reilly, M.D., L.R.C.S.I., was born at Ballinlough, County Meath, Ireland, August 11, 1806, and died at Hamilton, February 26, 1861, in his 55th year. He was the seventh son of Gerald O'Reilly, of Ballinlough, whose ancestry is traceable to the old Irish princes of East Brefney, of the ancient family of Brefney O'Reilly, A.D. 611. The old homestead near Crossakiel, County Meath, where this branch of the O'Reilly family have lived for generations, has recently been rebuilt, and is now in the possession of, and occupied by, Lawrence O'Reilly, only surviving son of the late Peter O'Reilly, and nephew of Dr. Gerald O'Reilly.

Gerald O'Reilly passed his early years at Ballinlough, and was educated by a private tutor, the Rev. Mr. Halpin, rector of Oldcastle, County Meath. At the age of seventeen he was sent to Dublin to enter the medical profession, his father having previously died, and was apprenticed to Dr. James Cusack, of Stevens Hospital, May 14, 1823, and remained with him for five years and six months. Dr. Cusack was at the time the resident surgeon at Stevens Hospital, and subsequently became surgeon to the Queen. Dr. Charles Keane, Sir Charles Lever and Dr. Digby, of Brantford, were articled students of Dr. Cusack at this time, as also the venerable Dr. Ridgeway (F.R.C.S.I.), at present alive, and practising at Oldcastle, County Meath (1888). Dr. Ridgeway relates in "Fitzpatrick's Life of Charles Lever" an amusing incident, when Charles Lever succeeded in personating Dr. Cusack to the class. Dr. O'Reilly formed one of the principal actors on this occasion. It is given as related: "The late eminent Mr. Cusack, afterwards surgeon to the Queen, was the resident surgeon at Stevens Hospital. On this personage many a characteristic trick was played by Lever. Like his co-novelist, Dickens, he was full of dramatic talent, and one morning absolutely succeeded in personating Cusack to the class. This freak will be found recorded with due dramatic effect in "O'Malley"; but the scene is laid at Trinity College, instead of the hospital, while in lieu of Lever,

Frank Webber plays the prank, and Dr. Mooney takes the place of Surgeon Cusack.

Two of the students present on this occasion, and who have since attained high rank in the profession, have committed to writing their recollections of the incident. We allude to Mr. Cullihan, F.R.C.S.I., J.P., Ennis, and Mr. Ridgeway, F.R.C.S.I., Oldcastle.

"The circumstances attending Lever's personation of Mr. Cusack were as follows," writes Dr. Cullihan: "Mr. Cusack used to sleep at the hospital when there were important cases under treatment, and particularly after the performance of capital operations. When he entered the hospital at night, the porter would ring a bell to announce his arrival, and the resident pupils used to muster to see such cases as Dr. Cusack thought it necessary to visit. After making the usual round, Mr. Cusack directed the pupils to attend in his bedroom in the morning, to be examined on a subject which he had specified. On the morning referred to, I was going round the hospital at an early hour, and learned that Cusack had unexpectedly left during the night and had not returned. I met Lever on his way to Cusack's rooms, and told him he was not there, that he had left during the night; and we conspired together to have 'a lark.' Mr. Cusack's bedroom had a double door; the inner (a baize door) was acted on by a 'dumb porter,' which creaked when the door was opened or closed. Lever went into Cusack's bed, wrapped himself up in the blankets, and put on the red silk nightcap of his chief. I remained in the room. 'The bell boomed,' to quote Lever's words; the sound of feet was heard on the stairs, the door creaked, and gradually the room was filled with shivering students, some half asleep, and trying to rouse themselves into some approach of attention."

Dr. Cullihan continues:

"K., one of the apprentices, came in. Lever, in an admirably disguised voice, asked, 'Who is that?' 'K., sir,' was the answer. The next to arrive was O'R. (who was always called by his Christian name, Gerald), and the usual question was asked, 'Who is that?' The answer was, 'Gerald, sir.'

Others came in succession, and Lever, selecting the subjects for his mock examination, began. After a few queries, he asked,

"'What is the next subject, Gerald?'

"O'R.—'Cancer, sir.'

"Here a normal snore resounded from the bed.

"Lever—'Cancer, O'R.?' (interrogatively).

"O'R.—'What about it, sir?'

"Lever—'What about it yourself?' (Giving a yawn as though he would dislocate his jaw.)

"O'R.—'Cancer, sir, is a malignant disease.'

"Lever (after a few snores)—'Well?'

"O'R.—'Well, sir?'

"Lever—'You are a stupid ass, O'R. What do you know about it, K.?' (K. was not very brilliant, and spoke with a lisp.)

"K.—'Cancer, sir, affects the lower lip of males.'

"Lever—'What more? What colour is it?'

"K.—'Wed, sir.'

"Lever (doubtingly)—'Red?'

"K. (prompted by me)—'It is yellow, sir.'

"Lever (still more doubtingly)—'Yellow?'

"K. (after another prompt)—'Bloo, sir.'

"K. would probably have been led through all the colours of the spectrum before satisfying his preceptor as to the colour of cancer, but Lever could preserve his gravity no longer, and starting up, to the amazement of Gerald and K., and the glee of the others, flung his nightcap into K.'s face, and jumped out of the bed."

It is said that among the questions the sham Cusack asked was, "Where's Lever?" and the party answered, "Absent, sir." "Sorry for it. Lever is a man of first-rate capacity, and were he only to apply himself, I am not certain to what eminence his abilities might raise him."

The late Sir W. Wilde told us that he had often heard Lever describe this laughable adventure in presence of the great surgeon whom he had ventured to personate. Sundry small details, not given in the book, were added, such as Lever placing on the bed, ere the class arrived, Cusack's boot-jack and slippers, wherewith he wreaked summary chastisement on the heads of those who had failed to answer to his satisfaction.

The articles of apprenticeship in those days were certainly very unique and to the point, and will give some idea of how medical students at the commencement of their career were supposed to act towards their masters. The indenture was not a mere formality, as a fee of £170 12s. 6d. had to be paid for the privilege.

"This Indenture witnesseth that Gerald O'Reilly, of Little Ballinlough, in the County of Meath, of his own free will and accord, and with the consent of his mother, doth put himself apprentice to James Wm. Cusack, of Doctor Stevens Hospital, in the City of Dublin, Surgeon, to learn his profession, and with him, after the manner of an apprentice, to serve from the fourteenth day of May, 1823, until the full end and term of five years from thence next following, to be fully complete and ended. During which term the said apprentice his said master shall serve, his secrets keep, his lawful commands ever gladly perform. He shall do no damage to his said master, nor see it done of others, but that he, to his power, shall let or forthwith give warning to his said master of the same. He shall not commit fornication or contract matrimony within the said term. Hurt to his master he shall not do, or cause or procure to be done by others. He shall not play at cards, dice, tables or any other unlawful games whereby his said master shall sustain loss, with his own or others' goods during said term without license of his said master, J. W. Cusack; he shall not absent himself from his business, haunt or use taverns, ale-houses or play-houses, nor shall he be absent day or night unlawfully, but in all things, as an honest and faithful apprentice, he shall behave himself before his said master and all his, during the said term. And the said master, the said apprentice, in the same art which he useth, by the best way and means that he can, shall teach and instruct, or cause to be taught and instructed, the said apprentice during the said term (in consideration of the sum of one hundred and seventy pounds, twelve shillings and six pence, sterling, apprentice fees) according to the custom of the Royal College of Surgeons in Ireland; and at the end of said period the said master, J. W.

Cusack, shall and will exert himself to have the said apprentice admitted a licentiate of said College of Surgeons, and for the due performance of all and every the said covenants and agreements either of the said parties bindeth himself to the other by these presents.

"In witness whereof the parties above named to these indentures have interchangeably put their hands and seals the 14th day of May, in the year of our Lord one thousand eight hundred and twenty-three.

"Signed, sealed and delivered
in the presence of "(S'd) J. W. CUSACK, [L.S.]
"DAVID KENNY. GER'D O'REILLY, [L.S.]"

During his medical course of studies, Dr. O'Reilly resided four years and six months as interne pupil at Stevens Hospital, and had certificates from Dr. Cusack to that effect.

Also he had certificates on leaving Stevens Hospital, December, 1829, signed by Drs. Crafton, Colles, Wilmot and Cusack, of attendance for five years and six months.

He attended lectures on midwifery and diseases of women at the Rotunda Lying-in Hospital under Dr. Robert Collins, the master of the hospital. He had certificates signed by Richard Grattan, M.D. (King's professor of the practice of medicine) at Sir Patrick Dunn's Hospital, Dublin, in theory and practice of medicine, in 1828-29. He had lectures in chemistry delivered at the laboratory in Trinity College, Dublin, by Dr. F. Barker, professor of chemistry, in 1827; also certificate of having attended lectures at Stevens Hospital and practice of medicine as physician's pupil, signed by John Crafton and Sir Henry Marsh, A.B., M.D.

He also attended the lectures in the Park Street, Dublin, Medical School for 1824; the tickets are signed by Drs. Cusack, Porter, John Hart, Jacob Wilmot and James Applejohn.

He had a very flattering certificate signed by Dr. J. Wilmot, professor of theory and practice of surgery to the Royal College of Surgeons in Ireland, dated Stevens Green, January 23, 1830, and also from Robert Smith, surgeon, dated September 19, 1832, whose assistant he was for two years.

He had certificates of having attended lectures on anatomy,

physiology and surgery, in the University of Dublin, under Dr. James McCartney. He finally obtained the diploma of R.C.S., Ireland, and the diploma in midwifery, November 2, 1829.

After completing his studies in Dublin, Dr. O'Reilly was taken to England by his uncle, Dr. John O'Reilly, who then resided at Windsor, and was Surgeon in Ordinary to George IV. He continued his studies in London and became a licentiate of the Society of Apothecaries, London, July 4, 1833. Shortly after this, he made up his mind to emigrate, and in the year 1833 he said good-bye to his mother-land and sailed for Canada with his old friend, the late Alexander Milne, barrister, of Ancaster. He then remained only a short time in Canada, as on the death of his uncle, Dr. O'Reilly, surgeon to the royal family and household at Windsor Castle, he returned to Windsor for the purpose of bringing out the books, instruments and other effects left him by will, amongst which was a valuable gold watch (a present from George IV.), made in Paris, marking the seconds, hours, days of week and days of month. This old relic was left by special mention in Dr. Gerald O'Reilly's will, to his second son and namesake, Gerald, and is in his possession now.

On his return to Canada, Dr. O'Reilly commenced practice in Hamilton. In a few years he was able to build the old homestead, corner of King and Mary Streets, where he resided and practised, where his children were all born, and where he died. Until a few years ago, this house was continually occupied as a medical residence. It was one of the first brick houses in Hamilton, and among the first private houses where gas was used for illuminating purposes, and was in its day considered a very fine residence.

In 1835, Dr. O'Reilly obtained the Provincial license to practise physic, surgery and midwifery in Canada, under certificate of Drs. Christopher Widmer, Peter Deihl, John King and John Rolph, signed by Sir John Colborne, Lieutenant-Governor of the Province of Upper Canada, dated at Toronto, January 6, 1835.

Almost on his arrival in Hamilton, Dr. O'Reilly's success was assured. He was popular from the first, and counted amongst his early friends and patients Sir Allan Macnab, John O'Hatt,

Hon. Peter Hamilton, Hon. S. Mills, Dean Geddes, Judge O'Reilly, Thomas Stock, Æneas Kennedy, the Secords, Ryckmans, Beasleys, Winers, Wilson and Edward Browne, the Carpenders, Captain Stewart, Colonel Ainsley, the Rosseaux, W. F. Murray-Davidson, the Collector of Customs, the Ritchie family, the Spohns, and many others. He was now known as the "young Irish surgeon," and commanded a large and lucrative practice, extending over a large radius, reaching from St. Catharines to Brantford and from the Grand River to Oakville. For many years before his death, having cut off his country practice, he occupied a leading position as a consultant.

During his life in Hamilton, Dr. O'Reilly filled many offices of trust and position. He held a commission as surgeon to the 3rd Gore Militia, or "Men of Gore."

Some of his old monthly sick returns to Government (say per July 1 to 31, 1838), read as follows:

Strength of militia on duty—

Four companies, total strength..................	200 men
Four additional companies, from July 2 to 6, strength	200 "
One troop of cavalry for same period.............	60 "

Some very interesting and carefully prepared returns, giving the names of the men and the diseases for which they were invalided at the time, from 1838 to 1842, are still in good preservation.

Dr. O'Reilly held the position of surgeon to the united counties of Wentworth and Halton, and was surgeon to the county and Hamilton gaol at the time of his death, having occupied the office for nearly twenty years.

He was one of the first who administered chloroform in Canada for surgical operation, and he administered it to one of his own children for the purpose of extracting a broken needle imbedded deeply in the foot. The infant was only a few days old, and was reported at that time as the youngest aspirant for "anæsthetic fame."

During the cholera epidemic in 1854, Dr. O'Reilly showed zeal and physical endurance, and how much work one man can do day and night. He visited from house to house, never thinking of going to bed. At last, when overcome by fatigue, he was persuaded to take a short rest on the sofa; but as soon as sleep overtook him, his wife determined that he should not be disturbed by either patients or messengers during that night at least, so she placed servants at the front and surgery doors of the house, had the bells and knockers muffled, and so carefully did she carry out his idea of keeping a house quiet, that he obtained nearly twelve hours continuous sleep, and woke up refreshed and rested, saying, "The cholera must be abated very much, as I have not been disturbed during the whole night." By this successful ruse perhaps his life was saved, and he was enabled to continue his arduous work among the cholera patients until the fearful scourge had passed over. Dr. O'Reilly was amongst the first surgeons present at the frightful railroad accident on the G.W.R., at the Desjardins canal bridge, where so many passengers were killed and injured in 1857.

Dr. O'Reilly was evidently educated at a period when both social and professional insults were generally and equally dealt with by those interested, without the slow, expensive, and often unsatisfactory results of a trial by jury. The following clipping from the Hamilton *Argus* will convince anyone that Dr. O'Reilly had an idea of what an apology should be, and when convinced of insult, lost no time in demanding every satisfaction.

"ADVERTISEMENT.

"I, Richard Howell, having, on the 21st of January last, published a statement in the Hamilton *Argus*, reflecting on the professional character of Dr. Gerald O'Reilly, of Hamilton, inasmuch as in that statement I accused him of extortion in charging me with the sum of £1 1s. 6d. for one visit, and also in stating that I did not receive any medicine from him. Now, I hereby declare that the whole of that statement made by me was totally without foundation, as after circumstances convinced me, for Dr. O'Reilly did visit my house on two occasions, for professional purposes, and also administered medicine, and further, that these visits were consultation visits with Dr. McCarthy, and I have since ascertained that, according to the medical tariff of this town, ten shillings is the regular charge for a consultation visit. I have now to express my deep regret in having been the cause in any way of injuring Dr. O'Reilly, either in his personal feelings or professional reputation.

"(Signed) RICHARD HOWELL.

"Hamilton, 2nd February, 1843."

Dr. O'Reilly was one of the founders and original shareholders of the Canada Life Assurance Company, and his signature will be found on the Trust Deeds, or Deed of Settlement, under which the business of the Company was begun, and before the charter was granted, in April, 1849, by the Parliament of Canada. He was also the first and principal medical officer and adviser of the Company in 1847. Dr. W. G. Dickinson was afterwards associated with him as medical adviser of the Company. Dr. O'Reilly continued to hold the position until a few years before his death. He was also one of the first assured in the Company, his first policy being No. 47, taken out in the first year of the Company's history, December, 1847. His old and intimate friend, Dr. Craigie, gave the certificate of Dr. O'Reilly's death, and became his successor in office.

Dr. O'Reilly was examiner in Principles and Practice of Medicine in the University of Toronto, 1856.

He was a member of the Loyal Hamilton Lodge Independent Order of Oddfellows, having joined the order in July 30, 1844, and was elected Surgeon to the Lodge, August, 1845, holding the position continuously until the time of his death.

As a practitioner, Dr. O'Reilly was most conscientious and painstaking, attending both the rich and poor alike, and yet he always found time to keep up in his professional reading. He not only took all the leading periodicals of the day, but rapidly acquired a very extensive library of all recent publications of professional and other works, and, being fond of surgery, accumulated a most extensive assortment of surgical appliances and instruments. He had a good idea of mechanics, and usually made his own splints and other appliances, to suit the individual cases. He was a very quick and expert operator, a good surgeon for those days of suffering, when every minute had to be considered, before the days of chloroform. He was a genial and liberal man, fond of society, and enjoyed hunting and shooting. He was a good musician, and thoroughly understood the violin and flute, and entered into everything he undertook with great enthusiasm, but he remained, as he had begun, a devoted student of his profession to the last.

He died suddenly, at the age of 55, the result of pyæmia, following the removal of a small osseous tumour of the leg, which caused great pain at times. He was confined to bed for one week only after the operation, this being the first and only time during his professional career in Hamilton that he was prevented from attending to his daily work by illness.

He left a name, reputation and influence which even now, in and about Hamilton, are well remembered, and the name of Dr. Gerald O'Reilly will not easily be forgotten by many of his old friends and patients, who knew him so well and who have survived him.

His funeral will long be remembered in Hamilton, showing by the crowds of mourners the high esteem in which he was held by both rich and poor. A massive, but plain, granite monument marks his grave at the family plot in Burlington cemetery, and a memorial tablet, erected in memory of Gerald O'Reilly and his wife, occupies a space on the south wall of Christ Church Cathedral, Hamilton.

Dr. O'Reilly was married to Henrietta, youngest daughter of Henry Harcourt Waters, of Hailsham, Sussex, England, and sister of Mr. Thomas Waters, an old resident of Port Dover, now residing at Windsor, Ont. The widow resided in Hamilton, attending to the education of her children, until the time of her death, December 19, 1884. Dr. Gerald O'Reilly left six children, who are all living in Canada (1894)—four sons and two daughters.

The eldest son, Charles O'Reilly, M.D., C.M., McGill College, of Toronto, has devoted his professional life to hospital work, having held the position of Medical Superintendent of the Hamilton City Hospital and Toronto General Hospital for over twenty-six years. He married Sophia, youngest daughter of George Rolph, barrister, of Dundas, and niece of the Hon. Dr. John Rolph and grand-daughter of Dr. Thomas Rolph. Their only son, now thirteen years old, Brefney Rolph O'Reilly, is the youngest member of the Canadian branch of the O'Reilly family (1894).

The second son, Gerald O'Reilly, M.D., C.M., Trinity College, Toronto, is practising his profession at Fergus, Ont. (1894). He is unmarried.

H. O'Reilly, third son, entered the Bank of Hamilton, at head office, when the bank was first established.

The youngest son, Edward B. O'Reilly, M.D., C.M., Trinity College, having spent several years as surgeon on the Allan S.S. line, has settled in Hamilton. He was Medical Superintendent of the Winnipeg General Hospital in 1888.

The eldest daughter, Elizabeth, unmarried, resides in Hamilton, Ont.

The youngest daughter, Alice, married Dr. Graves Kiltson, of Hamilton, son of the late Collector of Customs and nephew of the late Commodore Kiltson, of St. Paul, Minn., U.S.

John O'Reilly, M.D., F.R.C.S.I., of Washington Square, New York, was a younger brother of Dr. Gerald O'Reilly. He went to New York in 1849 and died in 1868.

Miss Alicia T. O'Reilly, now residing at Rathmines, near Dublin, Ireland, is the only and youngest sister of the late Dr. G. O'Reilly.

DR. JOSEPH ORLANDO ORR

Was the son of Andrew Orr, of Millbank, his mother being Mary Ann, daughter of Capt. John Forster, County Tyrone, Ireland. He was born at Omagh, County Tyrone, 1809. Having received his primary education in his native town, he commenced the study of medicine under Dr. Osborne, of Newton Stewart, and then attended medical lectures in London, England. Coming to Canada, 1831, he completed his medical studies under Drs. Widmer and Deihl, and then remained with them as an assistant for some years. In 1840, he opened a drug business on Yonge Street. He passed the Medical Board, July, 1841, and was in practice on Yonge Street until 1848, when he removed to Bond Head. Here he commanded a large practice until his death, 1869. Dr. Orr married, 1837, Maria Elizabeth Carter, of Bond Head, by whom he had seven children, of whom only a son and a daughter survive him. The son lives in Toronto, the daughter married Richard Slee, and resides in Brooklyn, N. Y.; her son, Dr. Richard Slee, is a medical practitioner of the same place.

There are now (1894) five nephews of Dr. J. O. Orr practising medicine in Toronto. Dr. Rowland B. Orr is registered as M.B., Toronto University, and Member College Physicians and Surgeons, Ontario, 1877. He was a representative to the Medical Council, Ontario, 1885, 1890, 1895. In addition to practice, he is Manager and Editor of the *Ontario Medical Journal*. Dr. Joseph Orlando Orr is registered M.D., C.M., University Victoria College, and Member College Physicians and Surgeons, Ontario, 1884. He has filled the post of Alderman, but is at present sojourning in England engaged in special studies. Charles J. Caldwell Oliver Hastings is registered M.D., C.M., Victoria College, 1885, Licentiate King's and Queen's College Physicians, Ireland, and Certificate British Registration, 1886. Dr. Andrew Orr Hastings has M.D., C.M., Victoria College, 1886; Licentiate Apothecaries' Hall, Dublin, and Certificate British Registration, 1877. Dr. John Alfred Burgess, the fifth nephew, practising in Toronto, is M.D., C.M., University Victoria College, and Member College Physicians and Surgeons, Ontario, 1885.

DR. HENRY ORTON,

Of Leicestershire, England, came to Canada, 1835, and settled at Guelph. He married Mary Jerram, who died in England, 1858. Dr. Orton was the Coroner for the county for many years; he died at Fergus, 1869.

Dr. Henry Orton had four sons who entered the medical profession. In fact, the Ortons are a race of doctors; for several generations all the male members of the family have been medical men.

DR. HENRY ORTON, JR., studied medicine at Trinity College, Toronto, and Jefferson College, Philadelphia, and took the degree of M.D., 1857. He practised for a time at Hespeler, and then settled at Ancaster. He died from the effects of an injury caused by his horse taking fright, running away, and dashing him against a tree. A local paper said of him that he was "foremost in every public charity and philanthropic enterprise. The widow, the orphan, and all needy in any way, will miss a helper ever ready to assist and advise."

DR. T. J. ORTON, having acquired his profession in Canada, proceeded to England at the time of the Crimean War, and entered the army, of which he became a Surgeon-Major. He was connected with the the Royal Artillery, was in the trenches before Sebastopol in 1855, and at the assault of the Redan. He received a medal and clasp, also a Turkish medal. He was in India under Sir Hugh Rose in 1858, and was in many engagements, for which services he again received a medal and clasp. Returning to Canada, he practised for a time at Ancaster, in partnership with his brother, in 1861.

The following sketch is taken from the *Empire*, of January 4, 1892 :

"Dr. Orton, of Guelph, is dead. About a week ago he was suddenly seized with a serious and painful illness. His son, who is also a physician in practice at Winnipeg, was telegraphed for. Drs. Howell, Keating and McKinnon were unremitting in their attention, but the disease was beyond the reach of human skill to conquer. Yesterday afternoon death came to the relief of the sufferer. The deceased gentleman was widely and favourably known, and enjoyed a large practice. His father, who was one of the first medical practitioners in Guelph, was for many years a partner of the late Dr. Clarke. He was twice married, his first wife being a sister of Dr. Howell, of Guelph. His second wife, who survives him, is a daughter of the late Capt. Leslie, of Puslinch. He leaves four children by his first wife, and one by his second, to mourn his comparatively early demise, he being only about fifty years of age. Widespread sympathy is evinced for his sorrow-stricken widow and children."

DR. GEORGE TURNER ORTON studied at the College of Surgeons, Dublin, and University of St. Andrew's, Scotland, from which he took the degree of M.D. in 1860, and the M.R.C.S.E. subsequently. He practised with his brother at Ancaster for a time; settled at Fergus, and soon had a large and lucrative practice. He entered Parliament in 1882 as representative of Centre Wellington: removed to Winnipeg in 1883; was a Surgeon to the famous 90th with Gen. Middleton; made Surgeon-Major, and was at Fish Creek and Batoche; was Chief Medical Officer to the Canadian Pacific Railway, 1884-85. Going to British Columbia, he was made Coroner.

"The career of Dr. Orton has been an active and an extremely useful one."—*Canadian Biography.*

DR. RICHARD ORTON took his M.B. at Toronto University, 1863, and practised at Guelph. He died, January, 1891.

ROBERT JOHN PAGET

Was born at Exeter, England, 1799. He was a member of the same family as the Marquis Anglesey. Educated at Edinburgh University, where he took F.R.C.S. Ed., and practised for a time at Exeter. In 1838 he came to Canada for the benefit of his health and practised for a while in Toronto, then at York Mills, and finally at Thornhill for twelve years very successfully. Dr. Scadding says, "He was an element of happy influence in the little world of this region; a man of high culture, formerly a medical practitioner of great repute in Torquay. (See proceedings of Medical Department, King's College.)

Dr. Paget had ten children, five being boys. Two of these entered the medical profession. Arthur H. graduated at Victoria College, 1858, and has since practised at Elora.

DR. GEORGE HAMILTON PARK

Appeared before Upper Canada Medical Board, April, 1834. "The Board is (was) perfectly satisfied by his examination and grant him a certificate to that effect." Dr. Park was a native Canadian, the son of Captain Park, who was a veteran of 1812. Like most natives of that period, and even of subsequent times, he did not enjoy the opportunities of acquiring a good primary education. But in the study of medicine he was fortunate in having the instruction and guidance of that prince of Canadian medical teachers, Dr. John Rolph. After obtaining his license he practised at Simcoe for seven or eight years. He also practised at Ancaster. He married a sister of Dr. Rolph, and through the Doctor's influence was, in 1848, appointed superintendent of the Toronto Lunatic Asylum.

Dr. Park received a complimentary address on leaving Simcoe, signed by upwards of two hundred. It is dated August 28, 1848. The address says, referring to his appointment: "It is the respect and affection which your urbanity of manners, your liberality in the promotion of public improvements, your generosity and bounty to the poor, your honourable principles as a man, and your acknowledged skill as a physician, which have so universally gained for you this regard of the community."

But Dr. Park, before many months, found that his position was a bed of thorns.

Had Dr. Park had a fair chance, it is believed that he would have well succeeded in discharging the duties of the office. While there he was liked by the inmates, which is no mean criterion. Dr. Park, for a time, was lecturer on anatomy at Rolph's School. He finally settled at Ancaster, where he died.

DR. CORNELIUS JAMES PHILBRICK

Was born in Colchester, England, May 30, 1816, being the son of a surgeon. He pursued his medical studies in London, Dublin and Edinburgh. The writer has before him numerous certificates to Dr. Philbrick from surgeons and physicians who were noted in their day, and whose names are interwoven in British History of medicine and surgery. He was a student at the Royal College of Surgeons, in Dublin, during the session of 1836-37. Besides the usual certificates from the several professors, he carried away with him particularly flattering testimonials from his teachers. The following is a fair sample of all:

"DUBLIN, *April* 30, 1837.

"Mr. Philbrick has been engaged in professional study during last session in the College of Surgeons, in this city, as will appear by the several certificates he has received from that institution. In addition to these, however, I have no hesitation in stepping out of the usual course and bearing my sincere testimony to the great diligence and peculiar assiduity which this gentleman evinced through the entire course. His general conduct, too, has been most exemplary, and I can truly affirm that few students have ever left such favourable impressions on the minds of his several teachers as he has done.

"ROBERT HARRISON, M.D.,
"*Professor of Anatomy.*"

Mr. Philbrick attended lectures in Edinburgh on midwifery and diseases of women and children from May 9 to July 31, 1837. He remained a student there during the session 1837-38, and testimonials again are found of his zeal and industry. In August, 1838, he became a member of the R.C.S. Eng.

A certificate from Thos. P. Dennett, of Harrington, Sussex, dated August 23, 1839, informs us that Dr. Philbrick had been his assistant for six months, during which time he had "the medical and surgical care of eleven parishes, and that the zealous and efficient manner in which he executed his duties always gave great satisfaction." In October, 1841, Prof. Kemp writes: "As I understand that you have the intention of settling in practice at Kidderminster, I most gladly avail myself of the opportunity of testifying in the strongest manner possible to your general and professional character.

"I know that you have studied the medical profession with the greatest assiduity and success, and that you have a thorough knowledge of it, as well in its general principles as in its practical details. Whilst you attended my course of practical chemistry and pharmacy I had every reason to be perfectly satisfied with your progress, and I had then also ample means of judging of your other attainments, of which I deem very highly.

"To your gentlemanlike conduct, to your kind, obliging and humane disposition, I also bear my willing testimony. With my most sincere wishes for your success."

The following is from the renowned Prof. Ferguson: "2nd March, 1842. I have been acquainted with Mr. C. J. Philbrick for many years, and have had frequent opportunities of observing his great professional knowledge and zeal. In my opinion he is highly qualified as a medical practitioner, and in every way likely to give satisfaction to those by whom his services are required." In 1849-50, Dr. Philbrick was again a student at Edinburgh, where he attended lectures on natural history as well as those on institutes of medicine. He received this certificate: "I have great pleasure in stating that Mr. Cornelius Philbrick was well known to me during the winter of 1849-50, when he resided in Edinburgh, and that I formed a high opinion of his intelligence, capacity and accomplishments as a surgeon from the conversations I had with him on medical topics. I saw Mr. Philbrick daily for six months, and had, in addition, many interviews with him in reference to scientific or professional topics. I can accordingly recommend this gentleman, as known to me and many others, to be unusually well grounded in his profession, and to have had much experience, for his years, as a medical practitioner, and especially as a surgeon. His accurate knowledge of anatomy and acquaintance with operations, peculiarly qualify him for success in the practice of surgery, and his courteous, kindly manners and moral character largely add to his claims as a medical man. I would add that, in addition to his qualifications as a private practitioner, Mr. Philbrick is a tried and approved teacher of anatomy, including operative surgery. GEORGE WILSON, M.D., F.R.S.E." He also obtained, by examination (an honour of which Dr. Philbrick was always proud), this diploma: "Know all men by these presents, That Mr. Cornelius James Philbrick, of Kidderminster, is hereby admitted a Fellow of the Royal College of Surgeons of England. Dated this eighth day of August, in the year of our Lord, one thousand eight hundred and fifty. No. 1. JAMES MONCRIEFF ARNOTT, *President;* JOHN F. SOUTH and CÆSAR W. HAWKINS, *Vice-Presidents.*"

It seems that Dr. Philbrick was desirous of a situation as hospital surgeon, and received a letter respecting it from John Simon, a name associated with surgical and pathological science, and conspicuous as the name of the father of State Medicine and Public Health in Great Britain, and the adviser to the Privy Council for many years on sanitary matters. Dr. Simon says: "I have much pleasure in stating, from personal knowledge, that I believe him to be very highly qualified for such an appointment, and likely, by his personal character as well as by his professional attainments, to reflect credit on whatever institution may obtain his services."

Shortly after this, Dr. Philbrick came to Toronto. About 1852 he was Professor of Surgery, Trinity College.

Dr. Philbrick took up his abode in Yorkville, now a part of Toronto, and devoted himself to general practice, although, having no degree in pure medicine, he called himself on his door-plate, "Mr. Philbrick, Surgeon." He was, perhaps, a little eccentric, but he enjoyed the greatest respect of his fellow-practitioners, and his large practice was evidence of his standing in the eyes of the public. He was commissioned Surgeon to the Militia Troop of York County, 1857, and for many years held the office of Coroner for the counties of York and Peel. Dr. Philbrick married some time before leaving England, and had one child, a daughter, who died there. His wife died in England about 1863.

In January 1, 1876, Dr. Philbrick took into partnership Arthur Jukes Johnson, M.B., M.R.C.S., Eng.; F.R.M.S., F.O.S., London, who afterwards succeeded to his practice.

Dr. Philbrick, for some time before his death, suffered from an internal ailment, and on the morning of Dec. 2, 1885, he was found dead in bed. His death was attributed to rupture of the intestines from cancerous disease. In a quiet corner, under shading trees in St. James' cemetery, Dr. Philbrick sleeps his last sleep. A marble slab covers his grave, on which are inscribed the date of his death, and these words: "Having practised his profession in this city with credit and distinction 34 years," and near the foot, set in the marble, is the door-plate, with the words, "Mr. Philbrick, Surgeon."

DR. FRANCIS W. PORTER,

Was thus gazetted, October 24, 1828: "Francis Wm. Porter, M.D., University Edinburgh, and Licentiate of R.C.S., Edinburgh, he having complied with the terms contained in the second and third sections of VIII. George." He came from Montreal and settled at Niagara. It is stated that he had been an army surgeon. He acquired an extensive practice, and was a prominent figure in the place. The charming appearance of his daughter is still remembered. The standing of Dr. Porter in his profession may be learned from the correspondence from him, Muirhead & Telfer, to the Medical Board. (See Minutes, October, 1832.)

Dr. Porter died at Niagara, March, 1840. The Niagara *Chronicle*, April 1, says: "Endeared to both rich and poor by his kindness of heart and professional skill, a loss more generally felt could scarcely have been sustained by this community. His remains were attended to the grave by an immense concourse of sorrowing relatives and friends."

"Married, October 24, 1850, George Maxwell, Esq., Collector of Customs, Grimsby, to Maria Ann, only daughter of the late Dr. Porter, of Niagara."

DR. GRANT POWELL

Was born in Norwich, England, 1779, his father being William Dummer Powell, barrister-at-law, who afterwards became Chief Justice of Upper Canada, and his mother Anne Murray. He studied medicine at Guy's Hospital, with his uncle, Dr. Archibald Murray, and took his degree at Apothecaries' Hall. The same Dr. Archibald Murray took part in prison reform with the well-known philanthropist, Dr. Howard. In the early part of this century, between 1800 and 1804, Dr. Powell was surgeon of an East India merchantman which sailed from Salem for the Spice Islands. A practice prevailed in those days by which all officers on such vessels were allowed poundage on the home voyage. This consisted in bringing out such articles as each one might select, in certain quantities, for his own benefit. In the present case, the subject of this sketch chose tobacco. Some of the crew having run short of this luxury, owing to the prolonged voyage, got ill from using other materials to satisfy their cravings for the weed. For some time the cause of their illness, which was a serious matter, jeopardizing the safety of the ship, was a mystery. On Dr. Powell discovering the secret, he threw open his stores, and, as he often said, with an almost miraculous result, the crew rapidly regaining their health and wonted vigour.

Dr. Powell came to America in 1804 and settled at Ballston Springs, N.Y., remaining there till 1807, when he went to Montreal and there practised until the autumn of 1812. He was familiarly known there as "the little doctor with the gold spectacles, or oftener, in French, as "le petit docteur avec les lunettes d'or." He came to York during the war of 1812-13, and was engaged as surgeon in the Incorporated Militia at Chippawa, and for his services he derived a pension of £200 per annum till his death. He never was enamoured of the practice of medicine, though always taking a keen interest in professional matters and medical politics. To use his own expression, "The theory was beautiful, but the practice was damnable." He gladly availed himself of the advent of Dr. Widmer to Toronto, to whom he virtually handed over what practice he had, though he still continued to advise old friends till his death.

Dr. Powell was one of the first members of the Upper Canada Medical Board, in the formation of which he had a good deal to do, and always took a lively interest in its proceedings. He virtually retired from practice about 1817, and on the death of the Clerk of the House of Assembly he received that appointment, and also that of official Principal of the Court of Probate. About 1820 he was also appointed Judge of the Home District Court and subsequently became Clerk of the Legislative Council. He died in office, June 12th, 1838, in his sixtieth year.

Dr. Powell married, 1805, at Ballston Springs, N.Y., Eliza Bleecker, and had eleven children, as follows: Anne Jane, John, Charlotte, William Dummer, Charlotte Bleecker, Elizabeth Van Rensselaer, William Dummer, Grant, Margaret Bleecker, Mary Boyles, Mary Catharine. Of the seven who survived him were five daughters and two sons. Of these, Margaret died in 1840; Elizabeth died of plague, in Mauritius, in 1867; William Dummer became Judge of the united counties of Wellington, Waterloo and Grey. He died at Guelph, 1854. Those still living (1889) are, Anne Jane, widow of the late C. Seymour, of H.M.

Commissariat. She now lives in Ottawa and is aged 82 years. Charlotte Bleecker, wife of John Ridout, Esq., Registrar of the County of York, and now living in Toronto, aged 75 years. Grant, now living in Ottawa and holding the position of Under-Secretary of State for Canada, aged 69 years. Mary Catharine became the wife of the late Hon. A. McKellar, Sheriff of Wentworth.

The only descendant of Dr. Powell who followed in his professional footsteps is his grandson, Dr. Robert Henry Wynyard Powell, who graduated at McGill University, 1876, taking the Holmes Gold Medal, and who has since practised in Ottawa. He is the author of the valuable book, "The Doctor in Canada" (1890).

Dr. Scadding, speaking of the subject of this sketch, says:

"Dr. Grant Powell was a handsome reproduction, on a larger scale, of his father, the chief. It is found recorded that Dr. Powell was Surgeon to the General Staff of Militia of Upper Canada in 1822. He had most to do with the erection of the old hospital, and it was by his direction that the building was built with its sides due north and south, and east and west. We learn from a letter written by Sir Isaac Brock to Sir George Prevost that during the war Dr. Grant Powell had the confidence of the civil and military commanders. In a letter addressed to Col. Baynes from York, July 23, 1812, General Sir Isaac Brock writes: 'I wish very much something might be done for Mr. Grant Powell. He was regularly brought up in England as a surgeon. I intended to have proposed to Sir George to appoint him permanent surgeon to the marine department, but I now seriously think the situation would not answer. His abilities, I should think, might be more fully employed, now that so many troops have been called out.' As a result of that, he was appointed Surgeon, and had the oversight of the hospital on the Niagara frontier."

During the war, Dr. Grant Powell bore an important relation to the Governor-General, and perhaps the condition of affairs in York after the second attack of the Americans in July, 1813, cannot be better described than by quoting the communication made by Dr. Grant Powell and Dr. Strachan to the Governor-General on August 2, 1813, as follows:

"We beg leave to state, for the information of His Excellency the Governor-General, that about eleven o'clock on Saturday morning the enemy's fleet of twelve sail were seen standing for the harbour. Almost all the gentlemen of the town having retired, we proceeded to the garrison about two o'clock, and watched until three o'clock, when the *Pyter*, the *Madison* and *Oneida* came to anchor in the offing, and the schooners continued to pass up the harbour with their sweeps, the wind having become light, then coming to abreast of the town, the remainder near the garrison. About four o'clock several boats full of troops landed at the garrison, and we, bearing a white flag, desired the first officer we met to conduct us to Commodore Chauncey. We mentioned to the Commodore that the inhabitants of York, consisting chiefly of women and children, were alarmed at the approach of the fleet, and that we had come to know his intentions respecting the town; that if it were to be pillaged or destroyed we might take such measures as were still in our power for their removal and protection. We added that the town was totally defenceless, the militia being still on parole, and that the gentlemen had left it, having heard that the principal inhabitants of Niagara had been carried away captive, a severity unusual in war."

DR. JABEZ PROCTOR POWERS,

Of English descent, was born, February 17, 1803, in Vermont. Removed, in 1808, to the then wilds of New York State, St. Lawrence county, where he spent his boyhood. In early manhood he returned to Vermont, the residence of his mother's family, the Proctors, of some local note in Proctorsville. The Governor of the State was his cousin. He graduated in Arts at Hanover University in 1826, and in 1828 took his degree in the Medical College of Fairfield, one of the best medical schools in the United States.

His "thesis" was pronounced the best that had been given, up to that time, in the college. Very retiring in disposition, and most diffident in general society, the incidents of his life are necessarily taken from the voluminous correspondence he has left behind.

His father belonged to the Society of Friends, and the Doctor used sometimes to tell of his pitched battles with his schoolmates when they called his father "a Quaker," and him "a little Quaker." Though his father died when he was young, his Quaker parentage was shown in his avoidance of all public notice or public offices of any kind, or membership in any secret society, as well as in his simplicity of manner.

Dr. Powers came to Canada about 1832. The political ferment in Upper and Lower Canada, which finally culminated in the rebellion of 1837, was already beginning to operate, and his sympathies were soon enlisted with those hostile to the family compact. He contributed political articles which were published in the newspapers and periodicals of that period.

He first settled in Demorestville, Prince Edward county, as a medical practitioner. Dr. Power's views were more in accord with the scientific views and practice of the present time than with those of his own age, especially as to the extensive use of intoxicating liquors and alcohol in diseases. He married (1837) Louisa Ford, eldest daughter of Gilbert Ford, and sister of C. R. Ford, of Colborne. He moved to Colborne, 1846, in which village he spent the rest of his days. Dr. Powers sometimes spoke of his life as a failure because he had not accomplished all he had hoped to do in early years, but in his self-depreciation he remembered not that for more than half a century, while in the practice of his profession, he had never refused to go to sick people because they were poor, ill-conditioned or degraded; and, though expecting no recompense, he had always given them not only professional advice but such care and medicine as he thought would alleviate their sufferings or heal their diseases. Throughout his long, laborious life, reaching considerably beyond fourscore years, whether riding or driving, by day or by night, Dr. Powers never lost his pleasant smile, his genial, simple, modest manner nor his kindly welcome of all friends to his home and hearty hospitality.

Dr. Powers died, May 1, 1886, aged eighty-four. He left a widow and two daughters. The eldest daughter married Geo. Young, M.A., editor of the Trenton *Courier*. The youngest daughter, now a widow, married Robert Deans, druggist, of Colborne.

DR. JEDEDIAH PRENDERGAST

Was probably the first practitioner of medicine in the Niagara District apart from those connected with the military service.

The Prendergasts, of Duchess county, N.Y., at the time of the rebellion of 1776, were natives of Ireland. Several brothers were active U. E. Loyalists. One, William, the father of Dr. Prendergast, did not commit himself to either side. His son, Jedediah, the subject of this sketch, was born May 13th, 1766. His medical education was obtained at Albany. In 1804, he was one of a party who left Mayville, now Chautauqua, N.Y., bound for Brockville, by way of the head of Lake Ontario; but the journey was cut short. As the party was passing along the mountain road between Lundy's Lane and Hamilton, in the vicinity of De Cews, the horses took fright and ran away. The travelling equipments were so badly damaged that they could not immediately proceed. It resulted in the Doctor's settling near the present site of Thorold, where he practised his profession until about six months before the commencement of the war of 1812, when he removed again to Mayville. His practice took him sometimes a long distance away, even to Long Point, where he performed operations; he made his journeys on horseback. At that time there were no other doctors in the district except the army surgeons, and it is said they were unwilling to go far away from their stations. Dr. Prendergast was a large-sized man and a skilful physician, and very methodical in his habits. He died at Mayville, N. Y. State, in 1848, aged eighty-two. He had one child, a daughter, who became the wife of the Hon. W. H. Merritt, who had become acquainted with her while the family were living near St. Catharines.

DR. ABRAHAM VAN VLECK PRUYN,

Of Bath, appeared before the Medical Board, April, 1831. The Board was "perfectly satisfied with his examination."

Dr. Pruyn was a native of Kinderhook, N.Y. Born 1808, he received his education at the academy in that town, and also studied medicine there with an English physician, Dr. Barthrop.

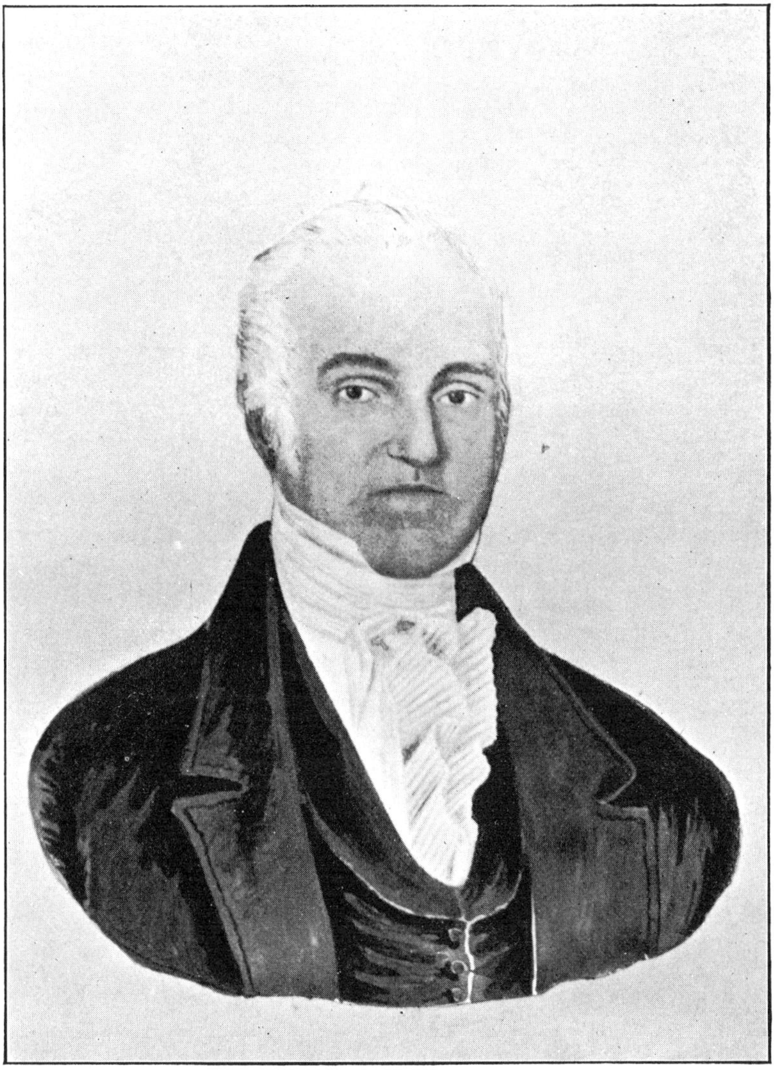

DR. JEDEDIAH PRENDERGAST.

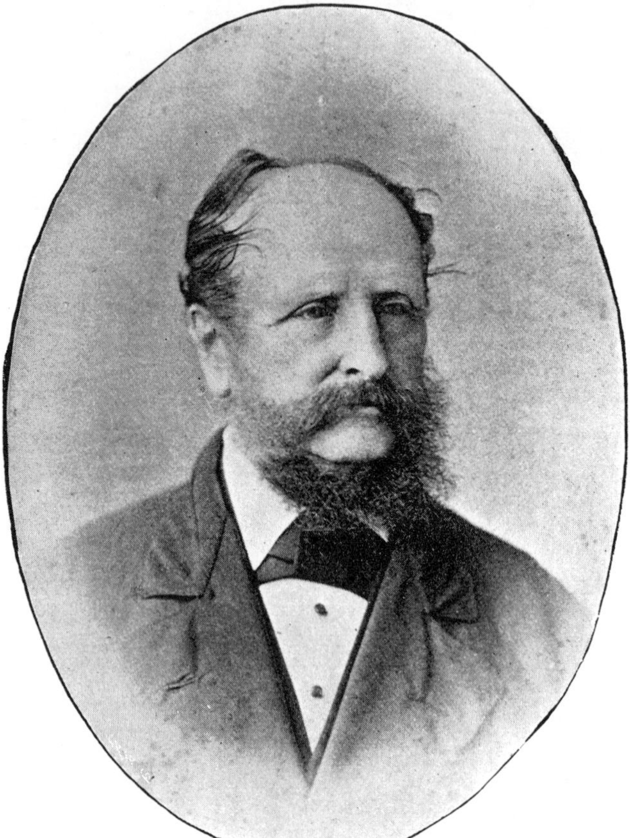

DR. THOMAS PYNE.

He received his medical diploma and license to practise surgery, physic, etc., from the Medical Society of Columbia County, N.Y., September 16, 1829. This only gave him authority for that State. He practised a few months at Oswego, N.Y., and then came to Canada and passed the Board a few weeks after his arrival. He soon after settled at Hallowell, now Picton, as this card indicates :

"Dr. Pruyn has opened an office in the dwelling-house of D. B. Stevenson, in the village of Hallowell, where he will attend to all calls in his profession.

"Hallowell, January 6, 1831."

He soon had a large practice, and continued to enjoy the confidence of his patients until his death.

In June, 1845, he married Clara Louisa M. Fairfield, youngest daughter of Benjamin Fairfield, of Bath. They had issue one son and two daughters: David John, born April, 1846; Emily Jane, born September, 1849; Annie Mary Louisa, August, 1853. Dr. Pruyn's children are now all dead but the son, who married the daughter of Rev. John Pape, Church of England minister. He lives at Napanee.

DR. THOMAS PYNE

Was born in the city of Waterford, Ireland, 1812, of English descent. He was one of a large family, and was left fatherless early in life. His father sailed for New Brunswick, and the ship and all were lost. He was educated at Graham's School, a noted institution at Waterford, and studied medicine in Dublin and London with a brother, Dr. George Pyne, who practised in London for years, and was at one time Professor of Anatomy in one of the London hospitals.

Dr. Pyne practised in the city of Waterford, Ireland, for a number of years, where he married the daughter of John Roberts, barrister. It may be mentioned that this family of Roberts are rather celebrated for their military and naval proclivities. Members of this family have risen to eminence in both branches of the service, viz.: Sir Samuel Roberts, at one time Commander of the flotilla on our Canadian lakes, and who commenced life as a cabin-boy in the merchant service; Sir Abraham Roberts, the oldest general on the British army list when he died, in 1874, and who was knighted for service in India; Sir Frederick Roberts, son of the former, the hero of the Afghan war—also knighted for service in India—the present Commander-in-Chief of the Indian army, and one of the most popular generals with the British nation at the present day. He is now (1894) Lord Roberts.

Dr. Pyne emigrated to the United States and settled in Princeton, Illinois, near Chicago, where he practised for a few years successfully, but his longing for British institutions and customs brought him to Upper Canada in 1849, and he settled in Newmarket, where he practised for sixteen years. He then removed to Hagersville, in the County of Haldimand, where he remained until 1871. Dr. Pyne represented the Erie and Niagara Division in the Medical Council of Ontario. He remained the representative of this division until his appointment as Registrar of the College of Physicians and Surgeons in 1872, when he removed to Toronto. This position he held until 1880, when he resigned.

He leaves two sons, Albert Roberts Pyne and Robert Allan Pyne, both physicians in Toronto. The latter succeeded his father as Registrar of the College of Physicians and Surgeons, and still holds this position (1894).

Dr. Thomas Pyne died at Belgrave, in the County of Huron, January 2, 1883.

DR. JOHN EDWARD RANKIN,

Of Ottawa, Licentiate of Lower Canada, 1828, before Upper Canada Medical Board, July, 1829. Examination "perfectly satisfactory." In 1845, received M.R.C.S. Edinburgh, also M.D., St. Andrew's University. He was in the British army service during the Crimean War. About 1854, he took up his residence at Picton, where he enjoyed a respectable practice until his death, August 5, 1878, at the age of eighty-one. He had two sons and one daughter. One son, Henry, became a captain in the British army.

There was a Dr. Rankin, possibly the same, in Toronto, 1847. The *Patriot*, July 20, 1847, says: "EMIGRANT HOSPITAL.—We understand that Dr. Hamilton has been appointed one of the physicians to the emigrant hospital, in place of Dr. Rankin, who demanded of the Medical Board that he should be placed at the head of the hospital, or at least be considered as senior physician, notwithstanding that Dr. Primrose and Mr. Henwood, sen., had been previously doing heavy duty there. The Board of Health most properly declined acceding to this request, on which Dr. Rankin threw up his appointment, leaving his patients at the hospital (about one hundred in number) unprovided for. Fortunately, the Board were able to have recourse to another gentleman, who did the duties until Dr. Hamilton was appointed."

DR. CHARLES RATTRAY

Was born at Dunkeld, Perthshire, Scotland, 1808. He studied medicine in Glasgow and in Edinburgh, and was admitted a member of the Royal College of Surgeons, Edinburgh, 1829. Immediately thereafter, he migrated to British Guiana, in South America, where he resided five years. In 1834, he came to Canada and took up his residence in Cornwall, where he continued until his death. He married a daughter of Peter Chesley, who, with four sons and three daughters, survived him.

The following tribute to the memory of Dr. Rattray appeared in the Cornwall *Gazette*, October 23, 1872: "When it became known this morning that Dr. Charles Rattray was no more, sorrow filled many a heart. A wise and a good man—one whose history was identified with that of the town, and whose place would not be filled in this generation—had been taken from amongst us. The trusted friend, the wise counsellor, the loved physician of many a household in this town and neighbourhood, had left us forever.

"Few of the old residents of this town have exercised so wide an influence as Dr. Rattray. Of decided individuality and force of character, from the day he first set foot in Cornwall until the hour of his death, he made himself felt socially, professionally and politically. A man of large brain, his mind well stored with general and professional learning, he attracted attention always. A great student, with keen powers of observation and a prodigious memory, he attained in the practice of his profession of medicine and surgery very great success—a success which earned for him the envy of some of his less gifted brethren, but the confidence of a large portion of the community. For many years he divided the honours and the emoluments of his profession here with our worthy townsman, Dr. Roderick Macdonald, and since that gentleman's retirement from active practice, he has stood at its head, and a couple of years ago was elected by his confreres to be President of the Counties' Medical Association.

"As a magistrate he was fearless, independent and just. During the many years he occupied the mayor's chair—he was the first elected by the people—he performed the duties impartially and well, and none but professional fault-finders ever cavilled at his acts. In private life, his many social qualities gained for him troops of friends, who for many a day to come will tell of his good sayings and of his good deeds. With his large and liberal views and a strong disposition to polemics, he was of necessity a strong politician, and lost no opportunity of urging the claims of the Reform party, with which he allied himself.

"It has been our good fortune to make the acquaintance of many men in our day, in the various walks of life, but among them all, a friend truer, firmer or more steadfast than Charles Rattray, there was not one. May he rest in peace!"

A son of Dr. Rattray, John, entered the medical profession, and having graduated at McGill College, went travelling abroad. Another son is a well-known electrician, living in New York. A daughter, Elizabeth, married James Bethune, LL.D., a well-known and popular lawyer in Toronto. He was made Queen's Counsel and had attained the highest standing in his profession, and would doubtless soon have adorned the Bench, had he not contracted typhoid fever, which resulted in his death, 1884. Another daughter married Wm. Drummond Hogg, Q.C., of Ottawa; and another, Helen, married John Drury, Esq., Toronto.

DR. READE,

Of the Royal Navy, with Dr. Connin, accompanied the immigrants who setted in Peterborough, 1825, under the guidance of the Hon. Peter Robinson. The Hon. Thomas A. Stewart, Member of the Legislative Council of Upper Canada, wrote: "Mr. Robinson has been particularly fortunate in his choice in the Medical Department, as the care, humanity and great attention shown by Dr. Reade could not be exceeded." In the winter of 1826, the Lieut.-Governor, Sir Peregrine Maitland, visited this section, and the new settlers, in an address to His Excellency, made use of these words in one paragraph: "Please Your Excellency, we are totally at a loss for words adequate to express the thanks and gratitude we owe Dr. Reade for his active, skilful and unremitting care, etc., for us."

A local writer says: "Dr. Reade, having fulfilled his engagement in reference to the immigrants, withdrew after their location on their lands," and returned to England.

DR. JOHN REED

Was before Medical Board, July, 1841; had diploma R.C.S. Ed.; received certificate for license. Dr. Reed, probably the same, issued the following notice:

"MEDICAL PROFESSION.—Understanding that Dr. Reid, of Moy, is about to remove from this country to British America, we avail ourselves of the occasion to express the very high degree of respect and esteem in which we hold him, not merely as a gentleman of excellent and unsullied character, but as a safe and judicious medical practitioner, so far as we have had an opportunity of witnessing his practice; and we respectfully recommend him to the favourable reception of our medical brethren in whatever district he may eventually take up his residence.

"W. L. KIDD, M.D., etc., etc.,
A. ROBINSON, A.M., M.D.,
THOS. CUMING, M.D., etc., etc., } Armagh.
ROBT. O. BOLTON, M.D., etc.,
WM. NEVILE, M.D., } Dungannon.

"Armagh, May 3rd, 1841."

"Doctor Reid, from Moy (Ireland), where he practised for the last twelve years, begs leave to announce to the inhabitants of the City of Toronto and the surrounding country, that, having obtained His Excellency the Governor-General's license, bearing date the 14th of July last, authorizing him to practise Physic, Surgery and Midwifery in this Province, he has opened an office in Richmond Street, a few doors east of Church Street, where he may be consulted daily.

"Richmond Street, August 18th, 1841."

Dr. John Reed, we presume the same, was a well-known practitioner at Thornhill for many years. He married Miss Mulholland. "Was a good man, professionally, religiously and in all the relations of life, and very highly esteemed." His son, John N., a fellow-student of the writer, both at Toronto and New York, passed Medical Board, October, 1853, and took M.D., New York, 1854. He succeeded to his father's practice at Thornhill. The writer was further associated with him as a co-lecturer in the Victoria Medical College. Dr. Reed held the professorship in Physiology for a good many years. He came to an untimely death from malignant disease of the tongue.

DR. WILLIAM REES

Came from England in 1819, and commenced the practice of his profession in Quebec. Toward the close of 1829 he came to York, and having passed the Medical Board, January, 1830, purchased the practice of Dr. Daly. This card appeared in the *Upper Canada Gazette:* "Dr. Rees has taken rooms, corner of Market Square, King Street. He will vaccinate and give advice gratis to the poor, Monday, Wednesday and Saturday." Subsequently he disposed of his practice to Dr. Grasett.

This card appeared in the Cobourg *Star:* "Dr. Rees, professionally educated in England; pupil of Sir Astley Cooper, and ten years a practitioner in the Canadas, respectfully tenders his services to the inhabitants of Cobourg and vicinity. October 21, 1832." But his stay at Cobourg was a short one.

Dr. Rees, it may be said, was a many-sided man. He conceived various projects of a scientific and benevolent character.

Dr. Scadding informs the writer that he was of a speculative disposition, and a man of unusual intelligence. We find in the public press, that on the 20th May, 1833, Dr. Rees received the thanks of the Home District Fair for seeds from the coast of Africa. He was a candidate for Parliament, First Riding of York, 1834. In the same year he established a Medical Dispensary, 74 King and New Streets, but he shortly after advertised it as for sale.

Mrs. Jameson, in her entertaining narrative of her sojourn in Canada, tells something interesting about Dr. Rees. It seems he entertained the idea of founding a house of reception for destitute female immigrants—a house where, without depending on charity, they might be boarded and lodged at the smallest possible cost, and be respectably protected until employment was obtained.

He presented a petition to Parliament in 1836, praying the grant of a sum of money for the erection of a provincial museum. He was acting in conjunction with Dr. Dunlop and Mr. Fothergill. It was intended to establish in connection with the museum, a botanical and zoological garden on a grant of land on the Government Reserve in the western part of the city. It, however, all fell through. Charles Fothergill was a well-known writer and publisher, and an influential person in Toronto. He was a nephew of the celebrated Dr. Fothergill, and died in May, 1840.

Dr. Rees was Surgeon to the 1st West York Battalion, 1837.

Another enterprise is indicated in the following:

"TO MEDICAL STUDENTS.—In pursuance of a plan for establishing a School of Medicine in this city, Dr. Rees proposes to deliver a course of lectures on Obstetrics and the Diseases of Women and Children, on the first Monday in November next. Anatomy, Physiology, Surgery, Materia Medica, the principles and practice of Physic, Chemistry and Medical Botany are the subjects which will be comprehended the ensuing season.

"Arrangements necessary with the other medical gentlemen will be determined by the 1st of October, when a prospectus and further particulars may be had on application as above (postpaid).

"Toronto, August 4th, 1834."

It is stated that Dr. Rees was also the originator of the present prosperous Toronto Club.

Up to 1841 no insane asylum existed in Upper Canada. In January of this year, the Provincial Asylum was first opened in Toronto, by virtue of an Act passed in 1839, and it was through the activity of Dr. Rees that this was accomplished. The provincial authorities had acquired the old gaol at the east side of Toronto Street, north of King Street, after the new gaol in the east end had been completed. Dr. Rees was the first Superintendent of the Asylum, and at first had seventeen patients. This building was soon densely filled, and it became necessary to procure further accommodation for the numerous applications for admission. The eastern wing of the Parliament buildings was appropriated to this purpose, and, subsequently, a still further addition was made, by the occupation of a vacant house near the old garrison. The three buildings were used until the present asylum was ready for occupation. Dr. Rees held the position until 1844, when he was succeeded by Dr. Telfer. The same year, the old gaol, with the two annexes, having become quite inadequate to afford accommodation for the increasing number of lunatics, commissioners were appointed to secure a proper site for a new asylum, and to superintend its erection. Fifty acres of land were acquired on what was then a part of the garrison commons, the site of the present asylum. The building was commenced in June, 1845. (For a further account of the asylum, see biography of Dr. Workman.)

Dr. Rees, unfortunately, notwithstanding the evident ability and enterprise he possessed, seems to have been wanting in a proper mental balance. A memorandum from Mr. C. Gamble to the writer, gives a brief succinct account of Dr. Rees and his connection with the Provincial Lunatic Asylum.

He says: "Dr. Rees was an Englishman by birth and education. I believe he was a learned man on some things, but an eccentric and most sanguine man—was always considered flighty, and never had much practice. Through his energy the first lunatic asylum was established in Toronto, and he was appointed to the superintendence and management thereof upon the principle, I suppose, of setting a madman to watch a madman). He was seriously injured by a blow on the head from one of the patients, the effects of which he felt to his dying day. Very properly after this he was removed from his position, and the asylum placed in other and, undoubtedly, more able hands, and it has continued to improve until there are none superior to it on the continent. But poor Rees never recovered from the effects of the step which, no doubt, the Government felt constrained to take. He brooded on the injustice that he thought had been done him, and never ceased to mourn over the neglect that the country had shown him. In all his madness he made several good speculations in land, but the benefit of these was reaped by others."

Dr. Rees repeatedly applied for some compensation for the time he had given in organizing the asylum and in the sacrifices he had made in connection therewith. As late as 1869, Dr. Rees memorialized the Government, but without success. That his application was considered a just one by some is shown by the following comments in the *Dominion Medical Journal:*

"We call the attention of the profession to the memorial of Dr. Rees, one of the oldest and most respected practitioners in this Province. His case is well known to a large number of medical men, who have at various times endeavoured to obtain justice for him from the Government. All he asks is a proper recognition of his services, and of the injuries which he received while discharging his duties as Medical Superintendent of the Asylum. He is now nearly blind from the formation of cataract, which is the consequence of injuries received by him while attending a lunatic in the Asylum. We hope that medical men will interest themselves in his case, and interest the representatives from their several constituencies to obtain justice for an old public servant, who well deserves a pension for his untiring efforts in behalf of a class of the community the most unfortunate and, until his efforts in their behalf, the most neglected in the country."

Opposite the old Parliament buildings, on what was called the "Broken Front," Dr. Rees constructed a wharf, which was long known as "Rees' Wharf." Near it, under the hill, he built a small but comfortable house, in which he passed his bachelor life, always ready to welcome any visitor and interest him with anecdote, of which he had a large fund.

DR. THOMAS REYNOLDS,

Born in Brockville, County of Leeds, October 17, 1820. His parents came from the north of Ireland in the previous year. He was educated at the District Grammar School in his native town, and at the age of sixteen went to study medicine with Dr. Stephenson, of Montreal. It seems that he desired to continue his studies at McGill, but the rebellion interfered with the college lectures. In 1839 he went to Scotland, and entered the University of Edinburgh as a medical student, where, passing his examination with credit, he received the degree of M.B. He then returned to Canada and entered McGill College, Montreal, where he received the degree of M.D.

He commenced practice at Williamsburg, now Morrisburg, or Matilda, now Iroquois, and subsequently removed to Brockville about 1846.

Dr. Reynolds took a great interest in all scientific and educational matters, and, in addition to contributing to the medical journals, contributed to the Canadian Institute and the Smithsonian Institute. In the *British American Medical Journal* for 1848-49, there are two of his contributions. He was an examiner in medicine for the University of Toronto. During the rebellion of 1837-38 he served as a volunteer, first in Montreal, and afterwards at the battle of the Windmill, near Prescott, November, 1838, having been instrumental in raising a company at Brockville of the Queen's Royal Borderers. At this time he was offered a commission in Her Majesty's regular army, and again when at college in Edinburgh. He was well known in Canada West from his connection with Oddfellowship, being the first Grand Master of the Grand Lodge of Canada West. In 1889 the Oddfellows in Brockville furnished a private ward in the Brockville General Hospital in his memory.

Dr. Reynolds married Eleanor Sarah Senkler, daughter of Rev. Edmund John Senkler, M.A., of Brockville, formerly of Dorking, England, and sister of Dr. A. E. Senkler, of St. Paul, Minnesota, who practised at one time in Toronto. His daughter, Frances Mary, became the wife of Dr. A. E. Malloch, of Hamilton. She died in 1890. One son, Edmund John Reynolds, of Brockville, now practising by himself, was a member of the la

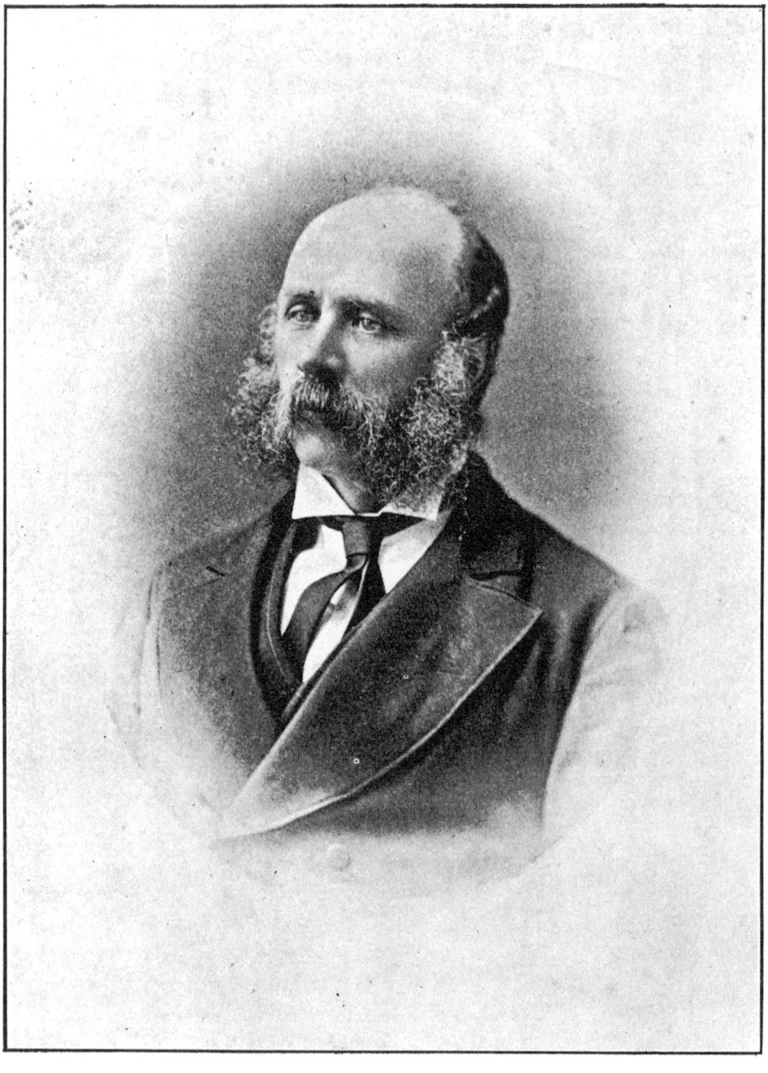

DR. JAMES H. RICHARDSON.

firm of Fraser & Reynolds, of which the senior member was Hon. C. F. Fraser, Q.C., Commissioner of Public Works for Ontario; another, Thomas William Reynolds, M.D., C.M., McGill University, 1881, M.C.P.S. Ont., 1881, is Assistant Superintendent, Asylum for Insane, Hamilton.

Dr. Reynolds died in Brockville, September 14, 1859. His widow died in 1886.

DR. JAMES HENRY RICHARDSON

Was born at Presqu' Isle, October 16, 1823. His grandfather had served in the British navy and came to Canada, 1785, when he received an appointment in the marine service. Dr. Richardson's father, James Richardson, for a long time bishop of the Episcopal Methodist Church, was born at Kingston. He married the second daughter of John Dennis, a well-known U. E. Loyalist, who came to Little York about the beginning of the century. His residence was on the north-east corner of King and Yonge Streets. He left large and valuable property in land, which is now in the heart of the city. James Richardson, afterwards bishop, served during the war of 1812 under Sir James Yeo, and in May, 1814, lost an arm at the shoulder, at the capture of Oswego by the British. He died at the advanced age of eighty-four, at Toronto, full of honours, and much beloved by all who had the privilege of knowing him.

James H. Richardson began his medical studies in 1841, with Dr. Rolph, then living in Rochester, N.Y., and remained with him two years. He then attended as a matriculated student the first course of lectures delivered by the medical faculty of King's College. In 1844, he proceeded to England and studied at Guy's Hospital for three years, spending the summer of 1846 at the hospitals and in attendance on lectures in Paris. He obtained his diploma at the Royal College of Surgeons, England, 1847, being the first Canadian, we believe, to receive that honour. He then returned to Toronto and commenced practice. In 1848, he took the degree of M.B. at King's College. In 1850, he was appointed to succeed Dr. Sullivan as Professor of Anatomy, in the newly constituted Medical Department of Toronto University, having discharged the duties during the previous year, in consequence of the illness of Prof. Sullivan. The same year he received the degree of M.B. He held the Chair of Anatomy in the University until the Medical Department was abolished, 1853. Some years later he accepted the Chair of Anatomy in the Toronto School of Medicine, and at the organization of the medical faculty of Toronto University, he was again appointed Professor of Anatomy, which position he still holds (1893).

Dr. Richardson has taken great interest in the volunteer force, and was successively surgeon of the Field Artillery, the Merchants' Company and in the 10th Royal Regiment. After twenty years of continuous service, he some years ago retired, retaining the rank of Surgeon-Major. During the time of his service, he was an enthusiastic and successful rifle shot, receiving, in 1861, the first prize ever competed for in Toronto at long range. The prize was presented to him by Gen. Williams, afterwards the hero of Kars. He has all his life been a lover of out-door recreation and amusement, as yachting, curling, bowling and fishing, and to this he attributes the good health which he continues to enjoy. In the last named sport he has passed his summer vacations from place to place at almost every noted fishing camp in the Dominion, from Cape Breton to the rivers and shores of Lake Superior.

Dr. Richardson, as an operator, has had usually well-appointed surgical appliances in his practice; but that he would have achieved success under less favourable circumstances is attested by an incident which occurred in 1859, when he was on one of his fishing expeditions up the Ottawa. On such occasions he never carried any surgical appliances, and it happened that a French-Canadian, whom he came across, was in the most urgent need of relief by the use of a catheter. While the doctor was troubled and anxious to give relief, his eye rested upon a goose's wing, used for dusting, and a happy thought came to him, upon which he promptly acted. He took the quills of the wing, cut them in convenient sections, and uniting them together, end to end, fixed the joints with shoemaker's wax. In this way he fashioned a catheter, and by it the suffering of the now fortunate Frenchman was removed, whose life was thereby doubtless saved and whose gratitude was unbounded.

The writer has lately seen this novel instrument, which is preserved by the Doctor as a memento, and which looks as if it might do similar service again.

Dr. Richardson stands in the foremost rank in his profession, especially as a sound surgeon and brilliant operator. He has for many years been on the staff of the Toronto General Hospital, also surgeon to the Toronto Gaol. He is an ex-President of the Ontario Medical Association, and has filled other important positions. He is one whom his medical confreres delight to honour, and one in whom a large circle implicitly trust as a physician.

Dr. Richardson married a Scotch lady, Miss Mary Skirving, who is now known as an active philanthropist. They have four sons and three daughters living (1893). One son, W. A. Richardson, entered the medical profession, and at the present time has charge of the Royal Jubilee Hospital at Victoria, B.C. The youngest son, G. H. Richardson, is a civil engineer. The other two are in business in Winnipeg.

DR. SAMUEL RICHARDSON,

Son of Euchmetty Richardson, of the County of Longford, Ireland, was born, February 31, 1809. He received his general education at Trinity College, Dublin, where he also studied medicine, and became M.R.C.S., Dublin, 1834. In the same year he emigrated to Upper Canada. He was before the Medical Board, April, 1835, and obtained a certificate to practise surgery. He settled at Guelph, where he practised for five years. He removed to Galt in 1839, at that time a mere hamlet, where he continued to practise. His field of labour was extensive and arduous; but he found time to act on the Town Council for seventeen years, and he has also filled the offices of Reeve and Deputy Reeve, as well as Justice of the Peace.

Dr. Richardson was twice married; in 1834, to Miss Mary Ann Brereton, of Dublin, Ireland, and in 1850, to Miss Annie Orr, of Galt. He had four children, two by each wife.

DR. GEORGE NEVILLE RIDLEY

Was born, February 22, 1794, at Kimbolton, Huntingdonshire, England. His father was a physician; and in fact, for generations the men of the family have been either doctors or clergymen. He studied at St. Thomas' and Guy's, and was a pupil of Sir Astley Cooper. He was always fond of surgery, although possessed in a remarkable degree of the faculty of diagnosing disease, and his opinion was seldom at fault. About the year 1818, while yet a student, he visited Canada. Arriving at Quebec, he proceeded to Montreal, and from Montreal he walked to Kingston, Cobourg, York, and visited Niagara Falls. He was much pleased at that time with the Niagara District and the vicinity of Grimsby. During this visit he became acquainted with many of the old families in the country, such as the Lesmesuriers, of Quebec; Moffatts, of Montreal; Dr. Sampson, of Kingston; the Boultons, of Cobourg, and Robinsons, of Toronto and Newmarket. One of his greatest friends was Mr. Peter Robinson, of Newmarket, whom he often used to mention when speaking of his early visit to Canada. Returning to England, he completed his studies, and received the degree of M.R.C.S. London. He soon after married and settled at St. Alban's, where he entered into partnership with his brother-in-law, Dr. Webster. This partnership was not a happy one. Dr. Webster became jealous of the success soon acquired by Dr. Ridley in his practice, and made it so unpleasant for him that he determined, rather than oppose his brother-in-law, to leave England and settle in Canada. In 1824, he returned to Canada with the intention of farming on an extensive scale, and purchased land near Belleville. He was, however, forced to practise his profession, as he could not refuse to visit those requiring medical aid. His practice extended eastward to Kingston and westward to Cobourg, and few serious cases happened in the neighbourhood of Belleville without his advice being sought, and he gave it ungrudgingly to the lowest and poorest as well as those better off. Often, in his earlier work, he placed his saddle under the seat of his waggon, or, as he called it, his grasshopper. He would go as far as he could in his waggon, then would leave it beside the clearing and mount his horse and go on horseback until he was stopped by the forest. He would there dismount and walk perhaps two or more miles through a blazed forest to get to the shanty and his patient. His remuneration would possibly be paid to him some years after in the shape of a load of potatoes or a few bushels of oats.

He never lost his anatomical knowledge. On one occasion, being asked by a brother practitioner to perform herniotomy, the medical gentleman sat down in the doctor's study to work up his surgical anatomy. Dr. Ridley quietly took his lunch, accompanied his friend and operated successfully.

His son, Dr. Henry Ridley, of Hamilton, says of his father: "When a student, I frequently accompanied him in his visits to his country patients, and he often on the journey put me through an anatomical grind, and I was too often aground before the journey was over. Dr. Ridley was appointed Surgeon to the 1st Hastings Regiment of Militia, July, 1826. In 1838, he was commissioned a member of the Upper Canada Medical Board. He was appointed by the Lieutenant-Governor, April, 1840, one of four to form a Board of Education for the District of Victoria.

"In politics he was a good old-fashioned Church and State Tory, and the most liberal-minded man to those who differed from him. I have heard him trying to persuade a Radical of those days to vote his way. He never lost his temper in argument, and if he could not convince an opponent he would scorn to try to compel him to vote his way, even if he had any power to do so. Honour with him was a part of his life. Hard, professional, never-ceasing work undermined a splendid physique and fine constitution, and before he reached his forty-eighth year he had a severe attack of diabetes, which, within three months, brought him down from a man of 225 pounds to a mere shadow of his former self. From this attack he never recovered, for, although he lived to the age of sixty-three, his life was one of suffering. During his long illness he was never heard to utter a word of complaint. Whatever suffering it pleased God to visit him with was borne with patient and Christian fortitude. At his death-bed, when all around him were filled with grief and sorrow, he spoke to them with such unbounded faith in his Saviour that left all fully impressed with the comforting belief that for him to die was gain."

The writer may be pardoned for indulging in some personal reminiscences. Dr. Ridley was for many years his father's family physician, and the writer knows not how much he owes the Doctor for introducing him into this world. But with the recollections of Dr. Ridley are associated an occasion of sadness, tears, a silent room, the looking-glass draped in white, the arrival of a coffin, the gathering neighbours, the minister's subdued voice, the way to the burying ground, the deep grave and the proclamation, "I am the Resurrection and the Life." There is another, a more pleasant remembrance—a pleasant sunny afternoon. In a one-horse carriage drive two gentlemen; as remembered, very much alike in appearance. Both past middle life, but possessing the looks of vigour, with something of a grand air about them. These two noble-looking men were Judge Hagerman and Dr. Ridley. They stop at the gate of the writer's parents, and enter the house. There were several such visits in the course of years—only one is remembered. Judge Hagerman, when at Belleville on his circuit, would have the Doctor drive him out to have a chat with his old Adolphustown schoolmates.

Two sons of Dr. Ridley became members of the medical profession—Charles Neville and Henry Thomas. Both had the advantage of the excellent medical training of their father. Charles became L.C.P.S., Canada, 1850, and practised his profession in Belleville, where he died, 1893. Henry graduated at McGill College, Montreal, obtained degree of M.D., C.M., and L.C.P.S., Canada, 1852. He chose Hamilton as his field of professional work, and soon acquired a first-class practice, which he still pursues with unabated vigour. He married the eldest daughter of the Hon. Edmund Murney, of Belleville.

Louisa Mary, daughter of Dr. Ridley, became the wife of Col. de Rottenburg, who has recently died (1894). The following notice appeared:

"The English papers announced the death during last month of a famous Canadian, Colonel Baron de Rottenburg. The deceased officer was a son of Major-General de Rottenburg, who was President of the Council of Upper Canada from June

19th, 1813, until December 13th, in the same year. He was born near Kingston in 1807, and entered the army in 1825. His first commission was in the 81st Regiment, from which he was transferred to the 60th Rifles, and later to the 49th Regiment.

"He served in Canada on the staff all through the rebellion of 1837-38, having then the rank of captain, but owing to his success 'on a particular service' during that period, he received the brevet rank of major in recognition of what he had done. In the first Carlist war in Spain, he, being then on the unattached list, joined the staff of General Sir de Lacy Evans, and did good service in the field. Later, having in the meantime become Lieutenant-Colonel, he again returned to Canada as Adjutant-General of the militia. While so employed, the 100th Prince of Wales Royal Canadian Regiment was raised here in 1858, and Colonel de Rottenburg was offered the command, which he accepted. He went with the 100th to England, and was quartered first at Shorncliffe, afterwards at Aldershot, and in May, 1859, again embarked on foreign service, going with the regiment to Gibraltar. He finally retired from the army by the sale of his commission in 1861, being succeeded by Major A. R. Dunn, V.C. Some few years later he became a Military Knight of Windsor, and in the quarters of that body, in the shadow of Windsor Castle, passed the remainder of his long and eventful life.

DR. ALEXANDER CHORLEY ROBINSON,

"Member of the Royal College of Surgeons and Licentiate of the Apothecaries' Hall, having received His Excellency's license to practise physic, surgery and midwifery in this Province, proposes to exercise his profession in this capital. Dr. R.'s residence is in Dr. Deihl's new house in York Street, near Osgoode Hall, where he will be ready to attend to all professional calls, and to visit patients either in town or the country. York, 6th January, 1835." The York directory for 1834 gives: "Dr. Robinson, Yonge St. Road;" "Steam Saw-mill, Kingston Road, near Windmill, on the Don."

The only further information at hand of Dr. Robinson is the following: *The Royal Standard* newspaper, Toronto, Dec., 1836, records: "Died.—Sarah, wife of A. C. Robinson, M.D., from fever." In 1837 the paper announced: "Married.—Alex. Robinson, M.D., to Miss E. M. Hains, both of Yonge St." It appears that he did not continue long to practise in Toronto.

DR. SAMUEL ROBINSON

Was a sojourner in Canada, 1832-33. He was one of a party who together chartered a vessel, the *Ann*, to cross the Atlantic. Among the company, beside Dr. Robinson, was William Hume Blake, well known in Upper Canadian history, as a man of legal eminence, a statesman, and more particularly as the first Chancellor of the Court of Chancery of Upper Canada. Chancellor Blake's wife was a stepdaughter of Dr. Robinson. Another of the party was Skiffington Connor, long known as Dr. Connor, also a well-known lawyer, statesman and judge, and likewise married to a step-daughter of Dr. Robinson. Others of the company were the late Archdeacon Arthur Palmer, of Guelph, and Bishop Cronyn, of the diocese of Huron.

The vessel sailed, July 11, 1832. The voyage was marked by adverse winds and the appearance of cholera on board, from which one of the passengers died. After six weeks on the Atlantic, they had to endure a long quarantine at Grosse Island. It may be supposed that the presence of Dr. Robinson on board was salutary in allaying the force of the disease, in preventing its spread, and in saving life. Dr. Robinson, with the Blakes, reached York in September. Dr. Robinson, we believe, spent some time in the neighbourhood of Lake Simcoe, where, although he did not desire to establish himself in practice, he found a good deal to do in alleviating intermittent fever, then very prevalent among the settlers. Dr. Robinson did not remain in Canada, but, after visiting relations in Maryland, returned to Dublin.

However, two of his sons became well-known citizens of the Province—Judge Robinson, of Sarnia, and Arthur G. Robinson,

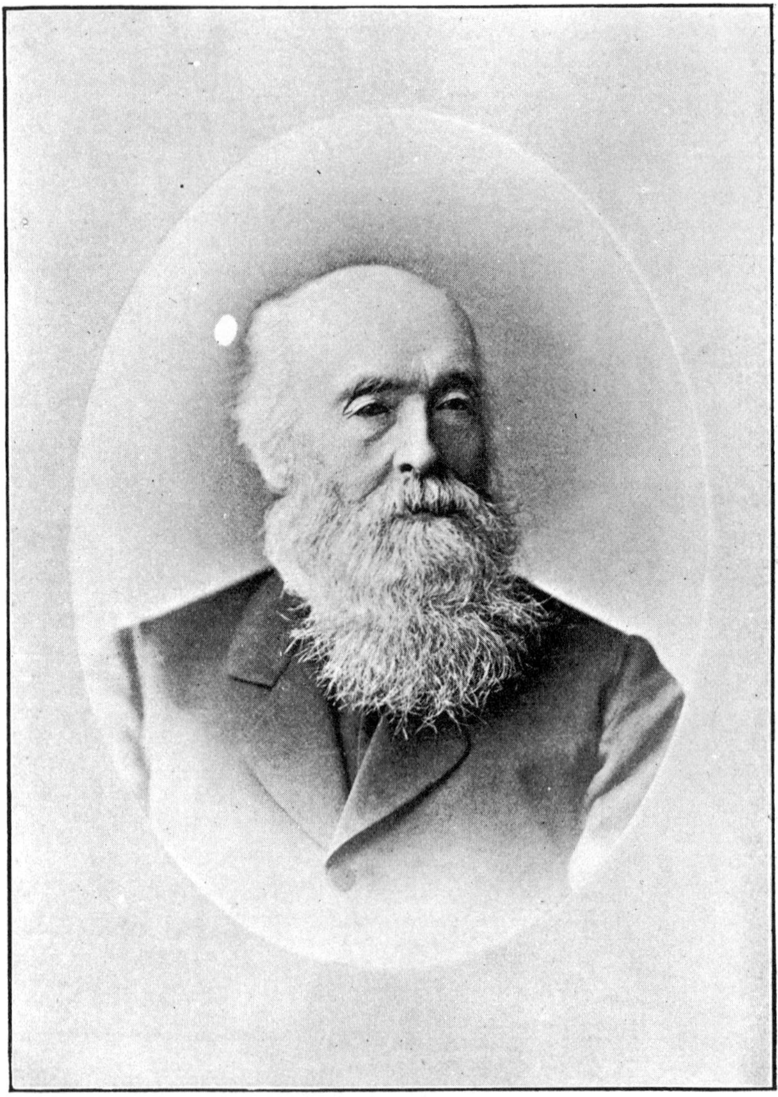

DR. T. SLADE ROBINSON.

C.E., residing in Orillia. The latter's son, Samuel Skiffington Robinson, is a well-known lawyer of that place.

Major William Robinson, of the British army, was a brother of Dr. Robinson. He was in Canada during the war of 1812, and was wounded at the battle of Lundy's Lane. He was voted a "Sword of Honour," by the Canadian Parliament for services rendered in disciplining the Canadian militia.

"The incorporated militia, now called by some the King's Canadian Legion, was taught the rudiments of war by the gallant Colonel Robinson, their late Commander. They have done ample justice to his instruction, and by their bravery, good conduct, and strict discipline, have equalled the best veteran battalions."—*Cameron's Almanac.*

DR. T. SLADE ROBINSON

Was born at Stone, Staffordshire, England, April, 1801; was educated in Wales, London and Dublin, and commenced the study of medicine, 1820, at Denby, Wales. He served an apprenticeship of five years, for which he paid £95. He was afterwards the pupil of the celebrated Abernethy and Sir Astley Cooper. He became a member of the Society of Apothecaries, London, 1825. In the years of 1824-25, he attended lectures at Royal College of Surgeons, Dublin; M.R.C.S. Eng., 1827. In 1828, he attended two courses of lectures given by Francis H. Ramadge, M.D., F.L.S., at the Central Infirmary and Dispensary, London. After receiving his degrees, he became the private physician of Lord St. Vincent's family, in England. He was afterwards physician to his Lordship's estates in the West Indies. Having suffered three attacks of fever in the last place, he decided, as soon as he had strength, to leave; and consequently, in 1831, came to New Orleans, and ascending the Mississippi, found his way to Montreal. Staying there a short time, he proceeded to Upper Canada, and spent a winter in Hamilton. He formed the acquaintance of Mr. (afterward Sir Allan) Macnab, and would have settled there had not a disastrous fire nearly destroyed the place, and as well had not inducement presented itself to go to Niagara Falls, where had been laid out a plot for a city, which was named the "City of the Falls." It was anticipated that the place would become a great manufacturing centre. He was led to invest largely in real estate there, and built himself a residence. He commanded a good practice while there, and among his patients was the son of Joseph Brant, in his last illness. The site of this "City of the Falls" is on the elevated ground on the old portage road, south-east of Drummondville, overlooking the Horseshoe Fall. It is now a common, and the ownership of the lots uncertain. A solitary tree on the highest point, where the cold north wind strikes the traveller with great violence, is known as the "North Pole." Friends of Dr. Robinson, in Quebec, persuaded him to go there. The expectations regarding the "City of the Falls" not having been realized, no doubt contributed to cause him to take this step. His professional life in Quebec was not quite agreeable. Several things combined to prevent his permanent settlement there, as the limited number of English-speaking people, the severe climate, and petty professional jealousy. Dr. Robinson had his friends, and his skill was appreciated. The most prominent druggist of the place declared that Dr. Robinson was the only medical man in Quebec who could write a prescription correctly. After a stay of five years, he decided, in 1842, to commence practice in Montreal. Here he remained also five years, enjoying a good practice and the warm friendship of many of the citizens. Some of these, however, removed to Toronto, and urged him to come also, which he began to prepare to do. But his friends in Montreal were equally assiduous in persuading him to stay. So he remained there altogether five years. In 1847, being still in the prime of life, and with a growing family, he thought he would join the throng who were then leaving the east for the great west, where many openings would present themselves for the family. He consequently sold out, and embarked, his place of destination being Milwaukee. His intention was to combine farming with practice. But one year's experience with the motley population, and the deadly malaria, which took off one of his children, was enough, and he resolved to seek a resting place again in Upper Canada, which he had long regretted leaving. Toronto was his choice, and here he found warm friends, who remained such for life. His remark to his son was: "I believe I have found a place that I feel satisfied to live and die in." And here he did spend the remaining thirty-seven years of his life; and here he died, rich in the love of his many friends, rich in his faith and trust in the God he had so faithfully served, and sure of the promise made to those who trust in their Saviour.

Dr. Robinson was a remarkable man. As a physician he possessed skill; in his practice he was judicious and successful. The last time cholera visited Toronto, he was particularly successful. But he will be remembered, by those who had the fortune to know him, as the Christian gentleman, the most devoted loyal follower of Him whom he served. The writer cannot forego the satisfaction of paying this tribute to one whom he found a kind friend, who gave professional care to the writer's family when he was absent from home.

This interesting testimony is given by Dr. F. C. Mewburn. He says: "Dr. Slade Robinson was at Niagara Falls in 1834, a very gentlemanly man (too much so for his benefit), well up in all the branches, neat in his appearance and perfect in manner. Many will remember the handsome turn-out of greys, driven tandem, and well driven, too. The Doctor was a good, consistent Christian in every sense of the word."

Dr. Robinson was married, November 7, 1833, to Mary Gillespie, a Scotch lady, by the Venerable Bishop Strachan. Eight children were born to them; six survived him. He died, November 6, 1885, at Toronto, aged eighty-four. His widow survived him six years, having died, November 16, 1891, in her eighty-first year. The writer, who has a keen recollection of the kind, gentle lady, the faithful friend, will not forego the satisfaction of making an extract from a communication to the Rev. Dr. Potts from the venerable and eloquent Rev. Dr. Douglas (lately deceased), on the occasion of Mrs. Robinson's death:

"Her personal self-sacrifice for the good of others was unsparing and tireless during her long life. No midnight darkness nor noonday sun ever held her back from the abodes of sorrow and despair. I have known her to tread weary miles amid winter storms to pour the wealth of her sympathy and the affluence of her prayers at the feet of outcast degradation, and countless are the fainting hearts that she has cheered as they advanced into the eternal. Her character was marked by great strength and vigour. With the advance of years she softened into a serene beauty, which surrounded her latter days with an indescribable charm. Ever green shall be her memory in the hearts of those who knew her. While the generation lives, the names of Dr. and Mrs. Robinson will abide as among the choicest examples of sustained and exalted devotion to God. Evermore shall the recollection of Mrs. Mary Robinson be enshrined in my heart, amid emotions soft and tender, until the twilight and evening star of earthly scenes have been exchanged for the eternal morn of heaven."

DR. THOMAS WEEKS ROBISON

Was the son of Richard and Mary Robison, who lived the first years of their married life at Kingston, and then returned to that place after a residence of some years at Napanee, where Thomas Weeks was born, November 10, 1810. A sister of Richard Robison was married to George O'Kill Stuart, afterward the Venerable Archdeacon of Kingston. Young Robison was educated at Kingston, then studied medicine in Dr. Sampson's office, and attended a course at New York Medical College, where he graduated. His last year of study was spent in London, England. He passed the Upper Canada Medical Board, July, 1833. Dr. Robison commenced practice in Kingston and there passed his life. He married his cousin, Elenora Cummings Robison, of Portland, Maine. They had no children.

Dr. Robison's life was an active one. He was surgeon to the 3rd Frontenac Battalion, organized at the time of the Mackenzie rebellion. He was at one time medical officer to the Penitentiary. He had charge of the fever hospital and sheds during 1847, when the "emigrant" fever raged. The following, taken from the Kingston *News*, relating to his death, which took place, May 6, 1866, pretty fully records the events of his life: "Dr. Robison, one of the most prominent citizens of Kingston, died in the fifty-sixth year of his age. He was elected Mayor, in August, 1844, and served the remainder of the year, which

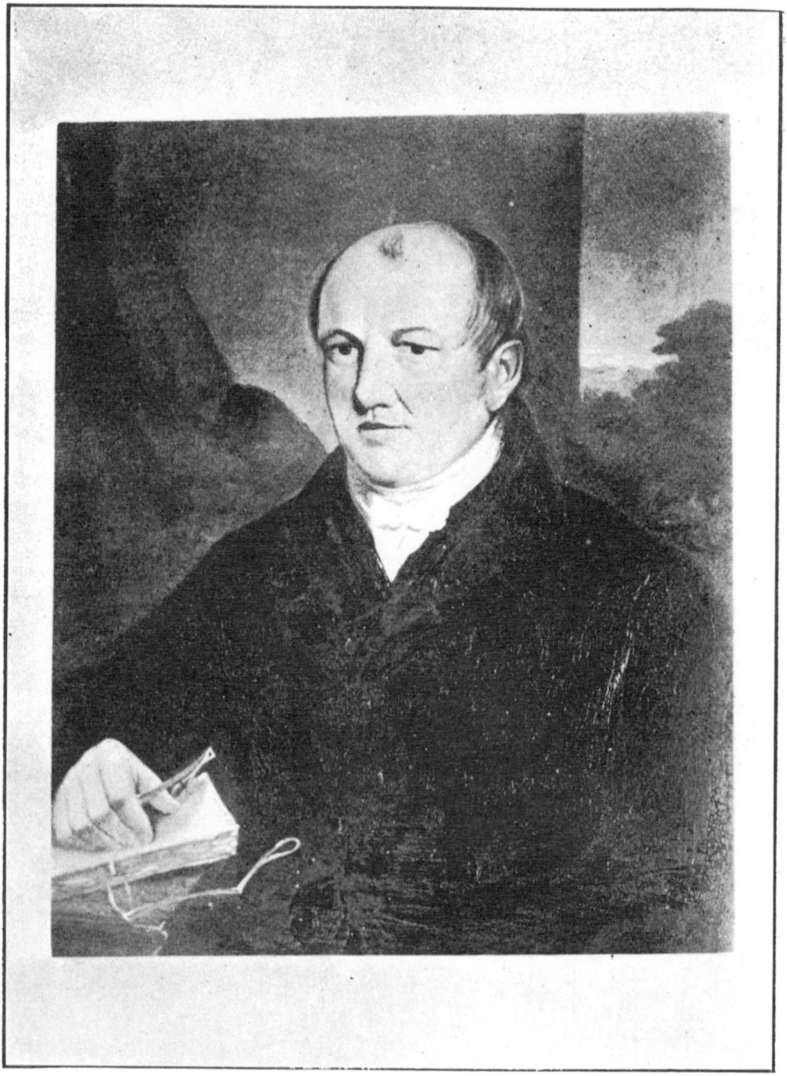

DR. THOMAS ROLPH.

ended in April, 1845, and was re-elected. His appointment as Police Magistrate was dated 1847, which office he filled for nearly nineteen years. He was always considered a just and faithful public servant.

DR. THOMAS ROLPH,

The father of the Hon. John Rolph, was the son of George Rolph, of Thornbury, Gloucestershire, England, Esquire, Attorney and Solicitor, and was born in Thornbury, April 29, 1768, where he received his early education. He afterwards removed to the Parish of St. Olaves, Southwark, Surrey. He married, when about twenty years of age, Frances Petty, only daughter of Ann Petty, of St. Mary's, Rotherhithe, Surrey, on the 25th February, 1788, at St. Margaret Pattens, Fenchurch Street, London, by whom he had seventeen children.

He became a member, April 21, 1790, of the "Corporation of Surgeons," London, England, now the "Royal College of Surgeons," and his name appears on the books of the college up to the year 1807. He practised his profession at Thornbury, Gloucestershire, until October, 1797, when he was succeeded by Mr. Edward Salmon, a cousin of the late Colonel Salmon, father of Judge Salmon, of Simcoe, County Norfolk, Canada, who had previously been articled, or apprenticed, as it was termed in those days, to him. Dr. Rolph was a personal friend of Dr. Edward Jenner, the discoverer of vaccination, whose residence was only nine miles from his place, and doubtless they were often in professional consultation. Dr. Rolph then practised at Camberwell and Peckham, Surrey, finally returning to his native place, where he had purchased the Grovesend Estate, about a mile from Thornbury, and in view of the beautiful river Severn, from Henry Stephen, Esq. (lately called Henry Willis), of Chavenage House, an old historical place in the Parish of Horseley, Gloucestershire, in 1803. After residing there some years, he came to Canada. The exact date is not known, but it was some time after 1807 and before 1810, and settled in the County of Norfolk, in the Long Point District. There is a deed registered in the Simcoe

Registry Office, conveying property in Charlotteville from David Secord to Thomas Rolph, dated September 27, 1810.

He acquired a considerable quantity of land, and we learn by a deed executed January 14, 1813, that he conveyed 1,218 acres of land in the Township of Malahide, County Middlesex, to his son John, in consideration of £800 currency. Dr. Rolph's property was situated between Normandale and Vittoria, County Norfolk. We have no record as to what extent he engaged in the practice of his profession in Canada, but the sparse population at that time necessarily limited the field of practice. He died at Charlotteville, March 24, 1814, leaving four sons and several daughters. Frances (Petty), the widow, died at the residence of her son George, at Dundas, on August 27, 1829, aged 57.

The sons of Dr. Thomas Rolph require some notice in these pages. The eldest, Dr. John Rolph, receives due notice in a separate sketch. (See page 590.)

GEORGE ROLPH, born in Thornbury, April 7, 1794, came with his father to Canada. He had, before leaving England, acquired a liberal education, and was qualified to become, as he did, a member of the Canadian Bar. But before this, Mr. Rolph took an active part in the war of 1812. Before the writer is the Commission received by him from General Brock, dated York, February 14, 1812, in the fifty-second year of George III.'s long reign, appointing him Lieutenant in the 1st Regiment of Norfolk Militia. Lieutenant Rolph accompanied General Brock's expedition to the West, which resulted in the surrender of Fort Detroit, August 16, 1812, by General Hull, by which the State of Michigan was ceded to the British. The writer has also before him the silver medal and crimson ribbon with blue edge, presented to Lieutenant Rolph. The medal bears these words: "1848—To the British Army, 1795-1814," while on the clasp above is engraved: "Fort Detroit." On the rim is also engraved: "G. Rolph, Lieutenant, Canadian Militia."

At a gathering of the veterans of 1812, at Hamilton, 1860, to meet the Prince of Wales, Lieutenant Rolph had the honour of wearing the medal (for the last time) when presented to the Prince.

A correspondent says that Lieutenant Rolph was present at

the battle of Queenston Heights, and took part in the engagement at Stony Creek, as well as other engagements with the enemy. Mr. George Rolph settled at Dundas, Gore District, in 1816.

He commenced the study of law at York, to qualify himself for the office of Clerk of the Peace, there being at that time no one learned in the law in the Gore District, and became the first Clerk of the Peace in the Gore District. Subsequently he was in partnership with his brother, Dr. Rolph. The firm had an office in Vittoria, at that time the district town of London District, and one at Ancaster. They had for some years the largest practice west of York.

He sat as member for the Gore District in the "last parliament of the King." It may be mentioned that Mr. George Rolph had no little public zeal and enterprise. Among other acts, he had constructed, at his own expense, a then very important public work, the Sydenham road, leading up the mountain from Dundas to Flamboro' Township. Mr. Rolph was Clerk of the Surrogate Court for about fifty-four years.

He died, at Dundas, July 25, 1875, aged eighty-one, leaving two sons and three daughters.

The eldest, the late Thomas Lawford, was educated in Canada, at Cheltenham College, Eng., and at Trinity Hall, Cambridge, where he gained a scholarship and obtained his B.A. degree. He was some time private tutor to the Marquis of Huntley, Aberdeenshire, and subsequently a partner in the law firm of Dawes, Son & Rolph, Throgmorton Street, London, Eng.

William M., the second son, is Lieut.-Colonel of the 1st Leicestershire, formerly the old 17th, Regiment of Foot, which was stationed in Toronto in 1866. On entering the army, he was commissioned in the 17th Regiment, which was then stationed at Quebec, in 1862, and he has remained with that regiment up to the present time (1894); passing through the various ranks to the command of the regiment, which he reached, February, 1890.

Of the three daughters, one is the wife of Dr. Allen Holford Walker, of Rotherham House (his private hospital); and another the wife of Dr. Charles O'Reilly, Superintendent of the Toronto General Hospital.

ROMAINE ROLPH, the third son of Dr. Thomas Rolph, was born May 7th, 1795, in Thornbury. He came with the family to Canada, and was a student of divinity under Dr. Strachan, at York. On October 10th, 1819, he was ordained Deacon by the Bishop of Quebec. He was the first missionary to Sandwich, Essex County, and became curate at Amherstburgh, for we find the first entry in the burial register there is signed, R. Rolph, with date 1820. He was ordained priest in the cathedral, Quebec, October 21, 1821; subsequently holding a parish at Innsbruck, then at March, near Ottawa, and finally at Queenston, where he died at the age of seventy-three. In St. Mark's church, Niagara-on-the-Lake, is a tablet to his memory, and the register states that "Romaine Rolph was interred, January 22nd, 1868." He left several children.

THOMAS ROLPH, the fourth son, born, September 16th, 1803, and baptized at St. Giles, Camberwell, Surrey, October 13, 1803, visited Canada several times. He received his early education at Peckham, Surrey, and took the degree of A.B., at St. John's College, Cambridge. He studied for holy orders, and was ordained Deacon, December 12, 1829, by the Bishop of Gloucester, and Priest, June 5, 1831. For many years he was a popular curate of Cirencester, Gloucestershire, and was appointed domestic chaplain to the Earl Bathurst, September 21, 1838; at the same time he was curate of North Cerney and perpetual curate of Baunton, Gloucestershire, November 8, 1841, being nominated to the same by the patroness, Jane Master, of the Abbey, Cirencester. Finally he became Vicar of Chiseldon, in Wiltshire, being appointed by the Bishop of Salisbury, April 26, 1866, where he died on March 14, 1887.

DR. JOHN ROLPH.

A full history of this most eminent member of the medical profession of Upper Canada remains to be written. The sketch for which room can be made in this volume must necessarily be comparatively brief, and consequently imperfect. We have endeavoured to gather up the facts relating to that portion of his life not generally known. Matters relating to

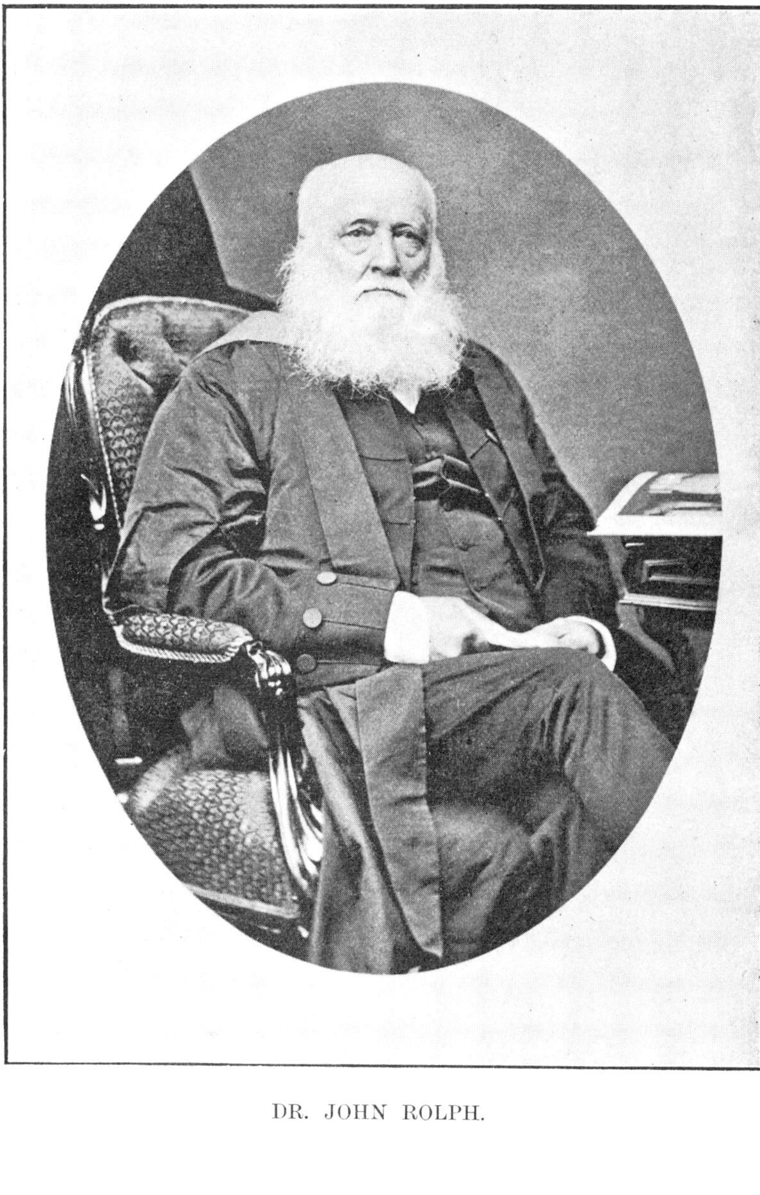

DR. JOHN ROLPH.

his middle life and advanced years are more familiar to the public, as they form an important chapter in the history of Upper Canada. Dr. Rolph was distinguished as a politician and as a successful practitioner of medicine, while he stood high as a member of the Bar. But his crowning glory was achieved in the lecture room of the Medical College. As a teacher of the Science of Medicine, it is doubtful if he had his equal.

Dr. John Rolph was born at Thornbury, Gloucestershire, March 4, 1793. Whether he accompanied his father to Canada is uncertain. Dent, who had access to many of Dr. Rolph's papers, says he did. But the writer has received information from Dr. H. H. Wright, who was for a long time closely associated with Dr. Rolph and living with him, also from Dr. J. H. Richardson, as well as from other sources, which strongly supports the belief that he remained in England to prosecute his studies, and did not cross the Atlantic until 1812. In the summer of that year he sailed from England to join the family in Canada, by way of New York. Before he reached New York, war had been declared by the United States against Great Britain, and it seems that the vessel in which he sailed became a prize. Dr. Rolph obtained a passport from President Madison to proceed to Canada. Reaching Buffalo, he was detained for a time, and while waiting, passed the time in solving a problem in Euclid. Being observed making unusual characters on a paper, he was suspected of being a spy and of making a sketch of the position of the United States forces, and was taken back by the authorities to Greenbush, and it was some time before negotiations could make it plain that he was not a spy. Shortly after the battle of Queenston, he was allowed to cross over into Canada. An informant says, "Up to his last years he would refer to the kindly way in which he was treated by the American surgeon and other officers, while he was detained a prisoner." He was at this time about nineteen years of age. Dr. Rolph served during the war as paymaster of His Majesty's militia forces in the London District. After the war he returned to England and engaged in the study of both law and medicine, probably concurrently. He was a student at Cambridge, where "he was recognized as a young man of very remarkable and precocious intellectual powers. He absorbed knowledge with marvellous facility, and never forgot anything he had learned."—*Dent.* He was a student-at-law in London, and in due time was called to the Bar of the Inner Temple. In medicine, he was a pupil of Sir Astley Cooper. Tickets of attendance at Sir Astley's lectures, dated 1818, are now in the possession of his son, Thomas Rolph, barrister, of Toronto. He was a student of Guy's and St. Thomas' Hospital, before they were separated into two institutions. He became a member of the Royal College of Surgeons, England. Dr. Rolph remained in England until 1821, as is shown by an entry in a Bible, now in possession of George Salmon, of Thornbury: "To Philemon Salmon, the gift of his Godfather and friend. (Signed) John Rolph, May 24, 1821." Returning to Canada, he made his residence in the township of Charlotteville, County Norfolk, at that time part of the Talbot District. He was called to the Bar of Upper Canada, 1821. He was the fourth Bencher in the Province. Dr. Rolph engaged in the practice of both law and medicine, and soon became a great favourite among all classes. He was the legal adviser and familiar friend of Col. Talbot, and one of the originators of the Talbot anniversary, kept up for more than twenty years in honour of the day of the Colonel's arrival, May 21, 1803. Subsequently their divergent political views caused an estrangement between them. It is related that Dr. Rolph at one time, being dissatisfied with law and medicine, turned his attention to divinity and applied for orders; but finding that he would be required to undergo some probation for this, abandoned the idea."—*Gamble.* In some reminiscences of medical men kindly furnished to the writer by Mr. Clarke Gamble, Q.C., he says: "My first introduction to Dr. Rolph was at the assizes in London, about the year 1827 or 1828, when he came into Court carrying a pair of saddlebags in his arms, one side being filled with surgical instruments, vials and package of medicine, etc., and the other with briefs and legal documents and books. He would attend to a case in Court, and, when through, would catch up his saddlebags, ascend the Court House steps, mount his horse tethered near by and ride off to visit a patient. He was not much of a lawyer, though an eloquent counsel." He became a prominent person in the London District. In 1823, he was a public school trustee and a member of the Board of Education; also a commissioner for taking affidavits.

The vast amount of energy which Dr. Rolph possessed was not exhausted in the two professions which he simultaneously followed, and he gave his attention to politics; and at the general elections of 1824, he was elected by the Reformers as member for Middlesex. About this time he removed to Dundas. Although he had practised medicine, he did not procure his license to practise in Upper Canada until 1829, as this announcement shows: "John Rolph, of the village of Dundas in Gore District, having complied with the provision of the statutes, was gazetted as a licentiate, July 10, 1829." In 1831, Dr. Rolph was a member of the Board of Education, also trustee for London District.

But Dr. Rolph's career, as a member of the Bar, was drawing to a close. In 1828, dissatisfied with a legal decision of Justice Sherwood, he, with Dr. Baldwin and his son Robert, threw off his gown and left the court. Soon after, believing, it is said, that he would never have justice, he resolved "to abandon the practice of law and to resume that of medicine," which latter, indeed, he had never wholly abandoned. This resolution was not fully carried out until more than two years after it had been formed, though he meanwhile accepted no new suits, and steadily prepared himself for the impending change. The decisive step does not appear to have been taken until 1832, when he transferred his legal practice to his brother George. Thenceforward John Rolph never again appeared in a Court of Justice in the capacity of an advocate. It was a momentous decision, for he had a fine legal practice and enjoyed the reputation of being the most eloquent man at the Upper Canada Bar. He had outlived the exuberance of youth, and was, at this time, nearly forty years old—an age at which few men would have had the courage to abandon a pursuit which had been followed with signal success for many years. He resumed the practice of medicine and surgery, and was thenceforward known as "Doctor Rolph." "He soon won a distinguished place in the ranks of his new calling, and reached a preëminence therein as great as he had ever attained at the Bar. There was no regularly organized medical college in Upper Canada, and the facilities for acquiring a competent medical training were few. In response to urgent requests from a number of influential persons in Toronto, he established a private medical class and gave instruction to a limited number of students. His teaching was eminently successful, and he made himself greatly beloved by his students. He seemed to have the whole round of medical literature at his fingers' ends, and his marvellous knowledge and graphic power of expression kindled in the breasts of the young men a love of knowledge for its own sake." "By no one were his attainments held in higher respect than by the Lieutenant-Governor. Sir John urged him to found a permanent medical college, and promised that Government aid for such an enterprise should not be wanting. But Dr. Rolph had other views." —*Dent.*

Dr. Rolph came to York, 1831, from Dundas. In the same year he was Vice-President of the Mechanics' Institute and one of the lecturers. He was commissioned a member of the Medical Board in 1832, and was present at the April meeting. In 1834 his name is given in York Directory as living in Macaulay Town, now near the site of the new Court House and City Hall. After the incorporation of Toronto as a city, Dr. Rolph was elected one of the first Aldermen. At that time the Aldermen elected one of their number to fill the Mayor's chair. Dr. Rolph aspired to the position and had expected that he would be elected, but Wm. Lyon Mackenzie was the choice. Mr. Mackenzie had recently received hard treatment from the Legislature, and his political friends in the City Council, who were in a majority, wished to show their sympathy in a marked manner, and resolved, at a caucus, to make him the first Mayor of Toronto. Dr. Rolph, although surprised and chagrined, acquiesced. He resigned before the election, thus paving the way for Mackenzie's election. Dr. Tims was elected to fill Dr. Rolph's place as Alderman.

October 30, 1834, this marriage notice appeared: "At Kingston, on Thursday, the 30th of October, by the Rev. Mr. Cartwright, Dr. John Rolph, M.A., of the city of Toronto, Member of the Honourable Society of the Inner Temple, London, barrister-at-law, to Grace, daughter of George Henry Haines, Esq., late of Leicester, England.

Dr. Rolph had been twice elected for Middlesex and once for Norfolk, and in 1835 he was appointed a member of the Executive Council of the Province with Drs. Baldwin, Dunn and Bidwell, but, in consequence of some act of the Lieut.-Governor, they all resigned. In 1836 Dr. Rolph was again elected for Norfolk. In the same year we find him delivering the closing lecture of the Mechanics' Institute.

In March, 1834, an address was publicly presented to Dr. Rolph, asking for the privilege of having his portrait painted. From this, and the various positions he occupied from time to time, it was evident that he was a very popular person.

During the period Dr. Rolph lived in Toronto he had received a number of pupils. He had already exhibited those qualities which subsequently made him famous, of imparting medical knowledge to students. The list of young men studying with him included Geo. H. Parks, James Mitchell, James Beatty, Barnhart, Frank Cameron, David Lee, J. W. Corson, J. W. Hunter, H. H. Wright and J. H. Richardson.

The year 1837 was one fraught with grave events. The Mackenzie rebellion had culminated in overt action on the part of the insurgents, and Dr. Rolph became involved in the outbreak. It is not our intention to enter into a discussion of the matter, but will give a statement from Dent. He says that at a conference at Dr. Rolph's house, Dr. Morrison, Mackenzie and one Lloyd, from Lower Canada, "a plan was discussed for seizing the arms in the City Hall, for taking into custody the chief officials, and for establishing a Provisional Government, with Dr. Rolph at its head"—the day fixed being December 7.

An account of his escape, after the collapse of Mackenzie's attempt to take Toronto, is of sufficient interest to merit a place in these pages. Dr. Morrison had been arrested on suspicion, and his arrest had been witnessed by H. H. Wright, then a house pupil with Dr. Rolph. "He lost no time in acquainting Dr. Rolph with what he had seen, and in advising him to seek safety in flight. Dr. Rolph speedily made up his mind. There was no longer any hope of success for the rebels. His own connection with the movement could not fail to become known, and he might count upon being prosecuted with the utmost rigour of the law. Dr. Morrison's arrest seemed to indicate that the Government had already become possessed of criminatory evidence—evidence which was quite as likely to compromise himself (Dr. Rolph) as the gentleman who had actually been deprived of his liberty. If so, no time was to be lost. In a very few moments one of his horses, a gray three-year-old colt, was saddled, and his young friend had mounted it and ridden westward along Lot Street. He himself followed leisurely on foot. A short distance up the street he encountered Chief Justice Robinson and two of his sons, who were probably on their way to the Lieutenant-Governor's headquarters in the Parliament Buildings. A grave salute was exchanged between them, after which each proceeded on his way. The Doctor continued his walk until he reached the spot where Dundas Street branches off northward from Queen Street, where he found his young friend awaiting him with the horse, from which he had dismounted. They exchanged quiet and undemonstrative farewells, after which Dr. Rolph mounted the horse and proceeded along Dundas Street, while the young medical student returned to the city.

"The Doctor made the best of his way to the United States. His journey was not unattended with peril, for any Tory whom he met on the way might possibly resolve to arrest him, and his complicity in the rebellion was susceptible of proof. He, however, rode westward about twelve miles without any misadventure, and was approaching the River Credit, when he encountered a company of loyalist volunteers *en route* for the capital. The gentleman in command was well acquainted with Dr. Rolph's political proclivities, but would probably not have suspected him of having any connection with the rebellion had he not thus met him far from home, and evidently prepared for a long journey. In reply to a demand as to his destination, the Doctor produced a letter which he had received on the previous day from his brother-in-law, Mr. Salmon, of Norfolk, acquainting him with the serious illness of his (Dr. Rolph's) sister, Mrs. Salmon, and requesting his presence at her bedside. This was deemed satisfactory, and the Doctor was allowed to proceed; but not long afterwards the officer, for some reason, became suspicious, and sent two volunteers in pursuit of the fugitive, who was soon overtaken, and brought back to Port Credit. He was greatly agitated, and a gentleman who was present at the time informs me that he trembled visibly. While he was still in detention, Dr. James Mitchell, of Dundas, a former student of Dr. Rolph's, arrived, and, doubtless with perfect sincerity, represented the absurdity of supposing that Dr. Rolph would really ally himself with such a one as Mackenzie for any purpose. The argument prevailed, and the Doctor was again permitted to resume his journey. Dr. Mitchell exchanged horses with him, remarking: 'Your beast does not seem equal to so long a journey—you had better take mine,' or words to that effect. Rolph directed his steps to the house of Mr. Asa Davis, on the outskirts of the village of Wellington Square, in the township of Nelson. Mr. Davis was an advanced Radical, and an old friend and client of Dr. Rolph, who, it will be remembered, had formerly practised the legal profession at Dundas, which is only a few miles distant from Wellington Square. He was cordially received, and invited to pass the night there, but he deemed it wisest to push on without delay. He, however, obtained an hour's rest and a fresh horse. He pursued his journey throughout the night, and early on the following morning reached the Niagara River, near Queenston. He soon placed the river between himself and danger. More than five years elapsed before his foot again trod Canadian soil." —*Dent.*

We are informed by Dr. C. W. Covernton that he was the physician attending Mrs. Salmon, and that it was he who wrote the letter to Dr. Rolph. That Dr. Rolph had good reason to make his escape soon is evident from the notice which appeared in the press, as follows:

"£500 REWARD.

"PROCLAMATION.

"By His Excellency Sir Francis Bond Head, Baronet, Lieut.-Governor of Upper Canada, etc., etc.

"Whereas, it appears that Doctor John Rolph, of Toronto, absconded hastily from his residence, on the breaking out of the insurrection.

"And whereas, from facts which have come to the knowledge of His Excellency the Lieutenant-Governor, it appears that he has been concerned in the traitorous attempt, which has happily been defeated, to subvert the Government of his Province, the above reward of Five Hundred Pounds is hereby offered to any one who will apprehend the said John Rolph, and deliver him up to justice, in the city of Toronto.

"December 11, 1837."

While in exile, Dr. Rolph engaged in practice at Rochester, where he remained until 1843, when the ban was removed by Act of Parliament, and those implicated in the rebellion were allowed to return.

It was subsequent to his return to Toronto that Dr. Rolph became so popular as a teacher of the Science of Medicine. We have seen that prior to 1837, he acquired a reputation in this respect, and had a number of students. While he was at Rochester he had Canadian students with him—H. H. Wright was one, and J. H. Richardson another. From 1843, it may be said, the formation of "Rolph's School" began. It rapidly grew in the number of students, and in popularity. So efficient was the instruction of Dr. Rolph that McGill College accepted the time passed with him as equivalent to attending lectures at a medical college. But many of the students went before the Upper Canada Medical Board.

The following notices appeared:

"Medical students, who do not intend to enter the university, will be, as heretofore, received by the subscriber, conducted through the usual course of medical studies, with such additional assistance as may be most desirable, and prepared for their diploma from the Medical Board.

"JOHN ROLPH.

"Lot Street, January 1, 1844."

"TORONTO SCHOOL OF MEDICINE.

"The session will commence on the last Monday in October, and end on the last Saturday in May, under Dr. Workman, Dr. Park and the subscriber.

"JOHN ROLPH.

"Toronto, September 25th, 1848."

As the number of students increased, Dr. Rolph obtained the assistance of other medical men to deliver lectures. Of these, Dr. Joseph Workman was by far the greatest acquisition. Rolph's School became a rival to the Medical Department of King's College; but as the staff of the latter controlled the Medical Board, Dr. Rolph's students were placed at a disadvantage—at least it was believed or feared that the ordeal before the Board would be to them more trying—nay, more, it was alleged that justice was denied to Rolph's students. In 1853 Rolph's School was incorporated under the title of the "Toronto School of Medicine."

It does not come within the scope of this work to enter fully into the history of the subsequent events in connection with this school. Having been an eye-witness of some of the events connected therewith, and, at a later date, to a certain extent a participant, the writer is in a position to furnish many particulars, and at a future time these may be given.

Dr. Rolph was too ardent a politician to remain out of Parliament, and his ability was recognized by the Hon. Francis Hincks, Premier of Canada. In 1851 he became a member of his administration and continued until 1854. Here may be given the estimate placed by John Charles Dent in the "Story of the Upper Canadian Rebellion:" "He possessed talents which, under favouring circumstances, would have made him a marked man in either professional or public life in any country. Chief among his qualifications may be mentioned a comprehensive, subtle intellect, high scholastic and professional attainments, a style of eloquence which was at once ornate and logical, a noble and handsome countenance, a voice of silvery sweetness and great power of modulation, and an address at once impressive, dignified and ingratiating. His keenness of perception and his faculty for detecting the weak point in an argument were almost abnormal, while his power of eloquent and subtle exposition had no rival among the Canadian public men of the times. . . . He was of full habit of body, even in comparative youth, and though he was rather under than above the middle height, there was dignity and even majesty in his presence that gave the world assurance of a strong man, while at the same time it effectually repelled unseemly familiarity. A pair of deep, clear blue eyes, surmounted by rather heavy eyebrows, glanced out from beneath his smooth and expansive forehead. He had light brown hair, a well-moulded chin, a firmly set nose, and a somewhat large and flexible mouth, capable of imparting to the countenance great variety of expression."

Dr. Rolph's School, as the Medical Department of Victoria University, enjoyed many years of prosperity. It was not until the latter part of the sixties that the Doctor exhibited any decay of his splendid qualities as a lecturer, and then it was more a loss of the clear, resonant tones of his voice than of mental grasp. He finally resigned his office of Dean in the early part of 1870.

The following account of the opening of the Medical Department of Victoria University (1870) is taken from the *Medical Journal*:

"The proceedings attending the opening of this institution during the past week have been of unusual interest. The Alumni residing in Toronto availed themselves of the occasion to entertain their brethren from the country, with several other gentlemen. The supper was given at the Queen's, on Tuesday evening, the 4th inst. In compliance with the particular request of the Committee of Arrangements, the Dean of the Faculty, Dr. Canniff, occupied the chair, and Dr. Agnew the vice-chair. Among the guests were the professors of the Medical Faculty; Dr. Hodgins, of the Education Department; W. W. Dean, barrister, Belleville; Drs. McGuire and Tuck, of Guelph; Corbett, of Perrytown, and others. Among the toasts of the evening was one of the late venerable Dean, the Hon. Dr. Rolph, to which Dr. Canniff was requested to respond. In doing so he expressed his sense of the honour conferred upon him by the committee in allowing him to respond. He referred to the many excellencies of the veteran teacher of medicine, whose ability to teach he had never seen equalled in the new or old world. He concluded by expressing not alone his personal regret, but that of his colleagues, that the hope always entertained by them that Dr. Rolph should continue to hold, as long as he lived, his position of Dean, had been unfortunately destroyed."

The death of Dr. Rolph took place at Mitchell, October 19, 1870, at the age of eighty-three. This sketch will be concluded by quoting from an obituary notice which appeared in a medical journal. After relating some of the events of his life, the medical journal concludes: "Two years ago, although he had undertaken to deliver his usual course upon the 'Practice of Medicine,' he was compelled from failing strength to cease his lectures. Indeed, during the previous year his feeble tones could not reach beyond the first seats of the class-room; yet the students were ever silent to try to catch the words of the 'old man eloquent.' Notwithstanding the waning physical strength of the old veteran, he retained much of his mental power, and continued to occupy the office of Dean until a few months before his death. When the fact of his death became known in Toronto, every respect was shown for his memory by the College over which he had so recently presided. The lectures were suspended for the week, and the students, after passing resolutions of condolence with the bereaved widow, resolved to wear mourning on the arm for a period of thirty days. Had the remains been interred in the city, the Faculty and students intended in a body to follow them to the grave."

The following address was presented by the students of Victoria College:

"*To Mrs. J. Rolph:*

"DEAR MADAM,—It is with profound feelings of sorrow that we, the undergraduates of Victoria College, learn of the death of our late and honoured Dean, Hon. Dr. Rolph.

"As it has pleased Almighty God, in His divine providence, to remove him from the cares and anxieties of this life, we feel it to be our duty to share, as far as possible, your great affliction and sad bereavement.

"By his removal you have lost a kind and devoted husband, we have been deprived of a great and faithful friend, and the profession to which we are aspiring of one of its ablest and most successful members.

"The kindness of his heart, the purity of his conduct, the urbanity of his manners, and the wisdom of his counsels, bound us to him by the strongest cords of affection.

"We have reason to be grateful that he has been spared so long to adorn the social and scientific walks of life, and to win for himself so many proud distinctions in science, arts and literature.

"The prosperity of Victoria College in the past, as well as its present proud and exalted position among similar institutions, is due, in a great degree, to the indefatigable energy, great ability, and untiring zeal of our late lamented Dean, whose name was almost synonymous with medical education.

"Although we will have him no longer in our midst, to cheer and assist us on, yet he has left a name and an influence that will encourage and inspire us in the acquisition of our profession.

"When *we* feel so keenly the loss of our esteemed friend and instructor, how much more keenly will *you* feel the loss of him who is torn from your bosom to be laid in the cold and silent tomb, whom you were wont to call by the tender and expressive name of husband.

"But God who called him from you, laden with the rich honours of a well-spent life, will be a husband to the widow and a father to the fatherless.

"We hope you may be strengthened and sustained in the midst of your sorrow and affliction by Him who can turn sorrow into joy, and grief into happiness.

"Dear Madam, accept our deepest sympathy and heartfelt condolence on your present sad bereavement; and we hope that when the cares of this life are over you may meet your dear husband in that brighter land that knows no parting.

"Signed on behalf of the students of Victoria College,

"R. McDONALD,
D. S. McCOLL,
F. D. ASTLEY,
L. C. CAMPBELL,
"*Committee.*

"Yorkville, 22nd October, 1870."

Dr. Rolph had three sons and a daughter: George Widmer, died at Rochester, 1840, aged eleven months. John Widmer entered the medical profession; received M.D. Victoria University, 1866, and L.R.C.P. London, 1867. He was for some time surgeon to the Mounted Police, N.W.T. He is at the present time practising at Kuanton, Pelang, in the Indian Ocean, and was for some time, by Government appointment, physician to the natives in the Straits Settlement. Thomas Taylor, the third son, educated at Toronto University, is a barrister, practising in Toronto. The daughter, S. Frances, became the wife of Lyster, eldest son of Alfred Hayward, of Port Hope, formerly of Buckingham, Bucks, Eng.

DR. THOMAS ROLPH,

Who first came to Canada, June, 1833, was not related to the family already spoken of. His home was in Ancaster, then an important village. He issued a card, which stated that he was "M.R.C.S.Eng. and Hon. Mem. of the Med. Society of London, and had commenced practising the three branches of the profession at Ancaster, August 13, 1835." He devoted much of his time in visiting the different parts of the Province, and in collecting facts relating to the condition and prosperity of the people, the character of the land, and what inducements existed for emigrants from the Old Country to make their home in the Province. As a result, he had published at Ancaster, 1836, a work giving a "Statistical Account of Upper Canada." He was in practice until the latter part of the thirties at Ancaster, and was succeeded by Dr. Dalton. He was gazetted Surgeon to 1st Gore Regiment of Militia, and was member of Board of Education, Dist. of Gore, July, 1838. His name is mentioned in the Act of Incorporation of the College of Physicians and Surgeons of Upper Canada in 1839. Dr. Thomas Rolph, unlike his namesake, was a strong Conservative, and intensely British at this time, when the Canadian rebellion had just been suppressed. In December, 1838, he addressed an open letter to Martin Van Buren, President of the United States, in which he dealt some hard blows to the United States Government for its conduct anent the Canadian rebellion. He became well-known in connection with a scheme to promote emigration from England to Upper Canada at that period. The following is taken from Charles Fothergill's almanac for 1839. Speaking of the necessity of some one visiting the Old Country to induce emigration, the writer recommended Dr. Thomas Rolph, of Ancaster. He says: "If an extensive knowledge of his subject, to which he has assiduously devoted his attention for several years; if vast collection of facts and references in regard to the present state and future prospects of this country, if talents of a very superior order, sound British principles, unwearied assiduity and a most surprising activity and readiness in any he undertakes, an able pen, and, above all, for our present cause purpose, a flow of eloquence that is always attractive and commanding, and sometimes inimitable and overwhelming; if these are requisites in a candidate for such a mission, we hesitate not to add that Dr. Thomas Rolph possesses them in an eminent degree."

Dr. Thomas Rolph was appointed Emigration Agent for the Government of Canada; was engaged in the work during 1839, '40, '41 and '42. He published the results of this mission in 1844, a volume of 376 pages, dedicated to Lord Stanley, Principal Secretary of State for the Colonies. The services of Dr. Rolph were evidently much appreciated. He says: "Immediately on my arrival at Toronto, I received a requisition signed by 171 persons, including all the judges, executive councillors, the Mayor (Dr. King), High Sheriff, and, indeed, by the chief respectable and moral and political strength of the city, without the slightest reference to party, to partake of a sumptuous banquet in the City Hall." The *Patriot* speaks of his "unremitting exertions through the United Kingdom, to bring before the British public the resources and capabilities of this Province." During the dinner, the Lieut.-Governor transmitted to him a highly flattering letter, recognizing Dr. Rolph's "zealous and able services" and "strenuous exertions." A few weeks later he was banqueted at Hamilton; then at Woodstock and Brantford and some other places. Having received an official appointment from Lord Sydenham, the Governor-General, he proceeded to Lower Canada. On arriving at Montreal, a large and influential meeting took place, thanking him for what he had already done. He was assisted by a powerful emigration association in Great Britain, and a Canadian Immigration Association was founded in Canada, with branches in most of the principal places. He sailed again the 1st January, 1841. On his return to Canada, a public meeting at Toronto commended his "eminent services," and hoped they would be continued by the Government. His services were recognized by Parliament. Dr. Dunlop, who declared to the House that Dr. Rolph knew more more about emigration than all of them put together, said that he had "rendered incalculable service to Canada."

Dr. Thomas Rolph seems to have been endowed with a large and educated brain, but he was of small stature. His wife, on the contrary, was of large size, but strikingly handsome. They had no children. He did not continue long at Ancaster after his emigration work had ceased, but returned to England and settled at Portsmouth.

The last chapter of Dr. Thomas Rolph's life is inexpressibly sad. The story of his death in England could hardly be credited did it not come from the most reliable source, and one could hardly believe that such a thing could occur in England. The facts have been given to the writer by Dr. C. W. Covernton. He relates that he was visiting at Portsmouth an old fellow-student, Dr. Wm. Engledon, the chief physician at the port. During his stay, when driving along a country road with his friend, and passing a churchyard, Dr. Engledon stopped, and directed Dr. Covernton's attention to a tombstone, the writing upon which could be read from the road. He then narrated that on a certain day, Dr. Rolph, as he was passing, caught sight of his name, and stopped to see what it meant. Perhaps only a medical man, especially a conscientious man, can conceive the terrible shock which would be experienced when he read the following awful indictment: "Sacred to the memory of the beloved wife of ————, who was killed by Dr. Thomas Rolph." This stone, with the execrable inscription, had been placed there for several months. The effect upon Dr. Rolph was that he went home prostrated, and within a short time died, the victim of malice. Dr. Engledon assured Dr. Covernton that Dr. Rolph was in no way to blame for the death of the woman. It was one of those unfortunate instances of unexpected hæmorrhage after childbirth.

DR. JOHN PARTINGTON RUSSELL,

The second son of Capt. R. H. Russell, of the Scots Fusiliers Guards, was born in Dublin, 1821, and came to Quebec with his father when quite young. He commenced and pursued his medical studies under Dr. James Douglas, of Quebec, a well-known and highly skilful physician of his day. Mr. Russell proceeded to Scotland and took a medical course at Edinburgh University, from which institution he graduated, 1846. He also became a member of the Royal College of Surgeons, England. Returning to Quebec, he engaged in practice with his elder brother, where he continued until 1860, when, on the death of his younger brother, practising in Toronto, he took up his abode there.

Dr. J. P. Russell continued in active practice in Toronto up to the time of his death, which occurred suddenly, May 14. 1890. During all these thirty years, Dr. Russell held a high position in the ranks of the medical profession, and justly enjoyed a reputation for possessing great skill and successful treatment of disease, which evidenced the thorough training he had received and the close application in pursuit of medical knowledge during his years of pupilage. Dr. Russell was greatly esteemed by his medical confreres, who frequently availed themselves of his services as a consultant. In that capacity he was often in demand throughout the Province.

Dr. Russell loved his profession, and took great pride in faithfully observing all the laws, written and unwritten, which govern the profession, He had a generous heart for those suffering from disease, and in alleviating that suffering he was not actuated by mercenary motives. Many a one in the poorer ranks of life had reason to regret his loss to the community.

Dr. Russell had one son and two daughters. The son, Dr. J. P. Russell, is a medical graduate of the University of Trinity College, Toronto, and also of Victoria University, and occupies the place where his father practised.

DR. ROBERT HENRY RUSSELL, the elder brother of the above, was also born in Dublin, 1819. Coming to Canada with the family, he also studied medicine with Dr. Douglas, of Quebec, then at the University of Edinburgh, and took the degree of M.D.,

1842, and as well M.R.C.S. Eng. He returned to Quebec, and commenced the practice of his profession, which he pursued there until his death, 1882. He held the position of President of the College of Physicians and Surgeons of Lower Canada, and was a Governor of that body for upwards of thirty years. He was also President of the Quebec Medical Society. The writer has a pleasant recollection of Dr. R. H. Russell as a brother charter member of the Canada Medical Association; his geniality, energy and zeal at the organization of that Association at Quebec, 1867, also his kindly hospitality and attention to the delegates from different parts of the Dominion. His services and worth were recognized by electing him the first Treasurer of the Association.

He left one son, now Dr. Henry Russell, practising in Quebec.

DR. FRANCIS M. RUSSELL, the youngest son of Capt. Russell, was likewise born in Dublin, 1825; studied medicine in Quebec with his brother, and likewise attended Edinburgh University, and graduated in 1855; also obtained M.R.C.S. Eng. On his return to Canada, he settled in Toronto, and soon acquired a large practice. He was appointed Professor of Surgery in the medical department of Trinity College, and occupied the chair until the department was discontinued. He died 1860.

DR. GEORGE RYALL,

Was born in County Tipperary, Ireland, August 9, 1797. His father was a man of unobtrusive habits, living quietly on his property. His mother was a lineal descendant of John Cumberland Hazlitt, who was a border knight.

In 1810, George entered Kilkenny College under the Rev. Andrew O'Callaghan, D.D., Principal of the College, and in 1811 matriculated in Trinity College, Dublin, getting first place out of one hundred matriculants. He was then under fifteen years of age. During his college course he was under the tuition of the Rev. Samuel Kyle, D.D., who was afterwards appointed Bishop of Cork. He also passed the best examination for scholarship, but the statutes of the College debarred him from getting one. He, however, was awarded an exhibition of £50 per annum for five years, while his name was entered on the books of the college.

As he was originally intended for the ministry, he took up the full Divinity course, and was ready for ordination when he received his degree of B.A. in 1818, but, according to the rules then existing, he could not be ordained until he was twenty-five years of age.

Shortly afterwards he was offered a high position in some Canadian College (probably in Montreal), by the then Bishop of London, Eng. He would have accepted it, but his parents were averse to his leaving them for so distant a country as Canada then appeared to be. There were no steamships in those days, and travel by sail was not so speedy as it has been in recent times.

He then commenced the study of medicine, three years of which were spent at the Royal Infirmary, Edinburgh. Dr. Herrick was also at that time a student there, being somewhat his senior. The remainder of his study was completed in Dublin, where he was Clinical Clerk to Dr. Barker, in Sir Patrick Dunn's hospital.

He received his degree of M.B. in Trinity College in 1825, and shortly afterwards settled in his native town, and received extensive patronage from the surrounding country. He was family physician to all the principal gentry of the neighbourhood, including Lord Gough and all his family connections; he also had medical charge of all detachments of military in barracks, when unaccompanied by a regimental surgeon.

Dr. Ryall was an excellent classical scholar. When at school, for some trivial offence, his teacher gave him fifty lines of Virgil to recite from memory. He did so, and then asked his teacher if he would like to hear him recite it backwards.

In his younger days he was very active, and could jump twenty-one feet on the level ground. He was also an excellent horseman, and very fond of horses. Often in practice, he would cross the country on horseback, saving several miles of road travel. When a student, he and another, out of a whole field of horsemen, cleared the lough of the bay near Dublin, which, at its narrowest point, was twenty-one feet wide, many of the others who attempted it getting pretty well soaked.

He was a man truly charitable, giving without ostentation, and never saw any deserving person in want when he could relieve them. He was a strict Low Church Episcopalian, and in politics was always Conservative.

Dr. Ryall was married twice, his first wife being Ellen, eldest daughter of James Brett, of Clebemon Hall, County Wexford, and granddaughter of Annesley De Renzie (now spelled Derinzy), of Whitehall House, Baltinglass, County Wicklow, and sister of the late Colonel the Honourable De Renzie James Brett, of the Upper House, Christ Church, New Zealand, who formerly served in the 31st Native Infantry, Madras Army, and was Brigadier-General in the Crimean War. Her father commanded the Wexford Yeomanry in the rebellion of '98, and was taken prisoner with a Mr. Pounden; sentenced to be shot on the bridge of Wexford, but whose lives were saved through means of a friendly priest, who delayed the sentence from time to time, until the British army came in sight, when the rebels decamped, without effecting their object. She was then a baby in arms, and her mother had to fly with her, concealed in a coal barge plying between Wexford and Enniscorthy. By her he had five sons and two daughters, most of them dying in infancy. Two are now living, Dr. Isaac Ryall and his sister, both residents of Hamilton (1894). Their mother died in 1839 of typhus fever, caught while visiting the sick poor.

On August 5, 1846, Dr. Ryall married Anna Maria, eldest daughter of the late Thomas Lindsay, of Lindville, County Tipperary, Ireland, by whom he had three sons. One died in infancy; another died in Hamilton, 1889; the youngest went to the North-West Territory.

Dr. Ryall and family left Liverpool for Quebec on the 8th of August, 1850, and arrived at the latter place on September 12. Settled in Hamilton on November 1, 1850. He died August 9, 1876, being the seventy-ninth anniversary of his birthday.

DR. ISAAC RYALL, Medical Health Officer, Hamilton, Ont., was the fourth son and sixth child of George Ryall, M.D., by his first wife. He was born in Fethard, County Tipperary, Ireland. Received his education principally from private tutors, but was also at Kilkenny College. Passed the matriculation examination of Trinity College, Dublin, in 1847. He was always intended for the army, but came to Canada with his father in 1850. Not knowing what else to turn to in Canada, he commenced the study of medicine at Toronto University, and passed the matriculation examination there. Attended the school until it broke up, then went to Trinity College School of Medicine, and received the degree of M.B. in 1855. He then went to London, Eng., and spent six months in St. Thomas' Hospital, visiting the chief London hospitals, and seeing the most celebrated surgeons operate. It was the good fortune of the writer to be a companion of Dr. Ryall at this time. Dr. Ryall returned to Canada and commenced practice in Hamilton, 1856.

Dr. Ryall was appointed Medical Health Officer of Hamilton in 1876.

DR. JAMES MOON SALMON,

Born, February 14, 1824, was the son of the Rev. Geo. Salmon, and the grandson of Col. Salmon, who was an intimate friend of Dr. Thomas Rolph and accompanied the family to Canada, both coming from Gloucestershire, England. James began the study of medicine with Dr. C. W. Covernton in 1842, or a little later. He subsequently studied in Toronto with Dr. King. Passed the Medical Board, April, 1847. Had numerous tickets of attendance upon lectures in the University of King's College, Toronto. He at once settled in Simcoe, where he has continued to live (1894). He was considered an able man, and soon acquired a good practice. His reputation as a surgeon was good. Of late, Dr. Salmon's practice has been limited to consultations with other physicians. He has not confined his attention to the practice of his profession, but by buying and selling land has acquired considerable wealth.

DR. JAMES SAMPSON

Was born 1790, at Magherally, County Armagh, Ireland; was the son of William Sampson, rector of that place. His mother was Alicia, daughter of Rev. James Brush, rector of Garnaghy,

County Down. The Sampson family were descended from a long line of soldiers and ecclesiastics. An editorial notice, clipped from a paper without name or date, but doubtless a Kingston paper, says:

"This deceased gentleman requires at our hands a more than passing notice. After receiving a good education, he served his time with an eminent surgeon in Dublin. He matriculated at Trinity College, Dublin. He spent a year at Middlesex Hospital, in London, and during a part of that time he had the advantage of being House Surgeon. In 1811, after passing a most flattering examination, he entered the army as Assistant Surgeon to the 88th Connaught Rangers. The year 1812 found him in Canada, in the 104th Regiment. He was at the attack upon Sackett's Harbour. Owing to his skill in surgery, and to the distaste for operations of his two senior medical officers, he performed all the operations required upon the wounded who were sent to Kingston.

"Later in the American war he proceeded, with a detachment, to Penetanguishene. During their journey, an accident happening to the officer in command, he planned and executed a night attack upon two armed American vessels then lying on Lake Huron. Both were captured without the loss of a man. This exploit undoubtedly had much effect in saving Upper Canada to the British rule.

"In 1817, being on half pay, he settled in Kingston. Shortly after, he was again called into active service, but, owing to the urgent entreaties of his friends, he threw up his commission. For nearly half a century that he has resided in Kingston he has ever been one of the most useful, influential and prominent citizens. Ever liberal, hospitable and benevolent, he was the true friend of all classes. He took a lead in every useful enterprise. In his personal exertions, with those of the late Hon. John Macaulay, the erection of our fine hospital is due.

"During the rebellion, when Kingston, without a soldier, was in imminent danger of attack from a large body of American sympathizers, his energy, zeal and ability organized the citizens for defence with such efficiency that the attempt upon the town was never made.

"Dr. Sampson attained the highest civic honours that Kingston could bestow—being Mayor in 1839, '40, '44. His portrait, as Mayor of the city, graces the City Hall. He also attained distinction on the Bench, and was, for a time, Chairman of the Court of Quarter Sessions.

"His eminence as a practitioner of medicine and as an operator was of Provincial, or rather American, fame. His integrity and honour were never impeached. While the members of the medical profession in other towns were too often at loggerheads, and forgetting in their quarrels the character of gentlemen, he, as the acknowledged head of his profession here, contributed to maintain that harmony and courtesy which should exist among gentlemen.

"For two or three years past his health has gradually declined, which induced him to surrender the greater part of his practice. He still continued to perform his duties as Surgeon of the Penitentiary, which office he held from the first establishment of the prison, twenty-six years ago."

The quotation above required some modification. Through the favour of Mr. Jas. Bain, Librarian of the Toronto Public Library, the writer has had the perusal of a number of letters written by Dr. Sampson to Samuel P. Jarvis, Niagara, the first of which is dated at Queenston, February 24, 1820, the last at Kingston, November 23, 1823. By these letters it is learned that Dr. Sampson was engaged in practice on the Niagara frontier between 1817 and 1820, and probably from 1815, at the close of the war.

Dr. Sampson writes at Queenston, 1820: "I have discovered two persons who are practising the noble science which I profess, without license, and in this neighbourhood, and I can obtain sufficient proof to convict them of the offence. What I want is information how to proceed against them; and should you think that application ought to be made to the Attorney-General, may I beg you will ask him to favour me with the necessary instructions. One of the offenders is an apothecary living in Niagara, who does not confine himself to his lawful trade; the other is a fellow who offered $600 a year to Dr. Muirhead, to be allowed to practise as his apprentice: they are both equal to the fine." The next letter, dated Kingston,

September 10, 1820, informs us that he and family had arrived there, and were settled in their own house.

The intimate friendship subsisting between Dr. Sampson and S. P. Jarvis is manifested by a letter of September 30, 1820. In it Dr. Sampson says: "I consider your silence on the subject of your wife and child, that they are quite well; as to the latter, I feel proud that his good mother should consider me worthy of the charge she thinks of assigning me. Tell her I shall be most happy to act as sponsor for the young gentleman. . . . I am in as good practice as I could well expect for the time. . . . Why do you tantalize me with reports of the rich medical harvest now reaping in your country? I am told Messrs. Widmer and Pilkington have their hands full at York. We have no less than ten medical practitioners here, of all descriptions; therefore you may suppose we are not held otherwise than cheap."

September 23, 1820, Dr. Sampson writes, speaking of social matters: "I never did, nor do I think it likely I ever shall be an admirer of them (Kingston society); they are a cold and formal set of people. I shall endeavour to be on good terms with them all, and if they condescend to employ me when they are, or imagine themselves, sick, I shall be their humble servant at command." He says: "All house supplies are so very dear here that I wish to get some things from Niagara," and goes on to speak of butter, cheese, stock hams and apples. "You say I must come down a 'peg lower'; if you saw the affability which I put on to all the riff-raff here, you would accuse me of familiarity with my inferiors. As for the 'first society' (who are not those by whom I most thrive), I cannot aspire to their patronage till I own a wharf or have ten shares in the Bank of Upper Canada. I was asked, however, to dine with the Lieut.-Governor some days ago, and I went, it being a male feast." He goes on to reflect somewhat seriously on "the newly created aristocrats," and for them expresses hearty contempt, calls them "egregious brutes," who "do not know what is due to the laws of common good breeding." In a letter, June 20, 1821, he says: "My receipts here, by the way, are very steady, and indeed I think have been more so than my Niagara practice produced." Then he writes: "I am told Mr. Pilkington is doing wonders at York; what a blockhead I was not to take your advice about going there near two years ago. Fitzgerald will not yet allow that I did wrong. He says Mr. P. makes his money by selling perfumery, etc."

In the minutes of the Upper Canada Medical Board, April 1, 1822, it is recorded that "the commission was read appointing James Sampson, Esq., late Assistant-Surgeon in His Majesty's Service, on half pay, to be a member of the Medical Board, in room of James Macauley, deceased."

The dissatisfaction of Dr. Sampson with Kingston as a home, shown in his letters, was, it would appear, about to be removed. The writer has heard from several excellent sources that Dr. Sampson was induced to retire from the service and settle in Kingston, by the pledge of twelve of the principal families there to pay him £25 each a year for his life, thus securing him an annuity of £300. But from the letters quoted from, this is evidently a mistake, so far as leaving the service to engage in private practice. But it may have been that he contemplated removing to York, and it was to prevent this and keep him in Kingston that the twelve families entered into a contract as mentioned. From this time, Dr. Sampson had no cause to complain of want of patronage among the "aristocrats." It was not long before he had everything in practice his own way among all classes. Around the Bay of Quinte his name was a household word. Dr. Sampson was physically, as well as mentally, a large and strong man, which enabled him to respond to the numerous calls, far and near, made upon him.

The Kingston *Herald*, June 12, 1835, says: "The Kingston General Hospital, which has been in course of erection for almost two years, is now nearly completed. It presents a fine appearance. Eighty-nine feet, four inches in length; fifty-three feet, four inches wide; four stories high; rooms lofty and well ventilated; can accommodate about 120 patients. It has two fronts, and is approached by a handsome flight of stone steps. Dr. Sampson is appointed physician to the hospital."

Dr. Sampson took a great interest in the Provincial Penitentiary at Kingston, and the unfortunate inmates. A saying of one of the convicts at the time of his death is still remembered, regarding the deceased. "Leaning on his staff, his head of snow and heart of fire."

Dr. Sampson was twice married; first, to Miss Cuyler, who was a niece or daughter of General Cuyler; secondly, to Eliza Chipman, daughter of Judge Edward Winslow, of Frederickton, New Brunswick. He had four daughters, one of whom is Mrs. Fenwick, of Montreal.

DR. JAMES SCHOFIELD.

Born in Connecticut, U. S.; came to Canada, 1795, accompanied by his son Ira, and settled in the County of Leeds. They built an iron forge and manufactured the first iron made in Upper Canada. In 1812, Dr. Schofield was Surgeon to the Forces. Ira commanded a company of militia at Gananoque and Prescott. Another son, James, was in the Commissary Department at Cornwall.

DR. PETER SCHOFIELD, son of the above, came to Leeds, 1800; after a few years went to New York and obtained his degree from the College of Physicians and Surgeons of New York; was Surgeon in the United States army, 1812. After the war he settled in County Leeds; became a Justice of the Peace and a member of the Commissioners' Court. In June, 1828, Dr. Peter Schofield delivered a temperance address, the first, it is stated, given in Upper Canada, and which led to the organization of the first temperance society. The address was published, and gave an account of a case of spontaneous combustion which the Doctor had seen. The Doctor passed the Upper Canada Medical Board, July, 1829. The "Board was perfectly satisfied." He died, May, 1860.

DR. JOHN SCOTT

Was born 1816, at Strabane, County Tyrone, Ireland. In 1831 he was apprenticed to learn the business of an apothecary. He was a student at University of Edinburgh, and therefrom received certificate November 28, 1835; he became M.R.C.S., London, May 24, 1841. Coming to Toronto, he married, Feb.

14, 1844, Mary Anne, only daughter of Rev. John Roaf, a well-known and esteemed clergyman of the Congregational Church in Toronto, father of James R. Roaf and Wm. Roaf, ex-Alderman, both barristers, of Toronto.

Dr. Scott engaged in practice at Toronto until 1849, when he was commissioned Superintendent of the Toronto Lunatic Asylum. This position he held until 1853, when, according to the statement of a trustworthy witness, he found the position made so intolerable to him by the twelve magnates who were managers that he resigned, feeling that he did not receive fair play. Dr. Scott resumed practice, and was made Coronor of Toronto. He died, May, 1864.

DR. JOHN SCOTT.—Mr. Young, in his "History of Galt," speaking of the Asiatic cholera, 1834, says: "Most valuable assistance was given by Dr. John Scott, then a young man of about twenty-one years of age, who, with his father and other members of his family, had fortunately arrived from Roxboroughshire, Scotland, about ten days previously. He was a brother of Mr. Andrew Scott, of Galt, and afterwards became widely known in Berlin as a skilful practitioner and a public-spirited citizen."

Dr. Scott was one of the most fearless of the little band who fought the cholera inch by inch, with their lives in their hands, until it finally disappeared.

DR. WILLIAM JAMES SCOTT.

A newspaper obituary notice says:

"THE LATE DR. SCOTT, OF PRESCOTT.—Died in Prescott, on Thursday, October the 14th, in his eighty-third year, William James Scott, M.D., Registrar of the County of Grenville, and father of the Hon. R. W. Scott, Senator, and Secretary of State for Canada, descended from an influential family in the County of Clare. He received his education under the care of his grandfather, Dr. McLachlin, of Dublin. He served on the medical staff in the Peninsular War, being attached to Lord Hill's division of the army, and was present at Salamanca, Vittoria, Badajos, and other great battles of the campaign. In the year 1814, he came to Canada, and was stationed at Quebec, Kingston, and Fort Wellington, Prescott. In the year 1817 he retired from the army, and soon after married Sarah Macdonell, daughter of the late Capt. Allan Macdonell, of the King's Royal Yorkers, then living at Matilda. For fifty-seven years they have lived together in all the enjoyment of domestic bliss, and to-day the disconsolate widow and her family have the earnest and heartfelt sympathy of all, far and near. In May, 1818, Dr. Scott entered the employment of the North-West Company, and remained for four years in the 'great lone land,' spending a winter at Cumberland House. His memory of the interesting events of his early life remained fresh to the end. Having taken up his permanent residence in Prescott in the year 1824, he devoted himself with all the energy of his self-denying heart to the practice of his profession. The heart-rending scenes of 1832 and 1847, when thousands of poor Irish immigrants lay dying, were well calculated to try men's souls. The sterling Christian charity of Dr. Scott shone forth then. He laid aside all self, and devoted all his time to caring for the afflicted exiles day and night; and often, with no one to lend a helping hand, he nursed and cared for the strangers. Quietly and unostentatiously he passed through life, beloved by all. Without pain, and as if gently touched by the hand of a spirit saying, 'Come up higher,' surrounded by his loving wife and children, he gently yielded up his spirit into the hands of his Creator."

One who knew Dr. Scott, about 1834, says he was the best known doctor in that part of the country. His practice extended over a large district, usually from Matilda to Brockville, and northward to the limit of settlement. In appearance he bore a strong resemblance to the pictures representing Sir Walter Scott, although claiming no relationship. He was a genial, not to say jovial person, of medium size, and moderately stout."

Dr. Wm. J. Scott passed Upper Canada Medical Board, July, 1831. He had one son and two daughters at least. His son is R. W. Scott, Senator. Dr. Scott died, October 14, 1875.

DR. JOSEPH SCOTT.—The following is taken from the Kingston *Gazette*, May 19, 1817: "Mr. Joseph Scott, M.R.C.S., Dublin, late of His Majesty's Ship *Montreal*, on Lake Ontario, formerly Medical Attendant, Lying-in Hospital, Dublin, acquaints the inhabitants of Kingston and its vicinity that he resides near the South Gate, in part of the house occupied by Mr. Richardson, and intends practising the several branches of his profession in future. Every attention will be paid to patients on the most reasonable terms." A short time later he announces that he "has taken in partnership H. McGee, Member of the Dublin and Edinburgh Colleges." In February, 1818, Drs. Scott & McGee advertise that one of them will visit Ernesttown every Friday.

DR. EDWARD QUINCY SEWELL

Was born at Montreal, April 5, 1810; was the eldest son of Stephen Sewell, K.C., for some time Solicitor-General for the Lower Provinces (who died of cholera, 1831), and nephew of Chief Justice Sewell, of Quebec. About 1830 Mr. E. Q. Sewell, accompanied by his brother Charles Stephen, proceeded to Edinburgh and entered the University as a medical student. In due time he received the degree of M.D., and became a M.R.C.S. at a later date. His father's sudden death hurried his return to Canada. In 1835 he received license to practise in Lower Canada. The following year he took a degree from the Albany Institute, and qualified to practise in New York State. In 1841, he took out license to practise in Upper Canada. He was in practice in Montreal, 1846, and at Sorel from 1848 to 1853. He then removed to Perth, Upper Canada, where he practised until 1867, when failing health compelled him to retire. He removed to Toronto, where he died, November, 1873.

Dr. E. Q. Sewell married Susan, only daughter of Edward L. Hayden, Esq., of Sorel, by whom he had two children, a son and daughter, who, with their mother, reside in Toronto (1894).

DR. CHARLES STEPHEN SEWELL

Was the second son of the Solicitor-General for Lower Canada, and brother of Edward Quincy. He studied his profession with his brother in Edinburgh from 1830 with considerable distinction, being elected, during his pupilage, President of the Royal Medical Society of Edinburgh. After obtaining M.D., University of Edinburgh, and M.R.C.S., Edinburgh, he studied at Paris. Returning to Canada, he commenced practice at Montreal, 1836 or 1837. In 1842, he was elected Lecturer on Materia Medica, McGill University, and Attending Physician to the Montreal General Hospital, which posts he held until 1848, when he resigned and left Montreal, probably on account of severe family affliction, which impaired his health. After two years of absence, mostly in the South, Dr. Sewell returned to Montreal, and again became a member of the faculty of McGill College, and of the hospital staff, where he lectured on Clinical Medicine. In 1852, he removed to Ottawa. Dr. Sewell contributed several papers of value to medical periodicals, the result of his observations. As a lecturer, he was clear and painstaking; though, perhaps, not brilliant as a teacher, he possessed that gentlemanly deportment which endeared him to his pupils.

Dr. Chas. S. Sewell married Isabel, daughter of Dr. Geddes, at Kingston, and had issue nine or ten children, yet he died childless, all of them but one having died of scarlet fever.

DR. GRIFFIN SMITH,

Of Barton (April 20, 1831), "announces that he has employed Mr. Robert Mutten, of Hamilton, as an assistant, and who was a student of two years' standing, lately returned from Montreal from two courses of lectures." This marriage notice appeared: "Married, in Hamilton, November 26, 1835, Dr. Griffin Smith to second daughter of Dr. Charles Duncombe, M.P.P., of Oxford." In 1836, Dr. G. Smith, in a letter to the *Correspondent and Advocate*, defended his father-in-law against newspaper assaults, who had visited England, and presented a petition to the Imperial Parliament, on Upper Canadian matters. It was a political squabble, and Dr. Smith said he did not agree with his father-in-law's political views.

DR. HERMANUS SMITH,

The son of a United Empire Loyalist settler, was born in the township of Barton, near by where St. Catharines now stands. He was not physically strong as a boy, and early showed a studious disposition. In the time of the war of 1812 he was not considered sufficiently strong to take a place in the ranks of the militia. Fortunately for the delicate and studious young man, there was a very competent and educated physician, Dr. Allen, living near his father's, with whom he became a student, and from whom he acquired his knowledge of the profession, and doubtless at the same time a good deal of general knowledge. Like a few others who have been no mean medical practitioners in Upper Canada, he never attended a course of medical lectures, nor walked the wards of a hospital. Probably he received some information from Dr. Lafferty, if the supposition be correct that he was the Dr. Smith who, in partnership with Lafferty, had an apothecary shop in the village of St. Catharines in 1818. Dr. Smith appeared before the Medical Board in October, 1819, and obtained his licence to practise. Hamilton and the surrounding country was the field of Dr. Smith's practice during his life. He married Miss Philmon, of Ancaster. His practice was extensive, and he acquired considerable property. The valuable property on the mountain, owned by the Hon. Mr. Buchanan, was bought from Dr. Smith, who then purchased land in Ancaster, where he made his homestead and where he died. Dr. Smith was not only a successful doctor, but was honoured by being elected to represent in the Provincial Parliament the County of Wentworth, in 1834.

He had three sons, who are still living in Ancaster (1889). His only daughter married Dr. William J. H. A. Case.

DR. GEORGE SOUTHWICK.

Was born at Twelve Mile Creek, where now stands St. Catharines, 1808. The family settled on a farm in Yarmouth, 1818. He was a student first with Dr. Josiah Goodhue, of St. Thomas, brother of Hon. G. H. Goodhue, of London, and then with Dr.

Duncombe. He then attended one course of lectures at "the Western College of Physicians and Surgeons, at Fairfield, Herkimer County, New York, one of the most noted medical schools of that day on the Continent." It was established in 1812 and dissolved in 1840. Dr. Southwick passed the Upper Canada Medical Board, October, 1835, and "his examination was very creditable and satisfactory."

Dr. Southwick practised for some years in the States, first at Buffalo, and then at Paducah, Ky. He returned to St. Thomas, 1839, and there continued to practice until his powers failed. In addition to his practice, he had at one time a drug store in St. Thomas.

"In 1854, he was nominated by the Reform party for the old Parliament of Canada, for East Elgin, and was elected as the first member for the riding, the county having sent only one member previously. His course in Parliament was marked by an independence of spirit peculiar to the man, and which probably alienated the sympathies of the extreme party men. During the latter years of his life he was a supporter of the Liberal-Conservative party on general questions. The Doctor occupied the Mayor's chair for several terms in the early history of the town. He was an effective speaker in his day, though, perhaps, he could not be termed eloquent."

He was thrice married. His children are, one son in the North-West, and four daughters. One daughter married E. Jones Parke, Q.C., Police Magistrate, London, son of Thomas Parke, who represented the County of Middlesex in last two Parliaments of the Province of Upper Canada, and in the first Parliament of Canada after the Union. The three other daughters, Misses Alice, Florence and Inez Southwick are at home.

He was an invalid for many years, and finally passed away, May 6, 1891, in his 84th year. The announcement of his death, says:

"Dr. George Southwick, a notable figure in the public life of this district in other days, and one who did much to assist in the development of the country, passed peacefully away last night after a life full of years and honours. He had resided in Elgin for nearly seventy-five years, and in St. Thomas for over fifty years."

The Doctor was a most able practitioner, and in the public affairs of the country always took an active interest.

Dr. Southwick was a quiet, reticent man, but a close student. Physically, he was one of the finest forms to be seen.

DR. THOMAS SPAREHAM.

In the old "U.E. List" is found the name of Dr. "Sparam," whose residence was at Augusta, Eastern District. A "hospital mate reduced. Had been in the war of 1763," on the "Provision List, 1786." The name of his son Thomas also appeared in the List, residing in Kingston. The name is undoubtedly misspelt. It should have been Spareham. It will be seen by looking over the U. E. List that very many names are differently spelt from what they are now by their descendants.

There is every reason to believe that both father and son were surgeons.

In 1808, Dr. Spareham was practising in the settlement at the mouth of Myer's Creek, now Belleville. His stay here was short, as in 1809 he removed to Waterloo, near Kingston, where his relatives lived, and where he passed the remainder of his days. Dr. Spareham was a patentee of one of the lots in Kingston. The writer has been told that Dr. Spareham, with John Turnbull, organized the first Sunday School at Myer's Creek. The only further information obtained regarding Dr. Spareham is taken from the Kingston *Gazette*: "Died, Friday, 20th, 1813, Dr. Thomas Spareham, at Kingston, aged eighty-eight. He was one of the first settlers in the country."

DR. F. B. SPILSBURY

Was born in London, England, in 1756, and was the eldest son of Dr. Francis Spilsbury, who was a prominent physician, residing and practising at Soho Square, in the West End of London. He pursued his medical studies at St. Bartholomew's Hospital, obtained the diploma of the Royal College of Surgeons, and

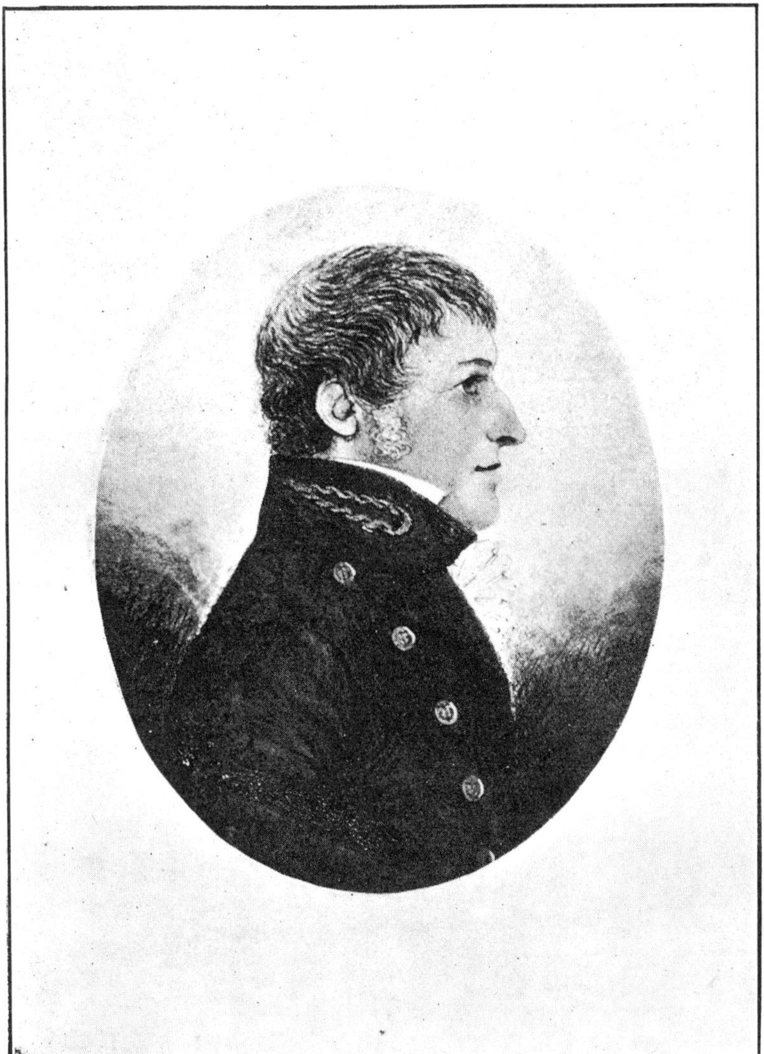

DR. F. B. SPILSBURY, R.N.

entered the Royal Navy as Assistant Surgeon, in 1778. From 1785 to 1807, he served in the Mediterranean Sea, where he was successively Surgeon to H. M. Sloop *Bulldog;* to the hospital at Beyrout, for the reception of the wounded during the siege of Acre; to the flotilla of French gun-boats, captured by H.M.S. *Le Tigre;* to the brigade of seamen serving on shore in Egypt; and Surgeon to the fleet under the command of Admiral Sir Sidney Smith. He served on English stations from 1807 until the spring of 1813, when he was sent to Canada as Surgeon to the fleet stationed at Kingston, on Lake Ontario, under the command of Admiral Sir James Yeo, during the war with the United States, and he was present at all the principal engagements between the fleets of Sir James Yeo and Commodore Chauncey, among which were that of Forty Mile Creek, June 8, 1813; off Niagara, August 8; off Genesee River, September 11; off Burlington Heights, September 28; at the sacking of Oswego, May 5, 1814; and at the blockade of Sackett's Harbour, in May, June and July, 1814. In 1815, after the close of the war, he retired from the navy on half-pay, and entered into private practice in Kingston, where he remained until his death in 1823. He wrote a number of small works on medical subjects, among them being, "Diseases of the Teeth and Gums," "The Treatment of Children during Dentition," both published in 1790; and, "Observations on the Origin and Cure of Ophthalmia of Egypt," published in 1802. He was an amateur artist of considerable merit, and wrote a book on "The Art of Etching and Aqua-Tinting," published in 1794. He was married in London, Eng., in 1783, to Maria Taylor, eldest daughter of Major Taylor, R.E., and had issue one son, Captain F. B. Spilsbury, R.N.; and two daughters, the eldest, Maria, married Lieut. Reed, R.N., and the youngest, Tryphina, died in early life.

Captain F. B. Spilsbury, R.N., only son of the above, was born at Plymouth, England, in 1784, and at a very early age entered the Royal Navy as midshipman, serving chiefly in the fleet under the command of Admiral Sir Sidney Smith, in the Mediterranean Sea, during the wars with the French, from 1798 to 1812. He was at the siege of Acre; and as a midshipman of H.M.S. *Le Tigre,* took part in the capture of a flotilla of French gun-boats taken by that ship, being promoted to the rank of Lieutenant for conspicuous bravery in this action. He also took part in Sir Sidney Smith's expedition to Egypt, as well as the various engagements of the British fleet in the Mediterranean, under that distinguished Admiral. At Malaga, on the south coast of Spain, when First Lieutenant of H.M.S. *Ajax*, Captain Usher, he was ordered to cut out and capture from under the batteries on shore, a French privateer, and for his bravery and success on this occasion he was promoted to the rank of Commander. At the close of this action he was wounded in the head by a spent musket-ball, which necessitated the removal of a portion of the skull, and the insertion of a silver plate. As a testimonial from the "Patriotic Fund" he was presented with a massive piece of silver plate, upon which was inscribed: "F. B. Spilsbury, Malaga, 29th of April, 1812. Patriotic Fund." During service in the Mediterranean Sea he rose very rapidly, having obtained the rank of Commander when only in his twenty-eighth year. In the spring of 1813, during the war with the United States, he was sent out with Admiral Sir James Yeo, and stationed at Kingston, Upper Canada. In this war he took part in all the engagements on Lake Ontario, between the fleets of Sir James Yeo and Commodore Chauncey, the chief of which are mentioned in the above sketch of his father's life. In Sir James Yeo's Lake Ontario fleet, Captain Spilsbury was first appointed to the command of the *Beresford*, twelve guns, and at Forty Mile Creek, June 8, 1813, was in command of the detachment of the fleet which captured the American batteries, camp equipage, stores, etc., at that point. The following is Sir James Yeo's official despatch to Mr. Croker, as given in "James' Naval Occurrences between Great Britain and America":

"H. M. S. *Wolfe*,
"KINGSTON, UPPER CANADA, *June* 29, 1813.

"SIR,—I have the honour to inform you, for the information of the Lords Commissioners of the Admiralty, that on the 3rd instant I sailed with His Majesty's squadron under my command from this port, to co-operate with our army at the head of the lake, and annoy the enemy by intercepting all supplies going to the enemy, and thereby oblige his squadron to come out for its protection. At daylight on the 8th, the enemy's camp was discovered close to us at Forty Mile Creek. It being calm, the larger vessels could not get in, but the *Beresford*, Captain Spilsbury, the *Sir Sidney Smith*, Lieutenant Majoribanks, and the gun-boats, under the orders of Lieutenant Anthony (First of this ship), succeeded in getting close under the enemy's batteries, and, by a sharp and well-directed fire, soon obliged him to make a precipitate retreat, leaving all his camp equipage, provisions, stores, etc., behind, which fell into our hands. The *Beresford* also captured all his bateaux, laden with stores, etc. Our troops immediately occupied the post. I then proceeded along to the westward of the enemy's camp, leaving our army in front.

"I have the honour to be, etc.,

"J. L. YEO,
"*Commander.*"

In the engagement off Genesee River, September 11, 1813, Captain Spilsbury was in command of the *Melville*, a frigate of twenty-one guns. In Commodore Chauncey's official account of this action to the American Secretary of the Navy, he says: "I got several broadsides from this ship (the *General Pike*) upon the enemy, which must have done him considerable injury, as many of the shot were seen to strike him, and people were observed over the sides, plugging shot-holes."

In answer to this, upon the authority of Admiral Yeo, James states in his "Naval Occurrences," "that the only shot received by the British fleet that wanted a plug, struck the *Melville*, and that so far under water, that Captain Spilsbury had to run his guns in on one side and out on the other, to enable him to stop it, after which he immediately came into action again." Upon the declaration of peace in 1815, Captain Spilsbury was promoted to the rank of Post-captain, and retired from the navy on half pay, having obtained this rank at the early age of thirty-one, and after twenty years active service.

Upon his return to England in 1815, immediately after the close of the war, he was presented at Court, and on the 20th of

December, in the same year, he was married at Deptford, County of Kent, to Fanny Bayly, daughter of Thomas Bayly, Esq., and had issue six sons and three daughters. He resided in England, at Newark, in Nottinghamshire, until the spring of 1819, when he returned to Canada, taking up his residence first at Kingston, for a short time, then at Cobourg, and finally purchasing a property near Colborne, District of Newcastle, Upper Canada, where he subsequently resided. In the autumn of 1819, he visited the township of Otonabee, Peterborough County, in company with the first actual settler, a Mr. George Kent, and purchased a block of 1,200 acres near Peterborough; at the same time he took up a Government grant of 800 acres, in the township of Monaghan, about three miles from Peterborough, which was given to him for his services during the war with the United States. In 1821 he took up his residence at his new place, Osmondthorpe Hall, near Colborne, where he remained until his death. He was the Tory candidate, in 1830, to represent the District of Newcastle, comprising the counties of Northumberland, Durham, Peterborough and Victoria, in the Legislative Assembly of Upper Canada, but was defeated, owing to his being too ardent a supporter of the Family Compact. He died at his residence, Osmondthorpe Hall, on the 6th of October, 1830, in his forty-sixth year.

Of his surviving sons, the eldest, F. B. Spilsbury, was born in 1818, at Osmondthorpe House, Newark, Nottinghamshire, England. In the spring of 1829, he entered the Royal Navy, at Kingston Naval Station, as midshipman, on H.M.S. *Cockburn,* under the command of Captain Barrie—Lieut. Holbrook being First Lieutenant. This was the only war-vessel in service on Lake Ontario at that time. In December, 1831, he sailed from Quebec, for Jamaica, to join H.M.S. *Racehorse,* as midshipman, under Captain F. V. Cotton. On the 5th of November, 1833, he sailed from Bermuda to England, in the same ship, to be paid off. In March, 1834, he retired from the navy and returned home to Canada to live with his mother, at Osmondthorpe Hall, near Colborne, that property, together with several hundred acres of land, having been left to him by will at his mother's death. He still resides at the family homestead, and during his active life has been largely identified with milling and agricultural interests. He has been a Justice of the Peace for many years, and holds a Captain's commission in the Reserve Militia. He was married, in 1852, to Selina Marks, niece and adopted daughter of Paymaster John Marks, R.N., and had issue three daughters, two of whom are still living.

Charles T. Spilsbury, the fourth son, was born at Osmondthorpe Hall, near Colborne, Upper Canada, in 1824. At an early age he settled in Peterborough, and commenced to improve the land his father received by Government grant. During his active life he was engaged in lumbering and agricultural pursuits. He retired several years ago, and is now residing in Peterborough, Ont. He still owns a portion of the original grant and purchase obtained by his father in the County of Peterborough in 1819. He was married, in 1854, to Caroline Attrill, eldest daughter of Thomas P. Attrill, Esq., Paymaster in the Royal Navy, and has issue two sons and one daughter.

DR. EDWARD A. SPILSBURY, eldest son of Charles T. Spilsbury, was born in Peterborough, in 1855. He received his education at the Peterborough Collegiate Institute; the Pennsylvania Military Academy, Chester, Pa., U.S.; the Rensselaer Polytechnic Institute, Troy, N.Y., and commenced the study of medicine at Trinity Medical College in 1878, and graduated with honours at the University of Trinity College, Toronto, in 1881, entering immediately into the practice of his profession, at Haliburton, Peterborough County, where he remained a little over five years. In the spring of 1887 he went to Europe and spent about a year and a half attending the practice of special hospitals, and on his way back to Canada remained for a short time in New York, observing the practice of leading men in that great medical centre. He commenced practice in Toronto, in September, 1888, and is now Lecturer on Laryngology and Rhinology in Trinity Medical College, Surgeon to the Throat Department, Toronto General Hospital, and Member of the Corporation of Trinity University.

DR. FREDERICK C. SPILSBURY, second son of Charles T. Spilsbury, was born in Peterborough, in 1863. He received his education at the Peterborough Collegiate Institute, and commenced the study of Pharmacy, in 1883, and graduated at the Ontario College of Pharmacy in 1886. He then entered upon the study of medicine at Trinity Medical College, in October, 1887, and graduated at the University of Trinity College, in April, 1891 —also in the same month taking the Fellowship Degree of Trinity Medical College. He is now (1894) practising in Buffalo, N.Y.

DR. ROBERT ST. PATRICK STEVENSON

Was born at Oakwood Farm, near Niagara-on-the-Lake, 1817. His father, John Andrew Stevenson, was an officer in the 100th Foot, stationed at Niagara, and his mother the daughter of the Rev. Robert Addison, the first clergyman to officiate in this part of Upper Canada, and the first incumbent of St. Mark's Parish. His records in the old St. Mark's register, now in the possession of the Venerable Archdeacon, Dr. McMurray, for many years the rector, contain a mine of local historical lore. The subject of this sketch was educated at Upper Canada College, being among the first pupils shortly after its opening. He then resided in the Old Country for several years, and on his return to Canada began the study of medicine under the instruction of Dr. Rolph. Subsequently, he took a course at Philadelphia and graduated. He settled at Lake Lodge, Niagara Township, on the farm purchased by his grandfather, Mr. Addison, 1792. Here, in semi-retirement, he passed his life. He did not engage in active practice, but kept himself in touch with the advancement of medical science. His time was mainly devoted to agricultural pursuits. He possessed good abilities and considerable literary acquirements.

Dr. Stevenson continued to reside at Lake Lodge until his death, January, 1893, aged 75. He was the last surviving grandson of Rev. Mr. Addison, the first rector of the ancient St. Mark's Church, at Niagara, and also a grandson, on the paternal side, of Sir John Stevenson, the famous composer of the music of many of Moore's melodies. The deceased's brother, Judge Stevenson, of Haldimand, died about four years ago.

DR. ROBERT ADDISON STEVENSON, of Toronto, is a nephew of the above, and son of the late Judge Stevenson, of Haldimand.

He is a lineal descendant, on his mother's side, of Col. John Butler, of Butler's Rangers. He is M.D., C.M., of McGill University, Member Royal College Surgeons, Eng., and Member College Physicians and Surgeons, Ont.

DR. ISAAC STEPHENSON,

Of York, before Medical Board, January, 1832. "The Board perfectly satisfied by his examination." This minute appears July, 1833: "Mr. Isaac Stephenson, House Surgeon of the York Hospital, is appointed by the Board the Secretary of that body, *vice* Dr. Lee, deceased. Signed, C. Widmer, President." The following year, 1834, being still House Surgeon, he published a pamphlet on Cholera, which that year prevailed in Toronto. The *Patriot* of August 2 says: "We have been assured it has already saved three lives." But it seems that it could not, or did not, save himself, as he became one of the victims. Dr. C. F. Mewburn says, "he died of cholera—the death of honour."

DR. JOHN STEWART

Became a licentiate of R.C.S., Edinburgh, 1833. In 1839 was licensed to practise in Upper Canada by the College of Physicians and Surgeons, Upper Canada. He settled in Kingston soon after, where he became a prominent figure. The following appeared in the daily press, 1891:

"Kingston has lost another noted citizen in the death of Dr. John Stewart, which occurred yesterday, after a few hours of unconsciousness, terminating a long season of weakness and suffering, which has for two or three years laid him aside from active duty. An enthusiastic Scotchman, Dr. Stewart was a native of Perthshire, and was educated in Edinburgh, to which his heart always affectionately clung. He settled in Kingston about half a century ago. He was public-spirited, and took an active part in founding the General Hospital and Royal College of Physicians and Surgeons, being for many years Dean of the Faculty. He was a man of great kindness of heart under a somewhat brusque manner, and won the grateful affection of many patients. During the fatal visitation of typhus fever, in 1847, he attended a great number of sick and dying immigrants, himself performing the last offices for the dead in the absence of the usual assistance, and having them interred in the hospital grounds under a mound still visible. For some years he conducted the *Argus* for the exposure of what he deemed abuses. In politics he took a keen interest, and even ran as a member for the city. The discipline of weakness and suffering had, however, latterly much tempered the keenness of his somewhat fiery spirit, and his gentleness and patience under the trying experience of confinement and inaction were very marked and impressive. He passed away in perfect peace. The Doctor's many legal battles are recalled. As his own counsel he amused judge and members of the bar, but sometimes his actions and words were very exasperating. He was a "thorn in the flesh" to various citizens, who had to pay, and some dearly, to counteract the legal complications the doctor would press upon them. He was quite vain, and the publication of his movements and words were prized."

DR. ELAM STIMSON.

For the following sketch we are indebted to James Stimson, M.D., of Watsonville, California:

The history of this early practitioner of Upper Canada well exemplifies the native pluck, energy, and determination to succeed, which characterized not a few of those who laid the foundation of the present prosperity, both of Canada and the United States.

The more remote ancestry of the subject of this sketch were English, and can be traced back several centuries. Many families of the name, sprung from a common stock, are to be found in England. His immediate ancestry were all natives of New England. To study and practise medicine seems to have been a family trait, so many Stimsons in tolerably regular succession in their families having been doctors. James Stimson, M.D., an eminent practitioner of Hartford, Connecti-

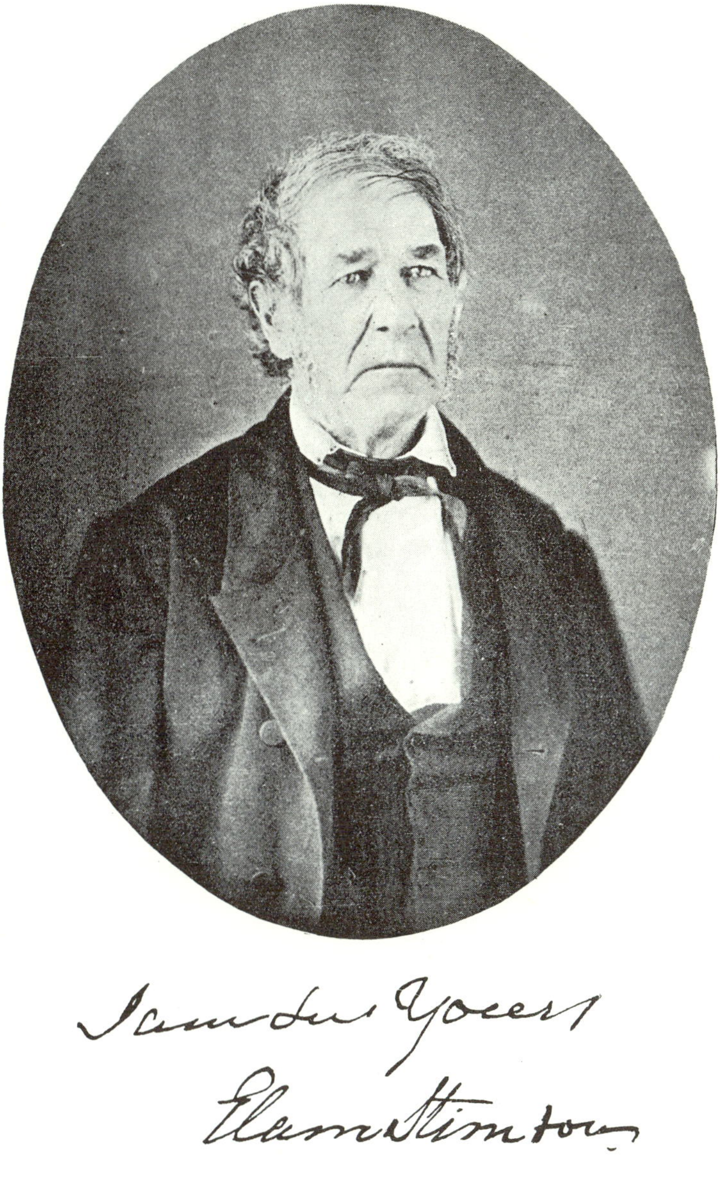

cut, was great-grandfather to this Elam Stimson. The one of whom we write, the youngest of a family of twelve children, was born at Tolland, Connecticut, October 4, 1792. When he was about ten years of age, his parents suffered severe reverses of fortune; and until they died, thirteen years after, his strong filial affection was shown by untiring and successful effort (seconding that of his next older brother, Joel) to provide for their maintenance.

Dr. Elam Stimson served in the United States army during the war of 1812, first, as substitute for a drafted man, for the term of three months, at New London, Connecticut; then as enlisted for one year, the greater portion of which time was passed on Staten Island, N.Y. He was third sergeant of his company. He thus wrote, concerning his army life:

"In everything but the time of enlistment we were *regular soldiers*, subject to the same rules and regulations. It was a year all but lost to me as regards usefulness (to any but the country) or preparation for it. Still, something was learned, *i.e.*, what to shun. The army is said to be a good school, but I believe few fathers who have been to that school would choose it for a son."

For his services in that war he received from the United States Government, about thirty years later, a bounty of one hundred and sixty acres of land, which he located in the prairie country of Northern Indiana, near Crown Point. His widow still surviving (February, 1894), receives a pension from the United States Government, by virtue of her husband's services as a United States soldier.

At the expiration of his term of enlistment he returned to his home and commenced the study of medicine. To obtain necessary means, he laboured on a farm or taught school.

A friend who owned a cranberry marsh gave him permission to make what he could from one year's crop. He hired help to pick the berries, marketed them in Hartford, and netted one hundred dollars by the operation. That hundred dollars, he remarked late in his life, seemed to him the greatest financial lift he ever had.

By dint of persevering effort, he gradually accumulated enough money to meet the expense of a course of lectures.

Meantime, while labouring or teaching, he had been reading medicine under the direction of Dr. Thompson, of Toland.

His first course of lectures was at Yale College, New Haven, Connecticut. The tickets read curiously, as compared with those of to-day, and give one a good idea of the comparatively narrow scope of medical teaching in the early part of our century, even at one of the then best seats of learning in America. There were but four lecturers—a "corporal's guard" as compared with the "full staff" of lecturers and teacher attached to each of the principal medical schools of to-day. Here is his matriculation ticket:

"*Medical Institution of Yale College.*

"Mr. Elam Stimson is matriculated into the Medical Institution of Yale College for the ensuing season.

"By order of the Faculty,

"J. KNIGHT.

"November 1st, 1817."

The lecturers were: On Chemistry and Pharmacy, B. Silliman; Anatomy and Physiology, J. Knight; Theory and Practice of Medicine, Surgery and Widwifery, Nathaniel Smith; Materia Medica and Diseases of Children, Eli Ives.

The summer following this course of lectures was spent in the office of an eminent medical man of Hartford, Connecticut, Mason F. Cogswell, M.D.

His next course of lectures was at Dartmouth, Hanover, New Hampshire. "Chymical" lectures were by J. T. Dana, and lectures on "Practice of Physick" and on "Obstetricks," by R. D. Mussey, M.D. At Dartmouth he graduated, Valedictorian of his class, August 18, 1819. The diploma is all *written* on heavy paper, but as to typography, bears a close resemblance to the diplomas now granted. The "Great Seal" attached to it is a fine elaborate specimen of the engraver's art.

While yet an undergraduate, he married, January 10, 1819, the eldest daughter of the Rev. Augustus Bolles, a man prominent in the Baptist Church—of superior ability as a preacher and editor.

He returned from Dartmouth to his native place and engaged

in the practice of his profession. An influential man in that community afterwards said to him: "You have served me faithfully and well in three different capacities, as a farm servant, as a teacher, and as my family physician."

Prospects of financial success not being brilliant in the East, with the pioneering enterprise characteristic of his ancestry he removed, with his family, to the then "far West," and settled in St. Catharines, Upper Canada, in the spring of 1823. St. Catharines was then but a hamlet, on the "Twelve Mile Creek."

Learning it was necessary he should be examined by a Government Board of Examiners and receive a license from the Governor before he could legally practise in Canada, he crossed, in a schooner, from the mouth of the Niagara River to York (now Toronto), and presented himself for examination before "C. Widmer, Grant Powell and R. C. Horne, Esquires," who expressed themselves as particularly well pleased with his proficiency, especially in anatomy—that of the brain. July 7, 1823, he was licensed to practise by Lieut.-Governor Sir Peregrine Maitland, of the Province of Upper Canada. On his license is this endorsement:

"Exhibited in the Gore District Court in the cause of Elam Stimson against James Dixon, the 12th day of April, 1827.

"JOHN LAW,
"*Clerk of Gore District Court.*"

It seems that even so long ago as 1827, there was a man who "kicked against paying his doctor bill." But little less than forty years after, this other endorsement was made, also necessary in order to collect his bills: "Registered, June 9th, 1866. H. STRANGE, M.D., *Registrar.*"

During his stay in St. Catharines, the Hon. Hamilton Merritt, then and afterwards prominent as the chief promoter of the construction of the Welland Canal, was his firm friend, and found in the doctor a hearty sympathizer and co-worker in furthering that great public enterprise.

Some time in 1824 he removed to Galt. His practice there was very extensive. Paris, Princeton, Drumbo, Ayr, Hamburg, Waterloo, Berlin, Guelph, Preston, East and West Flamborough, St. George, all are within the then sparsely settled country over which he travelled on horseback with capacious saddle-bags, green-baize leggings and heavy dark "surtout," ministering to the needs of the sick, poor or rich, oftener very poor than even moderately well-to-do, for those were pioneer days. Sometimes he was away from home for days together, sending word home where those needing him could find him. There was no bridge then, over the Grand River, between Galt and Brantford. Once, to see a very sick patient not more than two miles away from him, he had either to make a detour of many miles, to cross on a bridge, or ford the river on horseback. It was in the time of melting snows and spring rains. The river was unusually wide and deep, the waters cold and swift, but he was a good swimmer and his horse was powerful and sagacious. So, after arranging his saddle-bags and some of his clothing firmly on the pommel of the saddle, he plunged into the eddying flood, and after an exhausting struggle, clambered up the steep east bank of the river, grateful for deliverance out of danger. He remarked to the writer, as they were once passing the scene of this incident, that he "took too great a risk, and could never be induced to attempt so dangerous a feat again." Young practitioners of the present day can scarcely appreciate the easy conditions under which they acquire and practise their profession. Let them ponder upon the lives and revere the memories of those stalwart, brave veterans, who not only battled with disease, but also had to encounter and endure the trying disabilities of the "wilderness" state of the country. In the latter part of 1828 he removed still further west, to London, and continued the practice of his profession. Here his ride was as extensive and his labours as arduous as in Galt.

Among his documents is the following on heavy, gilt-edged foolscap:

"GOVERNMENT HOUSE, *May* 30th, 1831.

"SIR,—I am directed by the Governor to acquaint you, that a commission has been prepared appointing you a Coroner for the London District, and is now ready for delivering to any agent whom you may authorize to receive it.

"I have the honour to be, Sir,

"Your most obedient, humble servant,

"Z. MUDGE, *Secretary.*

"DR. ELAM STIMSON."

During the prevalence of an epidemic of Asiatic cholera, his wife fell a victim to that "Scourge of Nations," July 30, 1832, having been but twelve hours sick. Five days after, their youngest child, of two years, died of the same disease, and a daughter also was so low with it that she was robed in her grave-clothes ready to be coffined. But she regained consciousness and was restored to health. At his wife's death he had five children, the eldest of whom was aged but little more than thirteen years. In the fall of the same year, Dr. Stimson visited Hartford, Conn., and married Susan Bolles, his deceased wife's sister. Returned to Canada, he concluded to depart from the scene of so great affliction, so he wound up his affairs in London and settled late in August, 1833, at St. George, a pretty village—the centre of one of the most beautiful and fertile portions of Canada. Here, with the exception of a time spent in practice in St. Catharines, to afford better educational facilities for his children, he continued to reside and practise until his death, January 1, 1869.

Of his nine children, five grew to manhood and three to womanhood. Of his five sons he educated three as physicians—Edwin, James and William. His second son, Elam, became an Episcopalian clergyman. His fourth son, Augustus, received a thorough education by way of preparation for commercial life, but having a strong taste for agricultural pursuits, he came into possession of his father's homestead. Of his three daughters, the eldest, Susan, married Samuel T. Stanton, for many years a merchant and postmaster at St. George. The second daughter, Mary A., married Robert Christie, M.D., of Paris, Ont. The third daughter, Rebecca, married Nathaniel E. Mainwaring, M.D., of St. George, Ont.

There were in the family at one time six doctors—father, three sons and two son-in-laws; of all these, but one, the writer, survives. Edwin Bolles Stimson, graduate of the College of Physicians and Surgeons of New York City, was resident physician of the New York Lying-in Asylum, and brought chloroform into prominence in connection with parturition at that institution. He died of consumption, and he and his wife sleep side by side in the cemetery at Colchester, Connecticut.

William Stimson was a graduate of the Buffalo Medical

College. A letter dated October 31, 1889, says of him: "Dr. William Stimson was connected with the New York Eye and Ear Infirmary as house surgeon, and performed his duties faithfully and well; he was also one of the first members of the New York Ophthalmological Society. (Signed) D. B. ST. JOHN, Roosa."

He died of typhoid fever, contracted during too faithful attendance on a patient, and sleeps in the Evergreen cemetery at Lexington, Nebraska. Elam Rush Stimson, the clergyman, died at Hamilton, Ont., August, 5, 1888. He sleeps at his father's feet in the old cemetery at St. George.

James Stimson (the writer of this sketch) is a medical graduate of the University of the City of New York (1854), and of the University of Victoria College (1855). He is also a Member of the College of Physicians and Surgeons, Ont.; Member of the American Medical Association; Member of the California State Medical Society; Member of the American Microscopical Society; Member of the American Association of Economic Entomologists. For several years he was President of the Board of United States Examining Surgeons at Lexington, Nebraska. For the last three years he has resided and practised in Watsonville, the business centre of one of the very richest valleys in California.

To have seen Dr. Elam Stimson, was to remember him. He was a tall, large man, of fine physical proportions and commanding presence—a splendid specimen of vigorous, self-reliant manhood. His features were large and rugged, and the expression of his countenance, when in repose, was somewhat severe. His modest, honest, gentle, sympathetic nature fitted him well for his duties. He was a clear thinker, decided in his views, accurate in observation, careful and correct in his diagnosis, possessed of sound judgment, fertile in resources, a good operator, an ardent lover of his profession, and an able, skilful medical man. He was an investigator, a student, especially in his chosen work. Had his lot been cast in one of the medical centres, his abilities would have commanded superior eminence in medical ranks. But the anxiety incident to frontier life, the care and education of a large family and comparatively limited means, exposure, long rides and consequent great fatigue, were insuperable barriers to that close, continuous mental effort necessary to bring him into great professional prominence. He wrote a monograph on cholera, and contributions to the *Buffalo Medical Journal.* The burden of years and of cares prevented him completing a partly written brochure on " Longevity."

In his social relations, he was loved most by those most intimate with him ; only in the presence of such was he divested of a certain reserve of manner, beneath which was a hearty generosity, an affectionate disposition and a most tender heart. He was very fond of and much beloved by children. He was a faithful friend and a cordial hater ; he had most hearty scorn for whatever was not honest and true. He possessed a large fund of humour and anecdote, and was a good story-teller, his anecdote having always the merit of being *apropos* to the occasion. He loved a joke and had many a hearty laugh over a hit at himself. His home was always open for the entertainment of ministers of all denominations ; they and the interests they represented were all, when occasion required, the recipients of substantial tokens of his appreciation. Stumbled, in his youth, by the inconsistencies of some professors of religion, he neither united with any denomination nor made any profession of faith. His earlier and later years, however, were times of deep thought and much exercise of soul over Revelation and eternal interests. He was seventy-six years old on the 4th of October, 1868. One of the later days of the following December, he fell and injured his nose ; the weather was extremely cold, and erysipelas attacked the wounded part. Wife, children, and grandchildren forsook the Christmas dinner table for his bedside. The disease rapidly spread, involving in turn the face, head and throat. Soon after the bells rang the old year out and the new year in, he rested from his labours. His works follow him. His was a most useful and exemplary life—a life of love and labour, labour for love's sake. His record is one which, all in all, none need regret and all may emulate. More than a quarter of a century has passed away since that cheerless winter day when all of him that was mortal was laid in the grave. That lapse of time has but taught clearer, more love-inspiring appreciation of his great worth, and brought keener sorrow for our loss.

A massive monument, of simple lines, marks his last resting place, in the old cemetery at St. George. On the east face of the pedestal of the monument may be read :

> "God takes our loved ones, yet we lose not wholly
> What He has given.
> They live on earth, in thoughts and deeds, as truly
> As in His Heaven."

DR. THOMAS STOYELL

Had acquired a degree in medicine in the United States, and settled at York near the close of the last century. It does not appear that he engaged in the practice of his profession. His name appears as holding a minor municipal appointment in 1799. Dr. Stoyell is remembered as the owner of a tavern of some note at the time. About the time of the war of 1812 he graduated from a tavern-keeper to the position of a brewer. He was a person of some note. Dr. Scadding speaks of him as a "non-practising medical man with Republican proclivities." His name is found among the stockholders of the Desjardins Canal, in 1830. He died February 27, 1832, aged seventy-one, being one of the oldest inhabitants of York.

Dr. Stoyell at his death bequeathed his estate to the Methodist Conference. A Bill was before the Provincial Parliament to enable the executors to carry the will into effect. There was some opposition to this Bill ; and the *Christian Guardian*, in reference thereto, says :

"Apprehending that some erroneous impressions may be made in regard to the late Dr. Stoyell's Estate Bill, from the proceedings of the Assembly published in last week's *Guardian*, and as it is a matter in which the Methodist Church is directly concerned, we think it necessary to offer a few observations on the subject.

"As to the circumstances which gave rise to the Bill, it may be remarked that the late Dr. Stoyell, long a valuable member of the Methodist Church, and a highly respectable inhabitant of this town, having no heirs, bequeathed his property (in the hands of executors) to the Methodist Conference; one part to be applied to missionary purposes and the other part to the relief of worn-out and distressed preachers. His will, we understand, was made some time previous to his decease, and contained what Dr. S. had expressed his intention to do some years before that period. This Bill was to enable the executors (Mr. W. P. Patrick and Mr. Easton) to carry Dr. Stoyell's will into effect. Notice of it has been advertised in the *Upper Canada Gazette* a year and a half, and no heir or claimant has appeared. The only alternative is, that if the will of the testator be not executed, the property must go to the Crown; and upon this principle, it appears, Col. Burwell and Mr. George Boulton opposed the Bill, because the Crown ought to have the property.

"Dr. Stoyell had largely contributed to the ministry, missions and institutions of the Methodist Church during many years of his useful life; and when removed from his stewardship he left behind him an additional testimony that he still remembered the perishing heathen and the privations and infirmities of those who had worn themselves out in labouring in word and doctrine; and sorry shall we be, if, through bigotry, intolerance, prejudice or party spirit, his pious and benevolent intentions are defeated."

DR. JOHN STRATFORD,

Born at Penn Bucks, Eng., was an M.R.C.S. London. He was surgeon in Lord Grantley's regiment, Home Guards, and was connected with the army medical staff, with which he served during the Peninsular War. He came to Canada, 1833, and issued at Brockville, January 4, 1833, the following card:

"Dr. Stratford, Surgeon, Accoucheur and Oculist; thirty years a member of the Royal College of Surgeons, London; twenty years in His Majesty's military service in that capacity, and many years in extensive private practice. Dr. Stratford has extended his practice to the diseases of females and children with more than ordinary success in their treatment."

John Stratford, of Bathurst, passed Medical Board, April, 1833.

He obtained a large practice, and also acted as Military Hospital Steward. Visiting England, he was called to give evidence in favour of Lord Durham's report on Canada. Returning to Canada, he proceeded to Woodstock, where his son had commenced practice. Another son, William H., a druggist, was settled at Brantford, and Dr. John Stratford passed the remainder of his days between the two places. He died at Brantford, March, 1845, in his seventy-second year.

DR. SAMUEL JOHN STRATFORD, eldest son of the above, received his medical education at St. George's and Westminster Hospitals, London, being a pupil of Wm. Charles Bell. He was likewise a pupil of the famous Dr. Guthrie, at his eye infirmary. Having become M.R.C.S. London, he was commissioned Assistant-Surgeon in the 72nd Regiment Scotch Highlanders. After a time he disposed of his commission, and came to Canada, and for a time practised at By-town. He was gazetted Licentiate of Upper Canada, November, 1831. He removed to Woodstock, where he remained about twenty years, enjoying an extensive practice and the respect of the community. He was Surgeon to the 3rd Oxford Regiment Militia, 1837. He then took up his residence in Toronto, where he practised eight or ten years. He became a member of the Upper Canada Medical Board, Sept., 1838. Was editor of the *Upper Canada Journal of Medical, Surgical and Physical Science*, Toronto. He lectured on Anatomy at Rolph's for a while, and was also for a short time Professor at Trinity Medical College. He returned to Woodstock, where he practised until about 1868, when he went to New Zealand. On his arrival there, he met a British regiment starting for England without a surgeon, and he was engaged to accompany it home. They came by way of America. Dr. Stratford returned to New Zealand, where he died, leaving a large practice to his son-in-law, Dr. Wright, late of Toronto. Another daughter became the wife of Dr. Emery, at one time practising in Toronto.

WM. A. STRATFORD, brother of Samuel John, accompanied him to America, 1831, and lived in New York and Oswego until 1844, when he settled in Brantford. He had studied medicine in Dublin, but it does not appear that he took a degree. He engaged in the drug business until 1875. He is the founder of the General Hospital at Brantford.

DR. CYRUS SUMNER.

"An eminent physician, whose practice extended throughout the whole Niagara District."—*Dr. C. F. Mewburn.*

Dr. Sumner was a native of the United States, and belonged to the family of that name so well known in the annals of that country. In a "Genealogy of the Sumner Family," compiled by William Sumner Appleton, of Boston, from 1601 to 1880, it is recorded that Cyrus Sumner was born at Hebron, 1776, and that he studied his profession under Dr. Lyon, of Albany, N.Y., and that he came to Canada about 1800. He made his home at, or near, Newark, now Niagara, and was fortunate in winning the regard and friendship of Dr. Robert Kerr, a sketch of whom is given in this work. The following extract from a letter written by Dr. Sumner to his brother living at Saratoga, affords information respecting the first years of his life in Canada. The letter is dated "Clinton, Niagara District, October 10, 1804," and says: "I have not been idle since I came to this country, and have taken every advantage to gain information respecting my profession, and on Friday last, at York, I passed an examination before the Surgeon-General of York, Dr. Baldwin, Clerk of the Crown, and the Staff-Surgeon of Niagara, after which I received a very handsome letter from the Board, wishing me a great deal of prosperity and happiness, together with a license, on fine parchment, to practise physic, surgery and midwifery, in which several branches I have been closely employed ever since I came to this country. When I first came into this Province I put myself under the Staff-Surgeon at Niagara, Dr. Robert Kerr (my patron), who had shown me every mark of friendship that we can expect of our fellow-mortals, and has assisted me with books, medicine and instruments and his warm friendship, for which I feel myself extremely obliged." A letter from Dr. Kerr to A. MacDonell, Esq., casts additional light on the subject. It says: "Dear

Sir,—The bearer, Mr. Cyrus Sumner, I beg leave to introduce to you; he has been three years in this country, part of the time in my shop and the other part settled near the Forty Mile Creek, where he has been very successful in practice, especially fevers. He has passed the Medical Board at York. He is remarkable for sobriety, and very attentive and diligent to the studies of his profession. He had studied about four years in the United States before he came into this Province. Having heard a medical person was wanted on my Lord Selkirk's lands, he requested a letter of introduction to you. (Signed) ROBERT KERR."

From this time, Dr. Sumner was actively engaged in practice. His home was at Clinton, or Twenty Mile Creek. When the war of 1812 broke out, he had fully established himself as a leading physician of the old Niagara District, and was held in high esteem by all classes of the people. He still enjoyed the friendship of Dr. Kerr, and stood well in the sight of the public authorities. Although a native of the States, his loyalty to his adopted country was unquestioned; and from the first to the last of the struggle he was engaged in responsible service to the Crown, and intrusted with various important commissions in connection with the army medical service. This extract from a letter, May 9, 1816, to his brother will be read with interest: "A word of the war. At the commencement, General Brock requested me to go to Detroit with him, which I did, and was the only staff-surgeon on the expedition, and from that time until the end of the war was on the most active service and at almost every battle that was fought, but never wounded —though narrow escapes. The experience had was very great. We were run very hard at times, but finally acquitted with some degree of honour." This modest claim by Dr. Sumner to his brother, it is presumed, was not gainsaid. His brother, living at Saratoga, was in a position to know that the honours of the war were very largely on the side of Canada. The repeated attempts to conquer Canada by the United States forces during the war, had ended in their inglorious retreat. At the time Dr. Sumner wrote this letter, not a foot of Canadian territory was in their possession, except where they occupied "hospitable groves."

The writer has before him a number of interesting and valuable documents and letters, addressed to Dr. Sumner, which have been kindly furnished by his son, W. R. Sumner, Esq., of Ingersoll. From these, much is learned of the nature of the duties discharged by Dr. Sumner, besides not a few interesting historical matters, which we regret may not here be inserted.

The following is dated at Perth, Upper Canada, February 6, 1825:

"I certify that Cyrus Sumner was appointed temporary Hospital Assistant to the Army on the Niagara Frontier in the year 1812, and continued in the service till 1815, during which period he was diligent and zealous, and his conduct as a medical officer met my general approbation.

"ALEX. THOM,

"*Staff-Surgeon, N.P., then P.M. Officer of the Right Division.*"

Dr. Sumner was commissioned Surgeon to the 4th Lincoln Regiment Militia, January, 1822.

Dr. Sumner married, 1803, Mary, daughter of Benjamin Bell, of Grimsby, and a sister of Dr. Nathaniel Bell, of whom a sketch is elsewhere given. Dr. Sumner had ten children. Two sisters married nephews of the Hon. William McMaster; two others married sons of Col. William Nelles, of Grimsby. The youngest two were twins, a son and daughter—William Kerr, who was named after William J. Kerr, Chief of the Six Nations, and the daughter named after the Chief's wife, Elizabeth Brant. She became the wife of Dr. James Graham. (See sketch.) Of the ten children only two are now living (1893), Mrs. Captain McMaster and W. K. Sumner, of Ingersoll, who is an ardent, loyal Canadian, with a fine taste for historical lore. The writer is indebted to him for the foregoing interesting historical facts.

DR. HENRY SULLIVAN.

Concerning the family of which Dr. Sullivan was a member, while one became distinguished as a barrister and judge, Henry likewise became distinguished as a physician and professor in medicine, although an untimely death prevented the full development of his powers.

It may be stated that Dr. Sullivan's brother was the second mayor of Toronto, being elected in 1835. Henry began the study of medicine with Dr. King, of Toronto, and was a fellow-student with C. F. Mewburn. He then proceeded to the Old Country, and was a student at Dublin, where he became a licentiate accoucheur of the Dublin Lying-in Hospital, and at London, where he obtained the diploma of the Royal College of Surgeons. Returning to Canada, he obtained the license to practise in Upper Canada. He was appointed Surgeon to the Royal Foresters during the rebellion of 1837. In May, 1839, he became a member of the College of Physicians and Surgeons of Upper Canada, being No. 2 on the roll; and subsequently, February, 1840, was elected a Fellow, and the minutes of the College show that he thereafter took an active part in all of its proceedings while the College existed. In July, 1841, Dr. Sullivan was appointed a member of Upper Canada Medical Board. A new commission was issued in July, 1845, in which appears Dr. Sullivan's name as "Professor of Practical Anatomy," University of King's College, Toronto.

Dr. Sullivan died of consumption, February 6, 1850, at the early age of forty-five.

The Report of the Commissioners of Enquiry into the affairs of King's College says: "The salary of the late Professor Sullivan was increased by a subsidiary grant of £50 a year, for extra services, in 1847-48. This gentleman appears to have, for several years, pressed in vain for a regular increase of salary. In 1843 his case was recommended to the consideration of the Council by His Excellency the Chancellor." The Council, December, 1845, "could not accede to any augmentation of salary."

The extra services for which Professor Sullivan asked compensation were rendered in the dissecting room and in the Anatomical Museum, and his entire time was devoted to professorial labours. The Commissioners find "that Professor Sullivan's claims were not favourably entertained by the Council until 1847, when a gratuity of £50 was voted to him for his extra services in the current medical session; a second and last grant was made in 1848 of a like amount."

DR. HENRY TAYLOR,

One hundred years old, January 1, 1890. (*See Frontispiece.*) We are indebted to Dr. F. L. Howland, of Huntsville, Ont., who visited him January 10, 1890, for the following interesting sketch of a very remarkable man, who, of all spoken of in these pages, was alone a centenarian. His history supplies in many ways a most valuable lesson:

"Dr. Taylor is, we believe, the oldest medical practitioner in Canada, if not on this continent. He is still hale and hearty, and lives at Burk's Falls, Ont. The personal history of a doctor who has practised medicine for three-quarters of a century, must prove highly interesting. The subject of this sketch was born at Birmingham, Eng., January 1, 1790. His father, Samuel Taylor, M.D., had for many years a lucrative practice at Aylesham, Eng., and numbered among his patients Lords Suffield, Stratton, Kensington and the Earl of Oxford. The nineteenth century was ushered in with great rejoicings in England, and Henry Taylor, ten years of age, distinctly remembers dancing on the green with many other juveniles, to the tune of martial music. He was the youngest of a family of three brothers and three sisters. Two of his nephews are in the practice of medicine in England, one at Aylesham, the other at Coltishall. Henry mixed medicine in his father's surgery, when his height had to be extended by his standing on a stool. For seven years he was apprenticed as a medical student. Then for three years he attended Guy's and St. Thomas' Hospitals, taking his degree of M.D. when twenty-eight years of age. Dr. Taylor's countenance kindles with intellectual energy, as he proudly, yet reverently, speaks of his surgical tutor, Sir Astley Cooper. Blondil was the leading professor of midwifery. He knew Abernethy well. In manner Abernethy was the antipodes of Sir Astley. The latter was refined in manner, and gentlemanly to a degree. On lecturing, during the course, on a certain luxation of the hip-joint, over which he and Abernethy differed, he always drank an extra amount of wine, and rubbing his hands, 'piled' into Abernethy. Dr. Taylor had heard Abernethy use the most vulgar language, and a very nasty and unutterable expression was a favourite expletive. 'He was the most impudent man I ever saw,' said Dr. Taylor.

"On graduation, Dr. Taylor went into partnership with his father at Aylesham, where he remained until June, 1839, when he emigrated to Canada, and practised for a year in Montreal. During the summer season he had a paying practice waiting on English emigrants, but in winter he had little to do, and spent his summer earnings. He therefore determined to leave, and came to Ernesttown. Here, and in the adjacent villages of Camden, Wilton and Portland, he practised for twenty-six years, sixteen of which were spent in the latter place. He endured all the hardships incident to the practice of medicine in a Canadian pioneer settlement, and never refused to attend a poor patient. He was held in high esteem, socially and professionally. The poverty of his patrons bore hardly on him at times, and more than once his chattels were sold for debts contracted for medical supplies. He did not take out a Canadian diploma, and he was once hauled up for practising without a license, but the validity of his English diploma was maintained, and he was acquitted. For a time he kept three horses hard at work in making his professional calls. In earlier years he frequently travelled on foot, by the aid of a compass, between points where there was not even a foot-path. On one occasion, while waiting on a woman in confinement in a lonely house, a large pack of wolves crossed the door-yard in full cry.

"Dr. Taylor never took an active interest either in municipal or provincial politics. For three years, however, he was Master of the Orange Lodge in Portland, while for twelve years he was a member of the Sons of Temperance in Wilton. Rum and whiskey were the common beverage of the people, the former selling at 3s 6d per gallon, and the latter for 6d per gallon, in Kingston. In 1867 or '68, he removed to the township of Brook, Lanark County, where he remained a few years, but did not practise much. September 25, 1875, he settled in Ryerson Township, Parry Sound District, near to where a son was living. It is astonishing the amount of professional work, travelling for the most part on foot, he has done in Ryerson and vicinity. To-day, March, 1890, his memory is good, walks without a cane, and shaves himself. About seven years ago the writer met Dr. Taylor in consultation, he having walked that day fourteen miles to meet him. At that time, he frequently walked, in one day, from Ryerson to Rosseau, a distance of twenty-seven miles, and quite recently, he walked from Ryerson to Burk's Falls and thought nothing of it. He stands 5 feet 11¾ inches in height, and is nearly up to his average weight of 150 lbs. Until a year ago he could read ordinary print without spectacles, and his hearing is yet very fair. Dr. Taylor has always eaten in moderation of mixed plain food from the animal and vegetable kingdom, but avoided pastries, confectionery and such like. He has ever looked on the bright side of life; never desponded, and has decidedly kept, as he says, a 'stiff upper lip.' He drank moderately of wine and pure liquors in his earlier years, but latterly, for many years, has drank no alcoholic beverage. His wife died twelve years ago, at 58 years of age, and was thirty years his junior."

The following is taken from the Huntsville paper, April 18, 1890:

"It has fallen to the lot of very few journalists in Canada to record the death of a citizen as old as the late Dr. Henry Taylor, who passed peacefully away to his long home on Thursday, the 3rd inst., at the ripe age of 100 years, 3 months and 3 days. The last days of his life were spent in Burk's Falls with his daughter, Mrs. Snyder. He retained a wonderful degree of physical and mental vigour until the end. He was a member of the Methodist Church for over forty years, and was highly respected, both in his profession and private life, by all who knew him. He leaves to mourn his loss, four sons and one daughter, viz.: Mrs. Snyder and Walford Taylor, of Burk's Falls; Wm. Taylor, of Ryerson; Samuel Taylor, in western Ontario, and James Edward Taylor, in Michigan, U.S.A."

DR. WALTER TELFER,

A Scotchman by birth and education, from Niagara, appeared before the Upper Canada Medical Board, July, 1833. He had a diploma of the College of Surgeons of Edinburgh, and obtained his certificate. But a correspondence found in the minutes of the Medical Board between Drs. Telfer, Muirhead and Porter, and the Medical Board, in October, 1832, shows that Dr. Telfer was then in practice at Niagara. That he was there in 1828 is learned from the presentation of an address on October 16, of that year, to Sir Peregrine Maitland, the Lieutenant-Governor, on his departure. The first two names to this address were J. Muirhead, Chairman, and Walter Telfer. It seems that he settled here about 1826. On March 23, 1827, a meeting of the Presbyterians was held at Niagara, at which John Tannahill and Dr. Telfer were appointed a committee to collect funds for building a church. In September, 1828, Dr. Telfer was "at his home every morning from 8 to 10, to vaccinate the poor *gratis*." He continued in practice here until his removal to Toronto. This card appeared in the paper: "Mr. Walter Telfer, Surgeon, has removed from Niagara to No. 44 Newgate Street, Toronto. July 8, 1835."

Dr. Telfer at once took a prominent place in the profession at the capital. Among his countrymen he was a great favourite and soon commanded a large practice. He was considered skilful and attentive to his work; was highly respected by his confreres, and had the confidence of his patients. He loved his profession, not as a means of acquiring wealth, but for the aid and comfort he was able to give the afflicted.

Dr. Telfer succeeded Dr. Rees, as Superintendent of the Lunatic Asylum, in 1844, and held the office for three years. His removal from this office caused a good deal of newspaper controversy. It was alleged that the Government found an excuse for this action at the demand of Dr. Rolph, while, on the other hand, the organ of the Government declared that there was good cause for his removal. Dr. Telfer was one of the worthies the writer had the opportunity of following around the wards of the old Toronto Hospital, to which Dr. Telfer was an attending physician. In a new commission appointing members of the Medical Board, dated September 25, 1838, Dr. Telfer's name appears, and he continued an active member until his death in 1857. His widow returned to Scotland, where she died, October 9, 1880.

DR. WILLIAM TEMPEST.

The following obituary notice appeared in the *Canada Lancet*, September, 1871: "We regret to announce the death of Dr. William Tempest, of this city, on the 8th ult. He was born in Halifax, England, and settled in Toronto, in 1842. In 1844, he received his license from the Medical Board, and practised for some time in Trafalgar, and subsequently in Oshawa. In 1861, he obtained the degree of M.B., University of Toronto, and soon after commenced practice in this city, where he has remained since that time, and where he built up a comfortable practice, made many friends, and endeared himself to all who knew him by his kindness of manner and warmness of heart.

"In June, 1866, during the Fenian invasion, his son, a member of the volunteer corps, who was in his twenty-first year, fell at Ridgeway in defence of his country. This was a severe blow to the Doctor and the family, and an affliction that was not soon forgotten. Subsequently the Doctor held the position of Medical Health Officer for the city, for the period of two or three years; an office which he held with credit to himself and satisfaction to all concerned. He leaves a wife and five of a family (three daughters and two sons) to mourn his loss."

He died, August 8, 1871, aged 52.

DR. ALEXANDER THOM.

In an account of the funeral of William Weeks, barrister, who was killed in a duel, October 10, 1806, and whose body was buried at Niagara, it is stated that the funeral was attended by Dr. Thomas, of the 41st Regiment, and Dr. Muirhead. The name, it is believed, is a misprint of "Thomas" for "Thom." The next information at hand is contained in a marriage notice dated December 5, 1811, as follows: "Alex. Thom, Surgeon 41st Regiment, was married to Hannah Smith."

The official programme of the funeral procession of General Brock, dated October 16, 1812, has the name of Staff-Surgeon Thom, with Dr. Kerr and Surgeon Moore as "servants of the General."

Dr. Thom settled at Perth, prior to 1822, as we find from the "Civil List of Upper Canada," for that year, that he was Commissioner of the Peace for Johnston and Bathurst Districts, and for taking affidavits.

In 1826, an advertisement of the United Empire Life Association gives as its "physician and referee," at Perth, Dr. Thom, surgeon to the forces. In 1830, this notice appeared: "At Perth, 16th February, James Boulton, Esq., barrister-at-law, son of Judge Boulton, of Upper Canada, to Harriett, eldest daughter of Alexander Thom, Esq., Staff-Surgeon." Chief Justice Spragge married a daughter of Dr. Alex. Thom, Staff-Surgeon and Medical Superintendent of the military settlements on the Rideau."

"DIED.—At Perth, September 26, 1845, at an advanced age, Alexander Thom. Came to Canada, as Assistant-Surgeon of 41st Regiment, forty years ago. During the last war he was employed on Niagara frontier and Toronto, on the staff of Medical Department."

The "Code of Honour," so called, prevailed in the earlier years of the century in the higher class of society. Only two or three of the medical profession distinguished themselves on that field, of whom Dr. Thom was one.

"DUEL.—On Friday, the 11th inst., Alexander McMillan, Esq., and Alexander Thom, Esq., met in a field, on the Brockville Road, to decide an affair of honour—the former attended by Mr. Radenhurst and the latter by Mr. Cumming. After exchanging shots the seconds interfered, and, on mutual explanations being made, the matter terminated amicably. Dr. Thom received a contusion on the leg."

DR. OLIVER TIFFANY

Came from Schoharie, N.Y., to Canada, in the first decade of the present century. He was a student at Philadelphia Medical College, and when returning to his home, Schoharie, he tarried at Albany, where he met with a misfortune among the Dutch. Whatever it was, the course of his life was in consequence turned to Canada, and, sometime prior to 1812, he settled in

Ancaster, where he engaged in practice, and where he lived until his death. He was appointed Surgeon to 3rd Gore Regiment Militia, 1825. He never married. His death took place at his residence, near Ancaster, May 7, 1835.

DR. OLIVER G. TIFFANY

Was born at Schoharie, N.Y. He was the nephew of Dr. Oliver Tiffany, whom his father joined at Ancaster, after the war of 1812. When his father settled here, Oliver G. was but a boy. He probably studied medicine with his uncle. He attended at Fairfield Medical College at the same time as did Dr. W. J. A. Case. In 1822, he passed the Medical Board. He engaged in practice with his uncle for a time, and then went to Chicago and was appointed surgeon to the hospital there. He never married, and died at a comparatively early age.

Dr. Frederick W. Tiffany, probably a relative of the above, and a brother of George S. Tiffany, of Hamilton, died, February 3, 1842, aged 31.

DR. JOHN E. TIMS,

A native of Ireland, passed the Medical Board, January, 1828. He practised in York and became well known as a politician. Was Vice-President of the "Toronto Political Union Society," and was to some extent involved in the Mackenzie rebellion of 1837. He represented St. Patrick's ward as alderman in the first year of the incorporation of the city, 1834, being elected in place of Dr. John Rolph, who had declined to act after his election. He died, October 4, 1839, in the prime of his life.

DR. TOLMEN.

The following is taken from the York *Gazette:* "Dr. Tolmen presents his respects to the inhabitants of Yonge Street, and informs them that he has taken a room in the house of Elisha Dexter, in the Township of Vaughan, where he will attend to the commands of all those who may require assistance in the line of his profession as far as his health and abilities will admit of. He will likewise attend to the vaccine innoculation when required thereto by those who reside near him. Yonge Street, 3rd May, 1807."

In January, 1808, Dr. Tolmen appointed John Cameron to be his attorney to collect debts, and he gave notice that there must be immediate payment. He adds, "Grain of good quality will be taken in payment."

JOHN TURQUAND

Was for many years a well-known practitioner of Woodstock, and enjoyed a high reputation throughout the country. He was the son of a British officer. He commenced the study of medicine in Toronto, and in 1834 was a pupil of Dr. King. In July, 1837, "John Turquand, of the city of Toronto," appeared before the Medical Board. He "acquitted himself to the full satisfaction of the Board." Dr. Turquand was appointed Surgeon to the 2nd Oxford Regiment Militia, 1837. He became a Fellow of the College of Physicians and Surgeons, Upper Canada, 1840. He commenced practice at Woodstock, where he continued until his death, May 18, 1880, at the age of sixty-five; was Surgeon to the Great Western Railway for many years; was representative to the Ontario Medical Council for a number of years, of which he was an active and respected member.

DR. E. VAN CORTLANDT.

"This gentleman is well known in scientific and other circles as a mineralogist, geologist, botanist and physician of considerable repute in the Province, and as one who has done much to advance the interests of the Ottawa country, in the capital of which he has resided for many years.

"Dr. Van Cortlandt was born in Newfoundland, in the year 1805; he was the son of a retired military officer and a devoted Loyalist, who was connected with some noble English families.

His sister married Sir E. Buller, and her grandson is the present Lord Elphinstone. Dr. Van Cortlandt received his education at the celebrated school of the late Rev. D. Wilkie LL.D., Quebec, and at the early age of fourteen left to study medicine under Dr. Hacket, with whom he remained until he proceeded to England in 1825. In 1827, he passed his examination at the Royal College of Surgeons in London, having received on the occasion some very flattering encomiums from the celebrated Abernethy and Sir A. Carlisle, for the creditable manner in which he passed through the vigorous ordeal. In 1829, Dr. Van Cortlandt was chosen Librarian to the Royal Medical and Chirurgic Society of London, having ten or twelve English competitors; in preference to all of whom he was chosen, probably, in a great measure on account of the remarkably flattering notice of his examination at the Apothecaries' Hall. Here he had been asked to retire, after being examined only thirteen minutes, with these emphatic words: 'You may go, sir, for if you continue any longer here you will puzzle us.' Three years afterwards he came to Canada, and settled at Ottawa city (then By-town), according to the advice of Dr. Skey, a community in which he still lives, and which greatly benefits by his presence. He has been appointed Physician, and afterwards Consulting Physician to the Ottawa General Hospital, and Consulting Physician to the Protestant Hospital, Coroner to the City, Physician to the Gaol, and President of the Horticultural Society and Mechanics' Institute.

" Everyone must admit that he has been one of the most active and ardent promoters of the prosperity of Ottawa, and that district is not a little indebted to him for the numerous measures which he has originated and carried out in the furtherance of its interests. He is the chief promoter of exhibitions of Ottawa productions. He was the first to point out the locality of the stone with which the parliamentary buildings are being erected. To this he drew the attention of the Earl of Elgin, a circumstance which tended, perhaps more than anything else, to give to Ottawa favourable publicity. He has, at great expense, had constructed the best private archæological and geological museum in Canada, an object of great attraction to all who visit Ottawa; and he even, we believe, intends to reconstruct the edifice on a still grander scale. Dr. Van Cortlandt is the author of a pamphlet on Ottawa production, which has received great attention and been very favourably noticed; and also of another pamphlet, published by order of the City Council of Ottawa, on the building stones of the Ottawa, a publication which has done much towards drawing public attention towards the resources of that rich and beautiful country."—*Biography Celebrated Canadians.*

An early contemporary of Dr. Van Cortlandt describes him as rather eccentric, but during the "thirties," doing a large and lucrative practice at Ottawa. He imitated the manner of the great Abernethy, "but as always happens, a second edition is always a failure." He was a bold surgeon and a good operator. He was Surgeon to the Ottawa Field Battery, and was buried with military honours. His death took place at about seventy-six years of age.

DR. JAMES WALLEN.

We are indebted to Dr. T. K. Holmes, of Chatham, for the following account:

"Dr. James Wallen was born on the Island of Jamaica, August, 1809. He was educated at the University of Aberdeen, Scotland, and afterwards went to Paris University, where he graduated. Having resolved to devote himself to the medical profession, he took the diploma of the Royal College of Surgeons, England. After practising for some time in England, he came to Canada, 1834, and during the rebellion of 1837, he acted as surgeon to the volunteers on the Niagara frontier. The next summer he went to his native island, Jamaica, but returned in 1839 to Canada, where he thereafter continued to reside until his death, 1863.

He first settled in the county of Wentworth, but removed to Morpeth, in the county of Kent, 1844. At this village, and afterwards at Ridgetown, Wardsville, and finally at Chatham, he continued the practice of his profession with general satisfaction to the public and with credit to himself. At all the places mentioned he made many friends. His kind and sympathizing manner made him a favourite with his patients, while his intimate knowledge of his profession, together with his candid way of expressing his opinion on any subject, gained him the general confidence of all who knew him. Aside from his professional skill, his general manner and his scholarly attainments made him a model citizen, and his influence for good will never be lost.

DR. HIRAM WEEKS,

Of Fredericksburg, Midland District, appeared before Upper Canada Medical Board, July, 1820, and, being duly examined, was found fit to practise. But Dr. Weeks had been practising before the Board was established. He was born near Brockville, and studied medicine in New York. He had come to the Bay of Quinte about 1818. His field of practice extended along the bay on either side for many miles. Being a large, vigorous man, he was quite able to attend to his large practice on horseback. Dr. H. H. Wright remembers having seen him when young, about 1827, crossing the ferry from Adolphustown to Prince Edward County, equipped with his saddle-bags, containing drugs and instruments. He was the first doctor to use in this section the new medicine, quinine. Dr. Weeks was elected vice-president of a temperance society organized in Adolphustown, April 16, 1830. He died at his residence, Adolphustown, March 8, 1835.

DR. HENRY WHICHER,

A member of R.C.S. Eng., and Licentiate of the Apothecaries' Hall, was born at Petersfield, Hampshire, England, October 6, 1795, and was educated at the schools of his native town and in the Isle of Wight. He studied his profession in London, and was a pupil of Sir Astley Cooper, from whom he received many kindnesses in after-life. He practised in England about thirteen years, in London and at Hastings, near his native place, where he was very successful, and had among his patients some of the best families. In 1832, he emigrated to Fredericton, N.B., but not liking the country, came to Upper Canada,

September, 1834. After staying a few weeks in Toronto, and visiting different parts of the country, he settled twelve miles south of Hamilton, near what is now the village of Caledonia, where he continued to reside and practise till he died, 1865.

Soon after he had settled there, Sir John Colborne visited the Six Nations on the Grand River, and requested Dr. Whicher to take medical charge of the Indians at that place, which he consented to do; and was soon after regularly appointed their medical attendant, which appointment he held till his death, thirty years afterwards.

When the rebellion broke out, 1837, he was one of the first in that part of the country to volunteer his services. Was stationed at Drummondville and Chippawa, during the occupation of Navy Island by Mackenzie, and afterwards appointed Surgeon of the Battalion of Militia commanded by Colonel Martin, afterwards Sheriff of Haldimand.

During the two cholera visitations, and an outbreak of smallpox among the Indians, which was very fatal, he was constantly among them. It was difficult to persuade them to be vaccinated, which he took care to do, however. His professional talents were well known and recognized, and his kindly disposition and genuine honesty and integrity of character won the respect and confidence of all who knew him. He was married in 1818 to Matilda Enticknap, of the County of Sussex, England, and had five children, of whom four are still (1890) living: Henry Whicher, of Wiarton; John W., of Seneca, Haldimand; George W. and Mrs. Charles Hull, now of Woodstock, Ont.

DR. CHRISTOPHER WIDMER

Was unquestionably the Father of Surgery in Upper Canada. No more skilful surgeon than he has ever had a place in the ranks of the Canadian profession. His skill was equal in making a diagnosis, in deciding when operative procedure was necessary, and in handling the surgeon's knife or other instrument. These high qualities were manifested not only in private practice, but in the wards of the hospital. These qualities made him not merely a blessing to patients whom he

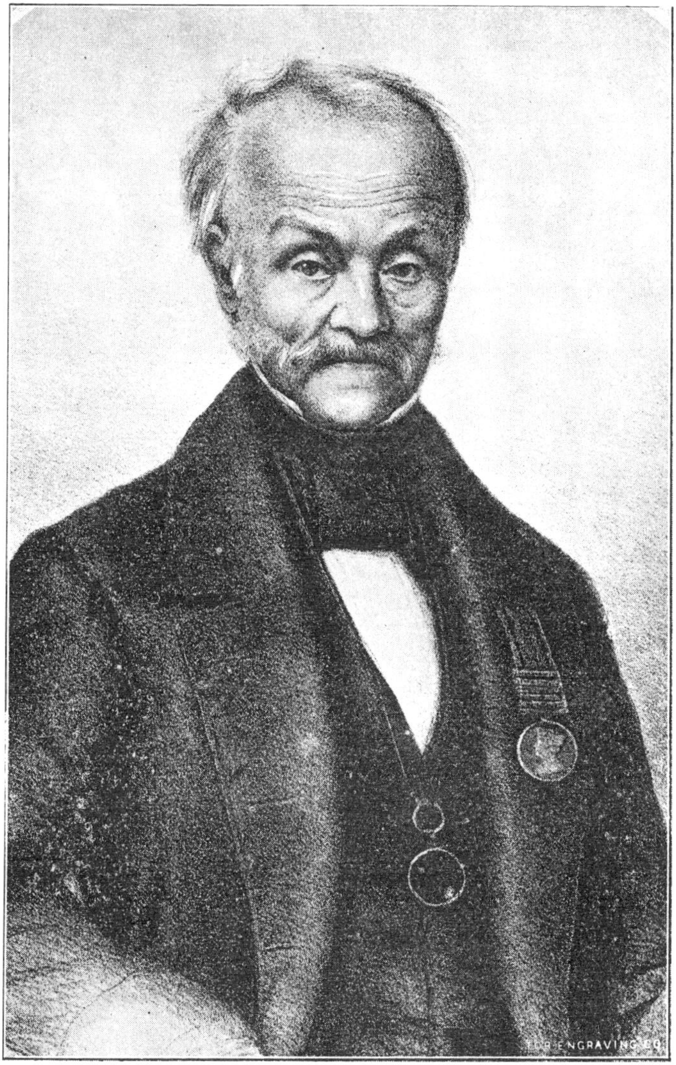

DR. CHRISTOPHER WIDMER.

treated himself, but to thousands treated by those whom he had educated by precept and example.

Dr. Widmer occupied a most prominent place in the history of the profession, equally as a practitioner, a member of the Upper Canada Medical Board from its first meeting in 1819 until his death, and chairman from 1823; and as the life and soul of the General Hospital from its beginning.

In the early days of York, the inhabitants were mainly dependent upon the military surgeons attached to the regiments stationed from time to time at the barracks. But after Dr. Widmer's advent as a private practitioner, outside skill was not required, although the army surgeons always enjoyed a certain amount of private practice, principally, however, as consultants. As a retired army surgeon, in the prime of life, Dr. Widmer at once commanded the confidence of the inhabitants of York.

Dr. Widmer was a Fellow of the Royal College of Surgeons, and formerly Staff-Surgeon, attached to the 14th Light Dragoons. He served through nearly the whole of the Peninsular campaign, and held the medal with five clasps, viz., for Vittoria, Salamanca, Fuentes d'Onoro, Busaco, and Talavera. He came to Canada towards the close of the war of 1812-15.

He probably commenced practice in York in 1815 or 1816. From that period until he retired from active work, every day of his life was given to the active duties of his profession, and during the first ten of these years he was the only qualified medical man in settled practice in York. Mr. Clarke Gamble says: "When I came to York, August, 1820, the only regular physician in practice was Dr. Widmer, a very skilful man and a practitioner of great experience."

That Dr. Widmer did not work for money merely, is evidenced by this notice in the *U. E. Loyalist* of May 5, 1827: "We are requested to state that the children of the poor will be vaccinated gratis, on their parents calling with them at Dr. Widmer's."

Mr. Gamble continues: "Several years after, Dr. Deihl commenced practice, and Dr. Widmer took him into partnership, and they had the whole practice of York and its neighbourhood for many years."

The Loyalist, of York, Nov. 15th, 1828, contains this announcement: "Dr. Widmer, finding his professional engagements much extended of late, and occasionally too arduous for one person, has been induced to enter into partnership with Doctor Deihl, a respectable practitioner, late of Montreal. It is expected that their united exertions will prevent in future any disappointment to Dr. Widmer's friends, both in town and country."

The partnership continued for nearly six years and a half, as the following notice shows, taken from the *Correspondent and Advocate*, and dated April 10, 1835: "The partnership between Messrs. Widmer and Deihl will terminate, by consent, on the 1st of May. Those persons who have long neglected to settle their accounts are requested to do so without delay. Dr. Widmer's office, after the 1st of May, will be in the house opposite the gate of his residence."

Dr. Widmer's residence was between King and Front Streets, the latter long known as Palace Street, near the lower end of Ontario Street. While the Doctor lived, this was a delightful location overlooking the bay, with the wooded peninsula in the distance, before the land, where is now the eastern gap, was washed away, thereby converting the western portion of the peninsula into an island. No factories or other industrial establishments then existed in the neighbourhood to mar the beauty or disturb the quiet home. Here Dr. Widmer passed his last days, and here he died.

The writer remembers with what profound respect he regarded Dr. Widmer, when he began the study of medicine. Dr. Widmer was as regular in his attendance at the hospital as had ever been his wont, and the students all venerated him, while they laughed at his brusque ways and too frequent expletives. The really destitute patients would receive the kindest attention; but if he thought anyone was seeking gratuitous relief who was able to pay for it, his words to him were such as only an old campaigner could utter. It was always a treat to follow him around the wards, for whatever he said or did relating to a patient was worth hearing and seeing. In the operating room he was the most brilliant. More than once the writer has seen him complete an operation with tact and precision over which another, although skilful, had become embarrassed.

As an examiner at the Medical Board, Dr. Widmer displayed his many-sided qualities, as an educated medical man, to advantage, although not always to the immediate advantage of the candidate. But if he ever erred in passing judgment, it was on the side of mercy to the trembling student.

The writer was examined by Dr. Widmer on midwifery, when before the Board on New Year's day, 1854, and the Doctor's kindness to him on that occasion has been a lasting remembrance, and made the preparation of this sketch a labour of love.

Dr. Widmer's public and private worth was recognized in many ways, by electing him to various offices of trust and responsibility. In 1826 he was appointed Medical Referee to the United Empire Life Association at York. In 1831, he was gazetted as a Director of the Bank of Upper Canada by the Lieutenant-Governor. In 1832, he was gazetted a Trustee of the General Hospital of Upper Canada. In 1834, he was one of the Committee of Management of the United Service Club for Upper Canada at York, with Dr. Grant Powell. He was one of the principal founders of the St. Andrew's Masonic Lodge, in Toronto. He was commissioned a member of the University of King's College, May 18, 1842, and was appointed a member of the Legislative Council of Upper Canada, 1849. These are only a few of the offices he was called upon to fill. In everything relating to matters affecting the well-being of the medical profession, Dr. Widmer was ever foremost. The high reputation Dr. Widmer possessed is evidenced by the fact that when Lord Sydenham, the Lieutenant-Governor residing at Kingston, unfortunately broke his leg, by the horse he was riding falling upon him, Dr. Widmer was sent for. This was before the days of the telegraph, and a messenger was sent post-haste to Toronto. Dr. Widmer set out forthwith, and by relays of horses, previously ordered to be in readiness, he was, without stopping, speedily conveyed to Kingston. The Governor's appreciation of his services on that occasion was manifested by presenting Dr. Widmer with a gold watch.

The following, taken from "Toronto of Old," by Dr. Scadding, who knew Dr. Widmer well, affords an excellent glimpse of the Doctor, as seen by the early inhabitants of York: "It is to be regretted that Dr. Widmer left behind him no written memorials of his long and varied experience. A personal narrative of his public life would have been full of interest. But his ambition was content with the homage of his contemporaries, rich and poor, rendered with sincerity to his pre-eminent abilities and inextinguishable zeal as a surgeon and physician. Long after his retirement from general practice, he was every day to be seen passing to and from the old hospital, on King Street, conveyed in his well-known cabriolet, and guiding with his own hand the reins conducted in through the front window of the vehicle. He had now attained a great age, but his slender form continued erect; the hat was worn jauntily, as in other days, and the dress was ever scrupulously exact; the expression of the face in repose was somewhat abstracted and sad, but a quick smile appeared at the recognition of friends. The ordinary engravings of Harvey, the discoverer of the circulation of the blood, recall, in some degree, the countenance of Dr. Widmer. Within the General Hospital a portrait of him is appropriately preserved. One of the earliest, and, at the same time, one of the most graceful lady equestrians ever seen in York was this gentleman's accomplished wife."

A tablet upon her grave, in the old St. James' graveyard, east of the Cathedral, tells us that she was the "third daughter of Richard Bignell, Esq., Banbury, Oxfordshire, Great Britain," and "Died, 31st August, 1833, aged fifty-three years."

Dr. Widmer was twice married. By his second wife he had a son and two daughters; the son, Christopher Rolph W., for whom his father had extraordinary love, died at the early age of twenty-three, April 19, 1857. The elder daughter, Annie, married Captain Clarke, of the 100th Regiment, and has been dead several years, leaving one son and three daughters, who live in Toronto. The second daughter, Charlotte, married Geo. M. Hawke, and is still living (1893). She has also one son and three daughters. The son, Widmer Hawke, is well known as an energetic partner in the firm of O'Keefe & Co., of Toronto.

An insight of Dr. Widmer's private character is obtained by an abstract from a letter written by him from Quebec to his daughter, Charlotte, now Mrs. Hawke, dated May 16, 1853. He writes:

"MY DEAR CHARLOTTE,—I have sealed this letter, and on my way to the post office, I bethought me that my dear little girl might feel a little jealous that I had written so long a letter to Chris., and not a word for you. I therefore opened it, and I desire you will believe that you are as much in my thoughts, and have as great a share of my affectionate love as your brother. I know you will continue to deserve this, by your conduct to Mamma, and by cultivating your taste by the acquisition of knowledge of all sorts, that will invigorate your intellectual faculties and enable you to pass through life with credit to yourself and satisfaction to all your friends. Light reading and trivial amusements ought not to constitute the sole object of a young woman's existence. She should strive to render herself conspicuous for enlarged and comprehensive views of matters connected with the sciences and mental operations. Not that I expect a woman to become a literary critic, or to profess high philosophical acquirements. She should, however, lose no opportunity by reading and study to make it appear that she is well acquainted with the topics of conversation, when she comes into the society of very clever people."

He concludes: "With many kisses to yourself, dearest Charlotte, and kindest love to dear Mamma, I remain your affectionate father, "C. W."

Dr. Widmer died on May 2, 1858, aged seventy-eight, and this sketch cannot be better completed than by quoting from the Journal of the Legislative Assembly of May 6, also an editorial note from the *Leader*:

"Prayers having been read, the Hon. Mr. Ross rose and spoke as follows: On entering this house a resolution was placed in my hands to which I will ask your unanimous concurrence. Most honourable gentlemen have no doubt heard of the sudden death of one of our brother members, Dr. Widmer. About twelve months ago his only son died. On Sunday Dr. Widmer walked from his house to the cemetery to visit his son's grave. The state of his feelings and the fatigue caused by the walk had no doubt produced its effect and caused him to faint at the grave of his son. He was removed to his residence and died about six o'clock this morning, without having rallied perceptibly, except to answer an occasional question. The circumstances, therefore, attending his death, are of a particularly affecting character. Dr. Widmer was one of the oldest inhabitants of Toronto. He had served with great ability during the Peninsular War as surgeon to the 14th Light Dragoons, and came to this country with his regiment during the war of 1812. At the declaration of peace he determined to remain in this country and practise his profession, and accordingly he settled in Toronto. This city was then a mere hamlet, containing but a few people, and with it Dr. Widmer had grown till it was a large and populous city. From his remarkable skill as a surgeon and a physician, he acquired large wealth, and enjoyed a most extensive practice in his profession. He was universally respected, and his death will cause regret throughout the entire city. Owing to the constant practice of the duties of his profession, Dr. Widmer did not take any prominent part in public affairs, as a member of either branch of the Legislature, until late in life. At the time of his death he was about eighty years of age. In 1843, during the administration of Messrs. La Fontaine and Baldwin, he was summoned by the Queen, together with his friend, the late Dr. Baldwin, to the Legislative Council, but owing to his infirmity and advanced age he had not been able to attend constantly in his place in the House, except during the period in which the seat of Government had been in Toronto, and upon some important public occasions, when he had invariably, notwithstanding his infirm health and great age, attended in his place at Montreal and Quebec, when the occasion required. Most members who were in the Legislative Council at the time would recollect one important occasion, in 1849, when he had but just recovered from a severe attack of illness, and had at the risk of his life attended the House, manfully taking part in the exciting legislation of that period—a period in which his presence was urgently demanded. He never shrank from duty, but performed it independently and honestly on all occasions. He was a devoted and sincere friend, and as such was universally respected. In his profession he was looked upon as one of the best, if not the very best, surgeons on the continent; and it was only to-day that, in conversation with a distinguished member of his profession, the gentleman with whom I was conversing remarked that, as an operating surgeon, he was a Sir Astley Cooper. He always made up his mind before operating, as to what was the best course to be pursued; and, having once settled on the course to be adopted, he performed his operation more quickly and skilfully than any other surgeon that gentleman had seen operate in the schools of Europe or America. I am sure that the House, as a mark of respect to the memory of their departed brother and colleague in the Council—Dr. Widmer—will unanimously join in the resolution of adjournment."

The *Leader*, of May 11, says: "The funeral of this lamented gentleman took place on Thursday, May 7. The corpse was followed to the grave by a very large number of the former friends of the deceased, all anxious to pay their last tribute of respect to his memory. After the return of the mournful cavalcade from the cemetery, a meeting comprising the most distinguished members of the medical fraternity of the city was held, and after discussion it was determined that a full-length portrait of the deceased should be painted, and placed temporarily in the Board room of the General Hospital, until such time as the contemplated medical college should be erected. A collection to defray the necessary expense was at once set afoot, and responded to with a liberality which showed the appreciation in which the deceased was held by the members of that profession of which the object of their tribute was in lifetime himself the brightest ornament."

DR. ROBERT WILSON

Was born at Niagara, and studied medicine with Drs. Melville and Grasett; attended lectures at McGill College, and took the degree of M.D. He was for a time in partnership with Dr. C. W. Covernton. He also practised at Cayuga and at Niagara for a time. He then went to the West Indies on account of ill-health, where he had a large practice and obtained improved health. He returned to Niagara, but some time later went to

Cobourg, where he carried on the drug business. He finally returned to Niagara, where he died.

DR. WILLIAM WINDER

Was licensed under 8 George IV. chap. 3. He was practising in Toronto at the beginning of 1836. It is related that he was a Lieutenant in the 49th Regiment in 1812, and was with the heroic FitzGibbon in the Niagara Peninsula, where he distinguished himself. He was gazetted a member of the Upper Canada Medical Board, but his name does not appear in the minutes of the Board. Dr. Winder was appointed to the position of Librarian to the House of Assembly when that body was at Quebec.

DR. ORLANDO SALATHIEL WINSTANLEY

Was born, December 5, 1823, at Wigginton, Oxfordshire, England. He was the son of the Rev. Charles Winstanley, M.A., of St. Edmund's Hall, Oxford, of the Church of England, then curate of parish at Wigginton; was educated at different schools conducted by clergymen of the Church of England. He commenced the study of medicine at Devonport about 1840; attended the London Hospital Medical School, as well as the London Hospital, from 1841 to 1844; passed examination of the Royal College of Surgeons, England, 1844; also the examination of the Apothecaries' Company, which was then necessary for those contemplating general practice in England, and which was the best general medical examination in England.

Dr. Winstanley came to Canada in the spring of 1845 to join his father's family, which had settled in Toronto, 1843. Before leaving England he had married Miss Andrews, daughter of Captain Andrews, R.N., of Cornwall, England. Dr. Winstanley did not then enter into practice, but remained in attendance on his father, who was in feeble health, till his death, which occurred at his house in the Scarborough Heights, called "Falling Brook," in 1847, whither he had removed. During the Doctor's residence at the corner of King and Peter Streets, his eldest son, Charles, was born. In 1848, he returned to Toronto, after visiting the United States, and commenced practice in Toronto, but he remained here only one year, preferring to live in the country. He moved out to a tract of fifty acres of land fronting on the Kingston Road and extending to Lake Ontario, which he had bought from his brother, Edward Winstanley, for the sum of $960, showing the relative value of such land at that time. This he afterwards sold to Peter Paterson, Esq., who built a handsome mansion and laid out the grounds which he called "Blantyre Park." The lake frontage he afterwards leased to the Victoria Park Company for park purposes, and it is now known as Victoria Park. Blantyre Park has recently been acquired as a site for an Industrial School for Roman Catholic boys. Dr. Winstanley practised here for two years, and then moved to Thornhill, 1850, to take care of the practice of Dr. Robert Paget, whilst he visited friends in England. In the spring of 1851, he removed to Bond Head, Simcoe County; thence, in 1852, to Willowdale, and continued in practice at various points on Yonge Street, from Thornhill to Eglington, until 1864 or 1865, when he again settled in Toronto, where he continued in active practice till 1883. From overwork and various ailments, Dr. Winstanley found it necessary to give up work. After living one winter in California, he found the equable climate suitable for his health. Consequently, early the following winter he removed to that country, where he continued to reside up to the time of his death. Whilst residing at Willowdale, Dr. Winstanley was requested to take a position as lecturer in Rolph's School of Medicine, several of the professors of that faculty having disagreed with Dr. Rolph and resigned. He came in from the country and delivered two lectures, but finding it impossible to devote the necessary time to that work, owing to a largely increasing practice, he was obliged to resign the position.

Dr. Winstanley had ten children—four sons and six daughters. Of these, one son and one daughter (an infant) are dead. The writer was fortunate to enjoy the friendship of Dr. Winstanley, whose unvarying kindness to him is a bright and pleasing remembrance. Dr. Winstanley died in May, 1893, in his seventieth year.

"At a meeting of medical men in St. George's Hall, May 23,

1893, called to consider the proposal to build a new city hospital, the following resolution, prepared by Dr. Canniff, and moved by Dr. Barrick, seconded by Dr. Palmer, was unanimously carried: 'Resolved, that the medical practitioners of Toronto here assembled have heard of the death of Dr. Winstanley, late of Toronto, with profound regret and sadness, and desire to express their high opinion of his professional worth, as manifested in his daily course of practice, by his uniform urbanity to all, combined with his skilful treatment of disease, by his honourable devotion to his profession and his courteous treatment of his confreres.'"

DR. JONATHAN WOOLVERTON

Was born in Grimsby, Ont., February 22, 1811. His ancestors, of English origin, came to America during religious persecutions under James II., and settled in New Jersey. His grandfather, Jonathan Woolverton, came to Canada, 1798, and settled where now is Grimsby. With him was his son Dennis, then a lad of eight years, who was widely known in the Niagara District and was universally respected for his integrity and honourable dealings, and at one time represented his county in the Legislature. Of his six children (three sons and three daughters), Mrs. Hough, of Lockport, N.Y., and Charles Woolverton, of Grimsby, survive.

Jonathan, the eldest son, the subject of this sketch, was born in the old homestead. In his early life there were but few settlements, and the roads connecting them were of the most primitive character. The inconveniences of to-day would have been deemed luxuries in those primitive times, and educational facilities were not easily obtained. He was fortunate, however, in having an Irish school-master who was exceptionally well educated, and taught him classics and enabled him to secure an education far above the average. He added year by year to his store of knowledge and became the possessor of a liberal education, which, from his natural modesty of character, was not obtruded on the world, but of which his friends secured the benefit, and learned to love him as he went in and out among them in his social and professional life during the fifty years he lived as a physician in their midst. Modesty and gentleness were the chief characteristics of his nature.

He studied medicine at Montreal, where he went in the autumn of 1832, and during the following summer he continued his studies under Dr. Rolph. In 1833, he entered the University of Pennsylvania, at Philadelphia, from which he received his degree of Doctor of Medicine. Within less than three years from commencing the study of his profession, he obtained his degree of M.D. and license to practise in Upper Canada. He left Toronto fully intending to return to establish himself in his profession, but while visiting his home he writes:

"I got into practice and found it difficult to leave. I have had diseases of various kinds to treat, as well as many cases of a very serious nature. I have had the good fortune to see the most of them reinstated in health; there are, however, a few exceptions.

"On the 15th January, my father came to attend the session of Parliament. My time was principally occupied either by the sick, the dying or the dead, chiefly the latter; and when I look back upon the scenes which were transacted in the cholera hospital during the winter, my mind almost recoils upon itself. I believe there were something like a dozen bodies mangled and dissected by James Mitchell and myself."

In the autumn of the same year (1835), he returned to Philadelphia for the purpose of visiting the one whom he expected to make his wife, and there he remained during the winter, "attending the lectures of both schools as much as time would permit, also the alms-house and hospital, and I think deriving much useful instruction, but not forgetting the main object of my visit." On the 22nd of February, 1836, he was married to Emmeline Bergmann. After a hymenial excursion, Dr. Woolverton, with his wife, returned to his native place to begin his labours. At the time of the Mackenzie rebellion he was out three weeks at the notorious siege of Navy Island, acting as Assistant-Surgeon. In 1855, he visited England, Ireland and France. His notes of his journeyings form interesting reading.

Educational interests were greatly aided by his support. For many years he was Superintendent of Public Schools in the County of Lincoln, and from time to time gave lectures before the School Boards, and was one of the foremost promoters in establishing the Grammar Schools in his county. A few years previous to his decease, April 12, 1883, Dr. Woolverton ceased from active practice. He and his wife (who died in 1872) lie side by side in the beautiful old English churchyard in Grimsby. A monument erected by his sons testifies that beneath it lie one of the noblest of fathers and best of mothers. But if you wish to find a greater monument, go ask the people among whom he dwelt for seventy-two years. You will find a memory of love and a remembrance of kindly deeds enshrined in the hearts of his people that speak louder than monumental structures, however grand. "*Si monumentum requiris circumspice*" was said of the great architect embalmed in St Paul's, London. So, in that beautiful old village of Grimsby he was the architect of a life whose fragrance dwells in the memories of its people.

He had six sons; one died in infancy, the rest are still living (1889). Theoron, a graduate in medicine, of Harvard University, has been for twenty-five years a surgeon in the United States Navy, and is now Medical Inspector, stationed at the United States Navy Yard at Washington, D.C. Edgar J. is a well-known fruit-grower; he lives upon the old place at Grimsby, being the fourth generation in direct descent to have possession. Algernon, a graduate in Arts of University College, Toronto, and in medicine of McGill College, Montreal, is a well-known physician in Hamilton. Solon practises his profession, D.C.L., in London. Delos, engaged in the banking business, resides in New York city. For the above information we are indebted to Dr. Algernon Woolverton, of Hamilton.

DR. JOSEPH WORKMAN.

Of all the names contained in this volume, and of all those whose life the writer is privileged to sketch, no one stands higher, and few, if any, so high, in the list of worthies who have adorned the medical profession of Upper Canada. He stands equally high as a physician, as a teacher, as a writer to the medical and secular press, as a critic, as a linguist, and especially high in that branch of medical science to which he gave the riper years of his active, practical life. The writer knows that Dr. Workman would prefer that only a brief notice of himself should find a place in these pages; but notwithstanding a desire to respect his wishes, a sense of justice impels the writer to give expression to what he believes would be the voice of all who have been privileged to know Dr. Joseph Workman personally, or by his writings. The extent to which he is known, and the estimate of his worth, is indicated by one long intimate with him, Dr. C. W. Covernton, who in a note to the writer, remarks: "Needless to allude to the distinguished rank he has ever occupied, and still occupies in his green old age, for it is not confined to Canada or the United States, but has extended to Europe, particularly with the advanced psychologists of Italy."

More might be said of Dr. Workman in a general way as a man of the people at large; but suffice it to say, that in all the relations of life he has held the greatest respect, and in his conduct, public and private, he has ever worn the white flower of a blameless life.

A sketch of Dr. Workman's family has recently appeared in the *Alienist and Neurologist*," published in St. Louis, and we are permitted to give the following extract taken from the proof: "Dr. Workman comes of a worthy and illustrious lineage. The Workmans of Ireland are descendants of an English ancestor, the Rev. William Workman, of St. Stephen's Church, Gloucester, England. He was deposed and excommunicated, by Archbishop Laud, for having preached against the setting up of images and pictures in churches. He had a numerous family. One of his sons, named William, joined the army of Cromwell, and came over to Ireland with that king-killer. As Cromwell was very liberal in rewarding his followers with the goods of other people, William received in compensation for his military services several tracts of land in the county of Derry, not far from Coleraine. All the Workmans of Ireland, Scotland, America and India are descended from this Puritan soldier. They all have been of a migratory tendency. The father of the late Dr. Wm. Workman, of Worcester, Mass., came to New England, before the conquest of Canada by the British, and fought at the siege of Ticonderoga. Joseph Workman, the father of the subject of our present memoir, was a native of Moneymore, in the county of Derry. He, in company with an elder brother named Benjamin, emigrated to the then new United States soon after the close of the War of Independence. He resided for three years in Philadelphia, and then returned to Ireland, where he married Catherine Gowdey, a girl of Scotch descent. By her he had nine children, eight sons and one daughter. Dr. Joseph Workman was the fourth of these sons. He was born near the town of Lisburn, in the county of Antrim, on the 26th of May, 1805. The eldest son, Benjamin, came to Canada in 1819; the second son, Alexander, followed in 1820; the three youngest, Samuel, Thomas and Matthew, came in 1827, and the rest of the family, with father and mother, in 1829. Only two of the sons now survive—Alexander, aged 91, and Joseph, aged 84. The father died past 88, and the mother past 102."

Dr. Workman was a student of medicine at Montreal during the epidemic of cholera in both 1832 and 1834, and when he completed his course at McGill College, in May, 1835, Asiatic cholera was the subject of his thesis. Five days later, May 30, he was married to Elizabeth Wasinge, daughter of an English manufacturer of cutlery, who had with his family come to Canada in 1829. Mr. Wasinge had established his eldest son in the hardware business, in Toronto, some time previous to 1835. In March Mr. Wasinge died, and it became necessary for the family to remove to Toronto to join the son. Dr. Workman was unwilling to have his betrothed go away, and hence a speedy marriage after he had obtained his degree of M.D.

Dr. Workman engaged in practice in Montreal, and continued for about a year. During this year his brother-in-law in Toronto met with an accident which resulted fatally. His mother, Mrs. Wasinge, continued the business; but, after a little, from adverse circumstances, it became evident that assistance was necessary to successfully carry it on. Dr. Workman having learned the state of affairs, came to Toronto with the view of putting matters right. But after a stay of five weeks, he decided to forsake for a time his professional work, and engage in business. He consequently removed his wife and infant child to Toronto, and became a partner in the hardware business. Although not bred for a business life, his ability to adapt himself to this calling, and achieve success, was soon apparent, and for four years the business continued to grow under his guiding mind. He then withdrew from the firm, and shortly after entered into the same business in Toronto, with his brother Samuel, who removed from Montreal. Six more years of his life were thus passed, when in 1846, he relinquished business, and returned to his first love. But Dr. Workman had never intended to devote his whole life to business. The year after his removal to Toronto (1837), he had procured his license to practise in Upper Canada ; and all the time he had maintained a *pseudo* connection with the profession by his writings, correspondence and reading of medical literature. Meanwhile he felt himself to be out of his natural element. He now resumed his place in the profession he loved, and in which, had he continued to follow it, in Montreal, he would already doubtless have secured a high position. While he was still in business, that astute observer, Dr. Rolph, had discerned the buried talent, and endeavoured to secure the services of Dr. Workman as a lecturer in his rising school of medicine. But Dr. Workman deemed it to be incongruous to deal in hardware and teach medical science at the same time, and therefore declined Dr. Rolph's invitation. When, however, he gave up business in 1846, he accepted the situation, and in the session of 1846-47, he delivered his first course on Midwifery and Diseases of Women and Children. He also began practice, and soon had a fair amount of patronage. He not only attended to his practice and delivered lectures (to prepare which he often remained up until two in the morning), but he was incessantly engaged in writing for the secular press. He was, indeed, a regular contributor to two papers. Needless to say, he wielded a keen weapon against those to whom he was opposed publicly, and was a tower of strength to the Reform party, of which he was an ardent member. During the second or third year of his connection with the Rolph School, he lectured, in addition to Midwifery, on Materia Medica. The strength and aid afforded by Dr. Workman had very much to do in making the Rolph School so generally popular.

Dr. Workman continued in practice until 1854, also to lecture. The writer attended the last two courses of his lectures.

The establishment of the Toronto Lunatic Asylum has been referred to in connection with Dr. Rees, and the circumstances attending his removal, as Superintendent. His successor was Dr. Telfer, who, although not regularly commissioned, held the position as temporary incumbent for three years, 1844 to 1847. He was followed by Dr. Parkes, who was Superintendent only six or seven months, in 1848. Following him was the temporary appointment of Dr. Primrose, who held it for eleven months (1848-49). Then Dr. Scott received the appointment, as regular Superintendent, who continued in office until 1853. (See sketch of Dr. John Scott.) To fill the position thus made vacant by Dr. Scott's resignation, there was no little manœuvring and intrigue. Dr. Workman was meanwhile in temporary charge. Candidates were called for by advertisement, both in Canada and elsewhere, and there were many applicants. Dr. Rolph, then an influential member of the Government, desired the appointment of Dr. Workman. Lord Elgin, then Governor-General, had a friend among the candidates, from his native town, Dr. John Hunter Robinson, and sought his appointment. But Dr. Workman was the choice by a large majority; and in July, 1854, he received his commission, and took up his residence at the asylum. It is not our purpose to follow the subject of this sketch during the years of his incumbency. The brilliant record of his work in that connection is well known; and some future pen will doubtless give to the world a proper account of his work. He retired from the position, July, 1875, to enjoy, in comparative retirement, the close of a distinguished career.

The writer cannot close this sketch of an esteemed friend without a personal reference. To him Dr. Workman has ever been a kind friend, from the period he became a student at Rolph's school to the present time. The lessons he learned from Dr. Workman's lectures were of incalculable value during the whole of his life as a practitioner. He does not forget the kind words of Dr. Workman on the day he passed the Medical Board. He is conscious of repeated kind acts of regard for forty years.

Since the foregoing was written, the death of Dr. Workman occurred died at his residence, 113 Mutual Street, Toronto, on Sunday, April 15, 1894, in his eighty-ninth year.

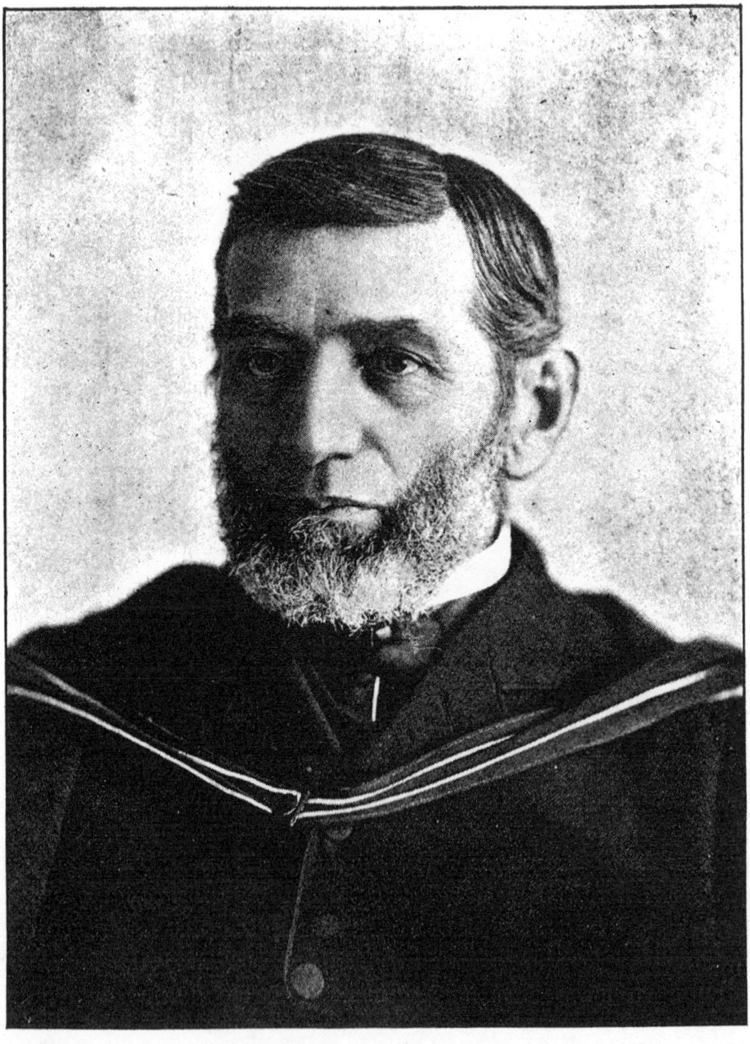

DR. HENRY HOVER WRIGHT.

DR. HENRY HOVER WRIGHT

A native Canadian, was born in Prince Edward County, 1816. His father, David Wright, also born in Canada, was a pioneer Methodist minister, being called to the work about 1820. He was much beloved by his people wherever he went as an itinerant minister of the Gospel. He had been a school teacher, and, considering the meagre advantages at that time, had a fair education. Henry Hover, as he grew up, had the benefit of his father's knowledge, and this, with such schools as existed where his father was stationed from year to year, formed the source of his general education.

In 1832, he came to York to commence the study of medicine with Dr. Rolph, and continued with him until Dr. Rolph went into exile in 1837. Young Wright was no unimportant actor on the occasion of Mackenzie's intended invasion of Toronto. The sympathizers of Mackenzie in Toronto were expecting the insurgent forces to enter the place to take possession, and, when they failed to appear, Wright, who had just arrived from Niagara, consented to go out on Yonge Street to learn the cause of delay and carry a message to Mackenzie that he was anxiously expected; but he had no conception it all meant rebellion. The task was duly accomplished, notwithstanding some difficulties and danger. The particulars of this excursion may be found in Dent's account of the "Upper Canadian Rebellion," Vol. I., pages 76-78. As may be seen elsewhere (page 595), Wright undoubtedly was the means of preventing the arrest of Dr. Rolph by giving him timely warning of Dr. Morrison's arrest and in aiding him to leave Toronto. Dent, in a foot-note respecting the messenger sent out by Dr. Rolph, says: "The messenger was a young man named Henry Hover Wright, who was then a medical student in the office of Dr. Rolph, but who is now (1885), and for many years past has been, one of the most eminent members of the medical profession in this country. Six months after Dr. Rolph's departure from Canada, young Wright followed him to Rochester, where he was for some time an inmate of his house, and where he pursued his studies under the Doctor's direction."

Dr. Wright obtained his license to practise through the College of Physicians and Surgeons, Upper Canada, January 28, 1839. The record says he "passed a very satisfactory examination in all of his profession."

Dr. Wright practised first in Dundas and then in Markham until about 1853, when he accepted a chair in Dr. Rolph's school. The writer was present, as a student, at the first of his lectures. Dr. Wright continued to be a lecturer from that time onward, and finally filled acceptably the Chair of Medicine in the Medical Department of Toronto University up to a recent date. He is not only known as a successful lecturer, but as a sound and scientific practitioner. He has enjoyed a large share of patronage, and pursues his daily work with unabated vigour.

Dr. Wright was a member of the Council of the College of Physicians and Surgeons of Ontario for many years, and President of the College, 1886 and 1887. He was Chairman of the Building Committee under whose directions the present local habitation of the College was erected; and the Registrar has often been heard to remark that "if the building had been his own private concern, Dr. Wright could not have manifested greater care or expended more time in the supervision of the work." He was also a member of the Public School Board for many years, and Chairman of the Board.

Dr. Wright was married in 1848 to Maria Phœbe Zwick, who died in November, 1893.

Dr. Wright's son, Frederick, entered the profession and graduated at the University of Toronto, 1872. He afterwards pursued his studies in Europe for two years. On returning, he commenced practice in Toronto, and was appointed Lecturer in Histology in the Toronto School of Medicine—a position he held until his death, 1882. A daughter of Dr. Wright is the wife of I. H. Cameron, Professor of Clinical Surgery in the University of Toronto, son of the late Sir Matthew Crooks Cameron, Chief Justice of the Court of Common Pleas.

DR. HORATIO YATES.

The following is taken from the *Queen's College Journal*:

"Dr. Horatio Yates, son of Dr. William Yates, of Sapperton, Derbyshire, England, was born in 1821, in Otsego County, N.Y., and came to an uncle in Kingston at twelve years of age. Five years later he was articled to the late Dr. Simpson as a medical student, attended the courses at the University in Philadelphia, and took his degrees there in medicine in 1842. Thence he went to London and spent a year at St. George's Hospital. Since then he has been employed here in an active and successful practice of his profession to the present time. He was much devoted not only to science, but to works of charity, and the poor always received medical services and medicine at his hands without stint. In 1854, he undertook a reform of the Kingston Hospital, which had become completely demoralized. He found, on his return to Kingston after a long absence from sickness, the building in a state of complete dilapidation, the fences gone and the little remaining furniture utterly worthless. The wards contained less than a dozen patients, and the medical services performed by an inexperienced young man at a petty salary. The hospital was being managed by a committee of the City Council, good men in their way, but who knew nothing and cared less for hospital work. In order to achieve his purpose, he became a city alderman, was placed on the Hospital Committee, and soon assumed full charge, medical and financial, assisted by Drs. Dickson and Strange, who cordially co-operated in the work. His first act was to advance from his own pocket many hundred dollars to pay off executions against the hospital and to purchase necessary supplies; next he sought and obtained a new charter, which he himself had drawn up, placing the charter in the hands of life governors and a few *ex-officio* governors. The new board relieved him of personal supervision, and has to this day managed the hospital with great success. He was for years chairman of the board. In the establishment of the Medical Faculty of Queen's University, in 1844, he took an active part, and chose for himself the chair of Science and Practice of Medicine. Until the change to the Royal College he had for some time been Dean of the Faculty. In the fall of 1873, he was appointed Surgeon in "A" Battery."

Dr. Yates married Jane, third daughter of the Rev. Joseph Bower, of Cheshire, England, September 8, 1846. His final illness was very short, as he lived only a few days after having been taken ill with pneumonia. His genial social qualities, combined with much ability, had made him very popular, and he will long be missed in his chosen city.

DR. OCTAVIUS YATES, brother of the above, was M.D. University Queen's College, Kingston, 1856. He practised in Kingston also. Was Surgeon to the Kingston Hospital. He died, November, 1876.

DR. HORACE YEOMANS,

Born at Colchester, Conn., U.S., September 27, 1789, came to Canada in 1805. Taught school for three years, and studied medicine at the same time; but during the period he attended a course of lectures at a college in New York State. After his marriage, in 1808, to Laura Fitch, of Edmonston, N.Y., he came to Waterloo, now Cataraqui, and commenced practice. Here he continued until his death, in September, 1854, at the age of 66. That he was well up in his profession, and remained so, is manifest from the fact that in 1823 he passed his examination before the Medical Board.

Like all the doctors at that period, he travelled the country on horseback. His field of practice was extensive—from Napanee on the west, and from Bath north to Sydenham. His practice was large and, in the end, remunerative, as he acquired considerable property.

Dr. Horace Yeomans had no children, but adopted his nephew, David P. Yeomans, and had him educated for the medical profession. In like manner the uncle provided for the son of David P., the present well-known Dr H. P. Yeomans, of Mount Forest, who has done such excellent work in connection with education and public health. He has now his uncle's copy of Cullen's "Practice of Medicine," which was his text-book.

Dr. Horace Yeomans was an intimate friend of Dr. Sampson, of Kingston, who "seemed to have a warm heart towards him."

DR. DAVID P. YEOMANS,

Nephew of Dr. Horace Yeomans, and father of Dr. Yeomans, of Mount Forest, by whom he was adopted and educated, graduated in Arts at Williams' College, Mass., U.S., in 1837. Some time after, he succeeded the subsequently famous surgeon, Samuel D. Gross, of Philadelphia, as Professor of Chemistry at Lafayette College, Pennsylvania. In 1847, having resigned this position, he came to Canada at the request of his uncle, who desired that he should succeed him in his practice. Before settling down to practice, Dr. D. P. Yeomans attended a course of lectures at McGill College, and procured his license to practise in Upper Canada.

Dr. D. P. Yeomans was married in 1839, and had three sons and three daughters. The eldest son was Dr. H. P. Yeomans, the next, John, is a druggist, and the third, George A., is a Presbyterian clergyman.

It is with deep regret the following obituary notice is added, taken from the *Canadian Practitioner*, January, 1890:

"It was a great shock to the many friends of Dr. H. P. Yeomans to hear of his death at his home in Mount Forest, December 22nd, at the age of 49. He was a graduate in Arts and Medicine of the University of Queen's College, taking the degree of M.D. in 1863. He was a man of more than ordinary ability, education and culture, and was highly respected by the profession generally, and greatly beloved by those who knew him intimately. He was a member of the Provincial Board of Health since its formation, seven years ago."

INDEX.

PART I.

PART II.

PART III.